ATLAS OF THORACIC SURGERY

VOLUME ONE

ATLAS OF

Thoracic Surgery

VOLUME ONE

EDITED BY

Academician Boris V. Petrovsky

Translated from the Russian by

Ludmila Aksenova

With a foreword to the English language edition by

Michael E. DeBakey, M.D.

810 figures, including 284 in color

The C. V. Mosby Company

ST. LOUIS • TORONTO • LONDON 1979

TWO VOLUMES

Originally published as *Atlas Grudnoĭ Khirurgii,* © 1974 by Meditsina Publishing House, USSR

Printed in the United States of America

The C. V. Mosby Company
11830 Westline Industrial Drive, St. Louis, Missouri 63141

Library of Congress Cataloging in Publication Data

Main entry under title:

Atlas of thoracic surgery.

Translation of Atlas grudnoĭ khirurgii.
1. Chest—Surgery—Atlases. I. Petrovskiĭ, Boris Vasil'evich, 1908- [DNLM: 1. Thorax—Surgery—Atlases. WF17 A881]
RD536.A7813 617'.54 78-23699
ISBN 0-8016-3832-1

GW/U/B 9 8 7 6 5 4 3 2 1 03/C/300

Foreword

This *Atlas of Thoracic Surgery,* originally published in Russian in 1974, is based on the extensive experience of Professor Boris V. Petrovsky, who has long been the Director of the Research Institute of Clinical and Experimental Surgery and is now Minister of Public Health of the USSR. A pioneer in this field of endeavor, Professor Petrovsky has developed this Institute into one of the great centers of thoracic and cardiovascular surgery. The experience gained in this Institute provides the basis of this *Atlas*.

The first portion of the *Atlas* is devoted to a detailed anatomic description of the thoracic wall and the organs of the thoracic cavity. This section is well illustrated with many color plates that are clear, precise, and well presented in terms of anatomic relationships. Although the actual anatomic presentations are fairly standard, emphasis is placed on the surgical approach to anatomy.

The subsequent chapters deal with technical principles of surgical procedures, first on the chest wall, including those related to trauma, thoracoplasty, and operation on the breast. Other chapters are devoted to technical consideration of various operations on the lungs, esophagus, and heart and great vessels. These are described in considerable detail, with extensive illustrations of each step of the operation. Several technical methods are presented for certain conditions, as exemplified in the approach to coarctation, consisting in resection and end-to-end anastomosis, resection and graft replacement, patch-graft angioplasty, and subclavian-artery bypass.

Although most of the operations described are based on the methods used by Professor Petrovsky and his associates, in general they represent surgical principles that are now fairly standard and universally employed. Accordingly, the *Atlas* serves a useful purpose as a general reference source for surgical anatomy of the thorax and for technical principles of surgical procedures that are applicable to this region of the body.

Michael E. DeBakey, M.D.
President and Chancellor,
Chairman of the Department of Surgery
Baylor College of Medicine
Houston, Texas

Preface to Volume One

The creation of illustrated works on surgery in the Russian literature dates back to the publication of the original atlases compiled by I. Buyalsky and N. Pirogov, eminent surgeons of the nineteenth century. They endeavored to provide physicians with visual aids demonstrating the anatomical and technical aspects of the performance of surgical operations.

The successes achieved in the development of Soviet surgery and the growth of specialized medical service called for the compilation of an authoritative practical atlas reflecting modern surgical techniques in such an expanding field as thoracic surgery. In creating such an atlas, the authors spared no effort to make not only a handy guide for experienced surgeons but, in equal measure, an indispensable manual for young surgeons just beginning to practice the specialty of thoracic surgery.

The *Atlas of thoracic surgery* we are offering to the reader comprises two volumes. The first deals with the surgical anatomy of the thorax and operations on the thoracic wall, the lungs, and the heart, and the second is devoted to operations on the major vessels of the thorax, on the esophagus, and on the diaphragm.

The material in the *Atlas* is based on the experience in the surgical treatment of diseases of the thoracic organs accumulated at the Institute of Clinical and Experimental Surgery, under the USSR Ministry of Public Health, headed by Academician Boris V. Petrovsky. This is why, from among the great variety of operations, preference has been given in the *Atlas* to modifications used by the authors. The modifications that are original are indicated in the text by an asterisk. Most of the drawings were made in the operating room. Drawings copied from other atlases or manuals are acknowledged in the legends.

The text accompanying the drawings explains the main principles of the methods and describes the techniques of the surgical operations as a whole.

The first volume of the *Atlas* was prepared for publication by specialists of the respective departments of the Institute (the section dealing with operations on the lungs by M. I. Perelman and V. A. Klimansky and the section concerned with operations on the heart by G. M. Solovyev) as well as by G. E. Ostroverkhov, Yu. M. Lopukhin, and N. S. Zheltikov, specialists in topographic anatomy and operative surgery, who have been closely collaborating with our Institute for many years.

The authors hope that the *Atlas* will prove valuable to all surgeons operating on the thoracic organs and will be grateful for any critical remarks in regard to this work.

Preface to Volume Two

The second volume of the *Atlas of thoracic surgery* is a continuation of Volume I which was published in 1971. This volume provides descriptions of surgical interventions undertaken in treating diseases of the major vessels of the thorax, the esophagus, and the diaphragm. Among the great variety of existing surgical techniques, the *Atlas* gives preference to those modifications that were elaborated at the Institute of Clinical and Experimental Surgery, under the USSR Ministry of Public Health, headed by Academician Boris V. Petrovsky. Most of the drawings were made in the operating room. This made it possible to reproduce the techniques of different stages of each operation as they were accomplished under the real conditions.

Contributions to the second volume of the *Atlas* were made by specialists of the respective departments of the Institute: the section dealing with operations on the major vessels of the thorax was contributed by N. N. Malinovsky and M. D. Knyazev, the section describing operations on the esophagus by E. N. Vantsyan and R. A. Toshchakov, and the section on operations on the diaphragm by N. O. Nikolaev and N. N. Kanshin.

Upon completing many years of work devoted to the *Atlas of thoracic surgery,* its authors hope that it will become a useful aid to surgeons operating on the thoracic organs. It is only natural that the first illustrated practical guide of this kind published in our country (USSR) will have its shortcomings, so the authors will be grateful for any critical remarks made by the readers of this work.

Contents

VOLUME ONE

VOLUME TWO

OPERATIONS ON THE DIAPHRAGM
N. O. Nikolaev and N. N. Kanshin

ATLAS OF THORACIC SURGERY

VOLUME ONE

The drawings in this volume were made by A. Medelyan (Surgical Anatomy of the Thorax), A. Gurevich and R. Dostyan (Operations on the Thoracic Wall), B. Shkuratov (Operations on the Lungs), and A. Gurevich, R. Dostyan, and V. Dedunik (Operations on the Heart).

SURGICAL ANATOMY OF THE THORAX

As a topographo-anatomical region the thorax is bounded cranially by a conditional line drawn along the edge of the jugular notch of the sternum, along the clavicles, and continued to the spinous process of the seventh cervical vertebra.

The caudal boundary of the thorax passes from the xiphoid process along the edges of the costal arches, through the ends of the eleventh and twelfth ribs, and then to the spinous process of the twelfth thoracic vertebra.

The thoracic region comprises the thoracic wall, the framework of which is formed by the bones of the thoracic cage covered with soft tissues, and the thoracic cavity containing the internal organs.

THE THORACIC WALL

The skeleton of the thoracic cage consists of the following structures: the thoracic vertebrae, twelve pairs of ribs, the sternum, the scapula, and the clavicles: it is covered with a musculoaponeurotic complex and forms a space for the thoracic organs, the thoracic cavity. Through the superior and inferior apertures of the thoracic cage the thoracic cavity communicates with the neighboring structures: the neck at the top and the abdominal cavity below. The superior aperture of the thorax (the inlet) is bounded by the first thoracic vertebra, the first pair of ribs, and the superior margin of the sternum. This aperture provides for the passage of the esophagus, trachea, vagus and phrenic nerves, the sympathetic trunk, carotid arteries, internal jugular veins, thoracic duct, and other structures.

The inferior aperture of the thoracic cage (outlet) is formed by the body of the twelfth thoracic vertebra, the lower borders of the twelfth ribs, the ends of the eleventh ribs, the costal arches, and the xiphoid process. The diaphragm, which is situated here, separates the thoracic cavity from the abdominal cavity. The aorta, esophagus, inferior vena cava, vagus and splanchnic nerves, thoracic duct, sympathetic trunk, and other structures pass through openings in the diaphragm. Two main shapes of the thoracic cage are distinguished: a wide and short, and a narrow and long shape. A wide thoracic cage is characterized by a large infrasternal (epigastric) angle reaching 120 degrees, a large circumference of the chest, and a width index (the ratio of the transverse measurement to the anteroposterior measurement multiplied by 100) of more than 140. In a narrow thoracic cage the infrasternal angle measures between 90 and 100 degrees, and the width index is under 130. The ribs extend more obliquely in a narrow thoracic cage than in a wide one.

The shape of the thoracic cage depends on the age, sex, and occupation of the individual, and the state of the internal organs.

Due to the relatively large dimensions of the liver, the thoracic cage of the newborn is characterized by a large anteroposterior diameter and horizontal position of the ribs. In adults the transverse diameter is larger than the anteroposterior, while the ribs acquire an oblique position.

The thoracic cage of females is relatively shorter and wider than that of males.

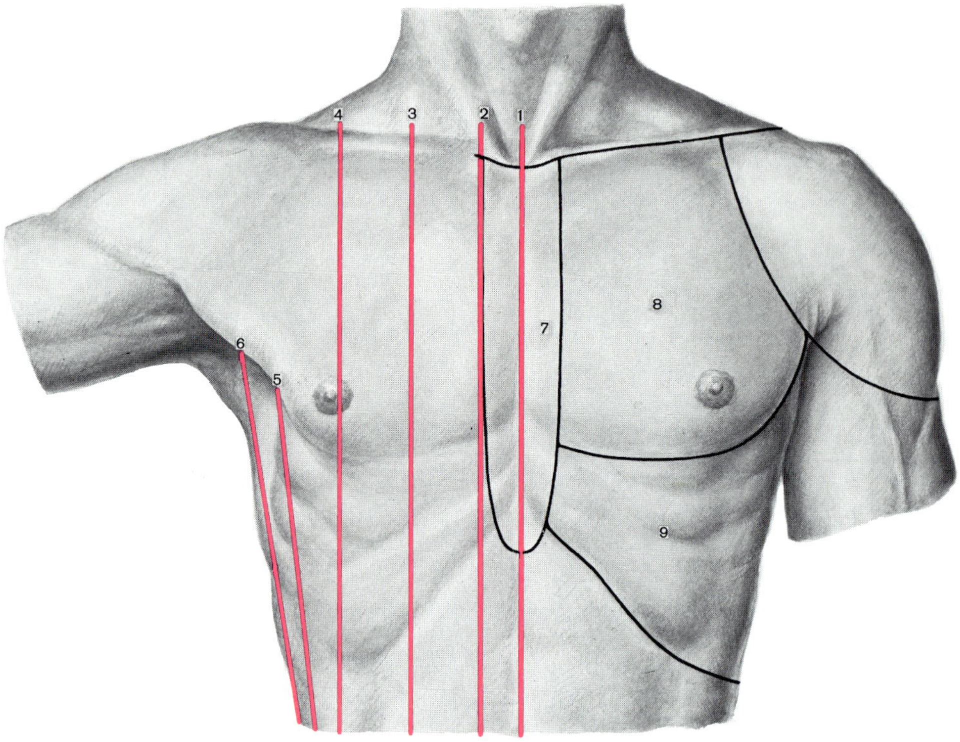

Fig. 1. Orientation lines and regions of the thorax (view from the front).

1 Anterior median line
2 Sternal line
3 Midclavicular line
4 Anterior axillary line
5 Midaxillary line
6 Posterior axillary line
7 Anteromedial region
8 Anterosuperior region
9 Anteroinferior region

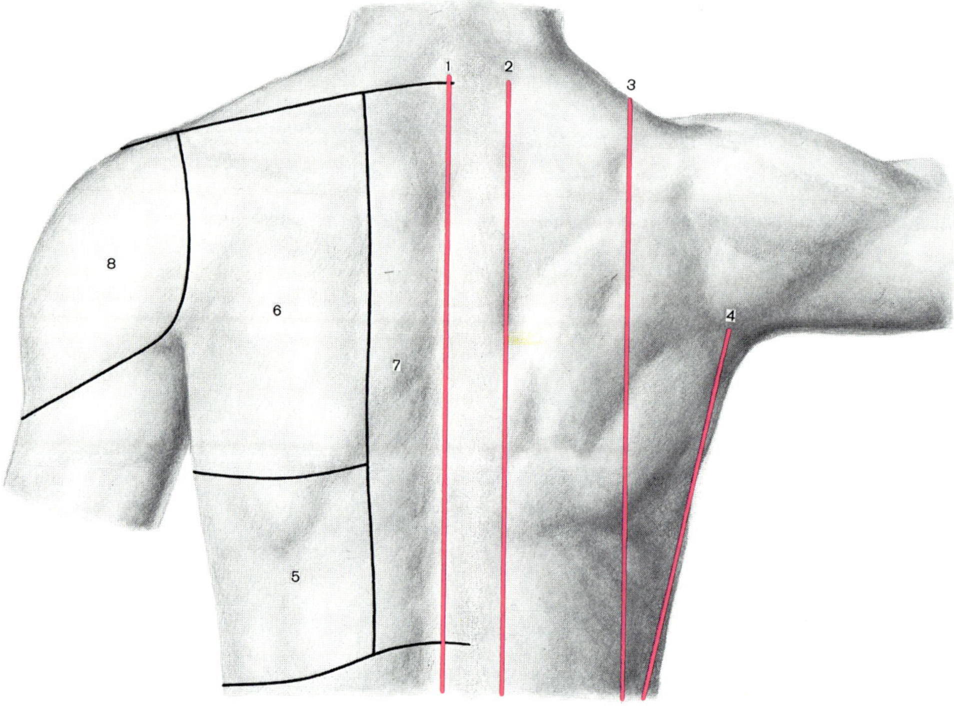

Fig. 2. Orientation lines and regions of the back.

1 Posterior median line
2 Paravertebral line
3 Scapular line
4 Posterior axillary line
5 Posteroinferior region
6 Posterosuperior region
7 Posteromedial region
8 Deltoid region

In most adults the thoracic wall is asymmetric because of the greater functional load experienced by the right shoulder girdle. Asymmetry of the thorax in athletes depends, to a definite extent, on the field of sports engaged in.

Pathologic processes in the thoracic wall, the skeleton in particular, as well as in the internal organs of the thorax or upper abdominal cavity may lead to considerable changes in the shape of the thoracic cage.

To determine the position of organs or the localization of pathologic processes, it is a common practice to draw vertical lines on the thoracic wall; the intersection of these lines with the ribs serve as precise topographic guides (Figs. 1 and 2).

The bone framework of the thoracic wall is covered on the outside with a musculoaponeurotic later, subcutaneous cellular tissue (subcutaneous fat), and skin.

The skin on the front and sides of the thorax is thin, and on the back it is thickened. The subcutaneous cellular tissue in the front is loose, while on the back it has a fine honeycomb structure and contains many connective tissue elements restricting the displacement of the skin.

In females the superficial fascia of the thorax is somewhat thickened along the upper margin of the mammary gland, acquiring the character of a ligament attached to the anterior surface of the clavicle. Arterial blood is supplied to the skin and subcutaneous fat by the branches of the internal thoracic, intercostal, and lateral thoracic arteries (Fig. 3).

The venous blood drains into the system of the axillary and subclavian veins. The veins of the anterolateral region of the thorax (vv. thoracoepigastricae and thoracicae internae) form wide anastomoses with the system of the superior vena cava and portal vein as the result of which they contribute to the development of collateral circulation in disturbed drainage along the portal vein system.

Innervation of the skin and subcutaneous fat of the thorax is effected by nn. cutanei colli, supraclaviculares, and thoracales laterales et intercostales. The lymphatic vessels extend to the lymph nodes situated in the axilla and behind the sternum.

The thorax, shoulder girdle, and part of the abdomen share a common musculoaponeurotic layer. In the anterior region, corresponding to the boundaries of the sternum, this layer is very fine and consists of just the fascia proper reinforced by tendon fibers that are firmly grown to the periosteum of the sternum.

In the anterosuperior region of the thorax (Fig. 4) the muscular layer is usually well developed and consists of the greater and smaller pectoral muscles, the former lying superficially and the latter deeper. In the upper part of the thoracic wall the subclavius muscle is found in the same layer as the smaller pectoral muscle, filling the space between the posteroinferior surface of the clavicle and the first rib. The four or five superior slips of the anterior serratus muscle arise from the lateral parts of the thorax.

The muscles of the thorax are invested in connective tissue sheets formed by the fascia pectoralis. Well-defined cellular spaces (known as superficial and deep subpectoral spaces) are found under the greater and smaller pectoral muscles; these spaces are continuous with the axilla (Fig. 5). The wide communication between the cellular spaces of the thoracic wall and the cellular tissue of the axilla provide favourable conditions for the spread of purulent inflammatory processes from one region to another.

The thoracic muscles are supplied with blood by branches of the intercostal, internal and lateral thoracic, and thoracodorsal arteries and are innervated by the anterior thoracic nerves.

Lymph drains into the axillary, clavicular, subclavicular, and retrosternal lymph nodes. Lymph nodes situated under the greater and smaller pectoral muscles collect lymph from the mammary glands. The fascia proper of the anteroinferior region of the thorax forms a sheath for the rectus abdominis muscle, which is inserted into the fifth, sixth, and seventh ribs. The cranial part of the external oblique muscle of the abdomen, arising from the anterior surfaces of the seventh and eighth ribs, adjoins the lateral surface of the rectus abdominis muscle. The fibers of the former muscle, interdigitating with the slips of the anterior serratus muscle, form a zigzagged line known as the Gerdi line. The fibers of the anterior serratus muscle also cover most of the lateral surface of the thoracic wall.

The intercostal, lateral thoracic, and thoracodorsal arteries contribute to the blood supply of the above-named muscles. Venous blood drains along the respective veins. Theregional lymph nodes are situated in the axilla. The muscles are innervated by n. thoracalis longus. On the back of the thorax (Fig. 6) the superficial muscles are the trapezius and the latissimus dorsi muscles, which are invested in a sheath formed by a superficial sheet of the thoracolumbar fascia. Next comes a group of muscles closely connected to the scapula (Fig. 7): the supraspinatus, infraspinatus, the teres major and minor, and rhomboid muscles. The last cover the posterior superior serratus muscle. The infraspinatus and supraspinatus muscles are situated in a well-defined osteofibrous space formed by the deep sheet of the thoracolumbar fascia and the posterior surface of the scapula.

In front of the scapula are the subscapular muscle lining the subscapular fossa and the anterior serratus muscle, which arises from the external surfaces of the

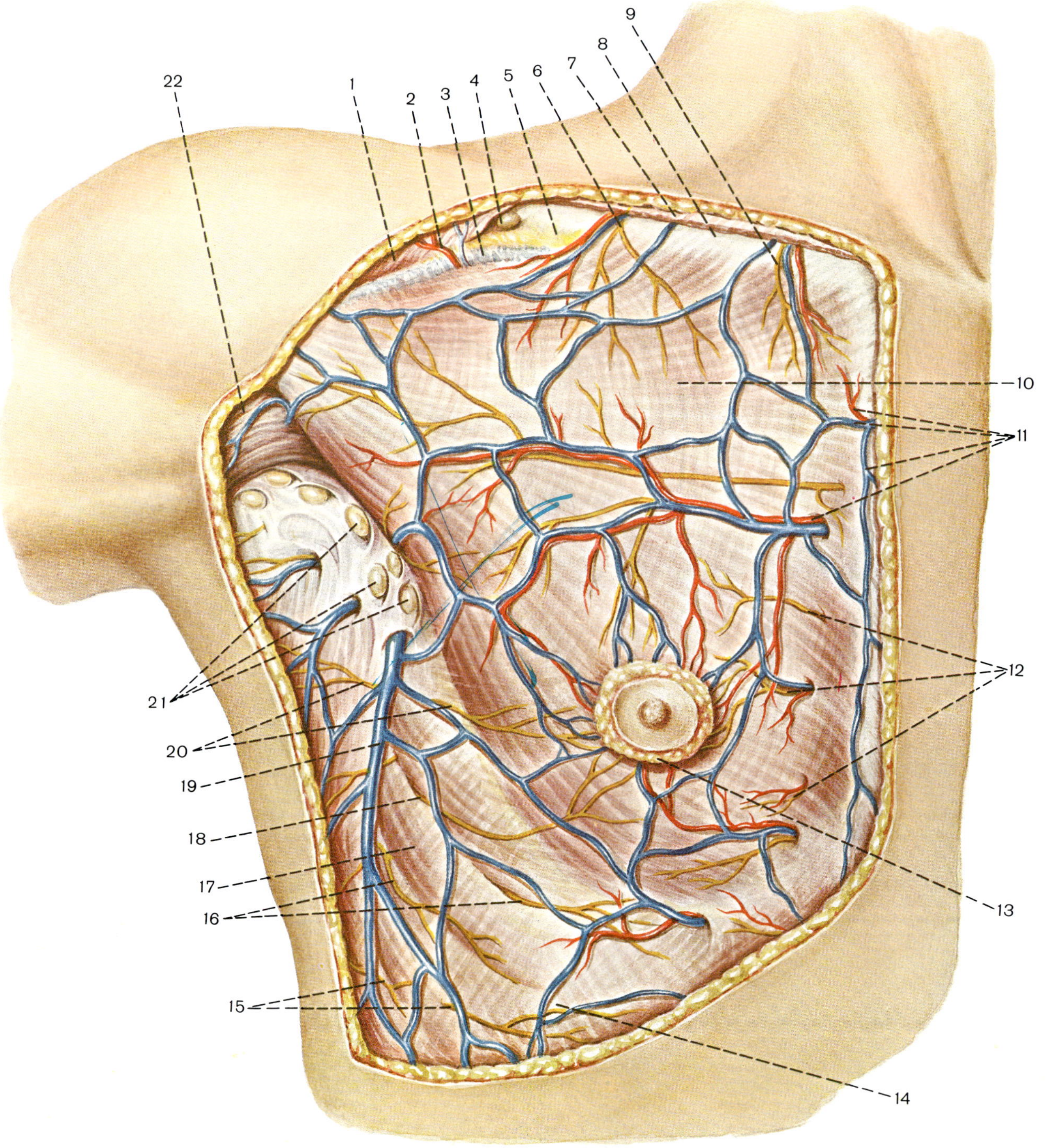

Fig. 3. Superficial vessels and nerves of the anterolateral region of the thorax.

1 Deltoid muscle (m. deltoideus)
2 Cutaneous branch (a. thoracoacromialis)
3 Cephalic vein (v. cephalica)
4 Subclavian lymph node
5 Infraclavicular fossa (fossa infraclavicularis)
6, 9 Supraclavicular nerve (n. supraclaviculares)
7 Platysma (m. platysma)
8 Clavicle
10 Greater pectoral muscle (m. pectoralis major)
11 rr. perforantes arterial thoracicae internae
12 rr. cutanei anteriores nn. intercostales
13 Mammary gland
14 External oblique muscle of abdomen (m. obliquus externus abdominis)
15 r. cutaneus lateralis n. intercostalis VII
16 r. cutaneus lateralis n. intercostalis VI
17 Anterior seratus muscle (m. serratus anterior)
18 r. cutaneus lateralis n. intercostalis
19 v. thoracoepigastrica
20 r. cutaneus lateralis n. intercostalis IV
21 Axillary lymph nodes
22 Biceps muscle of arm (m. biceps brachii)

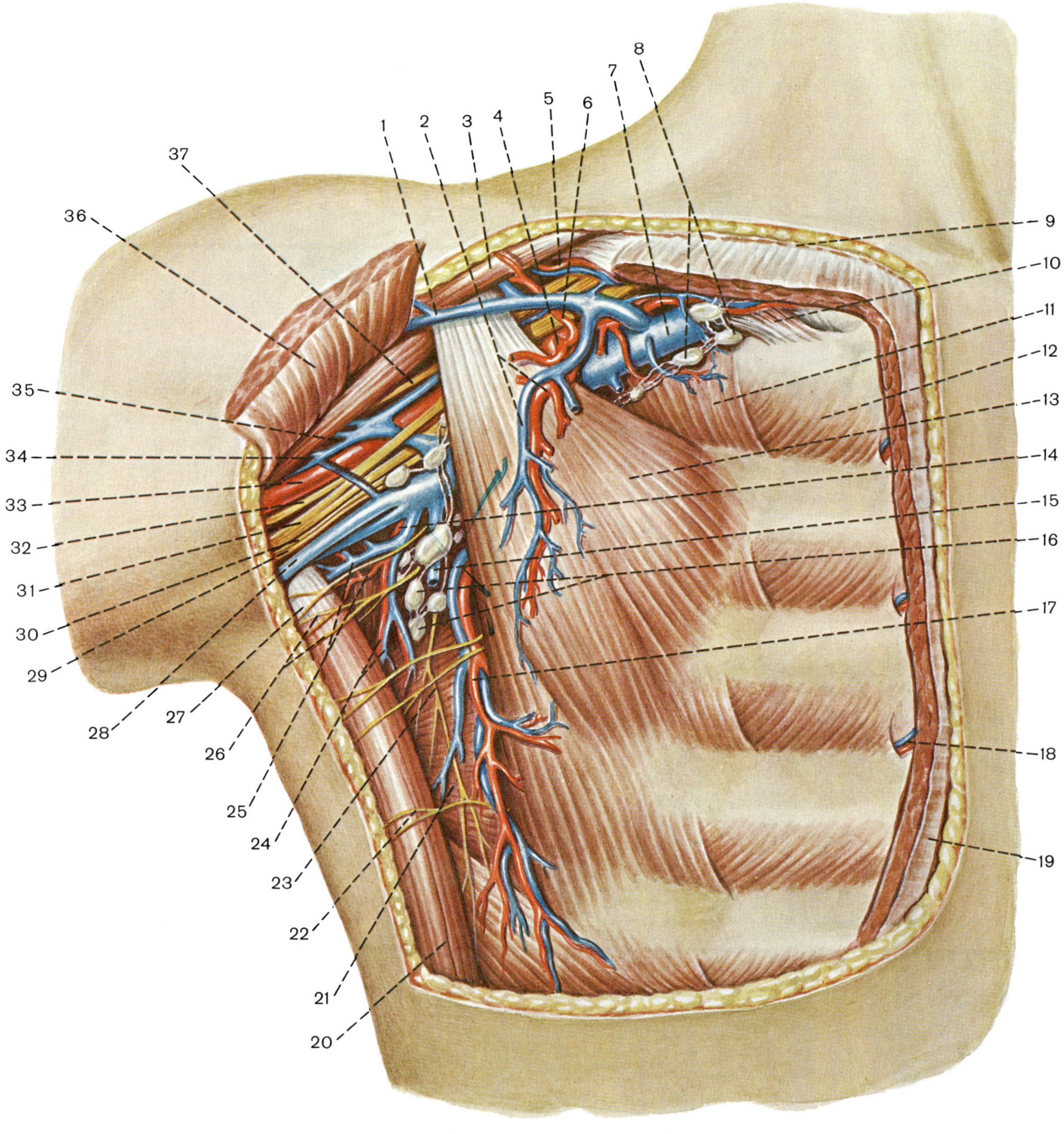

Fig. 4. Deep structures of the anterolateral thoracic region.

1 Cephalic vein (v. cephalica)
2 rr. pectorales a. et v. thoracoacromiales
3 Deltoid muscle (m. deltoideus)
4 a. thoracoacromialis
5 a. et v. suprascapulares, n. suprascapularis
6 r. acromialis a. thoracoacromialis
7 Axillary vein (v. axillaris)
8 Subclavian lymph nodes
9 Platysma (m. platysma)
10 Subclavius muscle (m. subclavius)
11 External intercostal muscle (m. intercostalis externus)
12 Internal intercostal muscle (m. intercostalis internus)
13 Smaller pectoral muscle (m. pectoralis minor)
14 a. et v. subscapulares
15 v. thoracoepigastrica
16 Deep axillary lymph nodes
17 Lateral thoracic artery and vein (a. et v. thoracicae laterales)
18 rr. cutanei anterioes nn. intercostales et rr. perforantes a. thoracicae internae
19 Greater pectoral muscle (m. pectoralis major)
20 Latissimus muscle of back (m. lattissimus dorsi)
21 Anterior serratus muscle of back (m. serratus anterior)
22 r. cutaneus lateralis n. intercostalis
23 Long thoracic nerve (n. thoracalis longus)
24 a. et v. thoracodorsales, n. thoracalis longus
25 a. et v. circumflexae scapulae
26 nn. intercostobrachiales
27 n. cutaneus brachii medalis
28 v. basilica
29 n. cutaneus antebrachii medalis
30 Ulnar nerve (n. ulnaris)
31 Median nerve (n. medianus)
32 Radial nerve (n. radialis)
33 Axillary artery (a. axillaris)
34 a. circumflexa humeri anterior
35 a. circumflexa humeri posterior
36 Greater pectoral muscle (m. pectoralis major)
37 Musculocutaneous nerve (n. musculocutaneus)

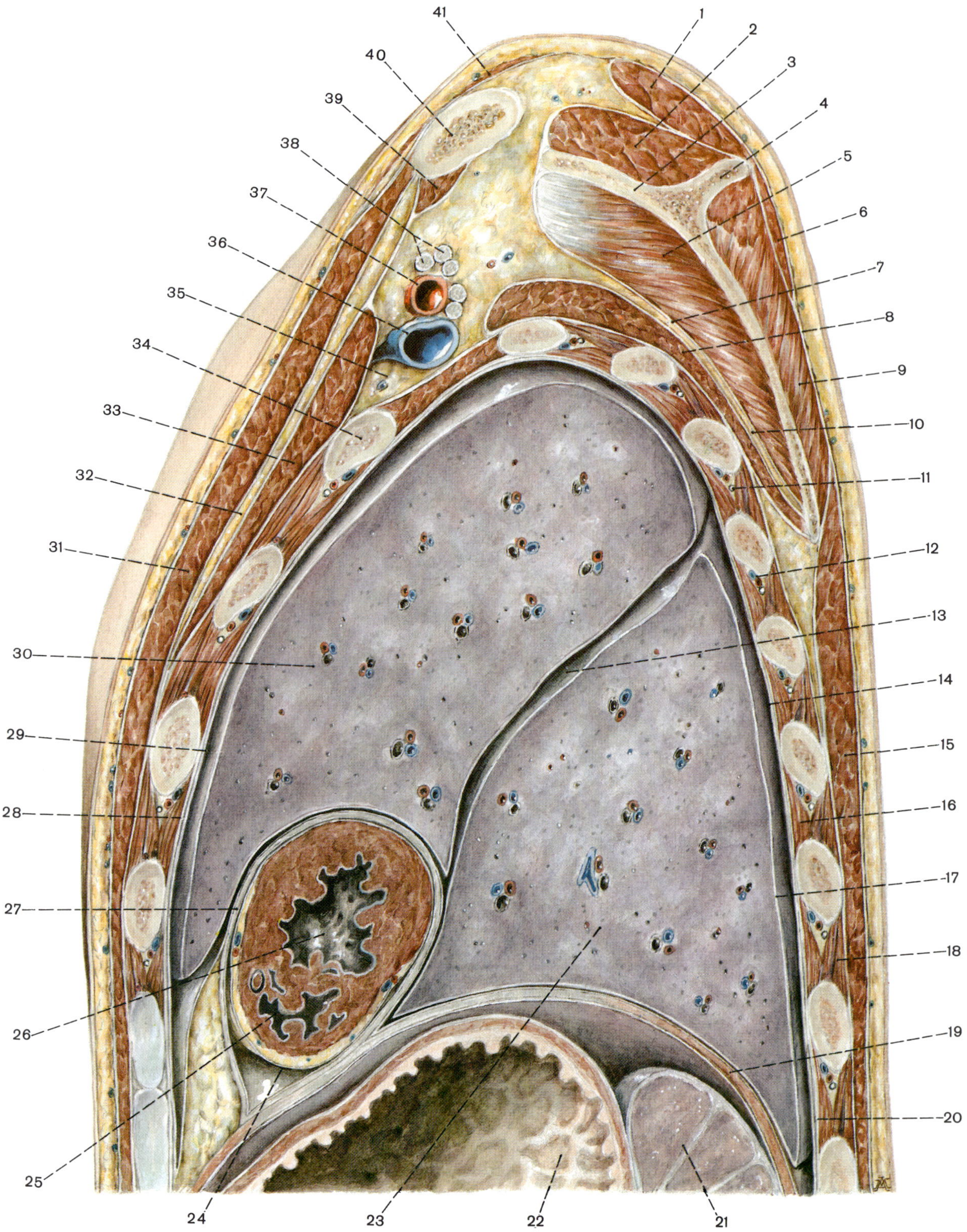

Fig. 5. Sagittal section of thorax through left scapula along midclavicular line.

1 Trapezius muscle (m. trapezius)
2 Supraspinous muscle (m. supraspinatus)
3 Scapula
4 Spine of scapula (spina scapulae)
5 Subscapular muscle (m. subscapularis)
6 Deltoid muscle (m. deltoideus)
7 Subscapular fascia
8 Anterior serratus muscle (m. serratus anterior)
9 Infraspinous muscle (m. infraspinatus)
10 Posterior prescapular space
11 Intercostal nerve (n. intercostalis)
12 Intercostal artery and vein (a. et v. intercostales)
13 Oblique fissure of lung (fissura oblique pulmonis)
14 Parietal pleura (pleura parietalis)
15 m. latissimus dorsi
16 Internal intercostal muscle (m. intercostalis internus)
17 Pulmonary pleura (pleura pulmonalis)
18 External intercostal muscle (m. intercostalis externus.
19 Diaphragm (diaphragma)
20, 28 Endothoracic fascia (fascia endothoracica)
21 Spleen (lien)
22 Stomach (ventriculus)
23 Inferior lobe of left lung (lobus inferior pulmonis sinistri)
24 Heart (cor)
25 Right ventricle (ventriculus dexter)
26 Left ventricle (ventriculus sinister)
27 Pericardium
29 Parietal pleura (pleura parietalis)
30 Superior lobe of left lung (lobus superior pulmonis sinistri)
31 Greater pectoral muscle (m. pectoralis major)
32 Superficial subpectoral cellular space
33 Smaller pectoral muscle (m. pectoralis minor)
34 Second rib (costa II)
35 Deep subpectoral cellular space
36 Left subclavian vein (v. subclavia sinistra)
37 Left subclavian artery (a. subclavia sinistra)
38 Brachial plexus (plexus brachialis)
39 Subclavius muscle (m. subclavius)
40 Clavicle (clavicula)
41 Platysma (m. platysma)

nine upper ribs and is inserted into the vertebral border of the scapula, securing it to the thoracic cage.

A space is left between the thoracic wall and the anterior surface of the subscapular muscle, which is divided by the anterior serratus muscle into two, anterior and posterior prescapular spaces.

The anterior prescapular space is located between the anterior serratus muscle and the fascia, which covers the ribs and intercostal muscles. It is relatively incommunicado, and therefore pus accumulating in it in purulent inflammatory processes may stay there for a long time without spreading to the neighboring region.

The posterior prescapular space is between the subscapular and anterior serratus muscles. The cellular tissue filling it is continuous with that of the axilla. The musculoaponeurotic structures of the dorsal surface of the thorax are supplied with blood by the transverse cervical, suprascapular, and subscapular arteries and other branches. The muscles are innervated by nn. subscapulares and suprascapulares.

The lymph drains into the system of the axillary lymph nodes.

The deep layer of the thoracic cage is formed of the thoracic vertebrae, ribs, sternum, clavicles, and the intercostal muscles (Fig. 8).

The external intercostal muscles fill the intercostal spaces along the distance from the tubercles of the ribs to the place where the ribs become continuous with the cartilages. From here the muscles are replaced by tendon fibers forming the external intercostal ligaments. The fibers of the external intercostal muscles extend downward, forward, and inward. The internal intercostal muscles stretch from the angles of the ribs to the lateral border of the sternum. The direction of their fibers is opposite to that of the fibers of the external intercostal muscles. Because of the opposite direction taken by the fibers of the intercostal muscles and the different levels of their insertion into the ribs, a space forms between the external and internal intercostal muscles filled with loose fatty cellular tissue in which the intercostal neurovascular bundle (the artery, vein, and nerve) is found.

The posterior intercostal arteries arise from the thoracic aorta, with the exception of the first two, which arise from the costocervical trunk.

The right posterior intercostal arteries cross the vertebral column ventrally, stretching behind the esophagus, thoracic duct, and the azygos vein and then behind the thoracic portion of the sympathetic chain.

The left posterior intercostal arteries stretch directly into the intercostal spaces, crossing the hemiazygos vein and the sympathetic chain on the dorsal surface. The posterior intercostal arteries have pronounced anastomoses with the anterior intercostal arteries, which are branches of the internal thoracic artery. These anastomoses are important in the development of collateral circulation in coarctation of the aorta and other abnormalities.

In the posterolateral parts of the thoracic wall the intercostal neurovascular bundle adjoins the costal sulcus, where it is covered with the lower borders of the ribs. To the back of the scapula and to the front of the anterior axillary line, the neurovascular bundle occupies a medial position in the intercostal spaces. In view of this, the vessels and nerves, unprotected by the ribs, may be injured when the thoracic wall is punctured dorsal to the costal angles, or ventral to the axillary line.

The transverse muscle of the thorax on the inner surface of the ribs arises from the lower half of the thoracic wall by means of three or four slips and is inserted into the cartilages of the second to sixth ribs.

The internal thoracic artery arising from the subclavian artery in the region of the scalenovertebral triangle stretches along the inner surface of the thoracic wall relative to the parasternal lines. To the level of the third rib the artery is located between the internal intercostal muscles and the endothoracic fascia. Below this level it is between the internal intercostal muscles and the transversus thoracis muscle. Then it passes through the intermuscular slits in the diaphragm onto the dorsal surface of the anterior abdominal wall, where it is continuous with the superior epigastric artery. Along its length the internal thoracic artery gives rise to branches to the intercostal spaces. At the level of the first rib the artery branches off the pericardiacophrenic artery, which accompanies the phrenic nerve and extends to the ventrolateral surface of the pericardium.

The cellular tissue around the intrathoracic vessels contains lymph nodes (four to five), which collect lymph from the medial parts of the mammary glands.

The inner surface of the ribs and intercostal muscles is lined with the endothoracic fascia, the strength of which is not the same in different parts. It is most conspicuous in the region of the cervical pleura because it is reinforced there with bundles of the costopleural and vertebropleural ligaments.

In the anterior parts of the thoracic cage the endothoracic fascia is also thicker and is called Rudnev's retrosternal fascia, which separates the retrosternal cellular space from the anterior mediastinum. The costal pleura lies directly next to the endothoracic fascia.

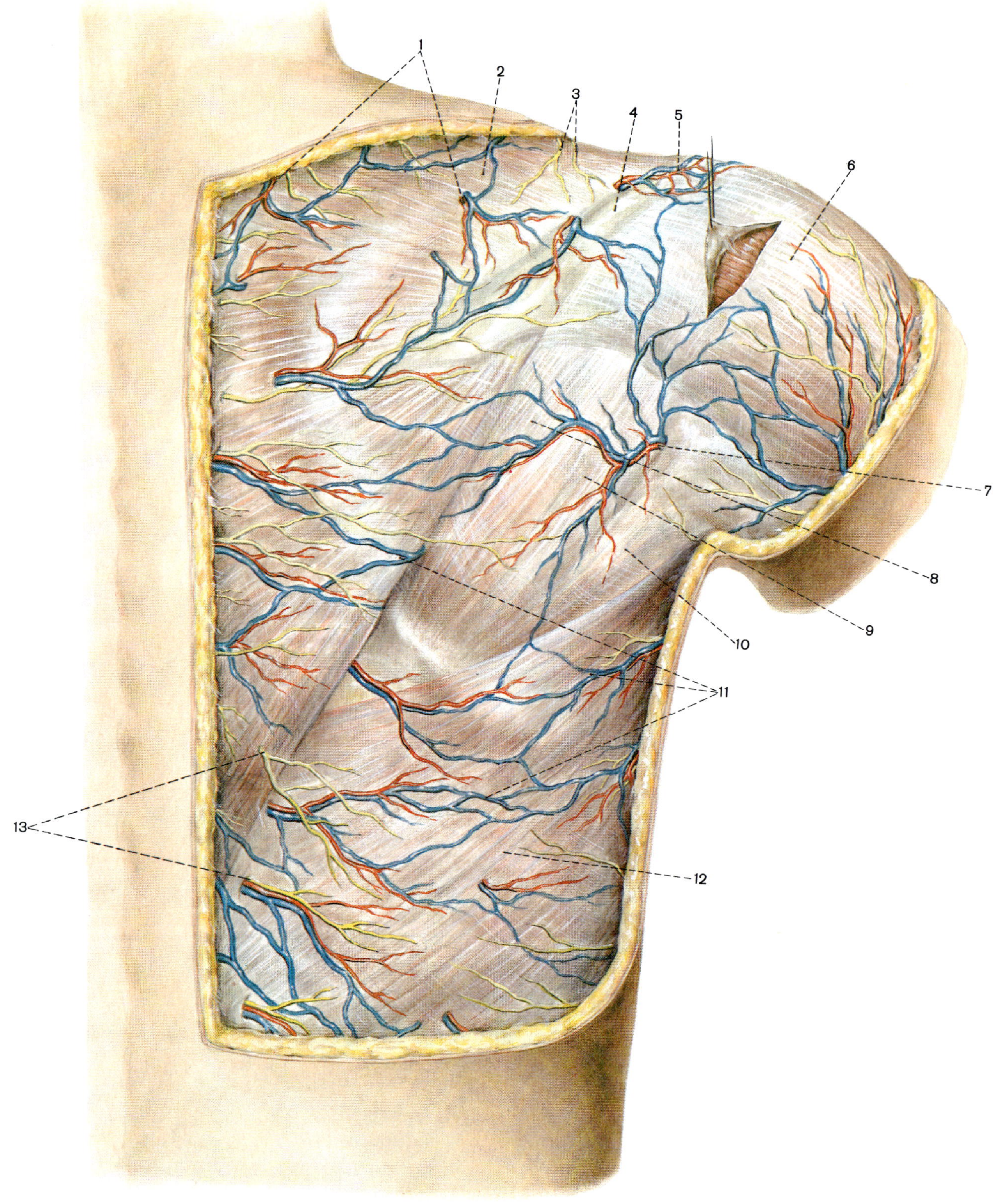

Fig. 6. Superficial structures of the back.

1 a. cervicalis superficialis
2 Trapezius muscle (m. trapezius)
3 nn. supraclaviculares posteriores
4 Spine of scapula (spina scapulae)
5 Rete acromiale
6 Deltoid muscle (m. deltoideus)
7 Superficial branch of a. circumflexae scapulae
8 Infraspinous muscle (m. infraspinatus)
9 Teres minor muscle (m. teres minor)
10 Teres major muscle (m. teres major)
11 Subcutaneous veins of the back
12 Latissimus muscle of back (m. latissimus dorsi)
13 rr. laterales, rr. dorsalium thoracicorum

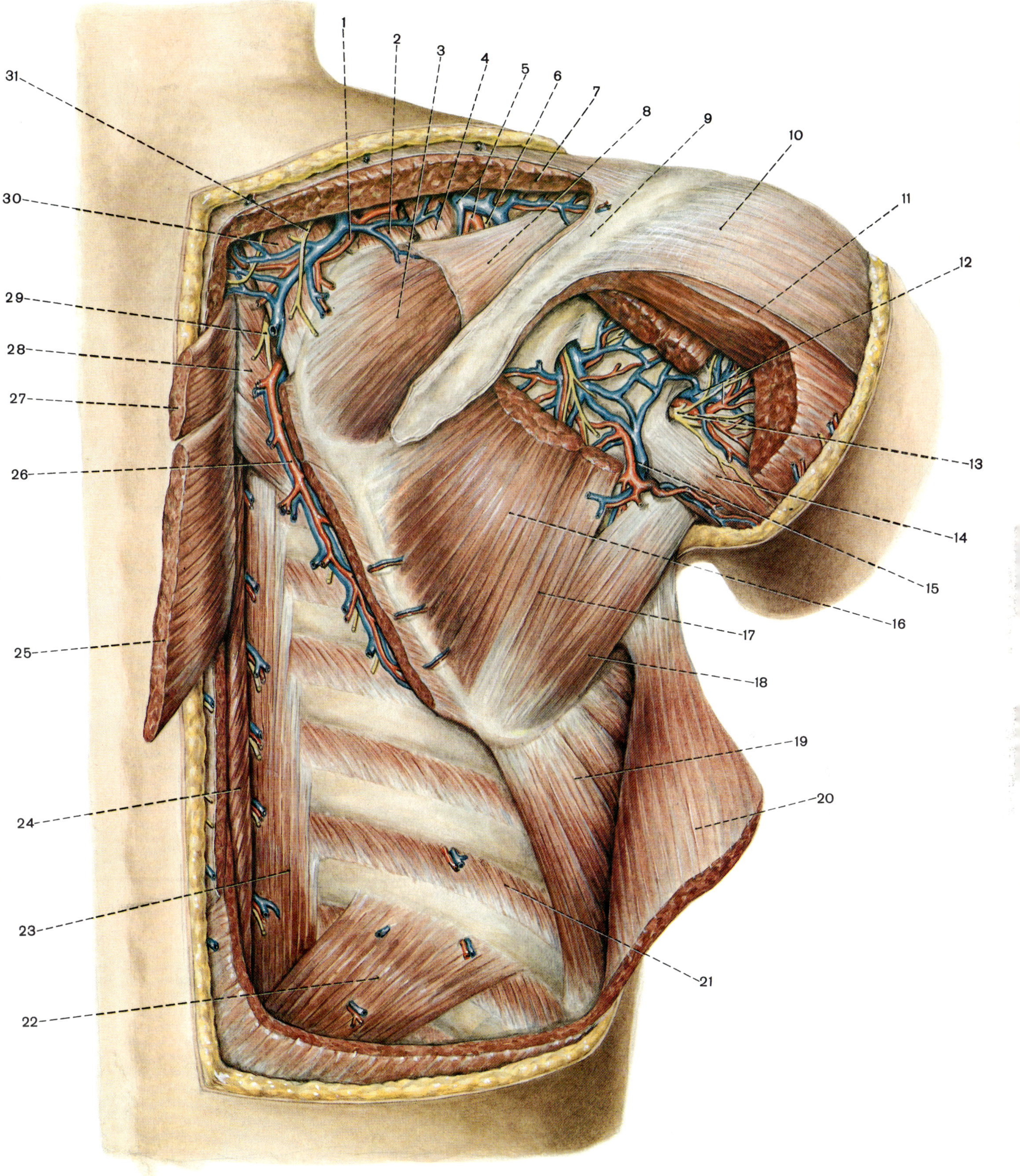

Fig. 7. Deep structures of the back.

1 Superficial branches of the transverse cervical entry (r. superficialis a. transversae colli)
2 Posterior scalene muscle (m. scalenus posterior)
3 Supraspinous muscle (m. supraspinatus)
4 Omohyoid muscle (m. omohyoideus)
5 Suprascapular artery and vein (a. et v. suprascapulares)
6 Suprascapular nerve (n. suprascapularis)
7 Trapezius muscle (m. trapezius)
8 Supraspinous fascia (fascia supraspinata)
9 Spine of scapula (spina scapulae)
10 Deltoid fascia (fascia deltoidea)
11 Deltoid muscle (m. deltoideus)
12 Circumflex humeral arteries and veins (a. et v. circumflexae humeri)
13 Axillary nerve (n. axillaris)
14 Triceps muscle of arm (m. triceps brachii)
15 Circumflex artery and vein of scapula (a. et v. circumflexae scapulae)
16 Intraspinous muscle (m. infraspinatus)
17 Teres minor muscle (m. teres minor)
18 Teres major muscle (m. teres major)
19 Anterior serratus muscle (m. serratus anterior)
20 Latissimus muscle of back (m. latissimus dorsi)
21 External intercostal muscle (m. intercostalis externus)
22 Inferior posterior serratus muscle (m. serratus posterior inferior)
23 Iliocostal muscle of thorax (m. iliocostalis thoracis)
24 Longissimus muscle of thorax (m. longissimus thoracis)
25 Greater rhomboid muscle (m. rhomboideus major)
26 Deep branch of transverse cervical artery (r. descendens a. transverae colli)
27 Lesser rhomboid muscle (m. rhomboideus minor)
28 Superior posterior serratus muscle (m. serratus posterior superior)
29 Dorsal nerve of scapula (n. dorsalis scapulae)
30 Levator muscle of scapula (m. levator scapulae)
31 Muscular branch of the cervical plexus (r. muscularis plexus cervicales)

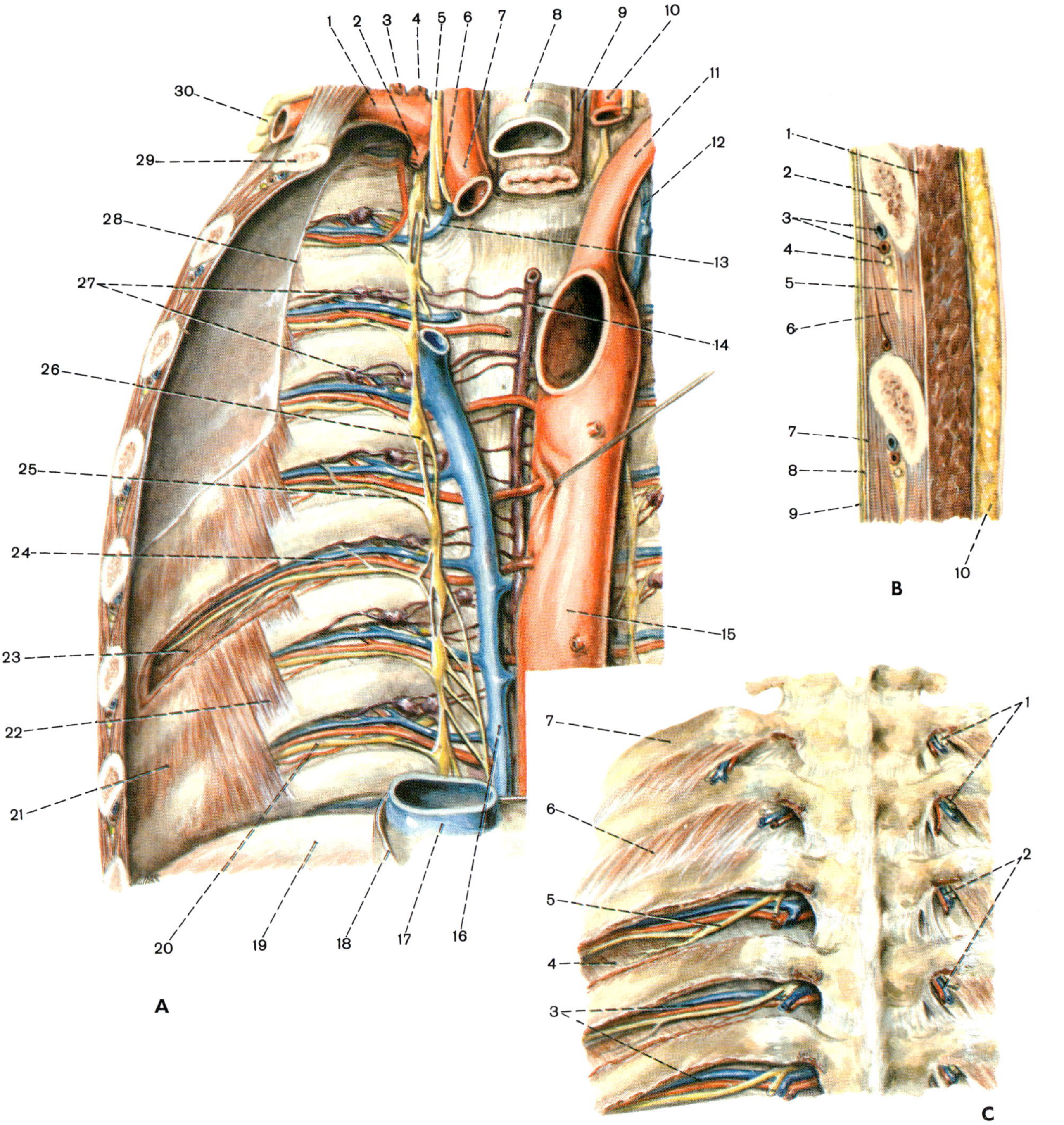

Fig. 8. Topography of intercostal neurovascular bundle.

A, ANTERIOR ASPECT:

1,11 Right and left subclavian arteries (aa. subclaviae)
2 Internal thoracic artery (a. thoracica interna)
3 Thyrocervical trunk (truncus thyreocervicalis)
4 Vertebral artery (a. vertebralis)
5 Right vagus nerve (n. vagus dexter)
6 Right recurrent laryngeal nerve (n. laryngeus recurrens dexter)
7 Brachiocephalic trunk (truncus brachiocephalicus)
8 Trachea
9 Esophagus
10 Common carotid artery (a. carotis communis)
12 Accessory hemiazgos vein (v. hemiazygos accessoria)
13 Highest intercostal vein (v. intercostalis suprema)
14 Thoracic duct (ductus thoracicus)
15 Aorta
16 Azygos vein (v. azygos)
17 Inferior vena cava (v. cava inferior)
18 Pericardium
19 Diaphragm (diaphragma)
20 Intercostal nerve (n. intercostalis)
21 Internal intercostal muscles (mm. intercostales interni)
22 Subcostal muscles (mm. subcostales)
23 External intercostal muscles (mm. intercostales externi)
24 Intercostal artery and vein (a. et v. intercostales)
25 Branch connecting the sympathetic trunk (r. communicans truncus sympathicus)
26 Sympathetic trunk (truncus sympathicus)
27 Intercostal lymph nodes
28 Costal pleura (pleura costalis)
29 First rig (costa I)
30 Brachial plexus (plexus brachialis)

B, CROSS-SECTION:

1 Pectoral fascia (fascia pectoralis)
2 Ribs (costae)
3 Intercostal artery and vein (a. et v. intercostales)
4 Intercostal nerve (n. intercostalis)
5 External intercostal muscle (m. intercostalis externus)
6 Internal intercostal muscle (m. intercostalis internus)
7 Endothoracic fascia (fascia endothoracica)
8 Prepleural cellular tissue
9 Costal pleura (pleura costalis)
10 Subcutaneous cellular tissue

C, POSTERIOR ASPECT:

1 Dorsal branches of intercostal nerves (rr. dorsales nn. intercostales)
2 Dorsal branches of intercostal arteries and veins (rr. dorsales aa. et vv. intercostalium)
3 Intercostal artery and vein (a. et v. intercostales)
4 Internal intercostal muscle (m. intercostalis internus)
5 Intercostal nerve (n. intercostalis)
6 External intercostal muscle (m. intercostalis externus)
7 First rib (costa I)

THE DIAPHRAGM

The diaphragm (Figs. 9 and 10) is located in the inferior thoracic aperture and separates the thoracic and the abdominal cavities. The diaphragm resembles a trifoliolate leaf in shape with a convex superior surface. Its central parts are formed of tendon structures, and the peripheral of muscular structures. The tendon and muscular areas have openings for the esophagus, aorta, vena cava inferior, azygos vein, nerves, etc.

The central tendon of the diaphragm is a dense plate of fibrous bundles. Three blades (leaves) are distinguished in it: two lateral (right and left) and an anterior blade. The medial part of the right blade has an opening for the vena cava inferior. Three parts are distinguished in the muscular area of the diaphragm: costal, sternal, and lumbar.

The costal part arises by separate muscular bundles from the six lower ribs. These muscular bundles are directed medially and are continuous with the central tendon.

The sternal part of the diaphragm consists of two small muscular bundles arising from the posterior surface of the xiphoid process. There are triangular spaces free of muscles between the sternal and costal parts which are known as Morgagni's triangle (on the right) and Larrey's fissure (on the left).

The lumbar part of the diaphragm forms three crura on each side: medial, median, and lateral. The right and left medial crura interdigitate to form the aortic and esophageal openings. The muscular bundles of the esophageal opening form a peculiar constrictor of the esophagus. In individual cases with developmental defects of the diaphgram, the esophageal opening may be the site of herniations of the diaphragm. The medial and median crura of the diaphragm form slits that transmit the splanchnic nerves and the azygos and hemiazygos veins. The sympathetic trunk stretches in the space between the median and lateral crura. A fissure left between the lateral crus and the costal part of the diaphragm is known as Bochdalek's foramen.

The diaphragm is covered on both sides with sheets of the endothoracic and endoabdominal (transverse) fasciae.

The diaphragm is supplied with blood by the internal thoracic artery, superior and inferior phrenic arteries, and branches of the intercostal artery. Venous blood is drained along the veins of the same name.

Innervation is accomplished by the phrenic nerves and branches of the intercostal nerves.

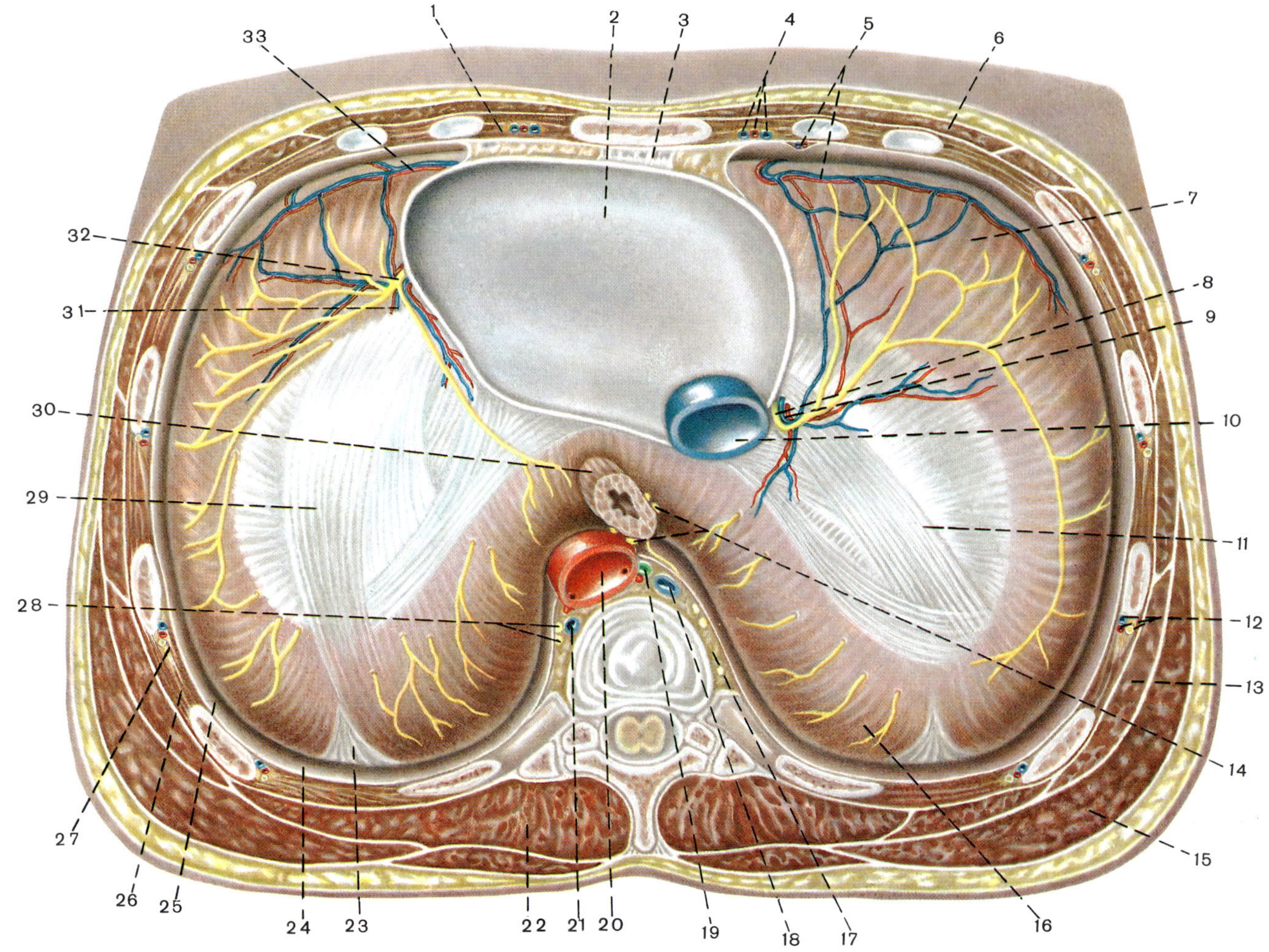

Fig. 9. Diaphragm viewed from thoracic cavity.

1 Transverse muscle of thorax (m. transversus thoracis)
2 Pericardium
3 Sternopericardiac ligament (ligamentum sternopericardiaca)
4 Internal thoracic artery and veins (a. et vv. thoracicae internae)
5 Right musculophrenic artery and vein (a. et v. musculophrenicae dextri)
6 Greater pectoral muscle (m. pectoralis major)
7 Costal part of diaphragm (pars costalis diaphragmatis)
8 Right phrenic nerve (n. phrenicus dexter)
9 Pericardiacophrenic artery and vein (a. et v. pericardiacophrenicae)
10 Inferior vena cava (v. cava inferior)
11, 29 Central tendon of diaphragm (centrum tendineum diaphragmatis)
12 Intercostal artery, vein, and nerve) a. et v. intercostales, n. intercostalis)
13 Anterior serratus muscle (m. serratus anterior)
14 Trunks of the vagus nerves (trunci nervorum vagalis)
15 Latissimus muscle of back (m. latissimus dorsi)
16 Lumbar part of diaphragm (pars lumbalis diaphragmatis)
17 Sympathetic trunk (truncus sympathicus)
18 Azygos vein (n. azygos)
19 Thoracic duct (ductus thoracicus)
20 Thoracic aorta (aorta thoracica)
21 Hemiazygos vein (v. hemiazygos)
22 m. erector spinae
23 Trigonum lumbocostale
24 Costodiaphragmatic sinus, or recess (recessus costodiaphragmaticus)
25 Parietal pleura (pleura parietalis)
26 External intercostal muscle (m. intercostalis externus)
27 Internal intercostal muscle (m. intercostalis internus)
28 Greater and lesser splanchnic nerves (nn. splanchnici, major et minor)
30 Esophagus
31 Pericardiacophrenic artery and vein (a. and v. pericardiacophrenicae)
32 Left phrenic nerve (n. phrenicus sinister)
33 Left musculophrenic artery and vein (a. et v. musculophrenicae sinistri)

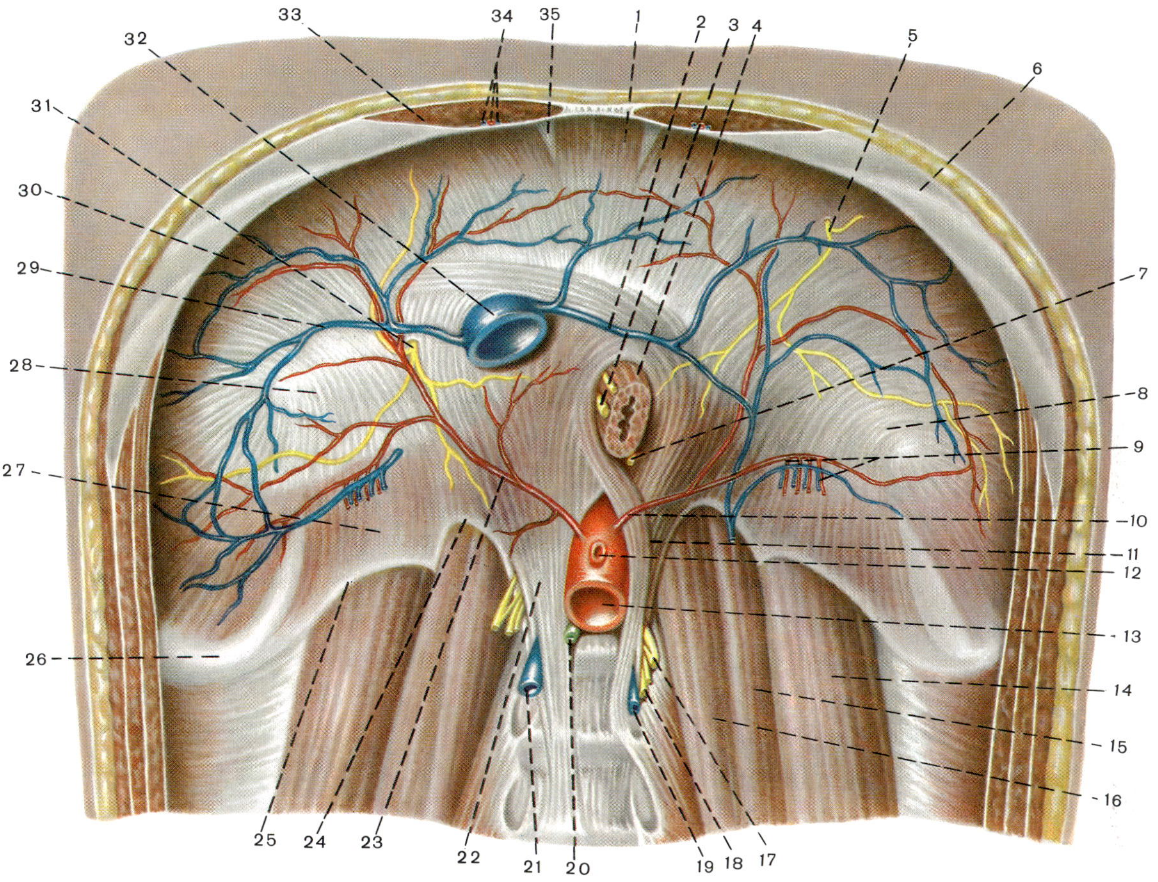

Fig. 10. Diaphragm viewed from abdominal cavity.

1 Sternal part of diaphragm (pars sternalis diaphragmatis)
2 Left phrenic vein (v. phrenica sinistra)
3 Right vagus nerve (truncus vagalis dexter)
4 Esophagus
5 Left phrenic nerve (n. phrenicus sinister)
6 Costal arch (arcus costalis)
7 Left vagus nerve (truncus vagalis sinister)
8 Central tendon of diaphragm (centrum tendineum diaphragmatis)
9 Superior suprarenal arteries and veins (aa. et vv. suprarenales superiores)
10 Left interior phrenic artery (a. phrenica inferior sinistra)
11 Left crus of diaphragm (curs sinistrum diaphragmatis)
12 Celiac trunk (truncus celiacus)
13 Abdomnial aorta (aorta abdominalis)
14 Quadrate muscle of loins (m. quadratus lumborum)
15 Greater psoas muscle (m. psoas major)
16 Smaller psoas muscle (m. psoas minor)
17 Sympathetic trunk (truncus sympathicus)
18 Greater and lesser splanchnic nerves (nn. splanchnici, major et minor)
19 Hemiazygos vein (v. hemiazygos)
20 Thoracic duct (ductus thoracicus)
21 Azygos vein (v. azygos)
22 Right crus of diaphragm (crus dextrum diaphragmatix)
23 Right inferior phrenic artery (a. phrenica inferior dextra)
24 Medical arcuate ligament of diaphragm (arcus lumbocostalis medialis)
25 Lateral arcuate ligament of diaphragm (arcus lumbocostalis lateralis)
26 Trigonom lumbocostale
27 Lumbar part of diaphragm (pars lumbalis diaphragmatis)
28 Central tendon of diaphragm (centrum tendineum diaphragmatis)
29 Right phrenic vein (v. phrenica dextra)
30 Costal part of diaphragm (pars costalis diaphragmatis)
31 Right phrenic nerve (n. phrenicus dexter)
32 Inferior vena cava (v. cava inferior)
33 Straight muscle of abdomen (m. rectus abdominis)
34 Internal thoracic artery and vein (a. et v. thoracicae internae)
35 Sternocostal triangle (trigonum sternocostale)

THE THORACIC CAVITY

The thoracic cavity is bounded by the plane of the superior aperture at the top, the diaphragm at the bottom, the dorsal surface of the sternum in front, the ventral surface of the vertebral column at the back, and the walls of the thoracic cage lined with the endothoracic fascia on the sides.

The thoracic cavity (Fig. 11) contains two pleural sacs with the lungs, and the mediastinum in which the heart with the pericardium, the large vessels, the esophagus, nerves, and other structures are located.

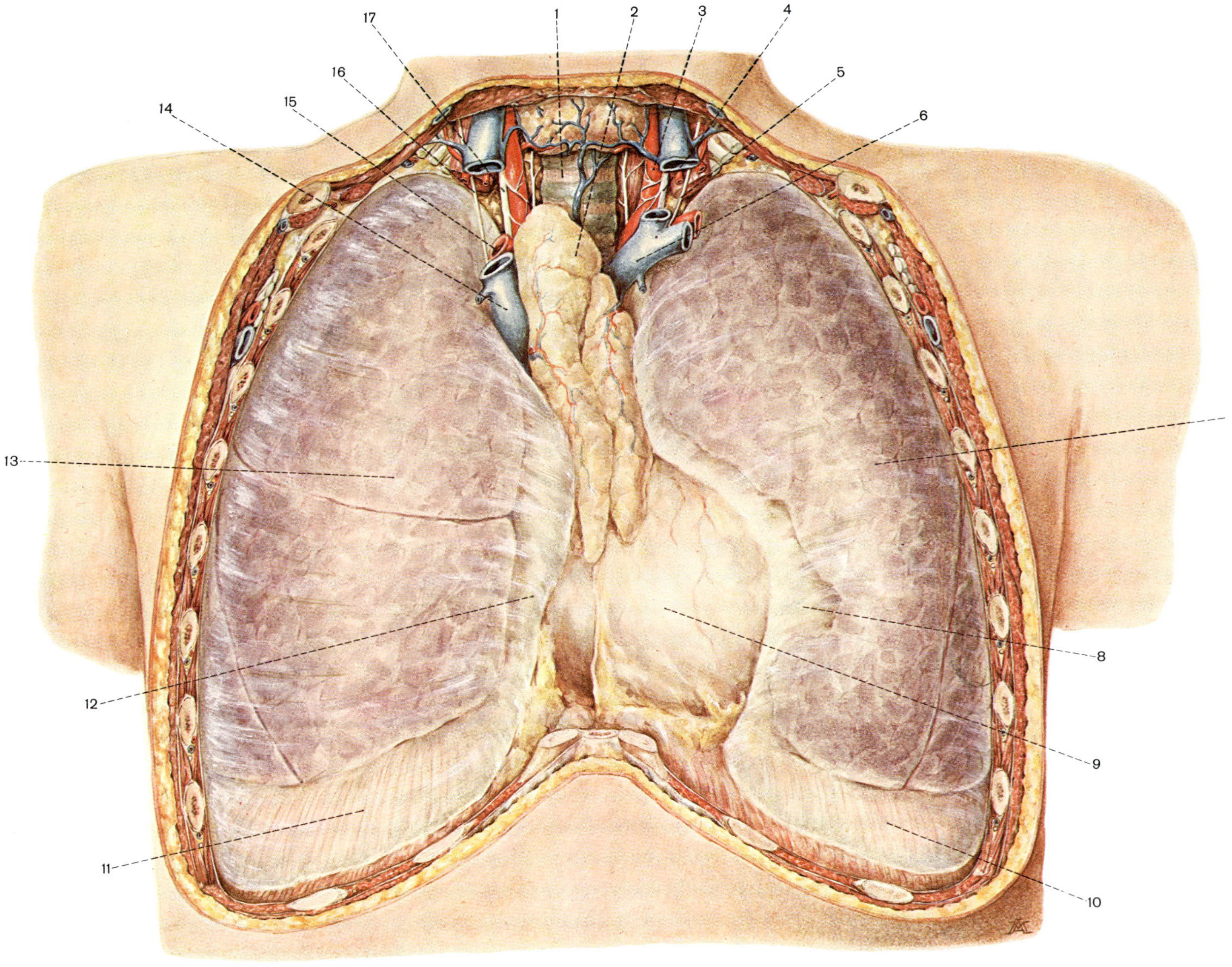

Fig. 11. Topography of thoracic organs. Anterior wall is removed, pleura is left intact.

1 Trachea
2 Thymus
3 Left common carotid artery (a. carotis communis sinistra)
4 Left vagus nerve (n. vagus sinister)
5 Left phrenic nerve (n. phrenicus sinister)
6 Left brachiocephalic vein (v. brachiocephalica sinistra)
7 Left lung (pulmo sinister)
8, 12 Costomediastinal sinus (recess) of pleura (recessus costomediastinalis)
9 Heart (cor)
10, 11 Costodiaphragmatic sinus (recess) of pleura (recessus costodiaphragmaticus)
13 Right lung (pulmo dexter)
14 Right brachiocephalic vein (v. brachiocephalica dextra)
15 Right subclavian artery (a. subclavia dextra)
16 Right phrenic nerve (n. phrenicus dexter)
17 Right vagus nerve (n. vagus dexter)

THE PLEURA

The parietal pleura, lining the inner surface of the thoracic cage, and the visceral or pulmonary pleura, covering the surface of the lungs, are distinguished.

The parietal pleura is continuous with the pulmonary pleura in the region of the pulmonary roots, as the result of which an isolated space, the pleural cavity, is formed (Fig. 12). Below the roots of the lungs the pleural fold forms a duplicate called the plumonary ligament. It is located in the frontal plane and descends to the diaphragm. The pulmonary ligament fastens the root and medial surface of the lung to the mediastinum and diaphragm.

The parietal pleura has costal, mediastinal, and diaphragmatic parts.

The costal pleura lines the inner surface of the ribs and intercostal spaces and, as is noted above, adheres to the endothoracic fascia.

The strength of fixation of the pleura grows in the dorso-ventro-caudal direction and depends on the extent to which the parapleural cellular tissue is developed.

The dome-shaped part, or the cervical pleura, and the paravertebral part of the pleura, extending for a distance of 5 to 6 cm along the sides of the vertebral column, are easily separated from the thoracic wall because of the presence of a well-developed parapleural cellular tissue.

It is more difficult to separate the pleura in the zone between the paravertebral and midaxillary lines.

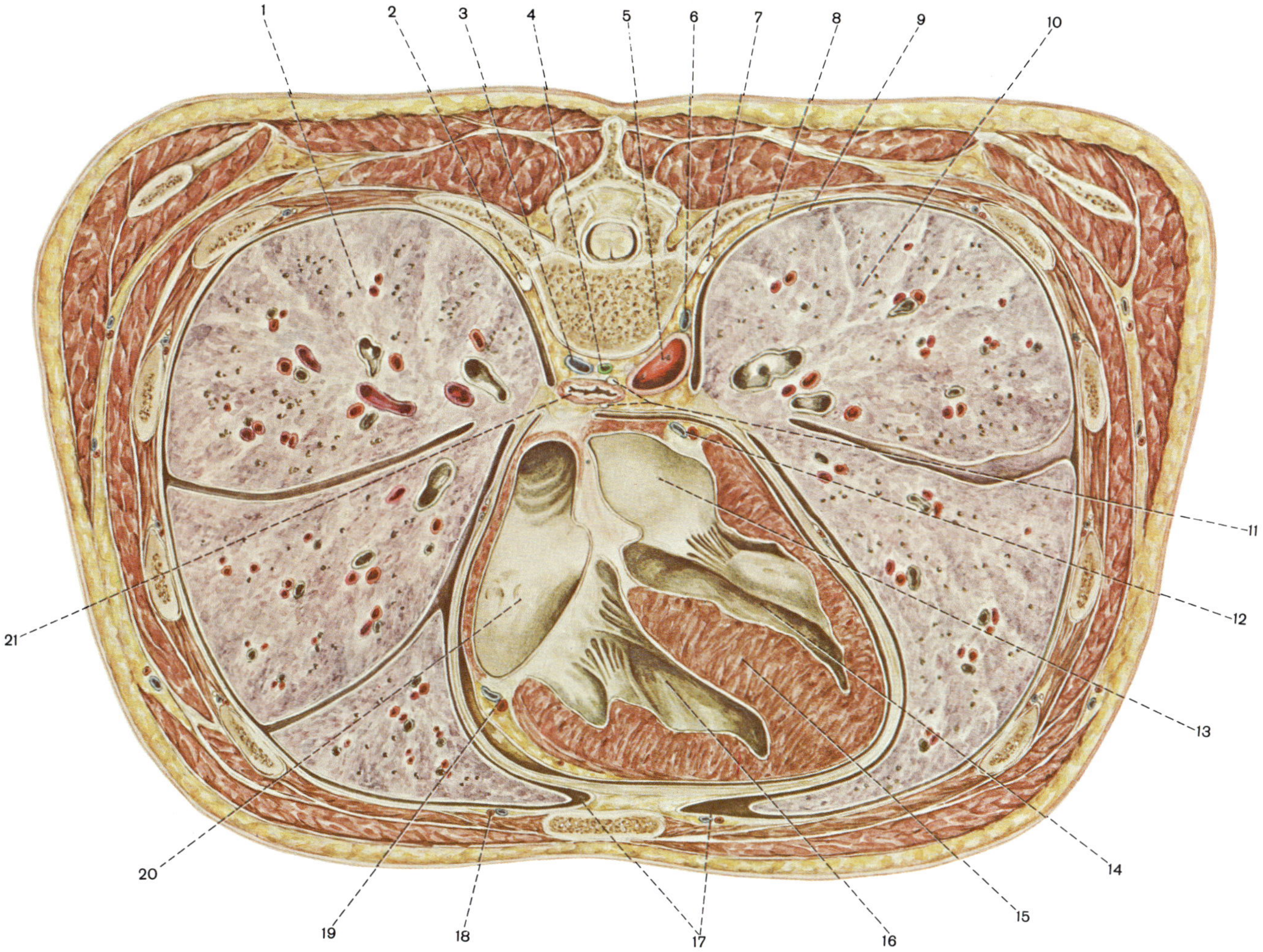

Fig. 12. Horizontal section through thorax at level of eighth thoracic vertebra.

1 Right lung (pulmo dexter)
2, 7 Sympathetic trunk (truncus sympathicus)
3 Azygos vein (v. azygos)
4 Thoracic lymph duct (ductus thoracicus)
5 Aorta
6 Hemiazygos vein (v. hemiazygos)
8 Costal pleura (pleura costalis)
9 Visceral pleura (pleura visceralis, pulmonalis)
10 Left lung (inferior lobe) (pulmo sinister)
11 Vagus nerves (nn. vagi)
12, 19 Coronary vessels (aa. et vv. coronariae)
13 Cavity of left atrium (sinus atrii sinistri)
14 Cavity of left ventricle (sinus ventriculi sinistri)
15 Interventricular septum (septum interventriculare)
16 Cavity of right ventricle (sinus ventriculi dextri)
17 Costmediastinal sinus (recess) of pleura (recessus costomediastinalis)
18 Internal thoracic artery (a. thoracica interna)
20 Cavity of right atrium (sinus atrii dextri)
21 Esophagus

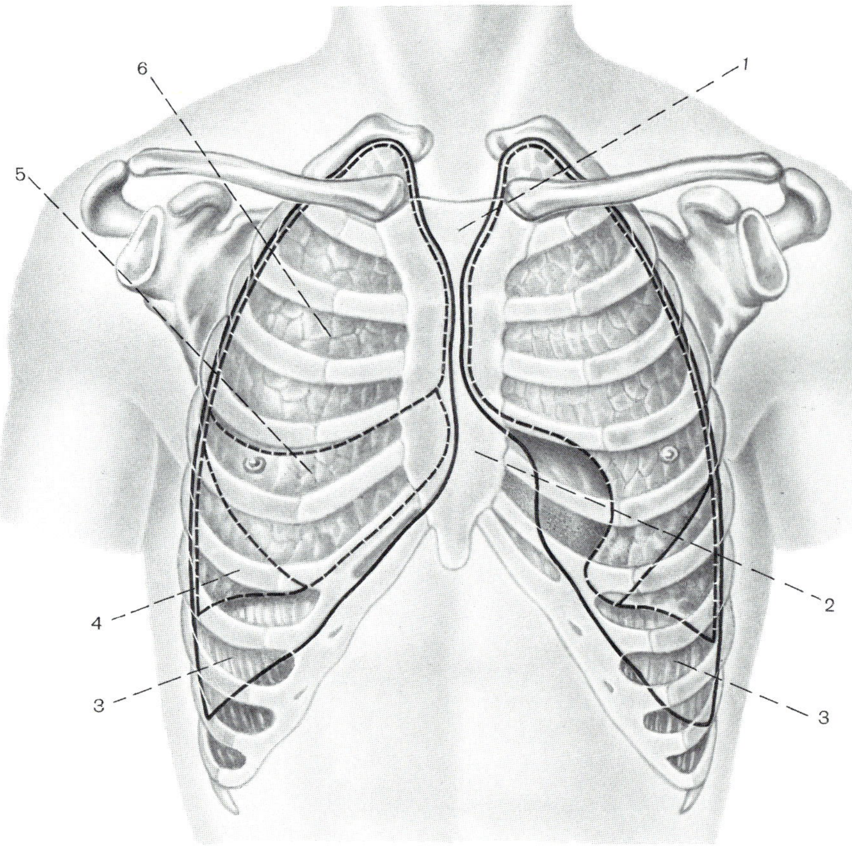

Fig. 13. Anterior pleural boundaries. Dashed line shows boundaries of lungs; continuous line shows boundaries of pleura.

1 Area thymica
2 Area pericardica
3 Costodiaphragmatic sinus (recess) or pleura (recessus costodiaphragmaticus)
4 Lower lobe (lobus inferior)
5 Middle lobe (lobus medius)
6 Upper lobe (lobus superior)

The costal pleura is fastened most securely in the ventral parts and in the costodiaphragmatic recesses, where there is practically no parapleural cellular tissue.

The mediastinal pleura forms the lateral boundaries of the mediastinal organs. It is situated in the sagittal plane and is continuous ventrally and dorsally with the costal pleura. At the bottom it is continuous with the diaphragmatic pleura. The sheets of the pleura embracing the root of the lung have a rich layer of cellular tissue, because of which the pleura is easily separated from the components of the pulmonary root.

The line at the junction of the right and left costal pleura with the mediastinal pleura (anterior pleural boundaries) varies in its projection upon the anterior thoracic wall (Fig. 13). The anterior (ventral) boundary of the right pleura extends from the space between the heads of the sternocleidomastoid muscle, crosses the sternoclavicular joints, and stretching caudally and and medially, reaches the midsternal line at the level of the second rib. It then passes vertically to the level of the attachment of the sixth costal cartilage to the sternum and turning laterally forms the lower (caudal) boundary of the pleura. The latter is projected upon the midclavicular line at the level of the seventh rib, along the midaxillary line at the level of the tenth rib, along the scapular line at the level of the eleventh rib, and along the paravertebral line at the level of the twelfth rib.

The ventral boundary of the left pleura is projected behind the left sternoclavicular joint, from where it extends along the left border of the sternum to the attachment of the fourth costal cartilage; it then deviates laterally, crossing the fourth intercostal space and the fifth costal cartilage, and reaches the lateral end of the sixth costal cartilage. Here the ventral boundary turns sharply to the side, forming the lower (caudal) boundary.

As the result of the asymmetric localization of the ventral pleural boundaries, two, upper and lower, interpleural spaces are formed in the ventral parts of the mediastinum; they are called area interpleurica superior

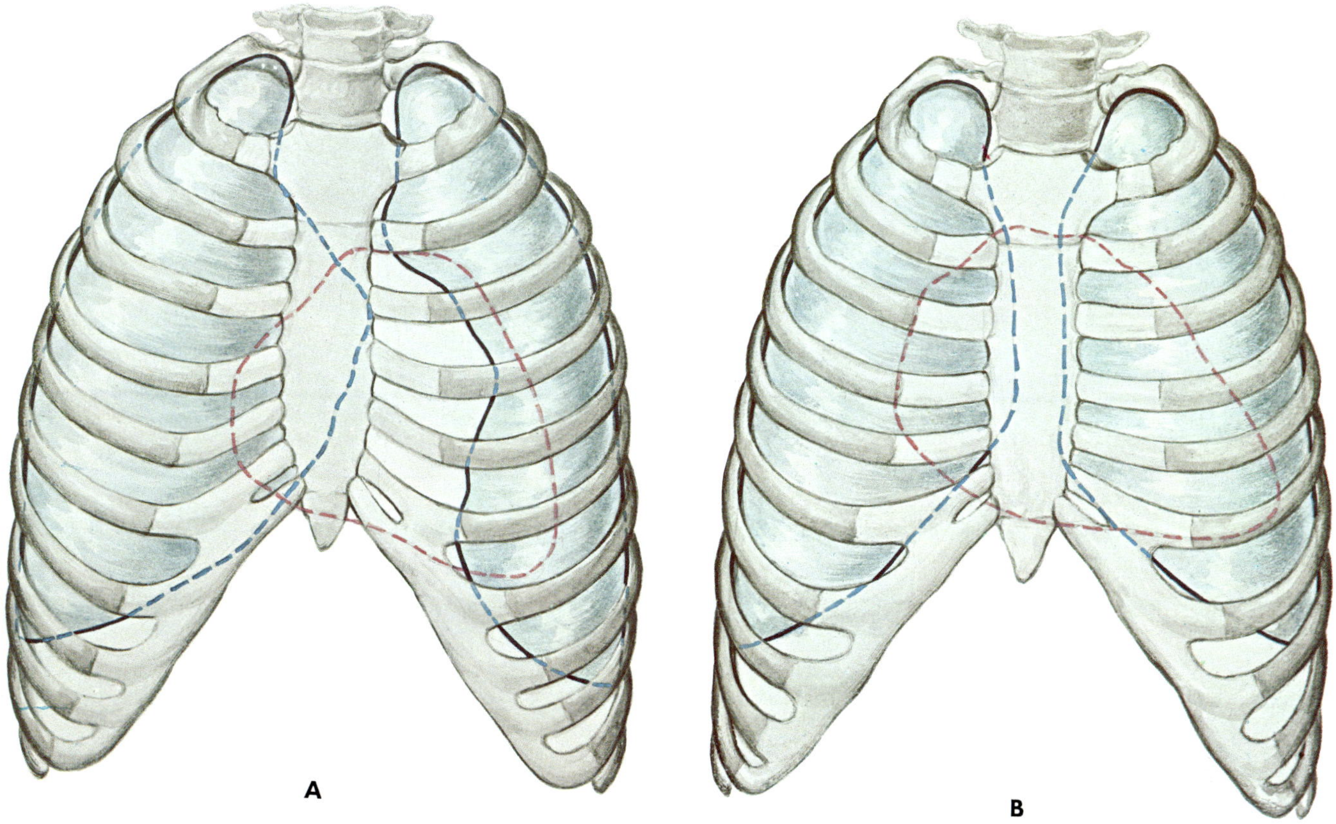

Fig. 14. Anterior pleural boundary in mitral valvular disease, **A,** and hypertensive disease, **B.** (After Yu. Lopukhin.) Blue line shows boundaries of pleura; red line shows boundaries of heart.

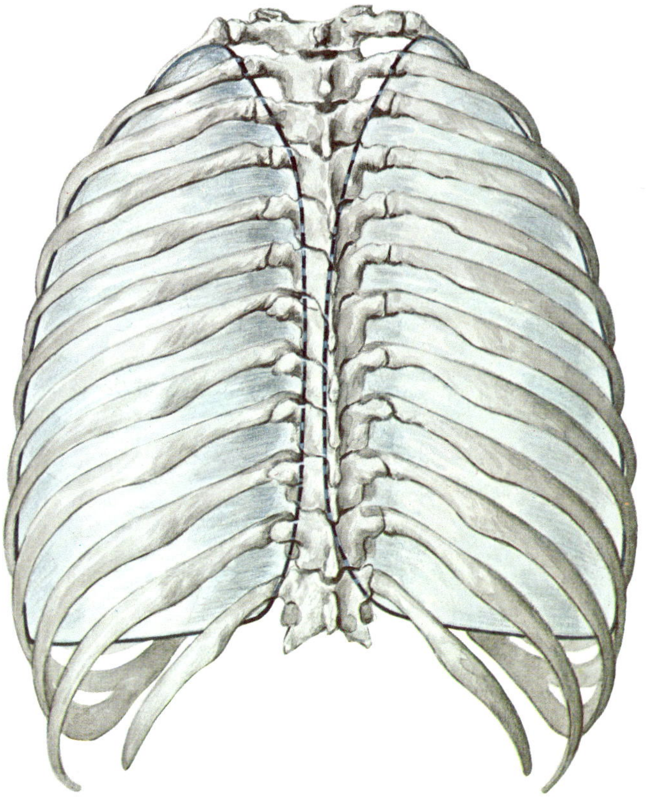

Fig. 15. Posterior boundaries of pleura. (After Yu.Lopukhin.)

et inferior and possess definite importance in extrapleural approaches to the heart and organs of the anterior mediastinum.

The position of the anterior pleural boundaries is characterized by considerable variability and is mainly determined by the peculiarities of the constitution.

In a narrow thoracic cage and weak development of the fatty cellular tissue, the ventral pleural boundaries lie close to each other, often touching at the level of the second and third ribs behind the sternum.

In a wide thoracic cage and well-developed fatty tissue, the ventral pleural boundaries are at a considerable distance from each other, forming a wide extrapleural field.

Morbid processes in the thoracic cavity cause a change in the position of the ventral pleural boundary.

In adhesion-forming processes in the pleural cavities the pleural boundaries are displaced laterally (i.e., in the direction of the adhesions). In pleural effusion and pneumothorax the boundaries are displaced medially.

In pathologic enlargement of the heart, the anterior interpleural space is distended (Fig. 14).

The posterior (dorsal) pleural boundaries, or the lines formed at the junction of the costovertebral pleura with the mediastinal pleura, are projected along the vertebral column with the formation of upper (cranial) and lower (caudal) interpleural expansions and a constricted part projected at the level of the fourth to ninth vertebra (Fig. 15).

The *diaphragmatic pleura* covers almost the entire cranial surface of the diaphragm with the exception of the area where the pericardium is attached to the diaphragm.

The pleural cavity is a narrow space no wider than 7 μm. Normally it contains about 2 ml of serous fluid, which promotes the sliding of the pleural layers.

In pathological conditions (exudative pleurisy, hemothorax, etc.) the pleural cavity may contain a considerable amount of fluid or air.

There are pockets and recesses in the pleural cavity which are also called pleural sinuses. The pleural recesses form where one part of the pleura is continuous with another (see Figs. 11 and 12).

Each pleural cavity has a costodiaphragmatic recess (sinus), two costomediastinal recesses (anterior and posterior), and a diaphragmaticomediastinal recess. Before he starts breathing, the newborn has two accessory recesses (recessus costathymica and recessus pericardiacothymica).

The costomediastinal and diaphragmaticomediastinal recesses are small and on inspiration are filled with the lungs. Because it is large, only the left costomediastinal recess is partly filled with the lung. In purulent inflammatory diseases of the pleura, incapsulated pleurisy-abscesses may be localized in these recesses.

The deepest costodiaphragmatic recess is formed by the costal and diaphragmatic pleura. It stretches for a distance of 6 to 8 cm along the midaxillary line and is projected on an area extending from the seventh to tenth ribs. The costodiaphragmatic recess is not filled with the pulmonary tissue even during deep inspiration. Below the level of the eighth intercostal space, the costal and diaphragmatic pleura touch, and the recess here is a narrow fissure. That is why it is recommended to perform pleurocentesis in the seventh to eighth intercostal space so as to avoid injuring the lungs or the organs located in the upper abdominal cavity.

The parietal pleura is supplied with blood by the intercostal, internal thoracic, pericardiacophrenic, and musculophrenic arteries.

The principal sources of blood supply to the visceral pleura are the pulmonary and bronchial vessels. The venous blood is drained along veins attendant to the corresponding arterial trunks.

The lymphatic fluid drains from the parietal pleura mainly along two routes: along the thoracic duct stretching next to the internal thoracic vessels, and along the posterior duct adjoining the vertebral column.

The lymphatic vessels of the visceral pleura are closely connected with those of the lung, forming a single network.

Sensory innervation of the pleura is effected by the intercostal and phrenic nerves.

THE LUNGS

The size and shape of the lungs differ with the individual and are closely dependent on the body build, age, and sex. The right lung is shorter but wider than the left and takes up more space.

On the average the length of a male's right lung is 27 cm, and of the left lung 29.8 cm; in females it is 21.6 and 23 cm, respectively. In males the base of the right lung is about 13.5 cm wide, and of the left lung 12.9 cm; in females these measurements are 12.2 and 10.8 cm, respectively. The smaller vertical measurement of the right lung is due to the higher position of the right diaphragmatic dome. Since the axis of the heart is displaced to the left, the transverse dimension of the left lung is larger than that of the right.

In shape the lungs (Figs. 16 and 17) resemble a cone transected along the axis. An apex, base, and three surfaces (costal, diaphragmatic, and mediastinal) are distinguished in the lung. The apex of the lung fills the cervical pleura and protrudes from the superior thoracic aperture to a level with the seventh cervical vertebra. On the ventral surface of the apex of each lung there is a groove corresponding to the direction of the subclavian artery.

The lateral surface of the lung forms an uneven convex fitting the walls of the thoracic cavity and is slightly curved at the back. The inferior surface of the lung is deeply concave and corresponds to the shape of the diaphragm. Along the entire distance of the mediastinal surface of the right lung there is a depression formed by the esophagus, and another formed by the azygos vein in the lower portion. There is a clearly outlined cardiac impression (impressio cardiaca) in the lower portion of the mediastinal surface of the left lung, corresponding to the position of the heart.

Three borders are distinguished in each lung: anterior (ventral), posterior (dorsal), and inferior (caudal), separating one surface of the lung from another. The oblique interlobal fissure arises on the dorsal surface of each lung at the junction of the upper and lower lobes. It extends along the lateral surface of the lung forward and downward to its anterior inferior angle. Here the fissure turns over to the mediastinal surface and terminates at the anterior border of the pulmonary hilus. The fissure is known for its constancy and is distinctly outlined in 82% to 97.4% of cases.

On the lateral surface of the right lung the oblique interlobular fissure is continuous with the anterior horizontal fissure, which extends to the ventral border. At the junction of the middle and lower thirds of the border it turns over to the mediastinal surface and reaches the middle of the pulmonary hilus. According to different authors, the anterior horizontal fissure can be clearly seen in 31.1% to 64% of cases, always shallower than the oblique interlobular fissure.

The anterior horizontal fissure is rarely encountered in the left lung (in 3% to 7% of cases).

The fissures of each lung divide it into lobes. The right lung has three lobes: the superior, middle, and inferior. The left lung has two lobes: the superior and inferior.

The development of pulmonary surgery and the advances made in topical diagnosis served as impetus for the detailed study of the structure of vessels and bronchi within the lung. The regularities revealed in the distribution of the bronchial tree formed the basis for the new division of the lungs into segments.

A segment is an area of pulmonary tissue ventilated by a bronchus of the third order (segmental bronchus) and separated from the neighboring structures by a connective tissue septum. The shape of the segment is that of a cone or pyramid with the base directed to the periphery of the lung. The stem of the segment, composed of the segmental bronchus, segmental artery, and, sometimes, a vein lies at the apex of the segment facing the hilus of the lung. The presence of an isolated bronchovascular stem makes it possible to resect a diseased segment of the lung in definite pathological conditions. In many cases this is prompted by the circumstance that such diseases as tuberculosis and suppurative processes in the lungs initially arise and develop within the limits of a single segment and only spread to the neighboring areas of the pulmonary tissue later.

The theory of the segmental structure of the lungs thus promoted the development of a new trend in pulmonary surgery confirming the scope of surgical manipulations to the minimum.

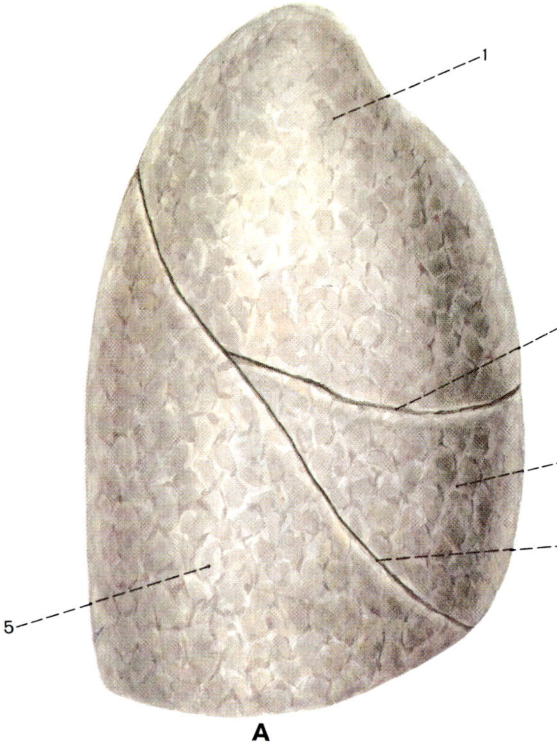

A

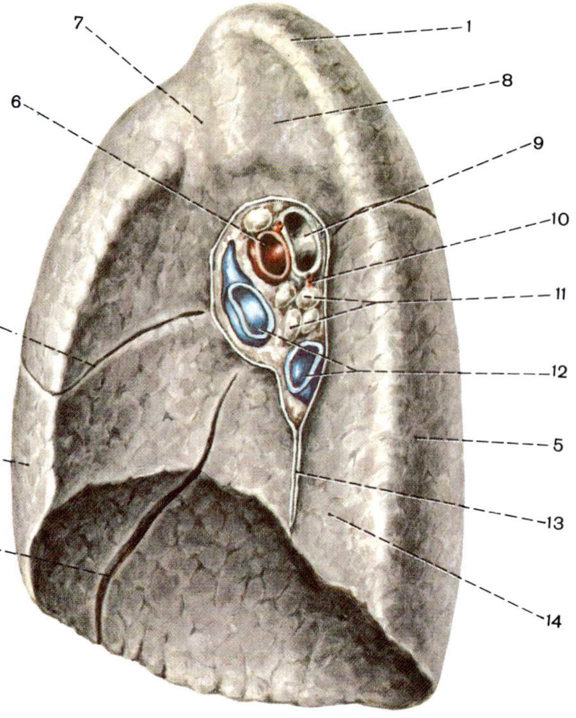

B

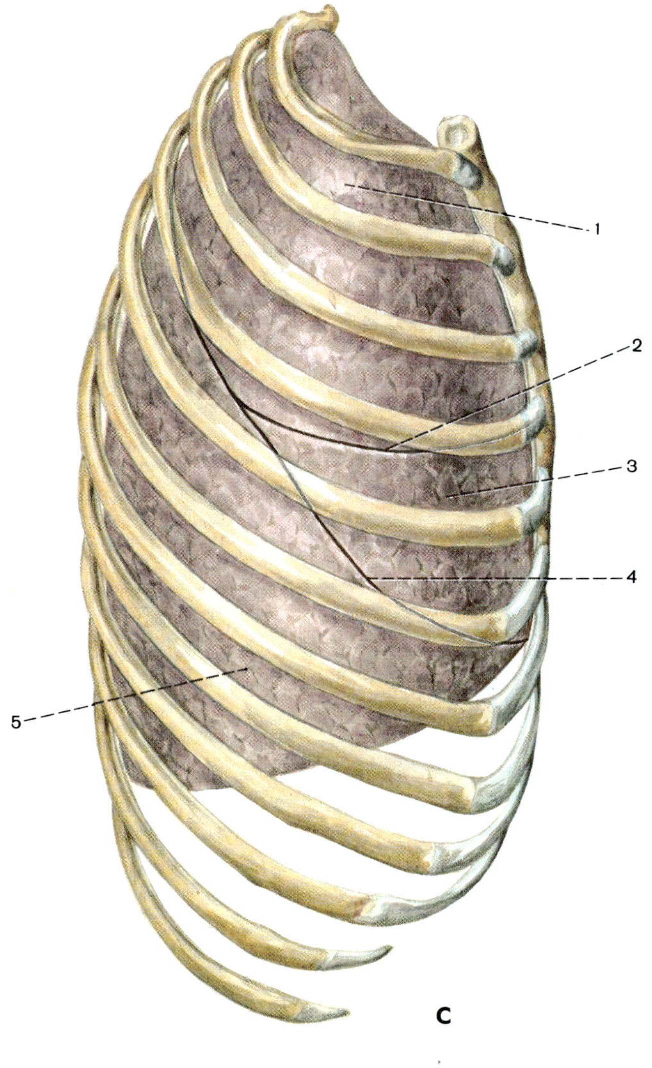

C

Fig. 16. Right lung. **A,** Lateral aspect. **B,** Medial aspect. **C,** Projection of pulmonary lobes on the thoracic cage.

1 Upper lobe (lobus superior)
2 Horizontal fissure (fissura horizontalis)
3 Middle lobe (lobus medius)
4 Oblique fissure (fissure obliqua)
5 Lower lobe (lobus inferior)
6 Right pulmonary artery (a. pulmonalis dextra)
7 Groove for brachiocephalic vein (sulcus v. brachiocephalicae)
8 Groove for subclavian artery (sulcus a. subclaviae)
9 Right primary (main) bronchus (bronchus principalis dexter)
10 Bronchial artery (a. bronchialis)
11 Lymph nodes (nodi lymphatici)
12 Pulmonary veins (vv. pulmonales)
13 Pulmonary ligament (ligamentum pulmonale)
14 Groove for inferior vena cava (impressio v. cavae inferioris)

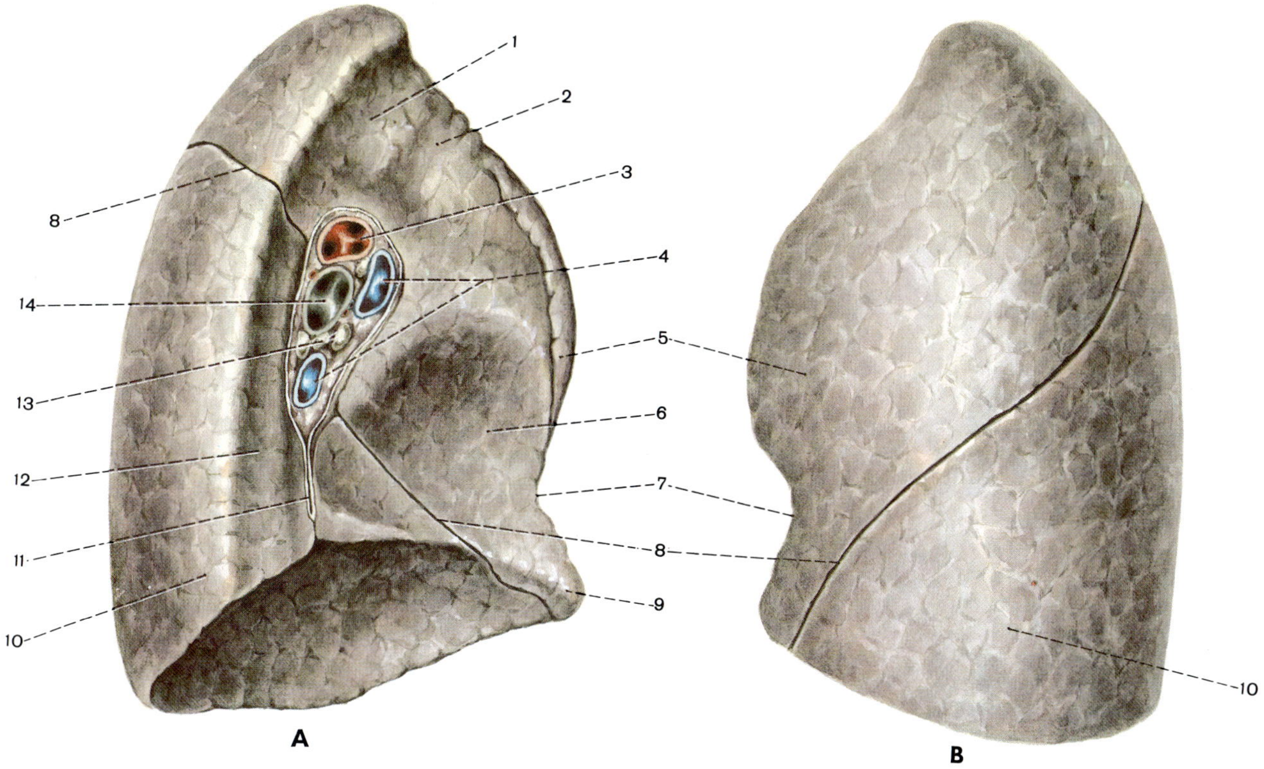

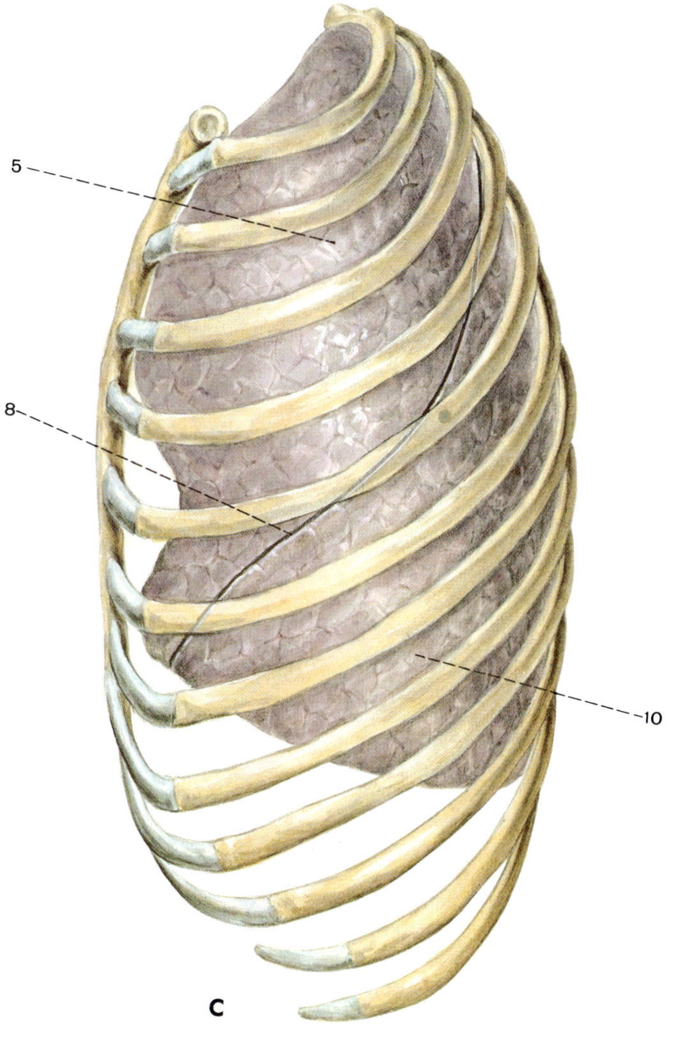

Fig. 17. Left lung. **A,** Medial aspect. **B,** Lateral aspect. **C,** Projection of pulmonary lobes on thoracic cage.

1 Groove for the subclavian artery (sulcus a. subclaviae)
2 Groove for the brachiocephalic vein (sulcus v. brachiocephalicae)
3 Left pulmonary artery (a. pulmonalis sinistra)
4 Pulmonary veins (vv. pulmonales)
5 Upper lobe (lobus superior)
6 Depression for heart (impressio cardiaca)
7 Cardiac notch of left lung (incisura cardiaca pulmonis sinistri)
8 Oblique fissure (fissure obliqua)
9 Lingula of left lung (lingula pulmonis sinistri)
10 Lower lobe (lobus inferior pulmonis sinistri)
11 Pulmonary ligament (ligamentum pulmonale)
12 Groove for aorta (sulcus aorticus)
13 Lymph nodes (nodi lymphatici)
14 Left primary (main) bronchus (bronchus principalis sinister)

The nomenclature now commonly accepted is that endorsed by the international congress of otolaryngologists, thoracic surgeons, and anatomists held in Paris in 1955. According to this diagram, ten segments are distinguished in the right lung and nine in the left (Fig. 18).

Right lung

Superior lobe

1 Apical segment
2 Posterior segment
3 Anterior segment

Middle lobe

4 Lateral segment
5 Medial segment

Inferior lobe

6 Superior segment
7 Medial segment
8 Anterior basal segment
9 Lateral basal segment
10 Posterior basal segment

Left lung

Superior lobe

1 and **2** Apicoposterior segment
3 Anterior segment
4 Superior lingular segment
5 Inferior lingular segment

Inferior lobe

6 Superior segment
8 Anterior basal segment
9 Lateral basal segment
10 Posterior basal segment

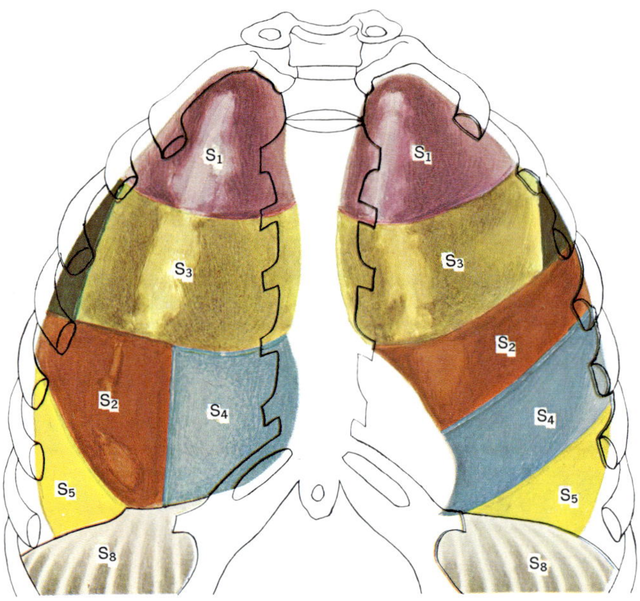

Fig. 18. Segmental structure of lungs (international nomenclature).

The right lung (Figs. 19 and 20)

The apical segment occupies the upper medial area of the superior lobe, protrudes from the superior thoracic aperture, and fills the cervical pleura.

The base of the posterior segment is directed laterally and dorsally, bordering upon the second to fourth ribs; the apex of the segment faces the superior lobar bronchus. The anterior segment adjoins the anterior thoracic wall with its base between the cartilages of the first to fourth ribs; its medial surface borders upon the right atrium and superior vena cava.

The base of the lateral segment is directed ventrally and laterally, while the apex points up and to the midline.

The medial segment of the middle lobe fits close to the heart, diaphragm, and the fourth to sixth ribs. The superior segment of the inferior lobe occupies the apex of this lobe and is located in the dorsal parts adjoining the paravertebral region. The medial segment forms, with its base, the mediastinal and partly the diaphragmatic surfaces of the lower lobe. It lies next to the right atrium and inferior vena cava.

The lateral surface of the anterior basal segment fits to the thoracic wall in the axillary region between the sixth and eighth ribs. Its base forms the diaphragmatic surface of the lower lobe.

The lateral basal segment of the inferior lobe is wedged between the other segments so that its base touches the diaphragm, while the lateral side adjoins the thoracic wall in the axillary region between the seventh and ninth ribs.

The posterior basal segment is situated paravertebrally, dorsal to all the other segments of the lower lobe, penetrating deep into the posterior part of the costodiaphragmatic recess of the pleura.

The left lung (Figs. 21 and 22)

The apicoposterior segment corresponds to the apical and posterior segments of the superior lobe of the right lung in shape and position. Its base touches the posterior parts of the third to fifth ribs. Medially, it touches the aortic arch and the subclavian artery.

The anterior segment is the largest and occupies a considerable part of the costal surface of the upper lobe from the first to fourth ribs and part of the mediastinal surface.

The superior lingular segment is an area of the upper lobe stretching between the third and fourth ribs ventrally and between the fourth and sixth ribs in the axillary region.

Caudally to the superior lingular segment is the in-

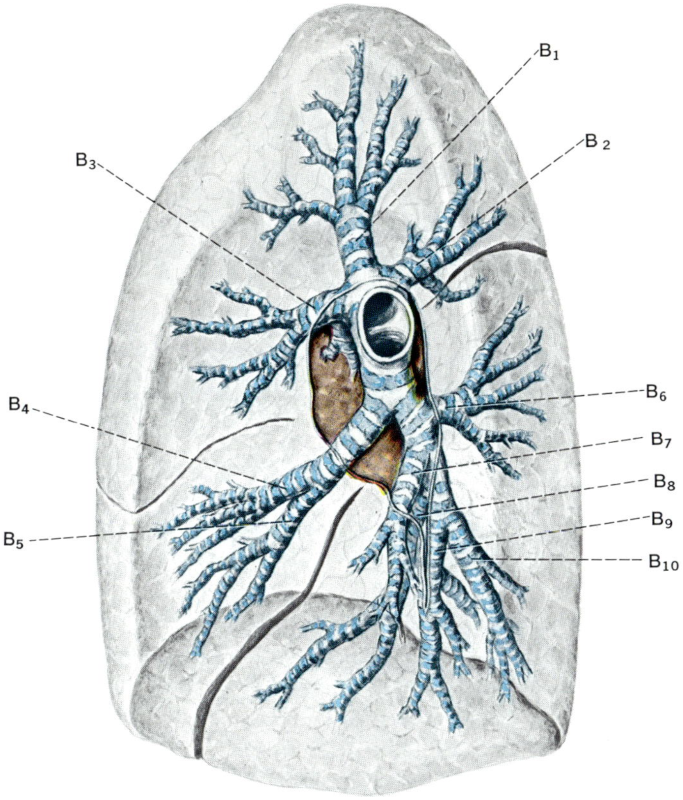

Fig. 19. Bronchial tree of right lung, medial aspect.

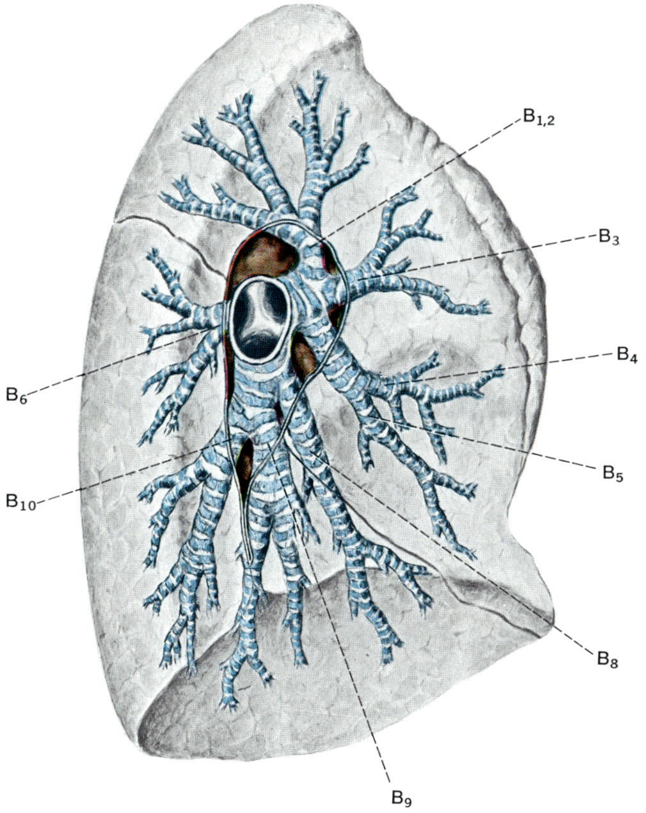

Fig. 21. Bronchial tree of left lung, lateral aspect.

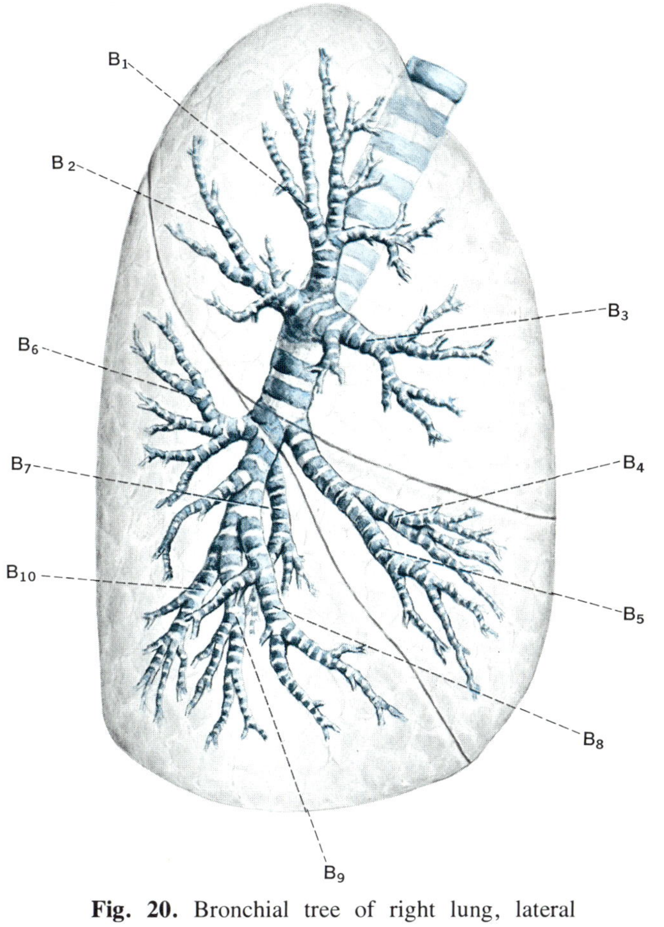

Fig. 20. Bronchial tree of right lung, lateral aspect.

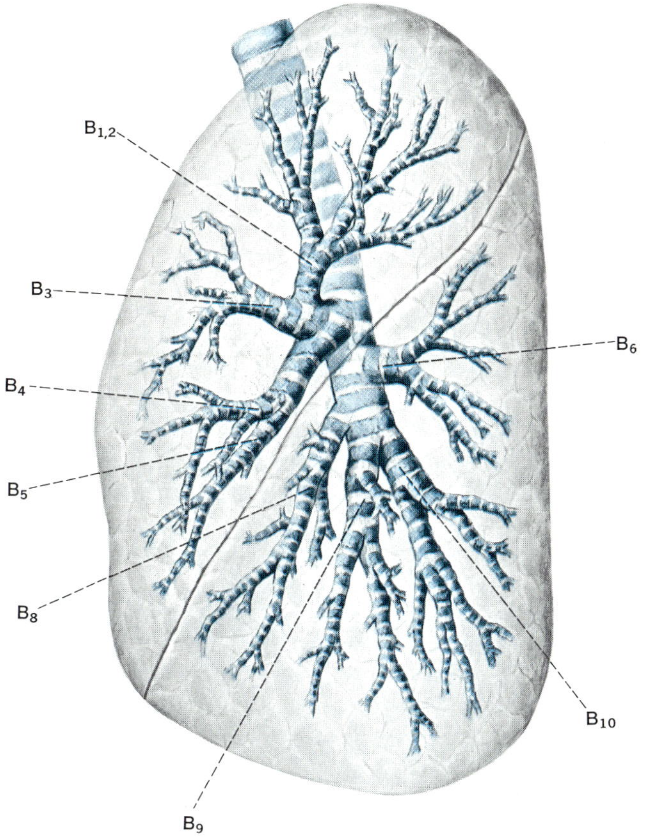

Fig. 22. Bronchial tree of left lung, lateral aspect.

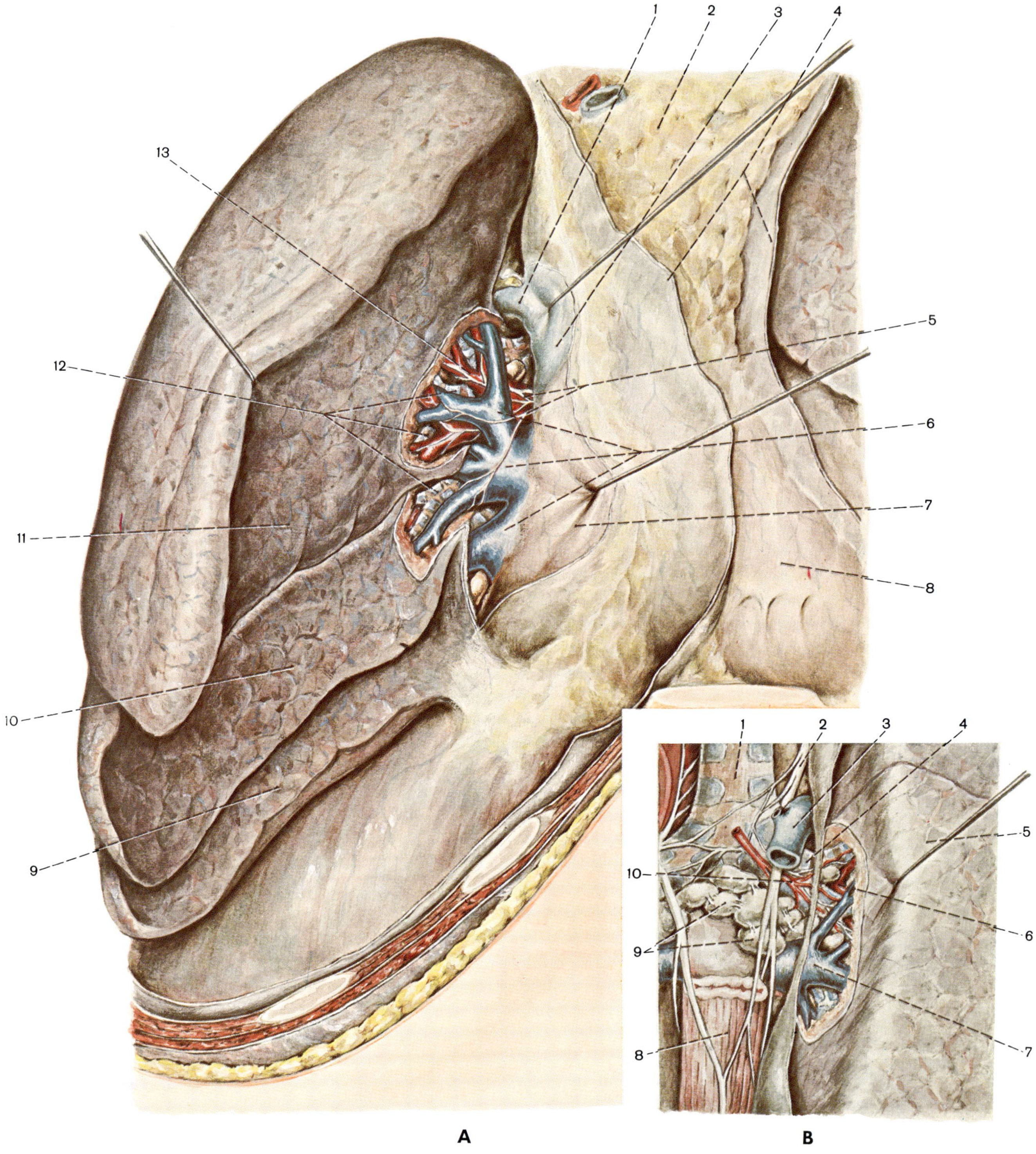

Fig. 23. Topography of components of root of right lung.

A, ANTERIOR ASPECT:

1 Azygos vein (v. azygos)
2 Cellular tissue of anterior mediastinum
3 Superior vena cava (v. cava superior)
4 Mediastinal pleura (pleura mediastinalis)
5 Anterior pulmonary plexus
6 Pulmonary veins (vv. pulmonales)
7 Right atrium (atrium dextrum)
8 Heart and pericardium (cor et pericardium)
9 Lower lobe of right lung (lobus inferior pulmonis dextri)
10 Middle lobe of right lung (lobus medius pulmonis dextri)
11 Upper lobe of right lung (lobus superior pulmonis dextri)
12 Segmental bronchi
13 Pulmonary artery (a. pulmonalis)

B, POSTERIOR ASPECT:

1 Trachea
2 Right vagus nerve (n. vagus dexter)
3 Azygos vein (v. azygos)
4 Right primary (main) bronchus (bronchus principalis dexter)
5 Lower lobe of right lung (lobus inferior pulmonis dextri)
6 Pulmonary artery (a. pulmonalis)
7 Pulmonary vein (v. pulmonalis)
8 Esophagus
9 Inferior tracheobronchial lymph nodes
10 Bronchial arteries (aa. bronchiales)

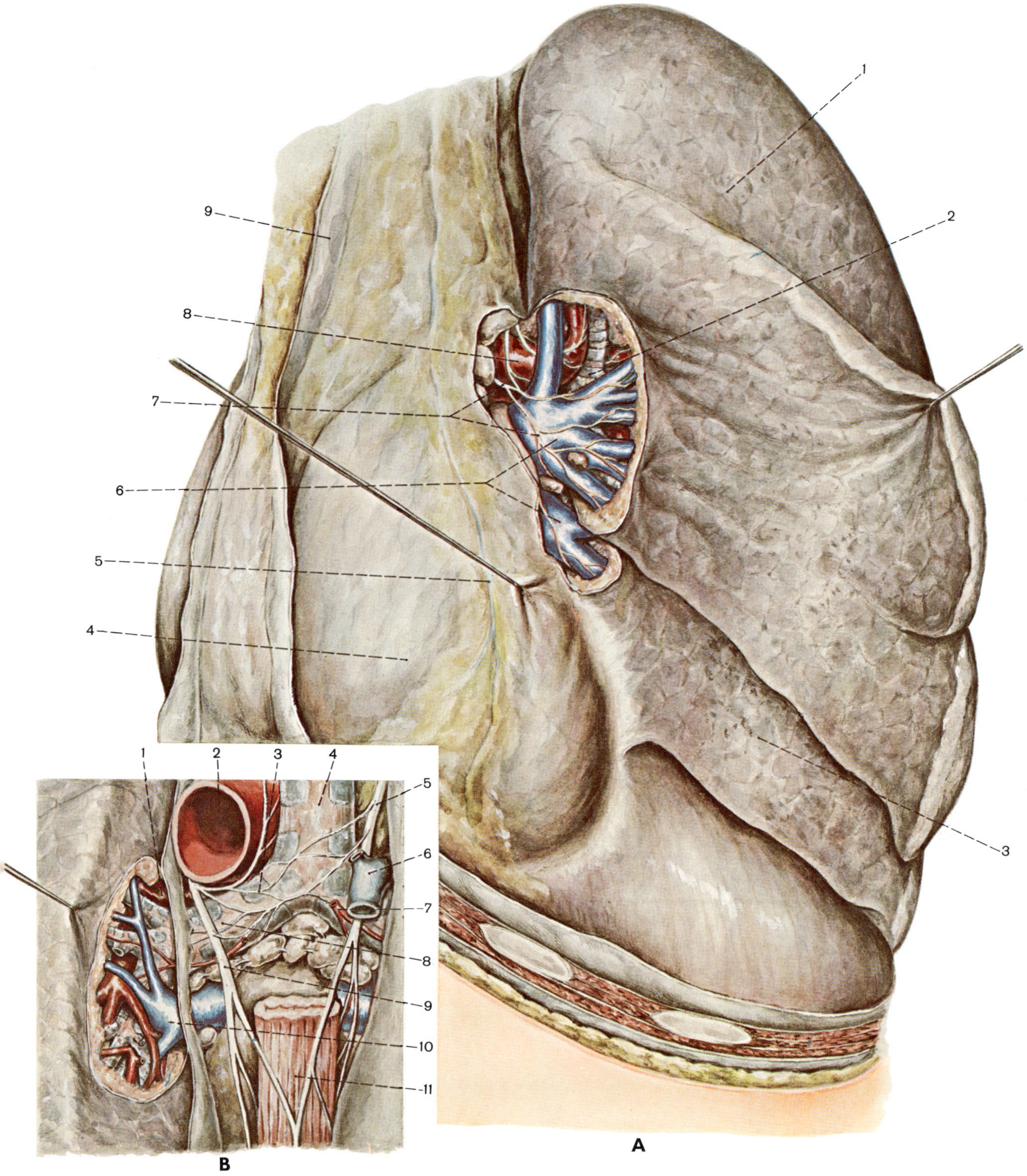

Fig. 24. Topography of components of root of left lung.

A, ANTERIOR ASPECT:

1 Upper lobe of left lung (lobus superior pulmonis sinistri)
2 Left primary (main) bronchus (bronchus principalis sinister)
3 Lower lobe of left lung (lobus inferior pulmonis sinistri)
4 Heart and pericardium (cor et pericardium)
5 Pericardiophrenic artery and vein (a. et v. periacophrenicae)
6 Pulmonary veins (vv. pulmonales)
7 Anterior pulmonary plexus
8 Pulmonary artery (a. pulmonalis)
9 Mediastinal pleura (pleura mediastinalis)

B, POSTERIOR ASPECT:

1 Pulmonary artery (a. pulmonalis)
2 Aorta
3 Posterior pulmonary plexus
4 Trachea
5 Right vagus nerve (n. vagus dexter)
6 Azygos vein (v. azygos)
7 Bronchial artery (a. bronchialis)
8 Left primary (main) bronchus (bronchus principalis sinister)
9 Left vagus nerve (n. vagus sinister)
10 Pulmonary vein (v. pulmonalis)
11 Esophagus

ferior lingular segment; these two segments correspond to the middle lobe of the right lung.

The superior segment of the inferior lobe of the left lung is a little larger than its analog on the right side.

The anterior basal segment is bounded laterally by the basal segment and dorsally by the dorsal basal segment. Its anterior surface faces the oblique fissure; the inferior is the diaphragmatic surface.

The lateral basal segment occupies the costal surface of the inferior lobe in the axillary region at the level of the seventh to tenth ribs. The posterior basal segment touches the seventh to tenth rib, the diaphragm, the descending aorta, and the esophagus. Apart from the name specifying its position in the lung, each segment has an ordinal number identical for both lungs.

The segmental arteries correspond to the bronchi, and their nomenclature, whether in full or abbreviated form, does not differ from that of the corresponding bronchi.

The anatomy of the venous system is complicated and variable. Central, segmental, and intersegmental veins are distinguished.

In the center of the medial surface of each lung, a little closer to the dorsal border, there is an oval slitlike depression called the hilus of the lung (see Figs. 16 and 17). Bronchi, blood and lymphatic vessels, and nerve fibers enter the lung tissue through the hilus. These structures are surrounded by loose cellular tissue and sheets of the mediastinal pleura and constitute the root of the lung.

The root of the lung is a short mesentery of the lung, no longer than 0.5 cm; its height is 5.7 to 6.6 cm, on the average. The hilus of the lung is projected on the ventral thoracic wall along the distance extending from the cartilage of the second rib to the cartilage of the third or fourth rib. Dorsally, the vertical diameter of the root extends from the level of the fifth to the level of the seventh thoracic vertebra.

The components of the roots of the right and left lungs are arranged asymmetrically (Figs. 23 and 24). In the root of the right lung the primary bronchus takes a cranial position; the pulmonary artery lies caudally and ventrally to it, while the pulmonary veins lie caudal to the artery. The right main (primary) bronchus arises from the bifurcation of the trachea at an angle of 25 to 35 degrees. It is shorter and wider than the left bronchus, its length measuring 2.3 to 2.5 cm and width 1.4 to 2.3 cm. Outside the parenchyma of the right lung the main bronchus gives rise to the superior lobar bronchus, the orifice of which is usually found 1 to 2.8 cm from the bifurcation of the trachea. Sometimes the superior lobar bronchus arises directly from the trachea. In such cases the branching of the trachea has the character of a trifurcation. The superior lobar bronchus extends laterally and somewhat cranially and usually divides into three segmental bronchi. The largest segmental bronchus of the upper lobe is that of the apical segment, which may be regarded to be continuous with the superior lobar bronchus. The anterior and posterior segmental bronchi are smaller than the bronchus of the apical segment. Each of the segmental bronchi mentioned most frequently divides dichotomously into subsegmental branches.

After giving off the superior lobar bronchus, the main bronchus is continuous with the intermediate bronchus, which extends to the level where the middle lobar bronchus, or the bronchus of the superior segment of the lower lobe, branches off.

The middle lobar bronchus arises from the ventral surface of the intermediate bronchus and extends in the ventrocaudal direction. In some cases its orifice may be on the lateral or medial surface of the intermediate bronchus. The middle lobar bronchus is 1 to 2 cm long and divides into the bronchi of the lateral and medial segments.

After giving off the middle lobar bronchus, the intermediate bronchus is continuous with the inferior lobar bronchus, which penetrates the parenchyma of the lower lobe at the medial margin of the interlobar surface and extends caudally, laterally, and dorsally.

The right pulmonary artery is about 4 cm in length and 2 to 2.5 cm in diameter. Having reached the ventral surface of the right main bronchus, the pulmonary artery gives off an anterior trunk ot the first and second segments. The artery of the second segment branches off below the orifice of the anterior trunk of the pulmonary artery. The middle lobar artery arises, as a rule, from the ventral surface of the artery at the level of the middle lobar bronchus and then divides into two segmental branches. The segment of the pulmonary artery between the orifice of the anterior trunk and that of the middle lobar artery is called the interlobar trunk.

After giving off the middle lobar artery, the interlobar segment of the pulmonary artery is continuous with the artery of the lower lobe and stretches along the ventrolateral surface of the inferior lobar bronchus. It then spirals along the length of the basal bronchus, giving off segmental branches one by one.

Blood from the right lung drains along the superior and inferior pulmonary veins.

The formation of the pulmonary veins is remarkable for its complexity and immense variability. The superior pulmonary vein of the right lung usually forms from the segmental veins of the upper and middle lobes. The length of its extrapericardial part varies from 0.8 to 1.4 cm. The inferior pulmonary vein is formed by the union of the superior venous trunk and the common basal vein. The superior venous trunk forms from the central vein of the superior segment and the intersegmental veins stretching between the superior and the adjacent segments. The central veins of the segment of the basal pyramid and the intersegmental veins form the common trunk of the basal vein. The extrapericardial part of the inferior pulmonary vein does not exceed 1 cm; it is shorter than the superior pulmonary vein and is situated dorsally and caudally to the latter.

The arrangement of the components in the root of the left lung is as follows. The pulmonary artery occupies the cranial position; the main bronchus is lower and to the back of it; while the pulmonary veins stretch along the anterior and inferior surfaces of the main bronchus and the artery.

The left pulmonary artery arises from the pulmonary trunk under the aortic arch. It is shorter and narrower than the right pulmonary artery (3.3 cm long, 1.8 to 2 cm in diameter), and approximately half of it is covered by the posterior sheet of the pericardium. Byeond the pericardium the left pulmonary artery penetrates the space between the aortic arch and the left bronchus, skirts the site of the origin of the superior lobar bronchus, and then extends caudally in the direction of the lower lobe. Its outline resembles a drawn-out arc stretching in the dorsocranial direction, from the peak of which the superior branch of the left artery arises. This branch is situated above the superior lobar bronchus and usually supplies the apicoposterior and anterior segments of the lung fully or in part. Arterial branches arising on their own from the pulmonary artery may contribute to the blood supply of the second segment. In most cases the fourth and fifth segments of the upper lobe of the left lung also have independent arteries located caudally to these. To be more precise, the pulmonary artery gives off a branch to the lingula of the left lung in the interlobar fissure; on reaching the lingula this branch divides into the superior and inferior lingular segmental arteries.

The inferior branch of the pulmonary artery (or the artery of the lower lobe) lies on the bottom of the oblique interlobar fissure and extends along the lateral surface of the inferior lobar bronchus.

The left main bronchus branches off from the bifurcation of the trachea at a sharper angle (40 to 50 degrees) than the right. It is up to 6 cm long, and its width varies from 0.9 to 2 cm.

The main bronchus of the left lung divides into two lobar bronchi within the hilus. They provide for the ventilation of the upper and lower anatomical lobes of the left lung.

The superior lobar bronchus arises from the ventrolateral surface of the left main bronchus and then extends ventrally dividing into two trunks, superior and inferior. The former measures 0.4 to 1.5 cm in length and is distributed in the superior and anterior parts of the upper lobe (in the apicoposterior and anterior segments).

The inferior, or lingular, trunk is the second branch of the bifurcation of the superior lobar branches. It stretches ventrally, caudally, and somewhat laterally and gives off branches to the superior and inferior lingular segments. It is from 0.3 to 2 cm long.

The inferior lobar bronchus, 0.6 to 1.4 cm long, arises below the origin of the superior lobar bronchus. The different lengths of the inferior lobar bronchus are determined by the level at which the bronchus of the superior segment branches away. When this occurs the inferior lobar bronchus becomes continuous with the basal bronchus, which is the segment of the inferior lobar bronchus extending between the orifice of the bronchus of the superior segment and the place where the basal bronchus divides into segmental branches.

The left superior pulmonary vein forms from the superior, middle, and inferior venous vessels collecting the blood from the apicoposterior, anterior, and lingular segments. Its extrapericardial part is 1.5 cm long, and the intrapericardial part 1.3 cm long. The vein adjoins the ventrocaudal surface of the superior branch of the pulmonary artery and drains into the left atrium at the level of the third costal cartilage.

The left inferior pulmonary vein forms from the superior venous trunk and the common trunk of the basal vein. The superior venous trunk forms from the central vein of the superior segment and intersegmental venous branches situated in a plane separating the superior segment from the adjacent segments of the basal pyramid. The total length of the left inferior vein does not exeed 2 cm. The vein stretches horizontally and drains into the cavity of the left atrium at the level of the fourth rib.

Besides the pulmonary vessels, the bronchial arteries also supply blood to the lungs (Fig. 25). Their number varies from two to six. Usually each bronchus has two arteries. These arteries form numerous anastomoses with the branches of the pulmonary artery, creating arteriovenous communications.

The innervation of the lungs is provided for by the vagus, sympathetic, and phrenic nerves (Figs. 26 and 27). In the region of the roots of the lungs these nerves form the anterior and posterior cardiopulmonary plexuses. The anterior nerve plexus is located on the ventral surface of the root components. The posterior plexus, of greater potential, lies on the dorsal surface of the bronchi. The fibers of the posterior pulmonary plexus are intimately fused with the bronchial adventitia

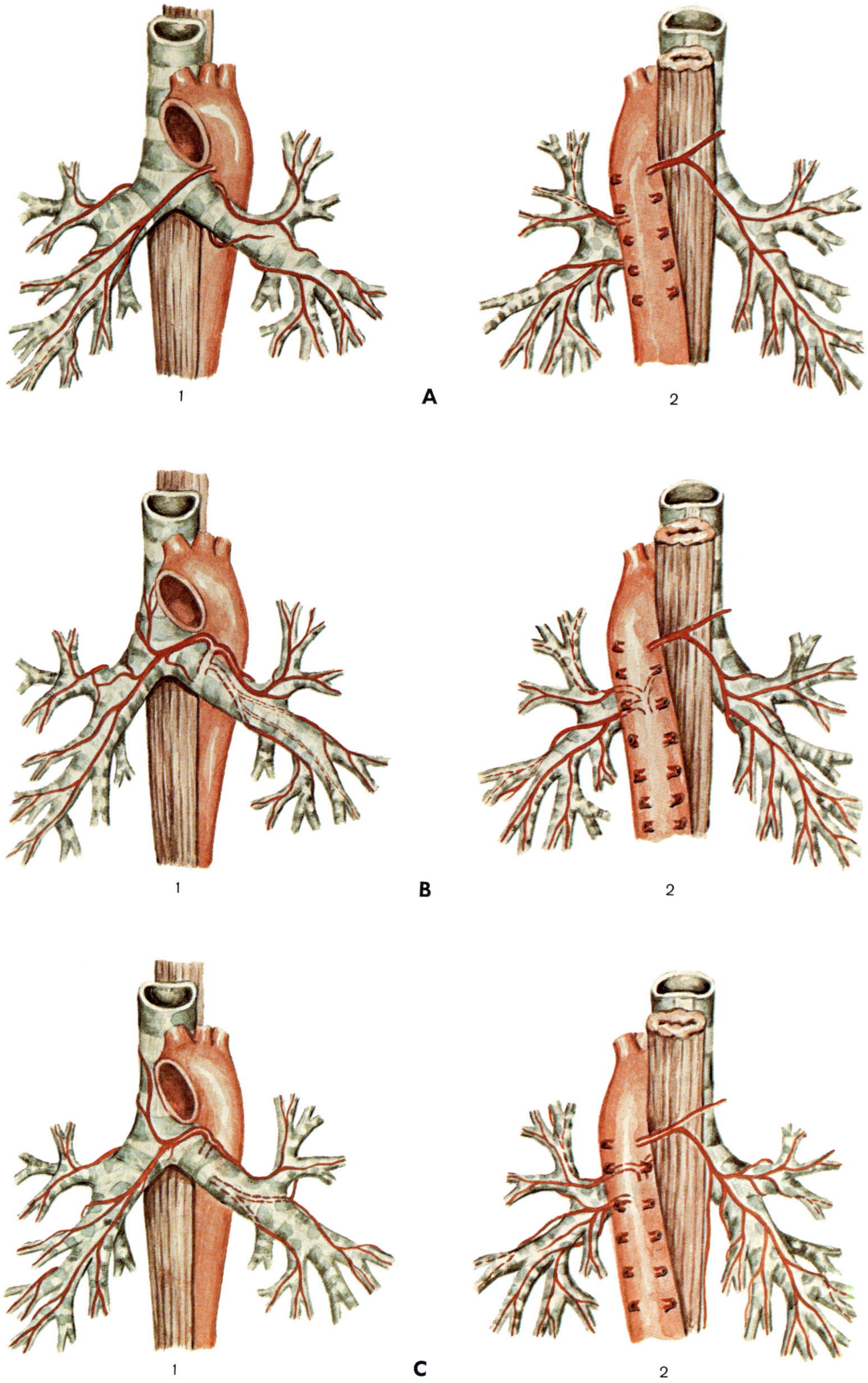

Fig. 25. Variants of branching of bronchial arteries. (After T. Fedorova.) **A,** first; **B,** second; **C,** third variant of branching of the bronchial vessels. **1,** Ventral view. **2,** Dorsal view.

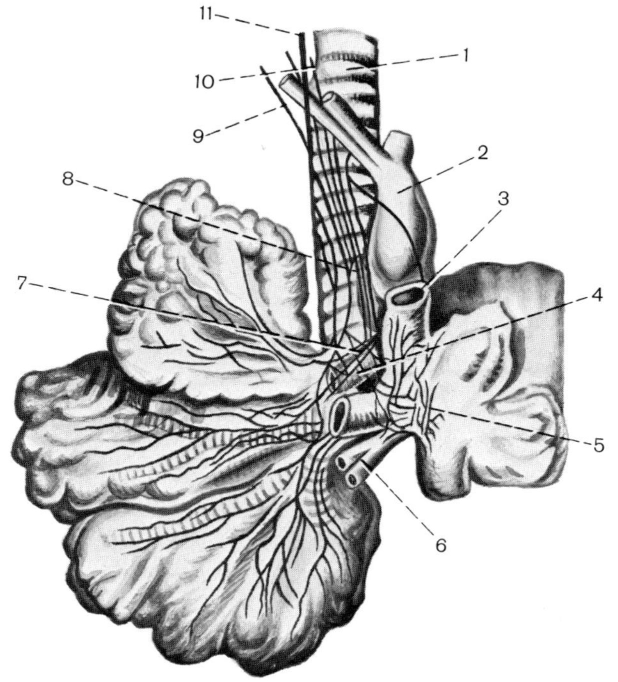

Fig. 26. Innervation of lungs. (After A. Taft.) Nerves of lungs on mediastinal surface of right lung (anterior aspect).

1 Trachea
2 Aorta
3 Superior vena cava
4 Pulmonary artery
5 Right posterior cardiac plexus
6 Segment of pulmonary veins extending outside of the organ
7 Anterior pulmonary plexus
8 Cardiopulmonary nerve
9 Sympathetic nerve, branch of inferior cervical ganglion
10 Recurrent laryngeal nerve
11 Vagus nerve

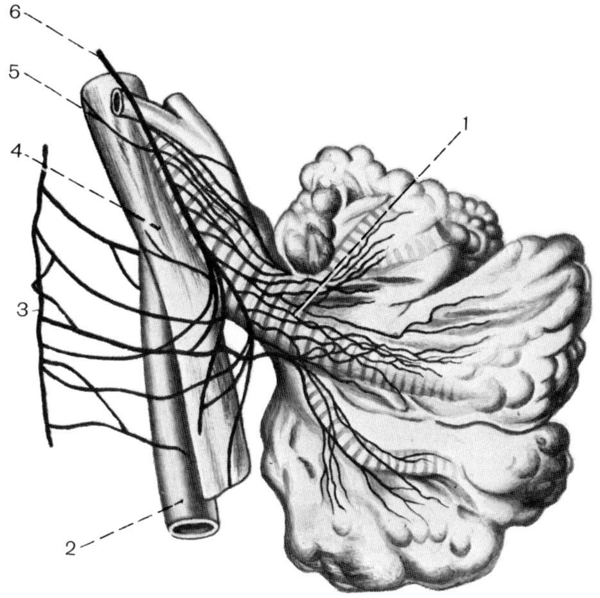

Fig. 27. Innervation of lungs. (After A. Taft.) Nerves on posterior surface of bronchus and lungs.

1 Posterior pulmonary plexus
2 Aorta
3 Sympathetic trunk
4 Esophagus
5 Sympathetic nerve, branch of inferior cervical ganglion
6 Vagus nerve

and penetrate the pulmonary tissue along its length. The nerve fibers of the anterior plexus spread into the lung parenchyma along the walls of the arteries and veins.

The lymphatic vessels of the lung (Fig. 28) form superficial and deep networks with an abundance of anastomoses between them. The superficial network is represented by lymphatic capillaries located in the visceral pleura. The vessels of the deep lymphatic network are situated inside the parenchyma of the lung between the aveoli and lobuli, in the submucosal coat of the bronchi, and around the blood vessels. The perivascular, peribronchial, and other lymphatic vessels extending to the root of the lung coalesce and form larger collecting vessels, which drain into the regional lymph nodes. Lymph is drained from the lung in three principal directions.

From the cranial part of the left lung the lymph flows into the left paratracheal (laterotracheal) lymph nodes. The lymph from the middle parts drains into the paratracheal and the bifurcation lymph nodes. The lymph from the caudal parts of the left lung is received by the bifurcation nodes. The lymph from the cranial parts of the right lung flows into the right paratracheal nodes and into the nodes of the anterior mediastinum. Lymph from the medial portions drains partly into the right paratracheal and partly into the bifurcation lymph nodes. The lymph from the caudal parts of the lung drains into the bifurcation lymph nodes. Besides, lymph from the lower portions of both lungs flows into nodes situated at the diaphragm behind the esophagus.

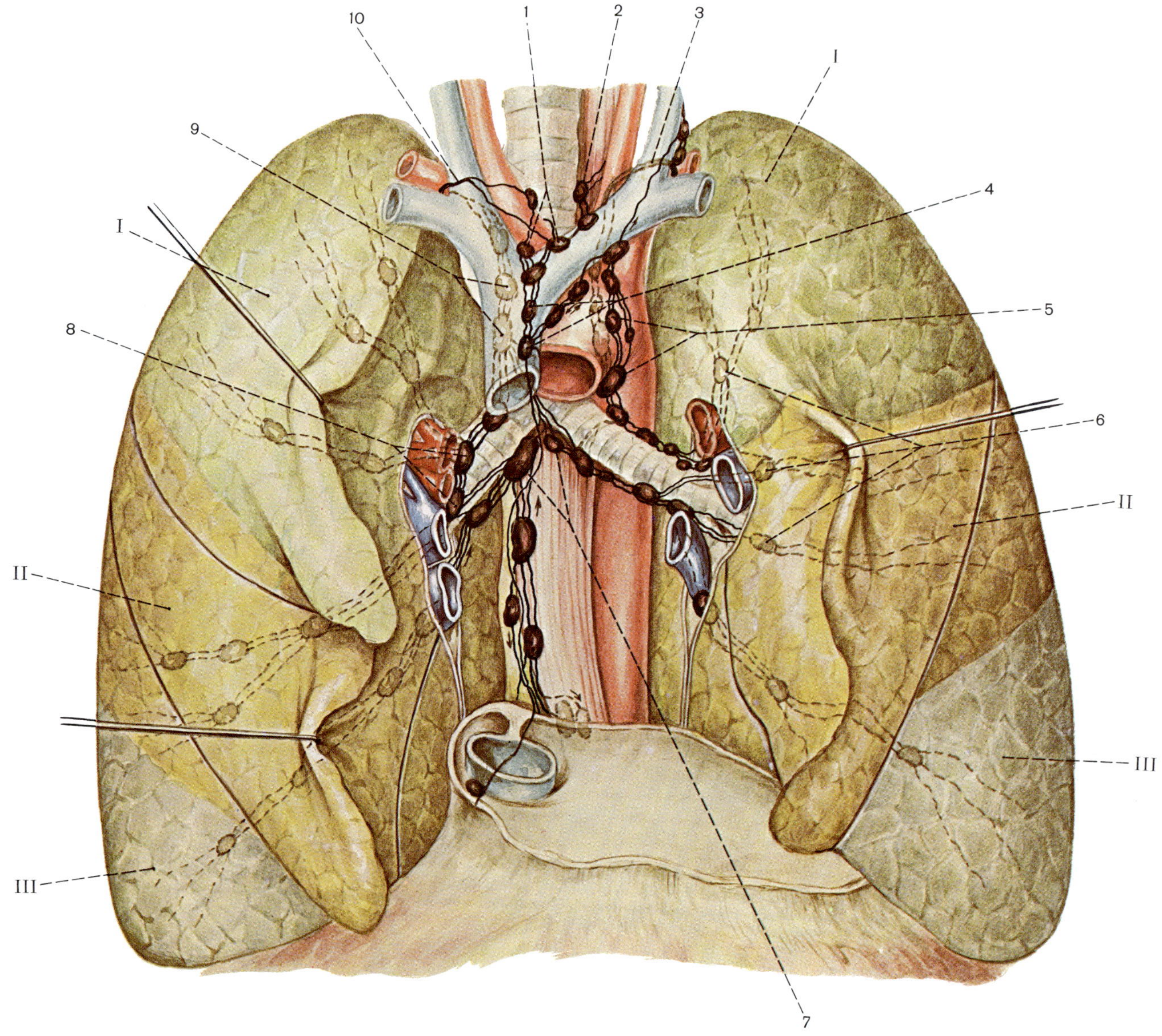

Fig. 28. Lymphatic system of lung. (After Rouvier-Zhdanov). **I,** upper area of lymph drainage. **II,** Middle area of lymph drainage. **III,** Lower area of lymph drainage.

1 Superior mediastinal lymph nodes
2 Left paratracheal lymph nodes
3 Ductus thoracicus
4 Prevenous chain
5 Preaortic chain
6 Intrapulmonary lymph nodes
7 Inferior tracheobronchial lymph nodes
8 Lymph nodes
9 Right paratracheal nodes
10 Right lymphatic duct

THE MEDIASTINUM

The mediastinum is the name given to that part of the thoracic cavity which is confined between the mediastinal pleurae and contains a complex system of organs and neurovascular structures surrounded by fatty cellular tissue (Figs. 29 and 30).

The boundaries of the mediastinum are the superior thoracic aperture at the top, the diaphragm at the bottom, the posterior surface of the sternum and partly the costal cartilages in front, the anterior surface of the thoracic spine at the back, and the mediastinal pleura on the right and on the left. In front, back of the sternum, the entrance to the mediastinum is bounded by the anterior reflections of the parietal pleura. At the back, and in front of the vertebral column, the entrance into the mediastinum is bounded by the posterior pleural reflections and by the line where the costovertebral pleura meets the mediastinal pleura. It is common practice to distinguish the anterior and posterior mediastina, the conditional borderline between which is a frontal plane drawn through the roots of the lungs.

In roentgenology the mediastinum is divided into three parts, which are clearly delineated in lateral-view chest roentgenoscopy: the anterior part called the retrosternal space between the posterior surface of the sternum and the anterior surfaces of the heart and major vessels; the middle part occupied by the heart and pulmonary roots; and the posterior part, or the retrocardiac space, between the posterior surface of the heart and the anterior surface of the spine.

The organs of the anterior and posterior mediastina are surrounded by loose fatty cellular tissue, which is of prime significance in the spread of purulent inflammatory processes. The fatty cellular tissue in the upper part of the anterior mediastinum located between the posterior surface of the sternum and the organs forms a cellular space communicating with the pretracheal space on the neck. This space of the mediastinum has two layers of cellular tissue separated at the back by Rudnev's sternal fascia. The first layer, the thinner one, lies directly next to the posterior surface of the sternum (Dyakonov's retrosternal space). The second deeper-lying layer, up to 0.75 to 1.5 cm thick, is bounded at the back by Meyer's fascial plate. Accumulation of pus in the retrosternal space may spread along the anterior surface of the pericardium to the diaphragm, and, from there, to the subperitoneal fatty cellular tissue. Besides, a pretracheal cellular space (''rhomboid'' according to Rudnev) is distinguished in the anterior mediastinum. It is bounded by the bifurcation of the trachea, the arch of the aorta, the branches of the pulmonary artery, and superior vena cava. There are also left and right paratracheal spaces.

The most pronounced in the posterior mediastinum is the retroesophageal cellular space communicating at the top with the retrovisceral space of the neck and at the bottom with the retroperitoneal cellular tissue through the aortic and esophageal openings.

The preesophageal cellular space is well developed in the zone of the bifurcation of the trachea (''glandular triangle'' according to Savvin) and also below between the anterior surface of the esophagus and the posterior surface of the pericardium.

The mediastinal cellular tissue contains a richly-developed network of arterial and venous vessels contributing to the vascularization of the organs. The sources of the arterial vessels are the aorta, the intercostal and subclavian arteries, as well as the internal thoracic and pericardiacophrenic arteries and the thyrocervical trunk. Among the arterial vessels of the mediastinum the most prominent are the bronchial vessels. which take part in the vascularization not only of the bronchopulmonary complex, but also of the trachea, esophagus, pericardium, the walls of the aorta and superior vena cava, the vagus nerves, the lymph nodes, and the cellular tissue of the mediastinum.

The bronchial arteries, numbering two to six, usually arise from the anterior surface of the aorta, where its arch is continuous with the descending part at the level of the superior and inferior margins of the left main bronchus. The bronchial arteries form numerous anastomoses with the arteries of the systemic (subclavian, internal thoracic arteries) and pulmonary circulation (pulmonary artery).

The venous network of the mediastinum represented by the peribronchial and periaortic veins, the veins of the nerves and lymph nodes, and veins carrying blood from the walls of the blood vessels and pericardium, drains into the venae anonymae and superior vena cava, into the system of the azygos and hemiazygos veins, into the inferior vena cava, and along the anastomoses with the veins of the retroperitoneal cellular tissue into the portal vein.

Besides that, the veins of the mediastinum communicate with the pulmonary veins. The mediastinal venous network, therefore, is a chain of anastomoses connecting various venous systems (superior and inferior venae cavae, veins of pulmonary circulation, the system of the portal vein).

The lymphatic system of the mediastinum (Fig. 31) consists of a large number of nodes that receive the lymph from the organs.

The parietal nodes are divided into anterior, or sternal, and posterior. The anterior nodes, four to five in number, are situated behind the sternum along the

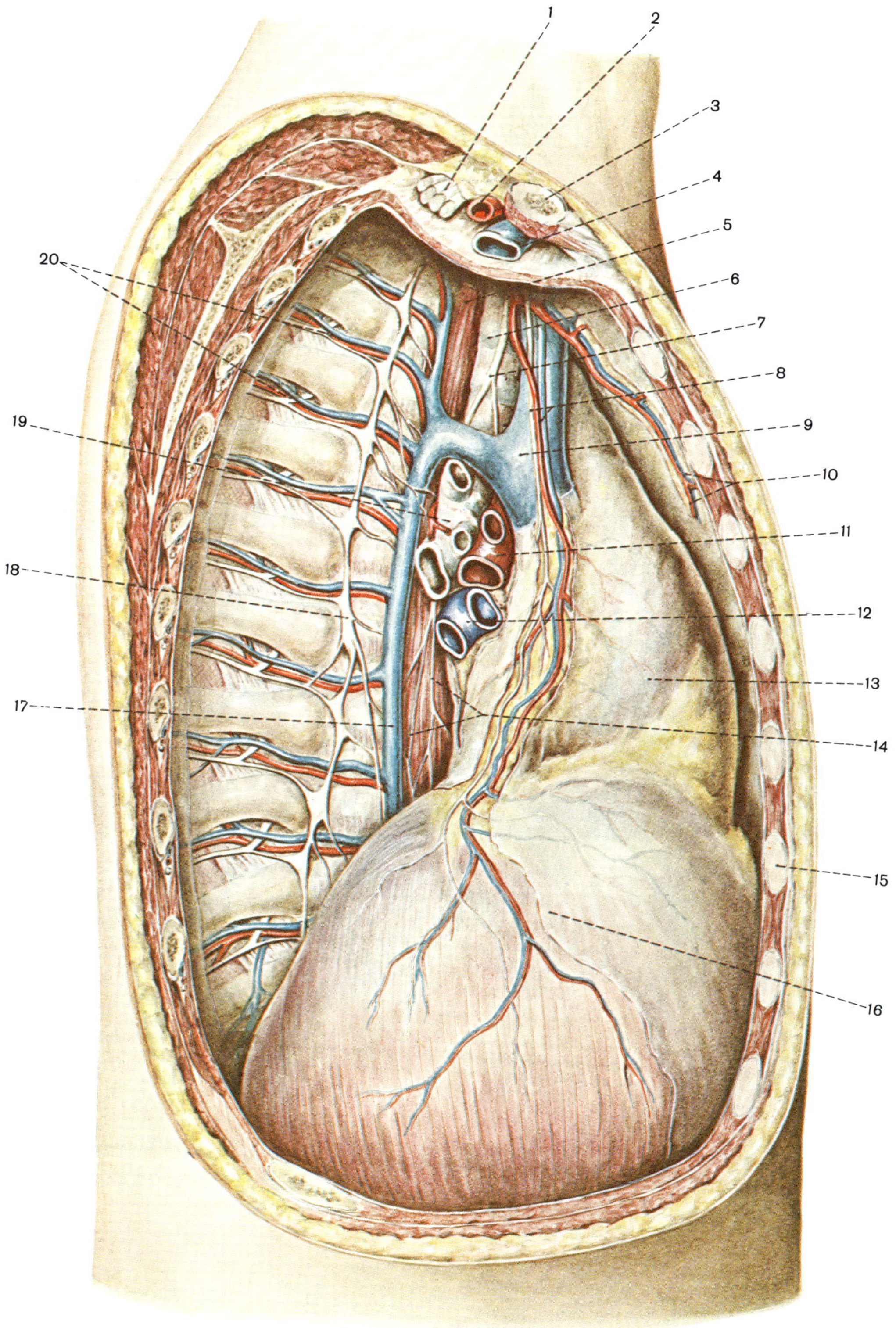

Fig. 29. Topography of organs of mediastinum, right view. (After E. Pernkopf.)

1 Brachial plexus (plexus brachialis)
2 Right subclavian artery (a. subclavia dextra)
3 Clavicle (clavicula)
4 Right subclavian vein (v. subclavia dextra)
5 Esophagus
6 Trachea
7 Right vagus nerve (n. vagus dexter)
8 Phrenic nerve and right pericardiacophrenic artery and vein (n. phrenicus, a. et v. pericardiacophrenicae dextrae)
9 Superior vena cava (v. cava superior)
10 Internal thoracic artery and vein (a. et v. thoracicae internae)
11 Right pulmonary artery (a. pulmonalis dextra)
12 Right pulmonary vein (v. pulmonalis dextra)
13 Heart and pericardium (cor et pericardium)
14 Right vagus nerve (n. vagus dexter)
15 Ribs
16 Diaphragm (diaphragma)
17 Azygos vein (v. azygos)
18 Sympathetic trunk (truncus sympathicus)
19 Right primary (main) bronchus (bronchus principalis dexter)
20 Intercostal artery, vein, and nerve (a., v., et n. intercostales)

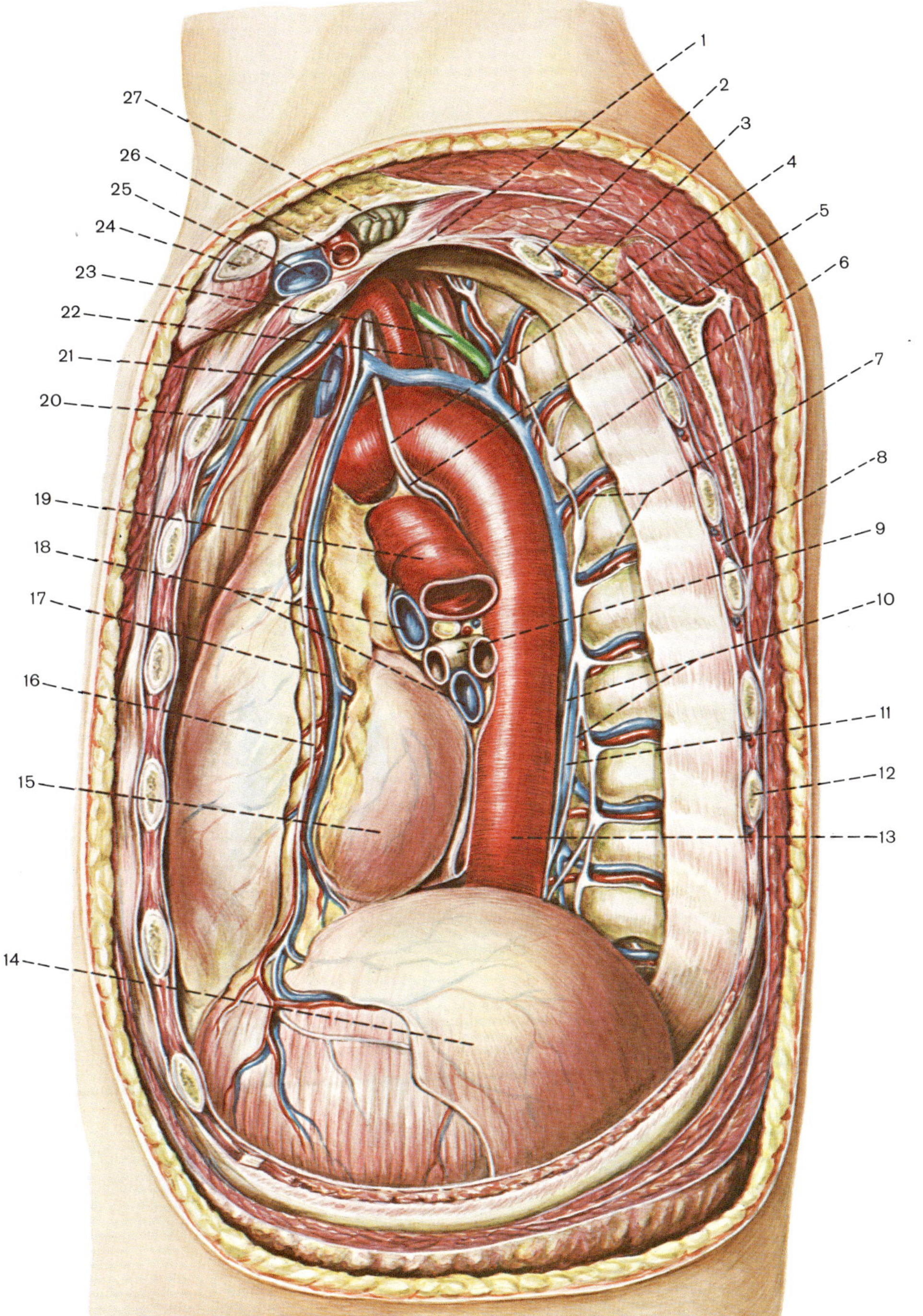

Fig. 30. Topography of organs of mediastinum, left view. (After E. Pernkopf.)

1 Cervical pleura (cupula pleurae)
2, 12 Ribs (costae)
3, 8 Intercostal muscles (mm. intercostales)
4 Left vagus nerve (n. vagus sinister)
5 Recurrent laryngeal nerve (n. laryngeus recurrens)
6 Sympathetic trunk (truncus sympathicus)
7 Intercostal neurovascular bundle
9 Left primary (main) bronchus (bronchus principalis sinister)
10 Greater splanchnic nerve (n. splanchnicus major)
11 Hemiazygos vein (v. hemiazygos)
13 Aorta
14 Diaphragm (diaphragma)
15 Heart and pericardium (cor et pericardium)
16 Phrenic nerve (n. phrenicus)
17 Pericardiacophrenic artery and vein (a. et v. pericardiacophrenicae)
18 Pulmonary veins (vv. pulmonales)
19 Pulmonary artery (a. pulmonalis)
20 Internal thoracic artery and vein (a. et v. thoracicae internae)
21 Superior vena cave (v. cava superior)
22 Esophagus
23 Thoracic duct (ductus thoracicus)
24 Clavicle (clavicula)
25 Left subclavian vein (v. subclavia sinistra)
26 Left subclavian artery (a. subclavia sinistra)
27 Brachial plexus (plexus brachialis)

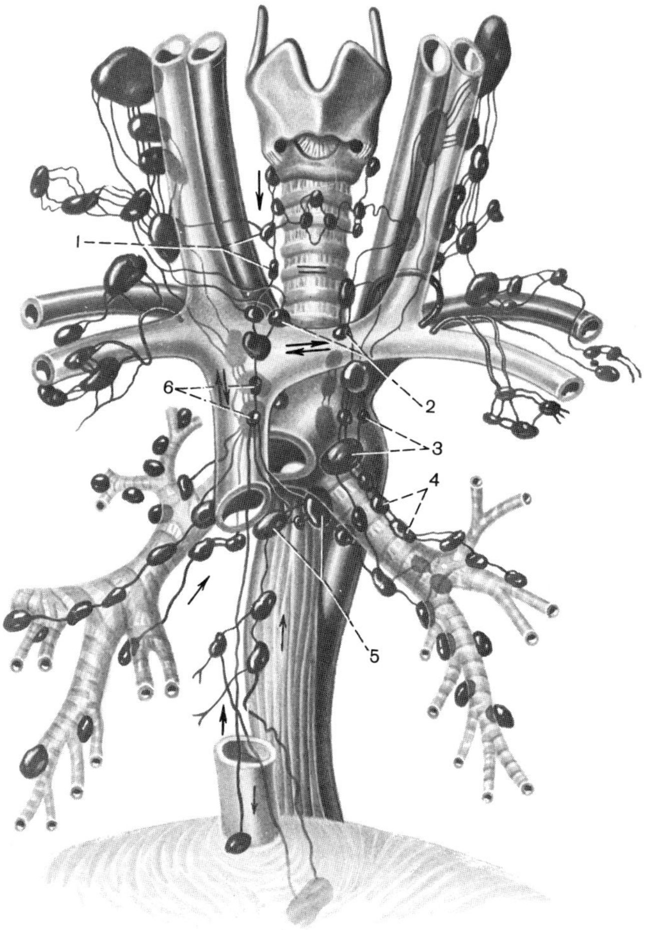

Fig. 31. Visceral lymph nodes of mediastinum. (After D. Zhdanov.)

1 Paratracheal lymph nodes
2 Transverse chain
3 Left vertical chain
4 Parabronchial nodes
5 Bifurcation nodes
6 Right vertical chain

length of the intrathoracic vessels. The posterior parietal nodes are represented by the paravertebral intercostal nodes. The paravertebral nodes are located on the lateral surface of the vertebrae mainly below the level of the sixth thoracic vertebra. One to six nodes are found in each intercostal space. The posterior intercostal nodes are constantly present, while the lateral nodes are less so.

The visceral lymph nodes of the mediastinum are divided into the anterior and posterior. Two groups of anterior visceral nodes are distinguished: superior and inferior.

The superior group is represented by chains extending along the length of large vascular trunks. There are two vertical chains, right and left, and a transverse chain linking them. The right vertical chain, prevenous, is located on the anterior surface of the superior vena cava and the right vena anonyma. It consists of two to five nodes among which the node in the angle formed at the junction of the venae anonymae is regarded as the most constant. The left vertical chain, called the preaortocarotid, begins as a large node situated at the ligamentum arteriosum. Then it ascends along the left vagus nerve, crossing the aortic arch. The transverse chain of nodes is situated along the superior and inferior margins of the left vena anonyma.

The prepericardiac and the lateropericardiac nodes belong to the inferior group of anterior visceral nodes. The former, two to three in number, are located behind the sternum at the xiphoid process where the diaphragm is attached to the seventh costal cartilage. The lateropericardiac nodes, one to three on each side, are grouped where the phrenic nerves enter the diaphragm.

The peritracheobronchial nodes form the main group of the posterior visceral nodes. Besides these, the paraesophageal (two to five) and interaortoesophageal nodes (one or two) are described in the posterior mediastinum, as well as a few lymph nodes inconstantly present immediately above the diaphragm, at the esophagus and thoracic aorta. The peritracheobronchial nodes are subdivided into peritracheal, bifurcation nodes, and nodes of the roots of the lungs.

The peritracheal nodes are situated to the right and left of the trachea as the right and left laterotracheal chains and to the back of the trachea as inconstantly present retrotracheal nodes. The right laterotracheal chain consisting of three to six nodes is located to the back of the superior vena cava at the right margin of the trachea and is bounded at the top by the subclavian artery and at the bottom by the arch of the azygos vein. The inferior node of the right laterotracheal chain is called "the node of the arch of the azygos vein." The left laterotracheal chain comprises four or five small nodes stretching along the length of the left recurrent laryngeal nerve.

The bifurcation nodes are located in the space between the primary bronchi and the pulmonary vessels. Their number varies from three to five.

The nodes of the root of the lung are subdivided into anterior, posterior, superior, and inferior in relation to the primary bronchi. The anterior nodes are situated to the front of the pulmonary veins, pulmonary artery, and bronchus. The posterior nodes are rarely encountered on the left. The inferior nodes are inconstant and are located between the sheets of the pulmonary ligament, most frequently on the left. The suprabronchial chain composed of two or three lymph nodes extends along the upper margin of the left bronchus.

The efferent vessels of the named lymph nodes are connected both with the thoracic duct and with the jugular and subclavian lymphatic trunks. The possibility of retrograde lymph flow has been established. This

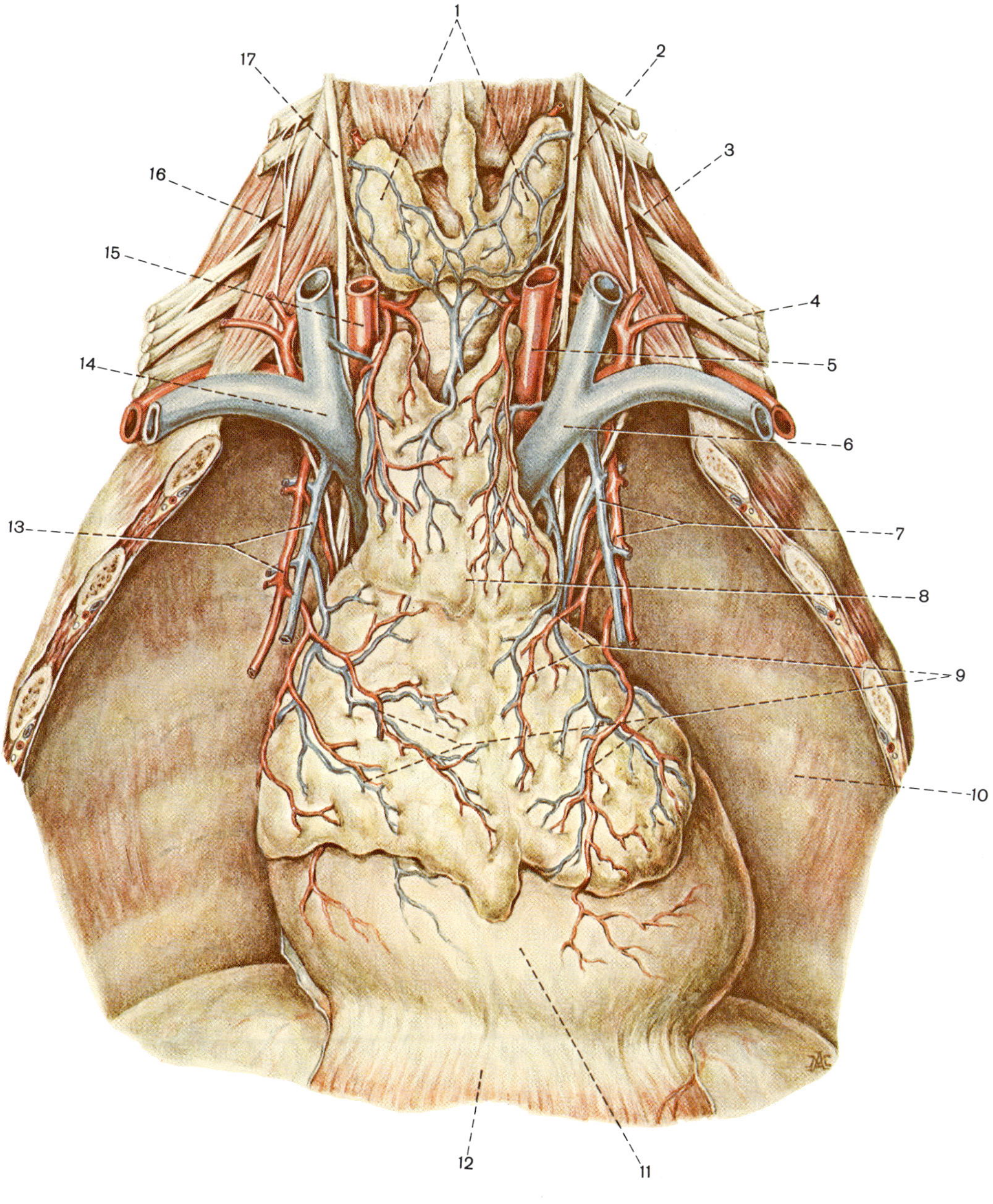

Fig. 32. Blood supply to thymus.

1 Thyroid (glandula thyroidea)
2 Left vagus nerve (n. vagus sinister)
3 Left phrenic nerve (n. phrenicus sinister)
4 Brachial plexus (plexus brachialis)
5 Left common carotid artery (a. carotis communis sinistra)
6 Left brachiocephalic vein (v. brachiocephalica sinistra)
7, 13 Internal thoracic artery and vein (a. et v. thoracicae internae)
8 Thymus (glandula thymus)
9 Vessels of the thymus (vasae glandulae thymicae)
10 Costal pleura (pleura costalis)
11 Heart and pericardium (cor et pericardium)
12 Diaphragm (diaphragma)
14 Right brachiocephalic vein (v. brachiocephalica dextra)
15 Right common carotid artery (a. carotis communis dextra)
16 Right phrenic nerve (n. phrenicus dexter)
17 Right vagus nerve (n. vagus dexter)

explains the cases with lymphogenous route of tumor metastases from the thoracic into the abdominal cavity.

Another specific feature of mediastinal lymph circulation is the presence of regional lymph nodes common to a number of organs, in which the streams of lymph merge. Lymph from the heart and pericardium, for instance, flows into the system of the right lymphatic chain into which lymph from the right lung also drains. The pathologic origin can thus be transferred from one organ to another within the thoracic cavity.

The mediastinum contains many nerve structures: nerve trunks, plexuses localized within and outside the organs, and nerve ganglia. The thoracic organs are innervated by the vagus and phrenic nerves and partly by the intercostal nerves and the sympathetic trunk. The branches of these nerves form a number of plexuses outside the organs, which also contain accumulations of ganglion cells.

Cardiac, pulmonary, aortic, tracheal, and esophageal plexuses are distinguished. They are localized in the fatty cellular tissue around the corresponding organs.

Thymus

The thymus gland (see Figs. 11 and 32) is a paired organ situated in the superior part of the anterior mediastinum. The primary importance of the thymus in the organism's immunologic reactivity, its participation in calcium metabolism, and its effect on the muscle tone have been proved to date.

The thymus attains maximum development by the age of 15, after which it gradually undergoes involution and is replaced by fatty and connective tissue. The average weight of the gland is 13 g in the newborn, 29 g in 15-year-old children, 21 g in adults between the ages of 20 and 25, and 14 g by the age of 60 to 75 (G. Ivanov).

The thymus is situated in the upper part of the anterior mediastinum. In children under 5 years of age it often protrudes above the jugular notch of the sternum, forming the cervical part. The upper pole of the gland in children is projected 1 to 1.5 cm above the manubrium of the sternum, the lower pole at the level of the third to fourth rib. Adults usually have no cervical part of the gland. In children under 3 years of age this part of the gland is localized behind the sternothyroid and sternohyoid muscles. Dorsally, the gland comes in contact with the trachea and touches the neurovascular bundle of the neck with its sides.

The thoracic part of the gland adjoins the sternum with its anterior surface. The posterior part of the gland adjoins the pericardium very tightly and touches the trunks of the superior vein and left brachiocephalic vein higher above. The anterolateral surfaces of the gland on the right and on the left are covered by the pleura. The thymus is supplied with blood by two or three main arteries of a small caliber arising from the right and left intrathoracic arteries. Besides this, the gland receives branches from the inferior thyroid and bracheocephalic arteries and the aortic arch. The veins of the gland drain into the intrathoracic, left brachiocephalic, and inferior thyroid veins.

The blood vessels enter the substance of the gland mainly from the top and lateral aspects, owing to which during operation the gland may be separated upward whenever necessary to expose the large blood vessels of the anterior mediastinum.

The parietal anterior retrosternal and visceral anterior transverse and prevenous nodes are the regional lymph nodes of the thymus.

The thymus is innervated by branches of the vagus and sympathetic nerves.

THE HEART

The heart (Fig. 33) is a hollow four-chamber organ with well-developed muscular walls. It is situated in the inferior part of the anterior mediastinum on the central tendon of the diaphragm, between the pleural cavities.

As a whole the heart is shaped like an irregular cone and is somewhat flattened in the anteroposterior direction. In newborn infants up to the age of 3 months, the heart is almost spherical due to the large dimensions of the atria and the large size of the right ventricle. By the age of 6 years the shape of the heart in a child hardly differs from that of an adult.

Two principal shapes of the heart are distinguished in adults: (1) a triangular-angulated or triangular-rounded, and (2) an egg shaped (''drop'') or cone shaped. The first shape is mostly encountered in a transverse position of the heart and brachymorphic body build, the second, in a vertical position of the heart and dolichomorphic body build. Besides these principal shapes there are intermediate shapes of the heart. The heart is displaced to the left in relation to the median body plane. In the oblique position of the heart two thirds of its bulk are located to the left of the midline and one third to the right of it.

The length of the heart (the distance between the base and the apex) varies in adults from 10 to 15 cm, the width (at the base of the heart) from 8 to 11 cm, and the thickness (anteroposterior measurement) from 6 to 8.5 cm. The circumference of the heart (maximum) is 28 to 30 cm, on the average.

The weight of the heart accounts for 0.5% to 0.57% of the body weight and varies from 200 to 440 g.

The heart has a base directed upward and to the back, an apex directed to the front, downward and to the left, and three surfaces: the anterior, or sternocostal; the inferior, or diaphragmatic; and the posterior, or vertebral. The heart surfaces are continuous one upon the other, forming the margins of the heart: the left, or upper, margin, which is rounded, and a sharper right, or lower, margin.

The anterior surface of the heart (see Fig. 33) is mostly formed by the anterior wall of the right ventricle and partly by the margin of the left ventricle and the left and right cardiac auriculae. The degree of the participation of these components in the formation of the anterior cardiac surface depends on the shape and position of the heart.

There are two grooves on the anterior surface of the heart: the coronary sulcus and the anterior interventricular (longitudinal) sulcus. The coronary sulcus stretches along the boundary separating the atrium from the ventricle. On the right it is located at the base of the right atrial auricula and then passes to the inferior surface of the heart. On the left in front the coronary sulcus is covered with the left atrial auricula. The right and left coronary arteries are accommodated in the coronary sulcus. The anterior interventricular sulcus corresponds to the central margin of the interventricular septum. At the apex of the heart this sulcus is continuous with the posterior interventricular (longitudinal) sulcus. The descending branch of the left coronary artery and the great cardiac vein stretch in the anterior interventricular sulcus.

The inferior, diaphragmatic, surface of the heart (Fig. 34) is formed mostly by the left ventricle and partly by the right ventricle and a small area of the right atrium. The trunk of the right coronary artery and the circumflex branch of the left coronary artery, as well as the coronary sinus of the heart and the small cardiac vein occupy the coronary sulcus. The posterior interventricular sulcus, which corresponds to the dorsal margin of the interventricular septum, contains the descending branch of the right coronary artery and the middle cardiac vein.

The posterior surface of the heart is formed by the walls of the atria and a small area of the left ventricle. The posterior interatrial sulcus stretching between the orifices of the venae cavae and the orifices of the right pulmonary veins is well discerned along the boundary between the atria.

The right atrium (Fig. 35) is bounded laterally by the coronary and the anterior and posterior interatrial sulci. The shape of the atrium with the auricula is greatly variable. A convex lateral and almost flat diaphragmatic and a concave medial wall are distinguished. Both venae cavae open on the dorsal wall of the atrium, the inferior on the boundary between the lateral and diaphragmatic walls, the superior between the lateral and medial walls. The cardiac auricula has two margins passing from the apex to the base. A shallow sulcus terminalis, which corresponds in position with the crista terminalis on the internal surface, stretches from the superior vena cava, along the lateral atrial wall, and to the anterior boundary of the inferior vena cava. The sulcus on the outside and the crista inside divide the atrium into two parts differing from each other in the structure of their walls. The posterior part, into which the venae cavae drain, is characterized by a smooth structure of its walls; it is called the venous sinus. Well-defined muscular ridges (pectinate muscles and trabeculae) are seen on the internal surface of the walls of the anterior part. An eminence known as Loweri's tuberculum is found on the posterior atrial wall between the orifices of the venae cavae.

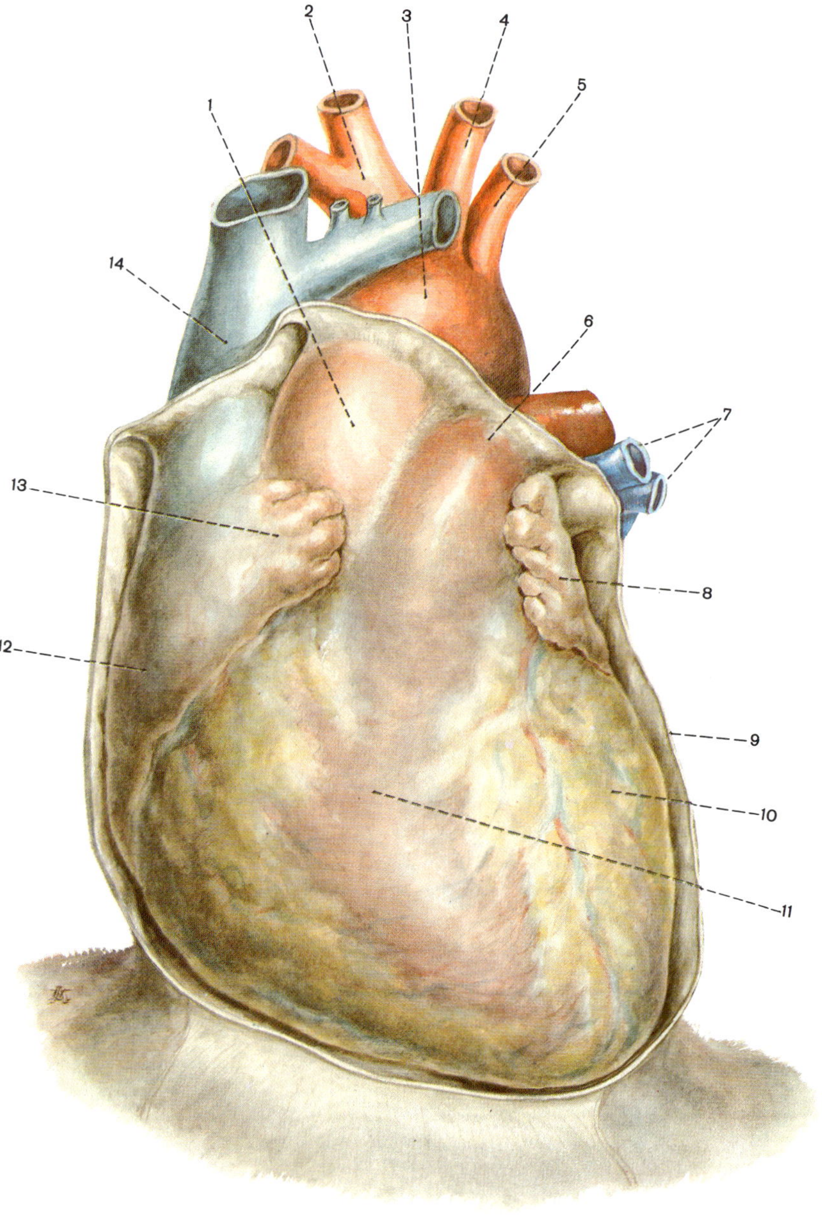

Fig. 33. Anterior surface of heart.

1 Ascending aorta (pars ascendens aortae)
2 Brachiocephalic trunk (truncus brachiocephalicus)
3 Arch of aorta (arcus aortae)
4 Left common carotid artery (a. carotis communis sinistra)
5 Left subclavian artery (a. subclavia sinistra)
6 Pulmonary trunk (truncus pulmonalis)
7 Pulmonary veins (vv. pulmonales)
8 Left auricle of heart (auricula atrii sinistri)
9 Pericardium
10 Left ventricle (ventriculus sinister)
11 Right ventricle (ventriculus dexter)
12 Right atrium (atrium dextrum)
13 Right auricle of heart (auricula atrii dextri)
14 Superior vena cava (v. cava superior)

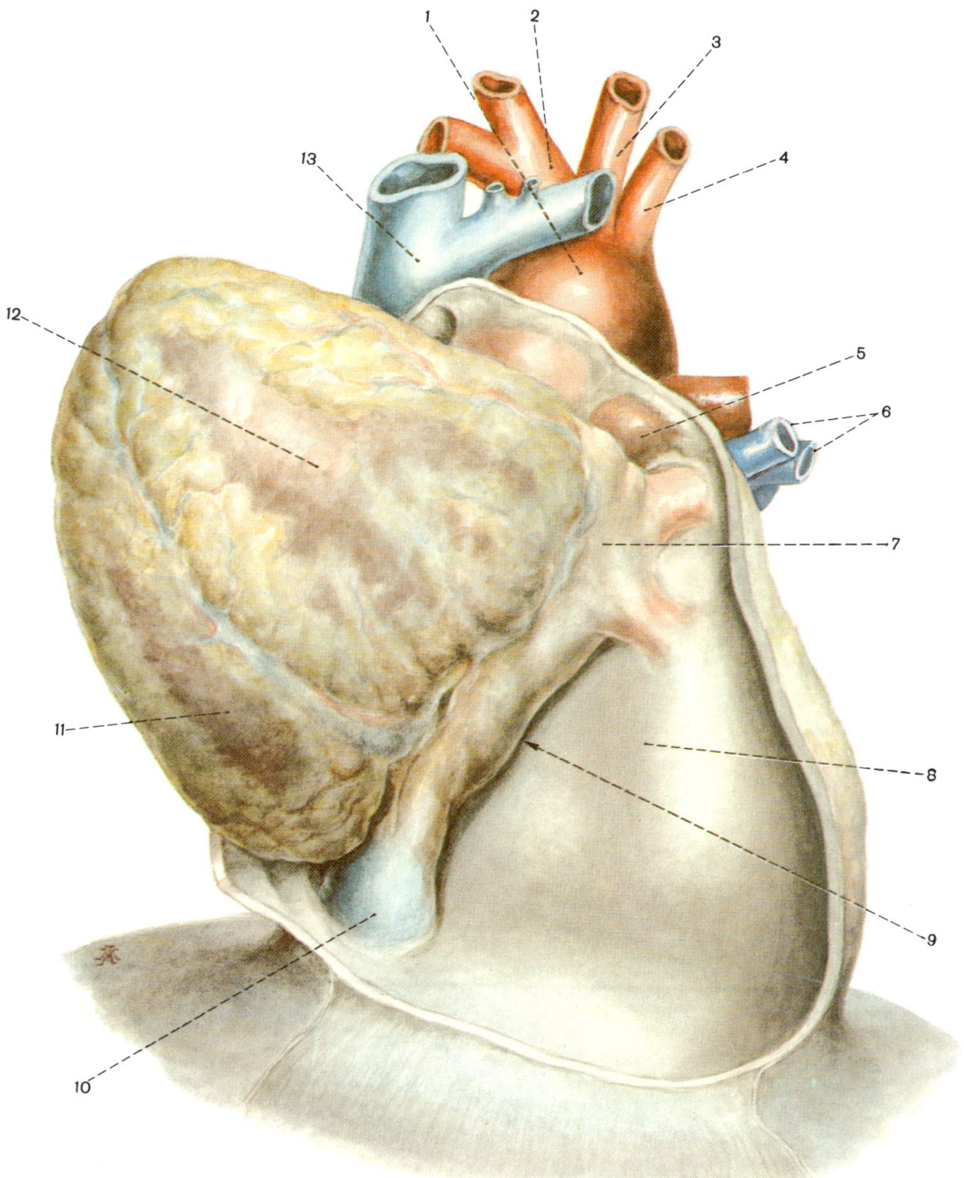

Fig. 34. Inferior surface of heart.

1 Arch of aorta (arcus aortae)
2 Brachiocephalic trunk (truncus brachiocephalicus)
3 Left common carotid artery (a. carotis communis sinistra)
4 Left subclavian artery (a. subclavia sinistra)
5 Pulmonary trunk (truncus pulmonalis)
6 Pulmonary veins (vv. pulmonales)
7 Left atrium (atrium sinistrum)
8 Posterior wall of pericardium
9 Oblique sinus of pericardium (sinus obliquus pericardii)
10 Inferior vena cava (v. cava inferior)
11 Right ventricle (ventriculus dexter)
12 Left ventricle (ventriculus sinister)
13 Superior vena cava (v. cava superior)

On the lateral wall the muscular bundles stretch almost parallel to each other and are called the pectinate muscles. In the atrial auricula they form a looped network, trabeculae carneae.

The orifice of the inferior vena cava is situated directly at the interatrial septum. The anterior margin of the orifice is 2 to 3 cm to the back of the atrioventricular orifice and is separated from it by the eustachian valve, the height of which varies between 2 and 15 mm. The orifice of the cardiac coronary sinus, usually covered with a fine endocardium fold (valvula thebesii), is located in the corner formed by the septum, inferior wall of the atrium, and the eustachian valve.

There is a depression on the inner surface of the interatrial septum, which is bounded by a muscular thickening (limbus) and is called the oval fossa. Its floor is a thin septum called the membranous part of the oval fossa. In 30% of adults there is a slitlike opening under the cranial margin of the limbus communicating with the left atrium. When the heart is in an in situ position, the right atrioventricular orifice is open downward, forward, and to the left.

The right atrioventricular orifice, 2.6 to 6 cm in diameter, is, in most cases, projected to the right of the midline behind the lower part of the body of the sternum. The center of the orifices is on the level of the sternal ends of the fourth, less frequently the fifth, costal cartilages.

The right ventricle (Fig. 36) on the whole is shaped like a trihedral pyramid, at the base angles of which the orifice of the pulmonary trunk is situated at the top and the right atrioventricular orifice at the bottom.

Three walls of the ventricle are distinguished: anterior, medial or septal, and posterior or diaphragmatic. The ventricle has two parts, the upper (conus arteriosus, or infundibulum), and the lower. The upper part serves as a route for the outflow of blood and the lower part for the inflow of blood. A large number of muscular trabeculae and papillae of muscles are found on the inner walls of the lower part. The walls of the infundibulum are smooth.

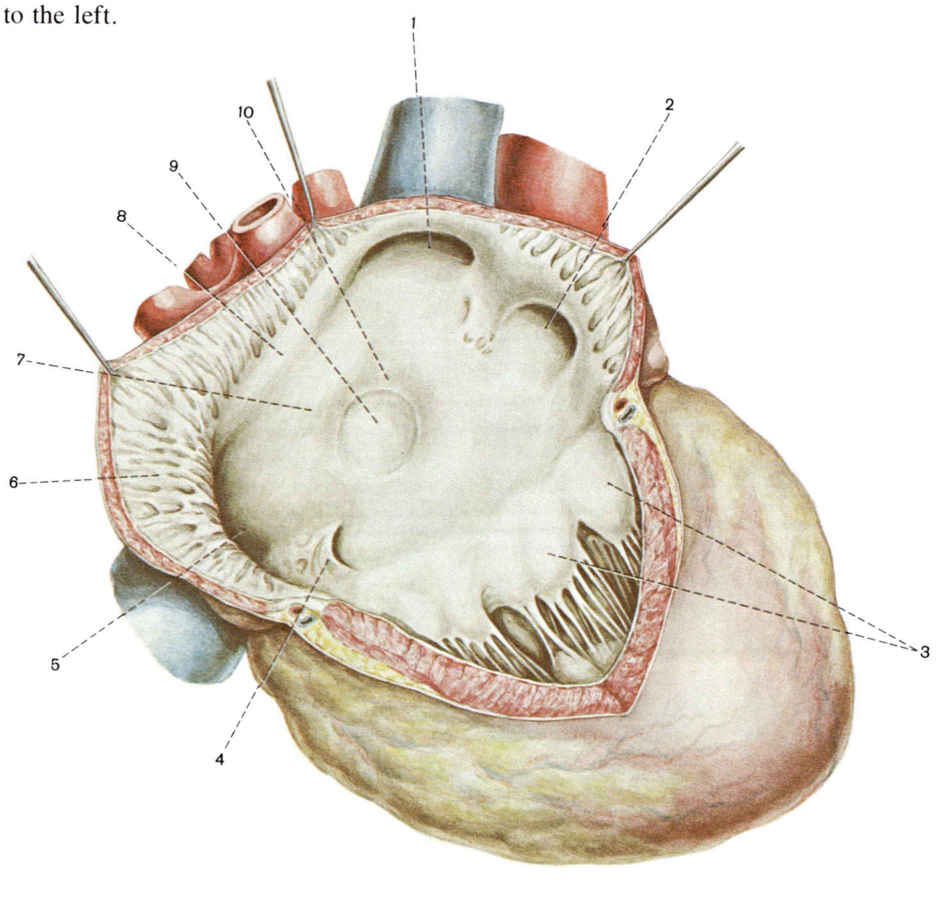

Fig. 35. Cavity of right atrium.

1 Orifice of superior vena cava (ostium venae cavae superioris)
2 Cavity of right atrial auricle (sinus aruiculae atrii dextri)
3 Cusps of the tricuspid valve
4 Valve of coronary sinus (valvula Thebesii)
5 Orifice of inferior vena cava (ostium venae cavae inferioris)
6 Trabeculae
7 Lower's intervenous tubercle (torus intervenosus Loweri)
8 Terminal crest (crista terminalis)
9 Oval fossa (fossa ovalis)
10 Limbus fossae ovalus

Three large papillary muscles are usually distinguished in the right ventricle: the anterior, posterior, and septal. The anterior muscle, the largest (1 to 3 cm long, and up to 1 cm thick at the base), arises from the anterior wall of the ventricle. In about 25% of cases, two or three anterior papillary muscles are encountered. The anterior papillary muscles give off three to ten chordae to the cusps of the tricuspid valve (mainly to the anterior and posterior cusps). The posterior capillary muscle arises from the posterior (diaphragmatic) wall of the ventricle. Sometimes two, three, and even four muscles are found here. The chordae from the posterior papillary muscle stretch to the posterior and medial cusps of the valve. The septal papillary muscle (most often one, but sometimes two) arises from the medial wall of the ventricle. Lancisi's papillary muscle is always found in the upper part on the border with the supraventricular crest. The infundibulum is continuous at the top with the right arterial orifice leading into the pulmonary trunk.

The right arterial orifice, 2 to 3 cm in diameter, is in most cases projected at the left margin of the sternum on a level with the lower border of the second rib, in the second intercostal space, 1 to 2 cm to the left of the midline.

The left atrium (Fig. 37) consists of three main parts: the left auricula, the atrium proper, and the sinus of the pulmonary veins. The inner surface of the left auricula has a well-developed network of muscular trabeculae. Its cavity is separated from the atrium by an interception 1 to 1.5 cm in diameter.

The sinus of the pulmonary vein is a depression between the orifices of the pulmonary veins. These are

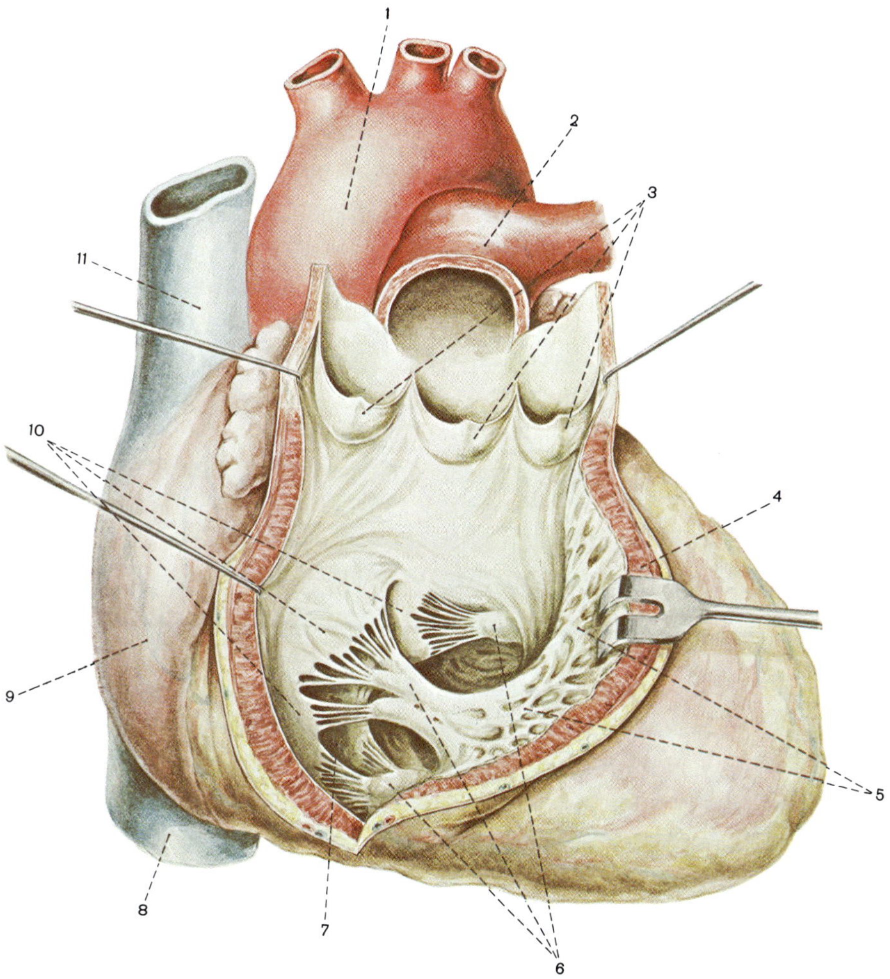

Fig. 36. Cavity of right ventricle.

1 Aorta
2 Pulmonary trunk (truncus pulmonalis)
3 Semilunar valves (valvulae semilunares)
4 Muscle of right ventricle (musculus ventriculi dextri)
5 Muscular trabeculae (trabeculae carneae)
6 Papullary muscles (mm. papillares)
7 Right atrioventricular orifice (ostium atrioventriculare dextrum)
8 Inferior vena cava (v. cava inferior)
9 Right atrium (atrium dextrum)
10 Cusps of right atrioventricular orifice
11 Superior vena cava (v. cava superior)

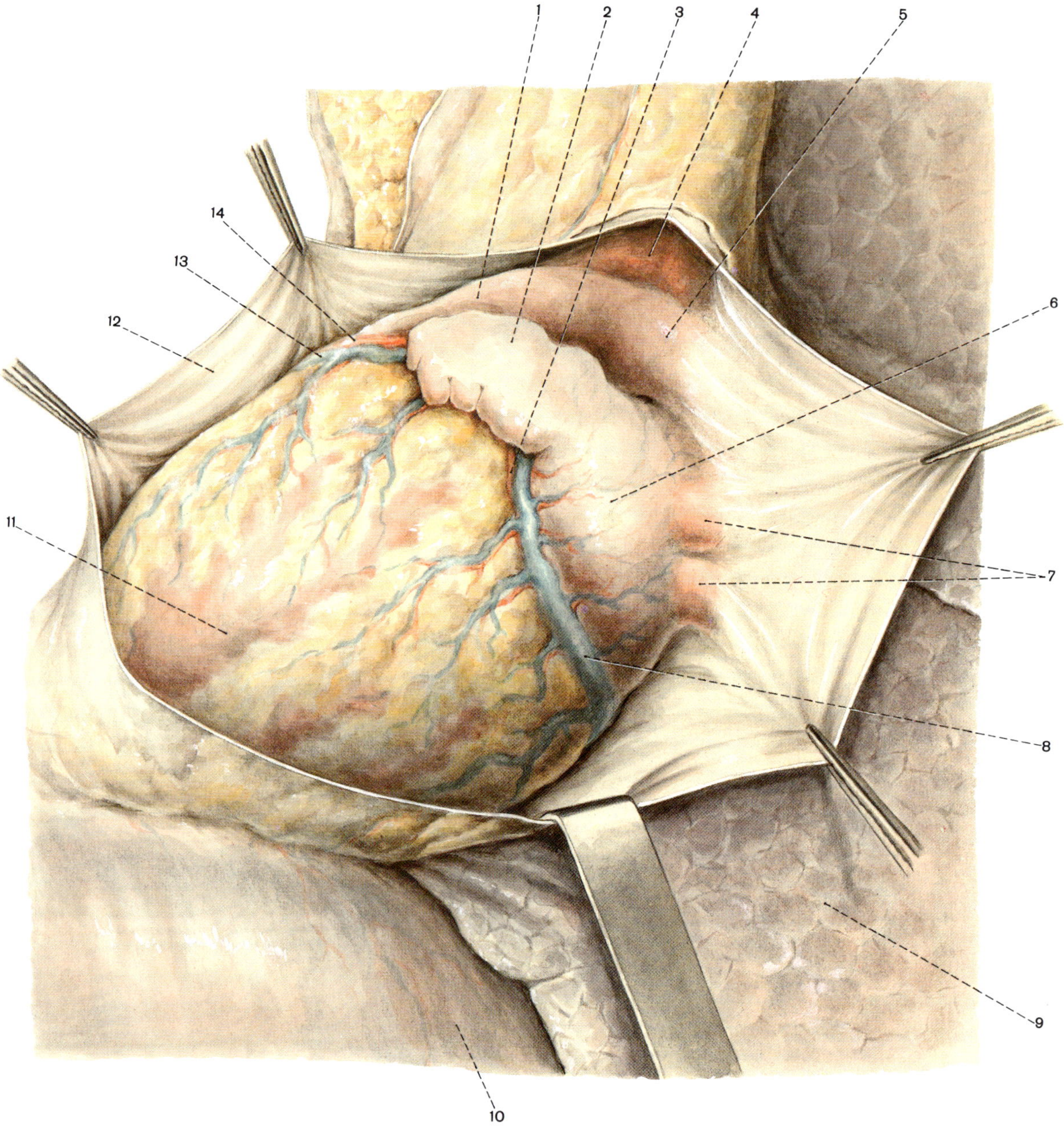

Fig. 37. Left ventricle and left atrium exposed after cutting pericardium.

1 Pulmonary trunk (truncus pulmonalis)
2 Left atrial auricle (auricula atrii sinistri)
3 Circumflex branch of left coronary artery (r. circumflexus arteriae coronariae sinistrae)
4 Aorta
5 Left pulmonary artery (a. pulmonalis sinistra)
6 Left atrium (atrium sinistrum)
7 Pulmonary veins (vv. pulmonales)
8, 13 Great cardiac vein (vena cordis magna)
9 Left lung (pulmo sinister)
10 Diaphragm (diaphragma)
11 Left ventricle (ventriculus sinister)
12 Pericardium
14 Anterior interventricular branch of left coronary artery (r. interventricularis anterior arteriae coronarie sinistrae)

usually four in number (two on each side); they open on the dorsal wall of the atrium. Before entering the atrium, the left pulmonary veins quite often join to form a common trunk. The inner surface of the left atrium is smooth. There is a valve of the foramen ovale on the interatrial septum; it is often hardly discernible. In incomplete closure of the foramen ovale this valve is well developed. The left atrioventricular orifice is open downward, a little to the left, and forward when the heart is in situ position. It has a diameter of 2 to 3 cm and is projected on a level with the third to fourth left sternocostal articulations, 1.1 to 2.5 cm to the left of the midline.

The left ventricle (Figs. 38 and 39) is conical with two openings at the base: the venous and the arterial.

The cavity of the ventricle is divided into two parts, the region where the papillary muscles are located, and the conus arteriosus. The first part corresponds to the route of the blood inflow, which stretches from the atrioventricular orifices to the inner surface of the heart apex, and contains the papillary muscles. These muscles are concentrated in two main groups. The apices of the muscles reach approximately to the midlength of the ventricular walls.

Two papillary muscles are usually distinguished, the posteromedial and posterolateral. A third papillary muscle, the posterior, is practically always encountered arising from the posterolateral wall of the ventricle. The number of papillary muscles is often greater.

The conus arteriosus is separated from the region of the inflow route by the aortic (anterior) cusp of the mitral valve. The three sides of the conus are bounded by muscular walls (the septum and the posterior and anterior walls of the ventricle), while the fourth is tendinous (the aortic cusp). Up and to the right, the conus arteriosus is continuous with the arterial orifice leading into the aorta.

The left arterial orifice, 2 to 3 cm in diameter, is projected 0.5 to 1.5 cm to the left of the midline on a level with the middle of the third rib (Fig. 40).

Heart valves and orifices. There are the atrioventricular valves (tricuspid and bicuspid) and valves of the arterial orifices (aortic and pulmonary).

Three cusps are usually described in the tricuspid valve, the anterior, posterior, and the medial, or septal. Quite frequently there are more cusps. According to T. Voropayev, most freqently there are four cusps (46.3%), less frequently three (23.6%), and rarely five (17.3%), six (8.2%), and seven cusps (4.6%).

The bicuspid (mitral) valve (see Fig. 39) consists of two large cusps between which there is often one small accessory cusp to the left (somewhat forward) and another to the right (in back). The number of cusps in the mitral valve varies from two to six; most common are three cusps. When the heart is in situ position, a large cusp located ventrally is called cuspis aortalis, and the large cusp located dorsally is called cuspis dorsalis. The aortic cusp is often called anterior, and the dorsal posterior.

The valves of the arterial orifices, both the aortic and the pulmonary, are each formed of three semilunar cusps. These semilunar cusps circumscribe the pouch-like dilatations of the vascular wall and the sinuses of Valsalva. The free margins of the cusps are thickened in the middle and form a nodule, which is most conspicuous on the aortic valve.

The aortic valve has a right, left, and posterior cusps. The orifice of the right coronary artery opens over the right cusp, and the orifice of the left coronary artery over the left cusp. With the heart in situ position, the right cusp is located in front, the posterior cusp on the right, and the left cusp somewhat to the back.

The pulmonary valve has anterior, right, and left cusps. When the heart is in in situ position, the anterior cusp is located in front and to the left, the left cusp on the left and to the back, and the right cusp on the right and in front.

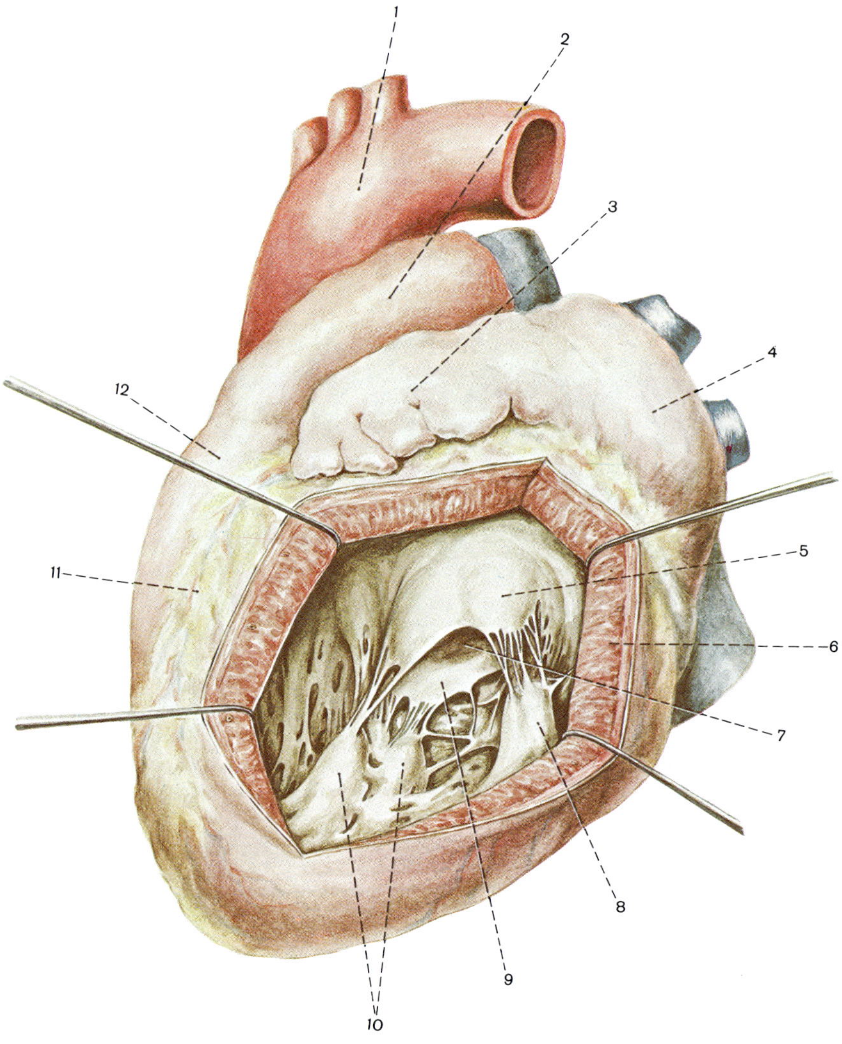

Fig. 38. Cavity of left ventricle.

1 Aorta
2 Pulmonary trunk (truncus pulmonalis)
3 Left atrial auricle (auricula atrii sinistri)
4 Left atrium (atrium sinistrum)
5 Anterior cusp (cuspis anterior)
6 Wall of left ventricle
7 Left atrioventricular orifice (ostium atrioventriculare sinistrum)
8 Posterior papillary muscle (m. papillaris posterior)
9 Posterior cusp (cuspis posterior)
10 Anterior papillary muscle (m. papillaris anterior)
11 Anterior longitudinal sulcus of heart (sulcus interventricularis anterior)
12 Conus arteriosus

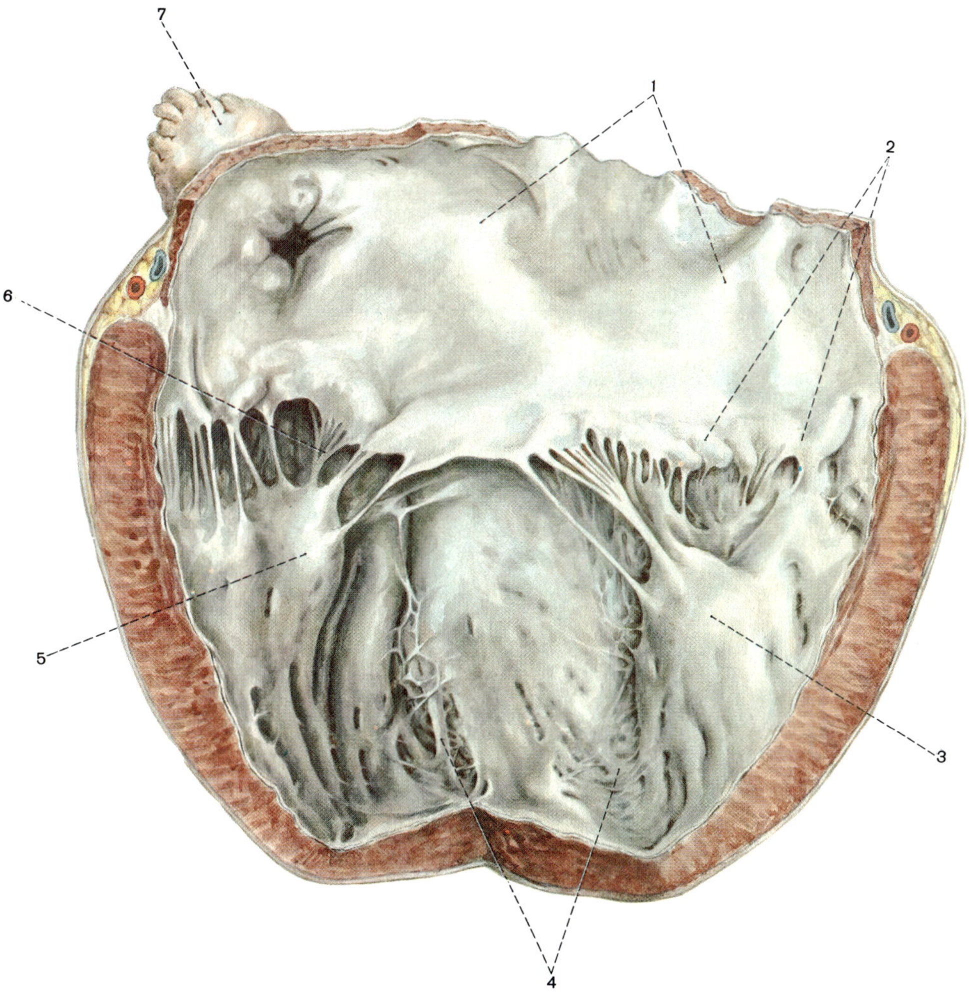

Fig. 39. Bicuspid valve.

1 Left atrium (atrium sinistrum)
2 Posterior cusp of mitral valve (cuspis posterior valvulae bicuspidalis)
3 Posterior papillary muscle (m. papillaris posterior)
4 Muscular trabaculae (trabeculae carneae)
5 Anterior papillary muscle (m. papillaris anterior)
6 Chordae tendineae
7 Left atrial auricle (auricula atrii sinistri)

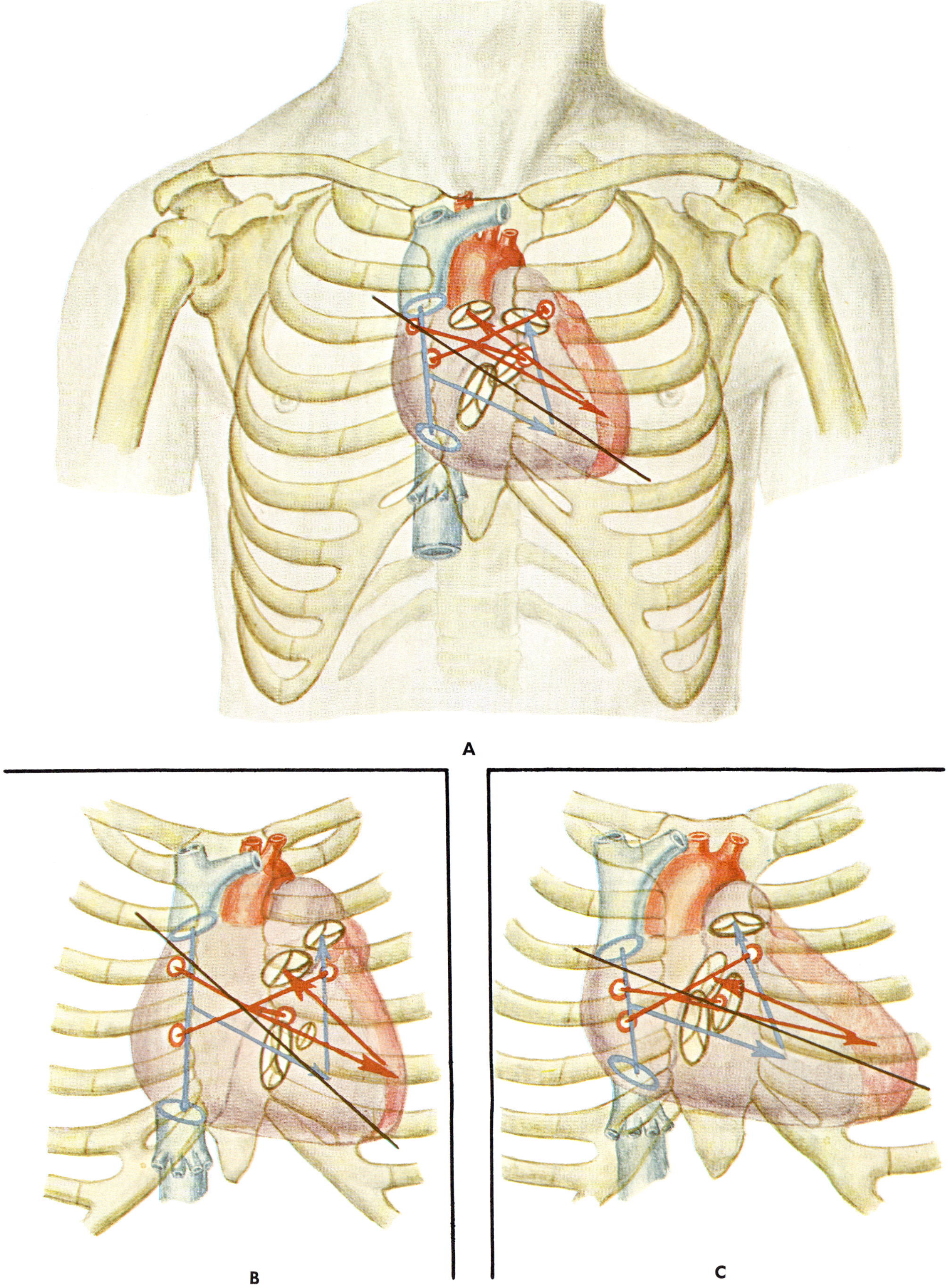

Fig. 40. Skeletopy of cardiac orifices and routes of blood flow. **A,** Normal, in oblique position of the heart. **B,** In mitral stenosis. **C,** In hypertensive disease. The black line represents the heart axis; the light blue lines show the flow of blood in the right heart; the red lines show the flow of blood in the left heart.

The conducting system of the heart (Fig. 41) is composed of muscle fibers that are of a special structure and can transmit impulses from the nerve apparatus to all groups of the heart muscles. The fibers are syncytially connected with one another and form ganglia and bundles of the conducting system of the heart.

The sinoatrial system consists of the Keith-Flack sinus node and two inconstant bundles called Wenckebach's and Schenberg's bundles. The Keith-Flack bundle, 1 to 2 mm in diameter, is situated in the wall of the right atrium under the epicardium between the right auricula and the superior vena cava. The bundles of this node embrace the orifice of the superior vena cava and spread in the wall of the right atrium. Wenckebach's bundle is located between the orifice of the superior vena cava and the interatrial septum. Schenberg's bundle passes in the posterior wall of the left atrium, and its fibers encompass the orifices of the pulmonary veins.

The atrioventricular system consists of the Aschoff-Tawara node and the atrioventricular bundle of His and its two branches.

The Aschoff-Tawara atrioventricular node is 2 by 5 mm in size and is situated under the endothelium in the posteroinferior part of the interatrial septum above the orifice of the coronary sinus. Lower down, the node is continuous with the bundle of His. This bundle, up to 8 mm long, penetrates the membranous part of the interventricular septum and at the superior margin of its muscular part divides into the right and left branches (limbs). Both branches descend to the apex of the heart along the septal surfaces, dividing into small terminal branches, Purkinje's fibers, which spread in the fibers of the myocardium.

The sinoatrial and atrioventricular parts of the conducting system are connected with one another by very many nerve pathways, which accomplish the complicated and versatile contact of the conducting system with all the nerve apparatuses of the heart.

The automatic rhythm of the cardiac contraction originates in the sinoatrial Keith-Flack node. Impulses from it spread in the musculature of the atria to the Aschoff-Tawara node and from there along the bundle of His to the musclature of the ventricles.

Blood supply to the heart (Figs. 42 and 43). The heart receives blood mainly from the coronary arteries. The Thebesian-Vieussens vessels and small branches of the mediastinal and bronchial arteries are also of definite importance.

There are, as a rule, two coronary arteries of the heart, the right and the left. In rare cases one coronary artery is encountered that divides into two at its origin.

The coronary arteries arise in the sinuses of the aortic bulb at the level of the superior margins of the right and left semilunar valves.

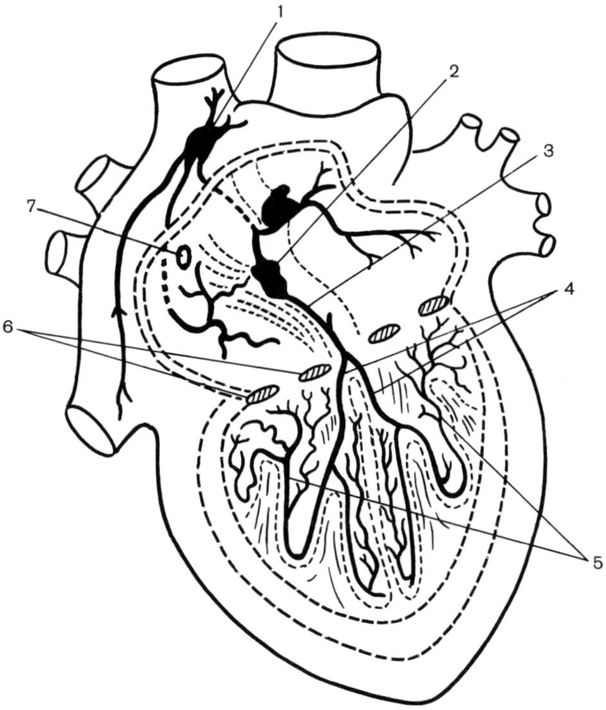

Fig. 41. Conducting system of heart. (After F. Volynskii.)

1 Sinoatrial node
2 Atrioventricular node
3 Bundle of His
4 Branch of bundle of His
5 Network of Purkinje's fibers
6 Coronary sinus
7 Heart valve

The right coronary artery adjoins the right semicircumference of the aorta at the beginning, then passes deeply in the coronary sulcus under the right atrial auricula, bends around the right margin of the heart, and passes to its posterior surface. Here the vessel also passes in the coronary sulcus to the posterior longitudinal sulcus, where it divides into two branches, the posterior descending and the left circumflex branches. The former stretches along the posterior longitudinal sulcus, giving off a number of small branches, and forms an anastomosis with the descending branch of the left coronary artery at the incisure of the apex. The circumflex branch of the right coronary artery forms an anastomosis with the branch of the same name of the left coronary artery.

The left coronary artery is located in the left semicircumference of the aortic bulb and then extends between the pulmonary artery and the left atrial auricula and divides into two branches, a large left circumflex and a thinner anterior descending branch.

The anterior descending branch passes along the arterial longitudinal sulcus to the incisure of the apex. The left circumflex branch is a continuation of the main trunk of the left coronary artery. It passes to the posterior surface of the heart, anastomosing with the circumflex

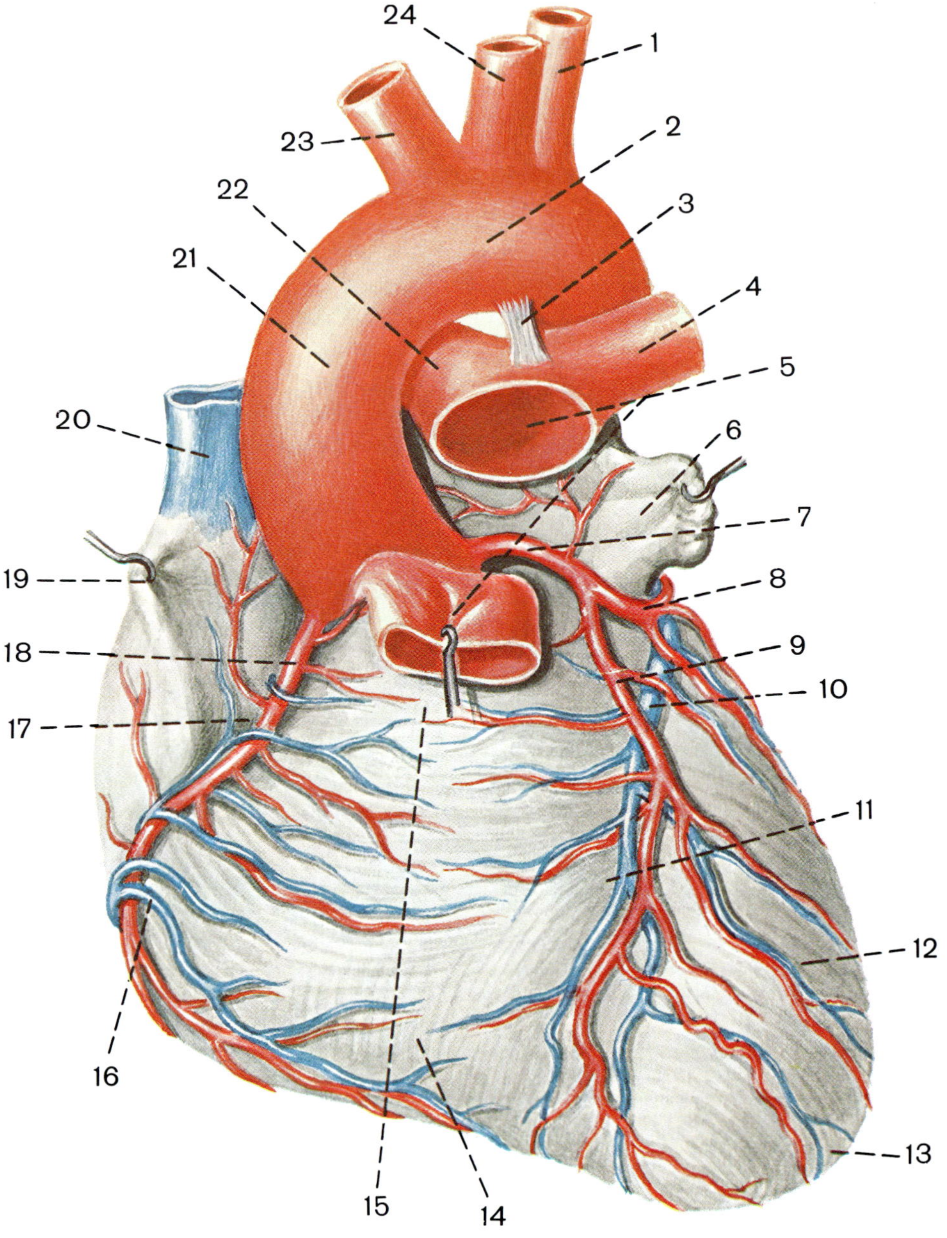

Fig. 42. Arteries and veins of heart, anterior aspect. (After R. Sinelnikov.)

1 Left subclavian artery (a. subclavia sinistra)
2 Arch of aorta (arcus aortae)
3 Ligamentum arteriosum
4 Left pulmonary artery (a. pulmonalis sinistra)
5 Pulmonary trunk (truncus pulmonalis)
6 Auricle of left atrium (auricula sinistra)
7 Left coronary artery (a. coronaria sinistra)
8 Circumflex branch of left coronary artery (r. circumflexus arterial coronariae sinistrae)
9 Anterior interventricular branch of left coronary artery (r. interventricularis anterior arterial coronariae sinistrae)
10 Great cardiac vein (v. cordis magna)
11 Anterior longitudinal sulcus (sulcus longitudinalis anterior)
12 Left ventricle (ventriculus sinister)
13 Apex of heart (apex cordis)
14 Right ventricle (ventriculus dexter)
15 Conus arteriosus
16 Anterior cardiac vein (v. cordis anterior)
17 Coronary sulcus of heart (sulcus coronarius)
18 Right coronary artery a. coronaria dextra)
19 Auricle of right atrium (auricula dextra)
20 Superior vena cava (v. cava superior)
21 Ascending aorta (aorta ascendens)
22 Right pulmonary artery (a. pulmonalis dextra)
23 Brachiocephalic trunk (truncus brachiocephalicus)
24 Left common carotid artery (a. carotis communis sinistra)

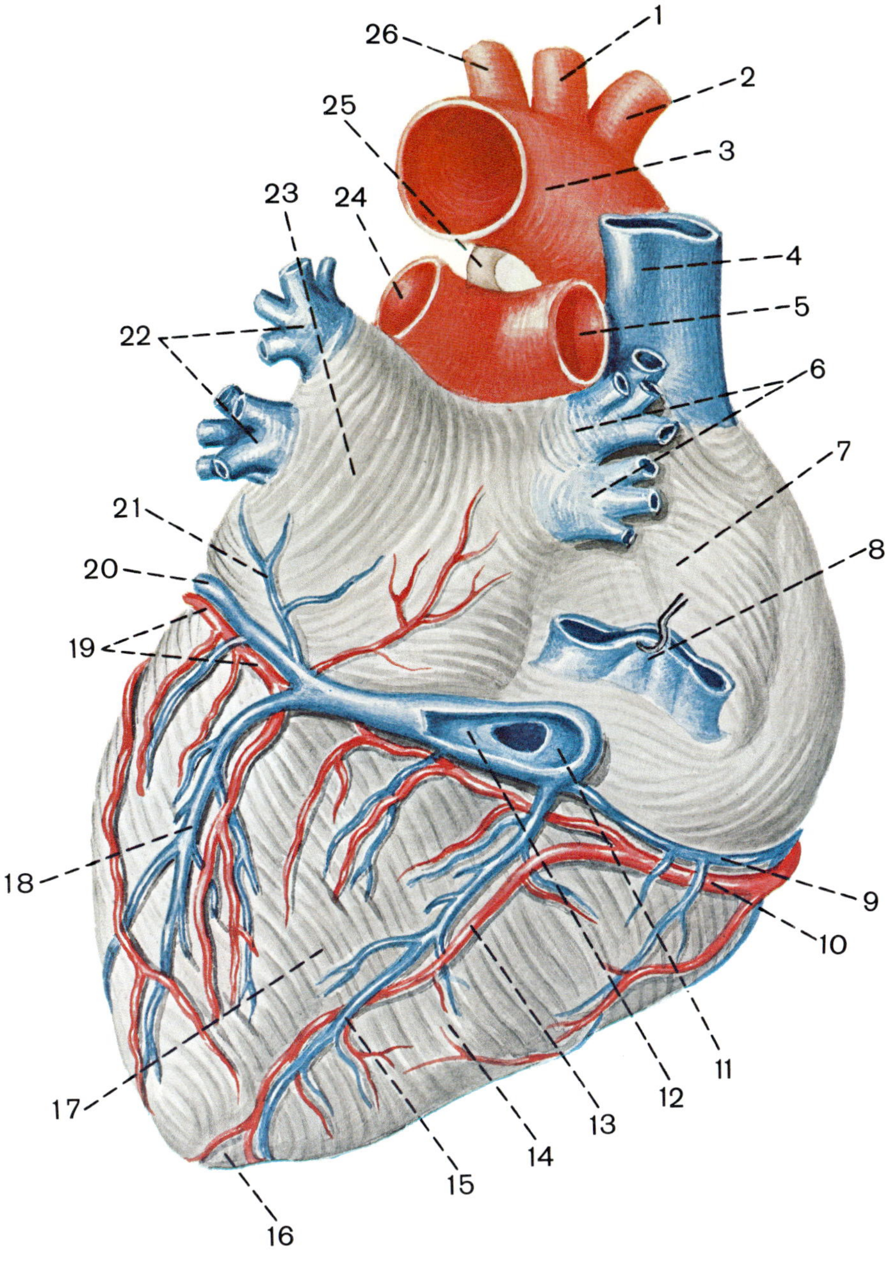

Fig. 43. Arteries and veins of heart, posterior aspect. (After R. Sinelnikov.)

1 Left common carotid artery (a. carotis communis sinistra)
2 Brachiocephalic trunk (truncus brachiocephalicus)
3 Arch or aorta (arcus aortae)
4 Superior vena cava (v. cava superior)
5 Right pulmonary artery (a. pulmonalis dextra)
6 Right pulmonary veins (vv. pulmonales dextrae)
7 Right atrium (atrium dextrum)
8 Inferior vena cava (v. cava inferior)
9 Small cardiac vein (v. cordis parva)
10 Right coronary artery (a. coronaria dextra)
11 Valve of coronary sinus (valvula sinus coronarii)
12 Coronary sinus (sinus coronarius cordis)
13 Posterior interventricular branch of right coronary artery (r. interventricularis posterior arterial coronariae dextrae)
14 Right ventricle (ventriculus dexter)
15 Middle cardiac vein (v. cordis media)
16 Apex of heart (apex cordis)
17 Left ventricle (ventriculus sinister)
18 Posterior vein of left ventricle (v. posterior ventriculi sinistri)
19 Circumflex branch of left coronary artery (r. circumflexus arterial coronariae sinistrae)
20 Great cardiac vein (v. cordis magna)
21 Oblique vein of left atrium (v. obliqua atrii sinistri)
22 Left pulmonary veins (vv. pulmonales sinistrae)
23 Left atrium (atrium sinistrum)
24 Left pulmonary artery (a. pulmonalis sinistra)
25 Ligamentum arteriosum
26 Left subclavian artery (a. subclavia sinistra)

branch of the right coronary artery. The right coronary artery vascularizes the right atrium, part of the anterior and the entire posterior wall of the right ventricle, a small area of the posterior wall of the left ventricle, the interatrial and the posterior half of the interventricular septa, the papillary muscles of the right ventricle, and the posteromedial papillary muscles of the left ventricle. A branch of the left coronary artery supplies blood to the other parts of the heart, namely, the left atrium, the entire anterior and most of the posterior walls of the left ventricle, part of the anterior wall of the right ventricle, the anterior two thirds (or half) of the interventricular septum, and the anterolateral papillary muscle of the left ventricle.

The Thebesian-Vieussens vessels originate in the left atrium and left ventricle and terminate as short veins in the right atrium and ventricle.

In those places where the cardiac wall is immediately next to the mediastinal cellular tissue (posterior surface of the left atrium, where the pericardium is continuous with the epicardium) it may be approached by several branches of the bronchial arteries. Such accessory arteries have also been described in the region of ligamentum arteriosum.

The vessels of the heart communicate through well-developed anastomoses with one another and partly with the arteries of the mediastinum.

The coronary sinus of the heart is situated on the posterior surface of the heart in the left coronary sulcus and drains into the right atrium between the valve of the inferior vena cava and the interatrial septum. Almost its entire length the coronary sinus lies in the thickness of the cardiac wall. The sinus is 3.5 to 4.5 cm long and 6 to 7 mm wide.

The coronary sinus of the heart receives blood from the great cardiac vein, oblique vein of the left atrium, the posterior vein of the left ventricle, the middle and small cardiac veins, and several inconstant veins (peripheral, right and left, and posterior veins of the right ventricle, and the marginal vein of the right atrium).

The great cardiac vein forms from the veins of the anterior walls of the ventricles, the interventricular septum, and partly from the veins of the left atrium. Its trunk is situated in the anterior longitudinal sulcus, then stretches in the coronary sulcus passing under the left auricula to the posterior surface of the heart, where it is continuous with the venous sinus of the heart. In some cases there is a special valve at the site where the great cardiac vein drains into the coronary sinus.

The oblique vein of the left atrium originates on the posterior surface of the left atrium and drains into the distal part of the coronary sinus and the great cardiac vein.

The middle cardiac vein forms at the apex, collecting blood from the anterior walls of both ventricles and from the interventricular septum. Its thick trunk, 4 to 7 mm in diameter, lies in the posterior longitudinal sulcus. In most cases it drains into the coronary sinus.

The small cardiac vein forms from the veins of the anterior and partly from those of the posterior surfaces of the right ventricle and the right atrium. It is situated in the right part of the coronary sulcus and passes in the sulcus to the posterior surface of the heart where it drains into the coronary sinus or into the middle cardiac vein.

The anterior cardiac veins, one to three in number, form from the veins of the anterior wall of the right ventricle and the region of the right conus arteriosus. In 20% of cases they drain by means of a common trunk directly into the right atrium, or less frequently (in 10%) into the right auricle or (in 1% to 2%) into the superior vena cava.

The small Thebesian-Vieussens veins, numbering 20 to 30, drain directly into the right atrium and ventricle without emerging to the outer surface of the heart.

The external structure of the cardiac veins is marked by considerable individual differences.

Lymphatic vessels of the heart. Four networks of lymphatic vessels are distinguished in the heart: subendocardial, intramuscular, intraepicardial, and, the most powerful, subepicardial network from which two principal collectors are eventually formed (the right and the left, extending along the length of the coronary vessels of the heart).

The left lymph collector forms from the draining ducts of the left half of the heart (from the anterior and posterior surfaces of the left ventricle and atrium). It empties into one of the paratracheal lymph nodes. The right lymph collector forms in the right part of the coronary sulcus from the draining vessels of the anterior and posterior surfaces of the right ventricle and atrium and drains into one of the left superior nodes of the anterior mediastinum.

Innervation of the heart. The nerve apparatus (Fig. 44) consists of two parts, extracardiac and intracardiac. The extracardiac part comprises nerve conductors connecting the heart with the central nervous system as well as with the nerve structures of other organs.

The components of the intracardiac part are the nerve plexuses and endings and also accumulations of glial masses localized in the heart itself.

The sources of cardiac innervation are the branch of the sympathetic trunk and the branches of the cervical and thoracic parts of the vagus nerve. Three cardiac nerves, superior, middle, and inferior, arise on each side from the ganglia and interganglionic connections of the sympathetic trunk.

The superior cervical cardiac nerve originates from

Fig. 44. Nerves of heart (After V. Vorobiev.)

1 Left superior cervical cardiac nerve (n. cardiacus cervicalis superior)
2 Left cervical plexus (plexus cervicalis sinister)
3 Left sympathetic trunk (truncus sympathicus sinister)
4 Left vagus nerve (n. vagus sinister)
5 Left phrenic nerve (n. phrenicus sinister)
6 Anterior scalene muscle (m. scalenus anterior)
7 Trachea
8 Left brachial plexus (plexus brachialis sinister)
9 Left subclavian artery (a. subclavia sinistri)
10 Left inferior cervical cardiac nerve (n. cardiacus cervicalis inferior sinister)
11 Brachiocephalic trunk (truncus brachiocephalicus)
12 Left common carotid artery (a. carotis communis sinistra)
13 Arch of aorta (arcus aortae)
14 Left recurrent laryngeal nerve (n. laryngeus recurrens sinister)
15 Anterior atrial plexus (plexus atriorum anterior)
16 Left pulmonary artery (a. pulmonalis sinistra)
17 Pulmonary veins (vv. pulmonales sinistra)
18 Left atrial auricle (auricula sinistra)
19 Pulmonary trunk (truncus pulmonalis)
20 Left coronary artery (a. coronaria cordis sinistra)
21 Left anterior plexus (plexus anterior sinistri)
22 Left ventricle (ventriculus sinister)
23 Right ventricle (ventriculus dexter)
24 Right anterior plexus (plexus anterior dexter)
25 Ganglion field in the region of conus arteriosus
27 Right coronary artery (a. coronaria cordis dextra)
27 Right atrial auricle (auricula dextra)
28 Aorta
29 Superior vena cava (v. cava superior)
30 Right pulmonary artery (a. pulmonalis dextra)
31 Lymph node
32 Azygos vein (v. azygos)
33 Right inferior cervical cardiac nerve (n. cardiacus cervicalis inferior dexter)
34 Right recurrent laryngeal nerve (n. laryngeus recurrens dexter)
35 Right inferior cardiac branch (r. cardiacus inferior dextra)
36 First thoracic ganglion (ganglion thoracicum I dextrum)
37 Inferior cervical ganglion of right sympathetic trunk (ganglion cervicale inferius dextrum trunci sympathici)
38 Right superior cardiac branch (r. cardiacus superior dexter)
39 Right phrenic nerve (n. phrenicus dexter)
40 Right vagus nerve (n. vagus dexter)
41 Right sympathetic trunk (truncus sympathicus dexter)
42 Superior cervical cardiac nerve (n. cardiacus cervicalis superior dexter)
43 Superior laryngeal nerve (n. laryngeus superior)

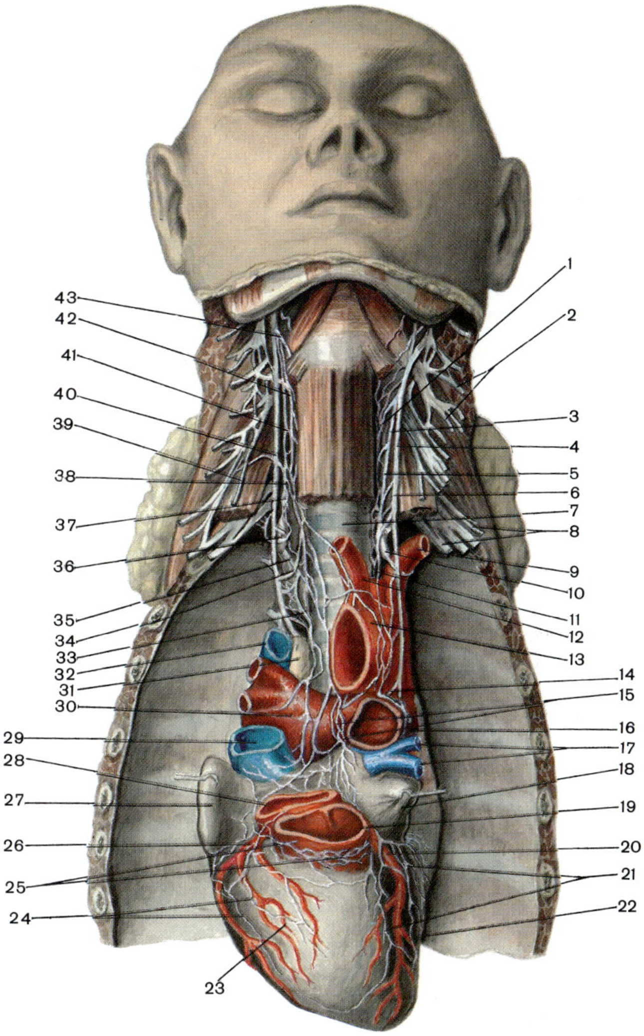

the superior cervical plexus. It always occurs as a small isolated trunk and is composed of several branches joined into a single nerve in the lower parts of the neck, or in the thoracic cavity.

The middle cervical cardiac nerve arises from the middle cervical ganglion or from the interganglion communications. It occurs in two thirds or four fifths of cases.

The inferior cervical cardiac nerve arises from the inferior cervical or stellate ganglion. It is represented by one or several trunks (up to four). Quite frequently it communicates with the branches of the vagus nerve.

Besides these, an innominate cardiac nerve is described (in 15.3% of cases, according to B. Erez), the right root of which originates from the superior cervical ganglion and the left from the left vagus nerve. The total number of cardiac nerves arising from the sympathetic trunk varies from three to fifteen.

The vagus nerves and their branches (the superior laryngeal and the recurrent laryngeal nerves) give rise to the superior and inferior cardiac branches.

The superior cardiac branches (one to three) originate from the trunk of the vagus nerve immediately below the ganglion nodosum and from the superior laryngeal nerve. The highest branch is called the depressor nerve (Zion's nerve).

The inferior cardiac branches (four to ten) form from the trunk of the vagus nerve and from the recurrent laryngeal nerve in the lower part of the neck and in the mediastinum. On the left the inferior cardiac branches arise from the recurrent laryngeal nerve on the level of the inferior margin of the aortic arch, on the right on the level of the subclavian artery (V. Vorobyev).

The above listed cardiac nerves and branches arising from the sympathetic and vagus nerves, repeatedly intertwining, form nerve plexuses along the length of the large vessels. There are two extracardiac plexuses:

a superficial plexus situated in front of the aortic arch and its branches, and a deep plexus located on the anterior surface of the lower part of the trachea. The plexuses communicate closely with one another and form a single anatomic structure on the grounds of which some authors consider them as a single cardiopulmonary (T. Lavrova) or pleurocardiopulmonary plexus (P. Petrov).

THE PERICARDIUM

The pericardium is a fibrous sac containing the serous cavity holding the heart, the initial parts of the aorta, the pulmonary trunk, and the orifices of the pulmonary veins and venae cavae. The pericardium has two layers, a parietal layer, or the pericardium proper, and the visceral, or the epicardium. These two layers are continuous on the large vessels of the heart.

The shape, position, and size of the pericardium are closely dependent on the individual, his age, and the constitutional features of the heart. The pericardium varies considerably in size. The normal height, the distance from the reflection on the aorta to the base, is 11.5 to 16.7 cm in adults; the greatest width 8.1 to 14.3 cm, and the anteroposterior measurement (at the base) 6 to 10 cm.

Three parts (or walls) are distinguished in the pericardium: anterior, inferior, or diaphragmatic, and posterior, or mediastinal. Some authors also distinguish two lateral parts. An area uncovered by the pleura and an inferior area directly next to the sternum and ribs are distinguished in the anterior part of the pericardium.

The dimensions of the extrapleural pericardium vary widely depending on the position of the anterior pleural reflections: the height from 10 to 15 cm, the width at the level of the pericardial base from 7 to 13 cm, and the area from 10 to 30 cm^2.

The sternocostal part of the pericardium is triangular in shape and bounded on the right and left by the pleural reflections almost converging at the level of the second and third ribs and on the bottom by the inferior margin of the pericardium. Part of this surface adjoining the left costal cartilages is called (according to A. Voinits-Syanozhentskii) the "safety" triangle. Irrespective of the variants in the shape of the sternocostal part of the pericardium and the position of the pleura in relation to the last (seventh or eighth) costal cartilage, it has an area free of pleura on the inner surface at the site where the costal cartilage is attached to the sternum.

The anterior surface of the pericardium is attached to the sternum by means of two ligaments: a superior ligament stretching from the manubrium of the sternum downward, and an inferior ligament passing from the inferior surface of the sternum upward.

The parts of the anterior surface of the pericardium covered with the edges of the lung and pleura are called partes pleuropulmonales, or lateral parts. The lower part of the pericardium fused with the central tendon of the diaphragm is either oval (55%), or round (18%), or shaped like an irregular triangle (27%).

The posterior wall of the pericardium (Fig. 45) adjoining the organs of the posterior mediastinum is divided into two parts: an upper part located above the transverse pericardial reflection, and a lower part, which is below this reflection.

The upper part is a small area of the pericardium behind the ascending aorta and pulmonary artery; a portion of it forms the posterior surface of the transverse sinus. The line along which the pericardium is continuous with the epicardium passes from the inferior vena cava upward, embraces both right pulmonary veins and the orifice of the superior vena cava, then crosses the posterior wall of the left atrium and embraces the orifices of both left pulmonary veins. Thus, two vertical (longer on the right side) and one transverse (horizontal, or connecting) reflection may be distinguished. The reflections are separated to a different degree on the posterior pericardial wall. There are sinuses in the pericardium, i.e., spaces between the pericardium and the wall of the heart or between different parts of the pericardium, and recesses or pouches, which are small slitlike spaces formed where the pericardium is continuous with the epicardium on the large vessels. Anteroinferior, transverse, and oblique sinuses are distinguished.

The anteroinferior sinus is an arched narrow space formed where the sternocostal part of the pericardium is continuous with the diaphragmatic. Its height (the distance between the inferior border of the heart and the inferior margin of the sinus on the midline) is 1 to 2 cm. This sinus is the lowest part of the pericardial cavity and the site of transudate and exudate accumulation.

The transverse sinus of the pericardium is a passage convex to the front situated behind the pulmonary trunk and ascending aorta. On the right the entrance to the sinus is located between the right auricula, the aorta, and the intrapericardial portion of the superior vena cava; on the left it is between the left cardiac auricula and the pulmonary trunk. Whenever necessary, fingers may be inserted into the transverse sinus for grasping and compressing the aorta and the pulmonary trunk.

Haller's oblique sinus (see Fig. 34) is situated behind the heart and bounded on the sides by the right and left,

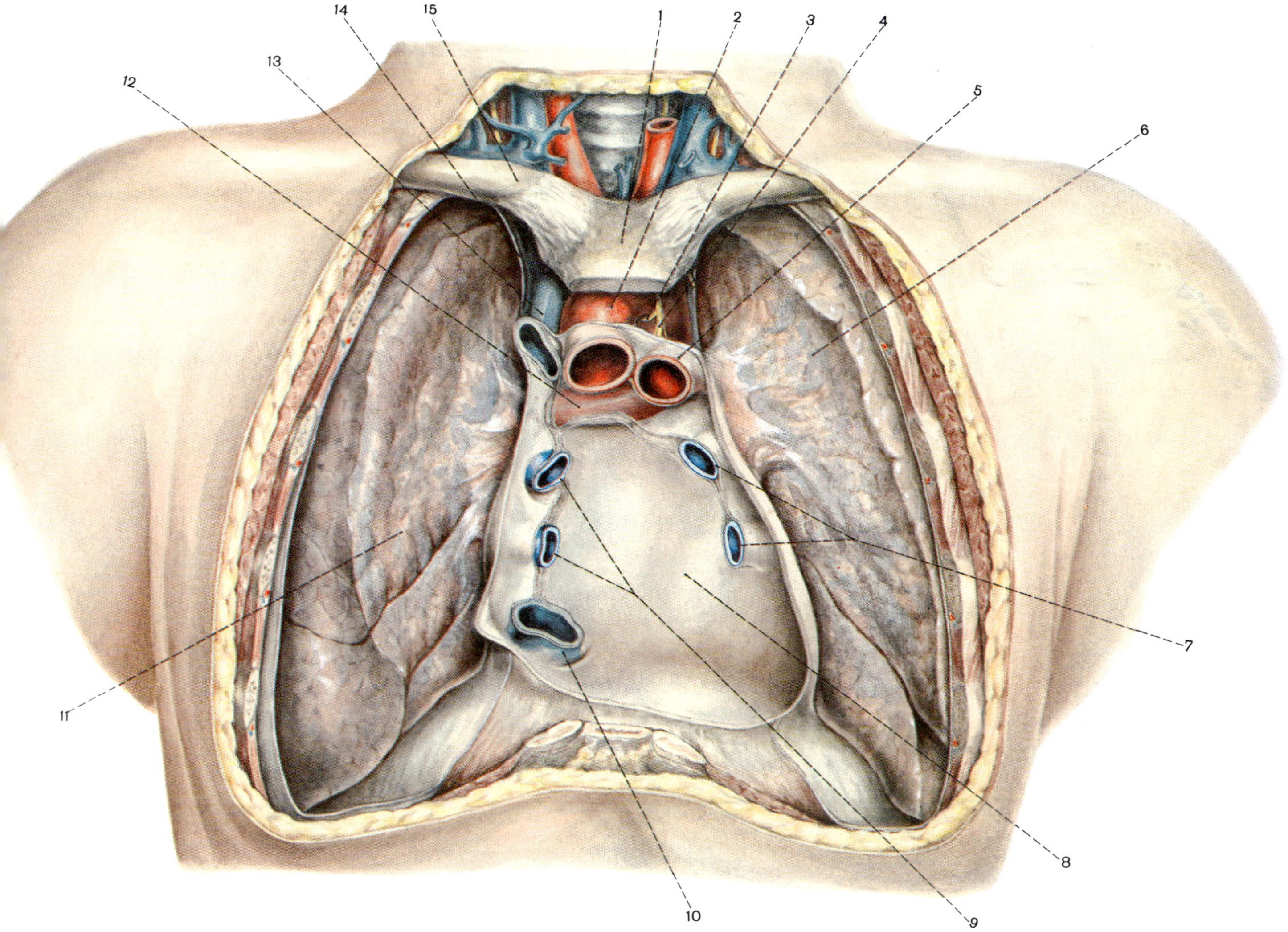

Fig. 45. Posterior wall of pericardium exposed after removal of heart.

1 Sternum
2 Ascending aorta (aorta ascendens)
3 Left recurrent laryngeal nerve (n. laryngeus recurrens sinister)
4 Left vagus nerve (n. vagus sinister)
5 Pulmonary trunk (truncus pulmonalis)
6 Left lung (pulmo sinister)
7, 9 Pulmonary veins (vv. pulmonales)
8 Posterior wall of pericardium
10 Inferior vena cava (v. cava inferior)
11 Right lung (pulmo dexter)
12 Right pulmonary artery (a. pulmonalis dextra)
13 Superior vena cava (v. cava superior)
14 Mediastinal pleura (pleura mediastinalis)
15 Right clavicle (clavicula dextra)

and on top by the transverse pericardial reflections. It is 6 to 8 cm high. The upper pole of the sinus is behind the posterior wall of the left atrium and often reaches the right branch of the pulmonary trunk.

Of the pericardial recesses, note should be made of the constantly encountered anterior aortic (anterosuperior) recess formed where the pericardium is continuous with the epicardium on the anterior surfaces of the aortic arch and the pulmonary trunk, a recess around the superior vena cava, and the retroaortic (posterosuperior) recess. The sources of blood supply for the pericardium are the branches of the internal thoracic artery and the branches of the thoracic aorta. Other contributing vessels are the branches of the arteries of the thymus (supplying blood to the upper portion of the anterior wall), branches of the intercostal arteries (to the lower part of the anterior wall), the pericardiacophrenic arteries (to the anterior and lateral walls), and branches of the superior phrenic arteries (to the inferior wall). Branches from the bronchial, mediastinal, and esophageal arteries pass to the posterior wall. Venous blood is drained along veins attendant to the arterial vessels. The pericardial wall contains a well-developed network of lymphatic vessels. The lymph drains into various groups of mediastinal lymph nodes (nodes of the roots of the lung, the superior and inferior nodes of the anterior mediastinum). Part of the lymphatic vessels of the lower wall of the pericardium descend through the diaphragm and drain into the nodes of the upper abdomen.

The pericardium is innervated by the vagus and sympathetic nerves, from the deep and superficial cardiac plexuses and from the anterior and posterior pulmonary, esophageal, aortic, and phrenic plexuses. It is also innervated by the phrenic, left recurrent laryngeal, and intercostal nerves.

THE MAJOR VESSELS

Intrapericardial parts. Three large vascular trunks are exposed when the pericardium is opened at the base of the heart: the superior vena cava on the right, the aorta in the middle, and the pulmonary trunk on the left.

The pulmonary trunk is covered with the epicardium for a distance of about 5 cm. It is at fist located to the left and to the front of the aorta. Then it deviates to the back and approaches the left lower surface of the beginning of the aortic arch, where it leaves the pericardium. The right pulmonary artery is continuous with the pulmonary trunk and passes behind and below the arch of the aorta, and in the region of the transverse sinus it is covered by the anterior surface of the epicardium. The left pulmonary artery is covered with the epicardium on a large area (0.5 to 1.0 cm) of the anterosuperior surface.

The ascending aorta (see Fig. 45) is covered with the epicardium on the right surface for a distance of 8 to 10 cm and on the left surface for a distance of 2.5 to 4 cm. The initial portion of the aorta (the bulb) is covered on the right and in front with the right auricula and in front and on the left by the pulmonary trunk. The ascending aorta forms an arch slightly curved to the right, touching the superior vena cava with its convex surface. The superior vena cava has a small intrapericardial surface (about 3 cm). In front and medially it is a little higher than in the back and laterally. Its posterior surface is not covered with the epicardium.

The inferior vena cava is covered with the epicardium for a distance not over 1 cm. In most cases the pulmonary veins are partly covered with the epicardium on the anterior surface. Often, particularly on the right, they are situated extrapericardially.

Extrapericardial parts. *The superior vena cava* is formed in the anterior mediastinum behind the right margin of the sternum where the first rib is joined to the sternal manubrium, by the union of the right and left brachiocephalic veins. The trunk of the superior vena cava, 4.0 to 6.5 cm long, enters the pericardial cavity, where its short intrapericardial part (described above) is located. In front of the superior vena cava are the thymus and the border of the right lung.

The right surface of the vein adjoins the mediastinal pleura and the right phrenic nerve passing here. On the left the vein adjoins the ascending aorta. The posterior surface of the vein is in contact with the lymph nodes and the root of the right lung. Dorsally, at the level of the upper border of the right bronchus, immediately before entering the pericardium, it receives the large azygos vein.

The brachiocephalic vein originates from the union of the internal jugular and subclavian veins. Each brachiocephalic vein forms at the level of the sternoclavicular articulation of the corresponding side. The right brachiocephalic vein is a short trunk directed downward nearly vertically. It is projected along the right border of the sternal manubrium. Its right surface adjoins the cervical pleura. The posterior is adjacent to the site where the brachiocephalic trunk divides and to the right vagus nerve.

The left brachiocephalic vein is twice as long as the

right and stretches horizontally or obliquely. In front it is covered by the thymus or its remnants (in adults). The posterior surface of the vein adjoins the arch of the aorta and its branches.

A double superior vena cava (right and left) is a congenital developmental variant of the venous system. It is encountered in approximately 1% of cases. The left superior vena cava is a nonobliterated embryonal Cuvier duct. It passes in the coronary sulcus behind the left atrium and, uniting with the venous sinus, drains into the right atrium.

The aorta. Three parts are distinguished in the thoracic portion of the aorta (Fig. 46): the ascending aorta, the arch, and the descending aorta. The ascending aorta stretches from the site where the aorta emerges from the left ventricle to the origin of the brachiocephalic trunk and corresponds to the intrapericardial portion of the vessel (described above). The arch of the aorta corresponds to the portion measuring from the origin of the brachiocephalic trunk to that of the left subclavian artery. Further, it is continuous with the descending aorta, which stretches caudally to the aortic opening of the diaphragm.

According to embryogenesis, the aortic arch is an independent portion (the fourth pair of the arterial branchial arches), although in appearance it does not differ from the ascending aorta, except for its shape. The lumen of the arch is almost the same along its entire length (21 to 22 mm). It is slightly narrower at the place where the arch of the aorta is continuous with the descending portion; this part is called the isthmus of the aorta. In developmental defects the lumen of the aorta at this site may be as small as 2 to 3 mm or totally obliterated.

The brachiocephalic trunk arises from the convex part of the aortic arch on the right; the left common carotid artery arises to the left and to the back of it; while the left subclavian artery originates even more to the left. The initial portion of the aortic arch is situated in the superior part of the anterior mediastinum, while its caudal part is in the posterior mediastinum.

Thus, the general direction of the arch is from right to left and from front to back. The initial portion of the arch of the aorta is projected on the thoracic wall at the right sternal border, at the level of the second sternocostal articulation. The junction of the arch with the descending portion is on the level with the body of the fourth thoracic vertebra, while the uppermost point of the convexity is at the level of the middle of the sternal manubrium.

The left phrenic nerve with the pericardiacophrenic vessels lies adjacent to the left anterior surface of the aortic arch, while the vagus nerve is somewhat to the back. The superior vena cava adjoins the right surface of the aortic arch partially; the trachea, esophagus, and thoracic duct are to the back; the concave inferior surface of the aortic arch is next to the bifurcation of the pulmonary trunk and to the left bronchus. The ligamentum arteriosum (or Botallo's duct) stretches between the arch of the aorta and the pulmonary trunk at the level of the origin of the left subclavian artery. The innominate (brachiocephalic) veins and the thymus are in front of the arch of the aorta and its branches.

The descending aorta extends from the level of the fourth to the level of the eleventh thoracic vertebrae and is situated in the posterior mediastinum. Its upper part is to the left of the vertebral column, while its lower part comes closer to the midline (between the seventh and eleventh vertebrae). In accordance with the shape of the posterior thoracic wall, it has frontal and sagittal curvatures. The diameter of the descending aorta is practically the same along its full length. The descending aorta gives off paired segmental intercostal arteries and a number of visceral (bronchial, esophageal, superior phrenic, mediastinal) arteries, which vary in number and topography.

The arch of the aorta is innervated by branches of the vagus nerve arising in the region of the neck, by branches of the cervical portion of the sympathetic trunk, and by branches of the spinal nerves (the anterior branches of the cervical plexus). The descending aorta is innervated segmentally by branches of the thoracic sympathetic trunk and branches of the intercostal nerve.

The superficial and deep cardiac nerve plexuses are situated in the region of the aortic arch with their branches as if embracing its circumference.

In the wall of the aorta there are nerve receptors (mechanoreceptors and chemoreceptors) differing in structure.

The greatest number of sensory nerve endings are found in the wall of the lower semicircumference of the aorta and also at the origin of the brachiocephalic trunk and common carotid and subclavian arteries (according to K. M. Bykov, the aortic reflexogenic zone). The ascending aorta and Botallo's duct contain a relatively small number of sensory nerve endings. Glomic structures (of the type of the carotid body) have also been described in the aortic wall. The supracardiac paraganglion (the supracardiac glomus aortica) is situated in the cellular tissue between the aorta and the bifurcation of the pulmonary trunk.

The Botallo duct. Normally, Botallo's duct connecting the pulmonary artery with the aorta, exists only in the uterine period. With the beginning of pulmonary respiration it is gradually obliterated and transformed into the ligamentum arteriosum. It usually closes completely by the sixth month of extrauterine life.

Botallo's duct is encountered in 0.2% to 0.7% of

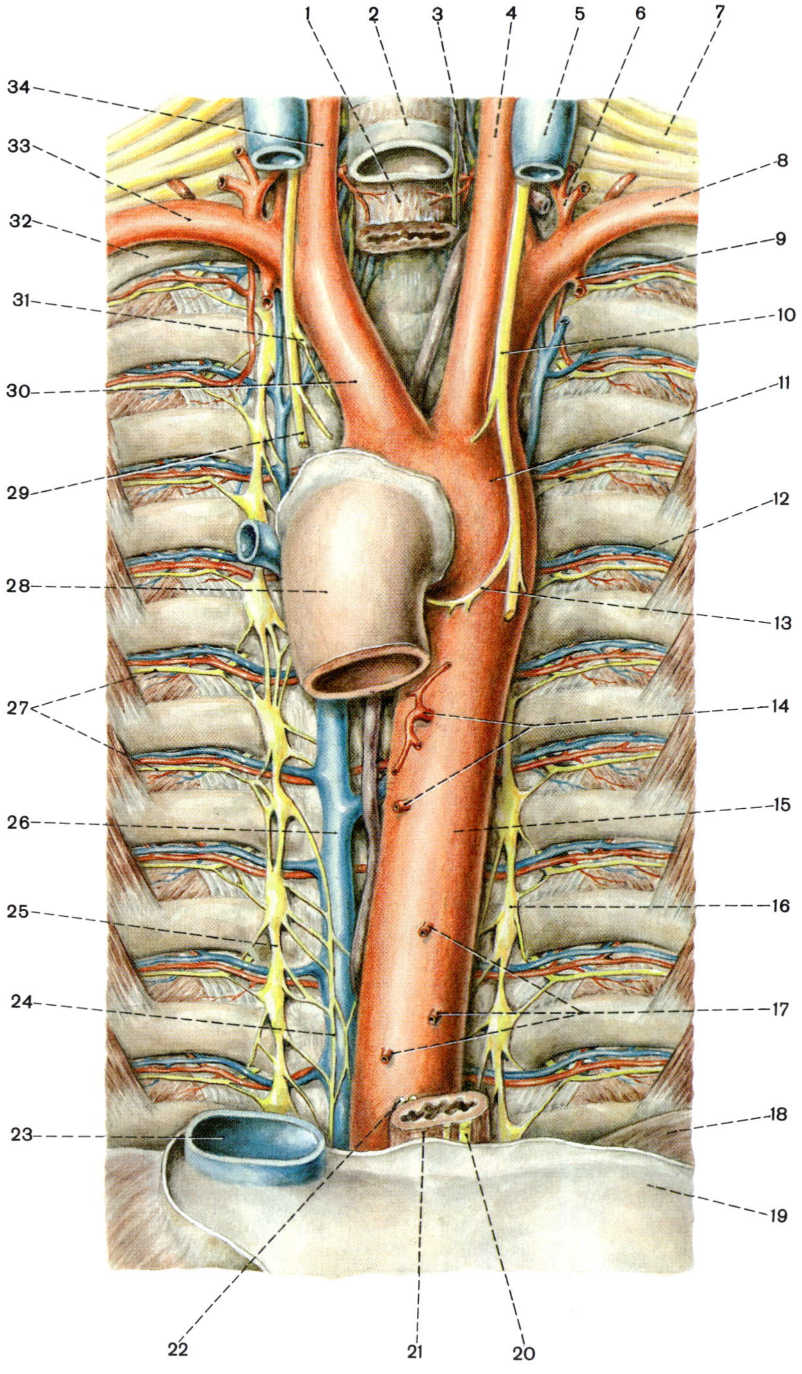

Fig. 46. Thoracic aorta.

1, 21 Esophagus
2 Trachea
3 Inferior thyroid artery (a. thyroidea inferior)
4 Left common carotid artery (a. carotis communis sinistra)
5 Left internal jugular vein (v. jugularis interna sinistra)
6 Thyrocervical trunk (truncus thyreocervicalis)
7 Brachial plexus (plexus brachialis)
8 Left subclavian artery (a. subclavia sinistra)
9 Internal thoracic artery (a. thoracica interna)
10 Left vagus nerve (n. vagus sinister)
11 Arch of aorta (arcus aortae)
12 Intercostal arteries and veins (aa. et vv. intercostales)
13 Left recurrent laryngeal nerve (n. laryngeus recurrens sinister)
14 Superior esophageal branches of thoracic aorta (rr. esophagei superiores aortae thoracicae)
15 Thoracic aorta (aorta thoracica)
16 Left sympathetic trunk (truncus sympathicus sinister)
17 Inferior esophageal branches of thoracic aorta (rr. esophagei inferiores aortae thoracicae)
18 Diaphragm (diaphragma)
19 Pericardium
20 Left vagus nerve (n. vagus sinister)
22, 29 Right vagus nerve (n. vagus dexter)
23 Inferior vena cava (v. cava inferior)
24 Greater splanchnic nerve (n. splanchnicus major)
25 Right sympathetic trunk (truncus sympathicus dexter)
26 Azygos vein (v. azygos)
27 Intercostal nerve (n. intercostalis)
28 Ascending aorta (aorta ascendens)
30 Brachiocephalic trunk (truncus brachiocephalicus)
31 Right recurrent laryngeal nerve (n. laryngeus recurrens dexter)
32 First rib (costa I)
33 Right subclavian artery (a. subclavia dextra)
34 Right common carotid artery (a. carotis communis dextra)

adults. It is a thin-walled vessel, 2 to 17 mm (usually 6 to 10 mm) long and 1.9 to 7 mm (in most cases 3 to 6 mm) wide. The duct is conical or cylindrical with the wider base (lumen) at the pulmonary artery. The wall of the duct is usually composed of two elastic membranes (external and internal).

The duct arises from the anterolateral surface of the pulmonary trunk at the place where the trunk branches out, and joins the aortic arch on its lower surface at the level of the origin of the left subclavian artery. In children it is projected on the thoracic wall on the left sternal margin at the level of the second rib, second intercostal space, or at the left surface of the third thoracic vertebra. The Botallo duct (ligamentum arteriosum) is usually located extrapericardially; about 0.5 cm away from and around it there is a small pericardial reflection.

Three nerves, the left phrenic, the left vagus, and the left recurrent laryngeal nerves, are located in the immediate vicinity of the duct under the left mediastinal pleura. The phrenic nerve usually passes 1 to 2 mm in front of the duct. The recurrent laryngeal nerve, which curves around the aortic arch below, is directly adjacent to the duct at the back. The vagus nerve crosses the aortic part of Botallo's duct. The posterior surface of the duct is adjacent to the anterosuperior surface of the left main bronchus.

The ligamentum arteriosum is a connective tissue structure 0.3 to 2.5 cm long and 0.3 to 0.6 cm wide. There is a small depression on the inner membrane of the aortic wall at the site where the ligamentum arteriosum is attached to it. On top, the ligamentum is covered with bundles of elastic fibers comprising the aortico-pericardial ligament.

THE PHRENIC NERVES

The phrenic nerves (see Figs. 29 and 30) are formed on the neck from the bundles of the fourth, and also, less frequently, from the bundles of the third and fifth cervical nerves. They enter the anterior mediastinum, passing both on the right and on the left between the subclavian artery and vein.

In the thoracic cavity the phrenic nerves are accompanied by the pericardiacophrenic blood vessels belonging to the system of intrathoracic vessels. Descending, the right phrenic nerve is first located between the lateral wall of the superior vena cava and mediastinal pleura, and then, caudally, between the pericardium and the mediastinal pleura, and in the inferior part of the mediastinum it runs between the inferior vena cava and the pleura.

The left phrenic nerve is located at the top between the lateral surface of the aortic arch and the mediastinal pleura in front of the vagus nerve; its lower portion runs between the pericardium and the mediastinal pleura somewhat to the back of the heart apex.

The right phrenic nerve enters the diaphragm a little nearer to the vertebral column than the left nerve. The left phrenic nerve enters the diaphragm more ventrally at the junction of the central tendon and the costal part of the diaphragm.

The phrenic nerves are motor and respiratory nerves; they innervate the musculature of the diaphragm. They also contain sensory and sympathetic fibers. The sensory fibers pass to the pleura, pericardium, and peritoneum.

THE ESOPHAGUS

The esophagus (Fig. 47) is a hollow muscular tube connecting the pharynx with the stomach. According to the topographic features, three parts of the esophagus are distinguished: the cervical, thoracic, and abdominal.

In males the esophagus is 24.5 to 25.5 cm and in females 23.5 to 24.0 cm long. The cervical part accounts for 5 to 8 cm of the total length, the thoracic for 15 to 18 cm, and the abdominal for 1 to 3 cm.

The cervical part of the esophagus begins at the level of the sixth cervical vertebra (in line with the cricoid cartilage) and stretches down to the level of the second thoracic vertebra.

In the thoracic part, terminating at the diaphragm, are an upper third (to the superior margin of the aortic arch), the middle third corresponding to the aortic arch and the bifurcation of the trachea (to the inferior margin of the root of the left lung, according to B. V. Petrovsky), and the lower third (from the bifurcation of the trachea to the level of the eleventh thoracic vertebra).

The abdominal part of the esophagus is situated in the esophageal opening of the diaphragm and below it and is marked by the greatest variability both in length and in topography.

In shape the esophagus is a tube flattened in the anteroposterior direction, more in the upper thoracic part. The shape of the esophagus is characterized by constrictions and dilatations, a spiral course in respect to the aorta, and by frontal and sagittal curvatures. The sagittal curvatures correspond to the curvatures of the vertebral column, while the frontal curvatures depend on the peculiarities of the syntopy of the esophagus with the organs of the neck and thorax and possess certain practical significance. In the initial part the esophagus is situated strictly along the midline, but it soon deviates to the left, and at the level of the third to fourth vertebrae, most of it is to the left of the trachea. In the middle part of the thoracic portion (fifth vertebra) the esophagus is again on the midline, being displaced slightly to the right of it by the closely adjacent aorta.

Lower, from the level of the eighth vertebra, the esophagus again passes 2 to 3 cm to the left of the midline. The esophagus has three constrictions with two dilatations between them.

The upper constriction is at the junction between the pharynx and the esophagus at a distance of 15 to 16 cm from the incisor teeth in males and 12 to 15 cm in females. In adults the width of the esophageal lumen in the region of the constriction measures 2.1 cm in the transverse direction and 1.3 cm in the anteroposterior direction. The lumen here is slitlike in shape.

The middle constriction corresponds to the bifurcation of the trachea where the aorta adjoins the esophageal wall. The lumen in adults at this point measures 1.4 cm and is rounded; it has an inward depression corresponding to the position of the aorta and the left bronchus, which is clearly visible on esophagoscopy.

The lower constriction is in the esophageal segment enclosed in the thickness of the diaphragm. It is 37 to 45 cm from the upper middle incisors in males and 37 to 41 cm in females. In a normal state the lumen here is closed; it is stellate and 2.0 to 2.2 cm in diameter. The esophageal lumen between the constrictions is 2 to 3 cm on the average.

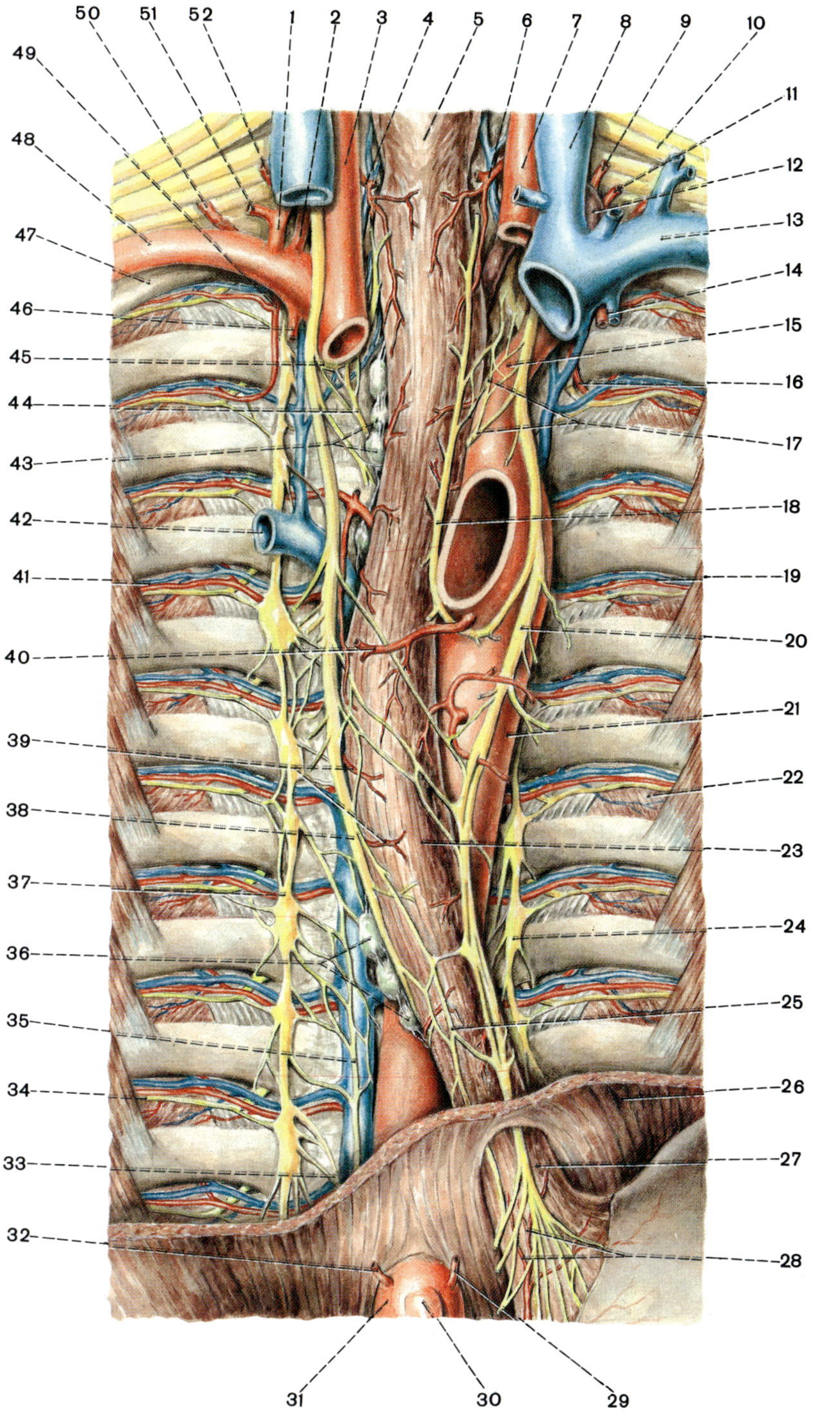

Fig. 47. Topography of esophagus. (After E. Pernkopf.)

1 Thyrocervical trunk (truncus thyreocervicalis)
2 Vertebral artery (a. vertebralis)
3 Right common carotid artery (a. carotis communis dextra)
4, 6 Inferior thyroid artery (a. thyroidea inferior)
5 Pharynx
7 Left common carotid artery (a carotis communis sinistra)
8 Left internal jugular vein (v. jugularis interna sinistra)
9 Ascending cervical artery (a. cervicalis ascendens)
10 Brachial plexus of the neck (plexus brachialis)
11, 51 Suprascapular artery (a. suprascapularis)
12 Thoracic duct, site of drainage (ductus thoracicus)
13 Subclavian vein (v. subclavia)
14 Internal thoracic artery and vein (a. et v. thoracicae internae)
15 Subclavian artery (a. subclavia)
16, 49 Highest intercostal artery (a. intercostalis suprema)
17 Inferior cardiac branches (rr. cardiaci inferiores)
18 Left recurrent laryngeal nerve (n. laryngeus recurrens sinister)
19, 41 Intercostal artery and vein (a. et v. intercostales)
20 Left vagus nerve (n. vagus sinister)
21 Thoracic aorta (aorta thoracica)
22 External intercostal muscle (m. intercostalis externus)
23 Esophagus
24, 37 Sympathetic trunk (truncus sympathicus)
25 Esophageal plexus of the vagus nerves (plexus esophagus nn. vagorum)
26 Diaphragm (diaphragma)
27 Abdominal part of the esophagus (pars abdominalis esophagi)
28 Esophageal branches of the gastric artery (rr. esophagei arterial gastricae sinistrae)
29, 32 Left inferior phrenic artery (a. phrenica inferior sinistra)
30 Celiac trunk (truncus celiacus)
31 Abdominal aorta (aorta abdominalis)
33 Lesser splanchnic nerve (n. splanchnicus minor)
34 Intercostal nerve (n. intercostalis)
35 Greater splanchnic nerve (n. splanchnicus major)
36, 43 Posterior mediastinal lymph nodes (nodi lymphatici mediastinales posteriores)
38 Right vagus nerve (n. vagus dexter)
39 Esophageal branches of the thoracic aorta (rr.esophagei aortae thoracicae)
40 Bronchial arteries of the thoracic aorta (a. bronchiales aortae thoracicae)
42 Azygos vein (v. azygos)
44 Inferior cardiac branch (r. cardiaci inferiores)
45 Right recurrent laryngeal nerve (n. laryngeus recurrens dexter)
46 Internal thoracic artery (a. thoracica interna)
47 First rib (costa I)
48 Right subclavian artery (a. subclavia dextra)
50 Deep cervical artery (a. cervicalis profunda)
52 Ascending cervical artery (a. cervicalis ascendens)

B. Petrovsky attaches particular importance to the two lower constrictions, since pathological processes (diverticuli, cicatricial stenosis, cancer, cardiospasm) are located there most frequently. The esophageal wall consists of three coats: connective tissue (outer), muscular (middle), and mucous coats. Neurovascular structures are found between the coats. The connective tissue coat is strongest in the lower portion of the thoracic part of the esophagus, in which the esophageal ligaments are situated. The mucous coat and the submucosa of the esophagus are the strongest from the mechanical standpoint.

The arterial circulation in the esophagus is segmental. The arteries of the cervical esophagus are branches of the inferior thyroid arteries descending from the neck and, less frequently, branches of the thryocervical trunk. The blood supply is not rich here.

In the middle third of the esophagus the arteries arise from the bronchial and also from the intercostal arteries. The esophageal branches of the bronchial arteries are located in the cellular tissue on both sides of the esophagus and penetrate its wall from the lateral and anterior surfaces.

The arteries of the lower third of the esophagus originate, as a rule, directly from the aorta at the level of the third to sixth right intercostal artery. The superior middle and inferior esophageal arteries arising from the aorta have quite a large diameter (the lower 0.8 to 1.2 mm) and are quite long (5 to 10 cm). Lying in the paraesophageal cellular tissue, they ender the esophageal wall from all sides and divide into ascending and descending branches.

The diaphragmaticoabdominal part of the esophagus receives blood from vessels that branch off from the left gastric and inferior phrenic arteries; some branches of the latter also contribute to the blood supply of the esophageal wall extending 1 to 2 cm above the diaphragm.

The esophageal wall contains a multilayer network of arterial vessels that is well developed along the entire length of the esophagus and located in the muscular and submucous coats and in the mucous membrane (B. Ognev). This network, situated within the organ, ensures the uniform distribution of arterial blood in the esophageal wall.

Four venous networks are distinguished in the esophageal wall. They are located subepithelially in the thickness of the mucous coat, in the submucous layer (the most developed), and in the connective tissue.

The submucous layer contains two venous plexuses, one of which is located at the junction between the pharynx and esophagus, and the other at the level of the diaphragmatic opening at the site of the lower esophageal constriction.

A. Maksimenkov believes that the venous plexuses play an important role in the physiology of the esophagus, particularly in the function of the "mouth of the esophagus" and the cardia. The venous plexuses, the lower ones especially, undergo varicosity. The character of these changes is similar to those observed in hemorrhoids of the rectum (esophageal "hemorrhoid," according to B. Ognev).

Blood is drained from the esophagus through the external venous (periesophageal) network along trunks stretching next to the arteries into the system of the azygos and hemiazygos veins. Besides, blood drains off through anastomoses with veins of the diaphragm into the inferior vena cava and by way of anastomoses with veins of the stomach into the system of the portal vein.

Blood from the upper parts drains into the system of the superior vena cava (internal jugular and superior thryoid veins, venous plexuses of the thyroid gland).

The intramural *lymphatic structures* of the esophagus are a network of plexuses situated between the layers of its tissues.

The draining lymphatic vessels pass through the regional lymph nodes. Some of them empty directly into the thoracic duct, by-passing the nodes (D. Zhdanov).

The regional lymph nodes in the cervical part are the paratracheal and partly the deep nodes situated behind the internal jugular vein.

Lymph from the upper third of the thoracic esophagus usually drains into the bifurcation nodes and into the tracheobronchial nodes.

From the lower third of the thoraric esophagus the lymph drains mainly in the direction of the stomach as well as into the mediastinal lymph nodes.

The regional lymph nodes for the lower third of the esophagus are the anterior and posterior nodes located around the cardia of the stomach (where the esophagus is continuous with the stomach; F. Stefanis, D. Zhdanov) and the left gastric nodes (on the lesser curvature of the stomach along the left venous artery and the gastropancreatic ligament; F. Stefanis).

The vessels that carry lymph to the mediastinum usually empty into the parapericardial node and, less frequently, directly into the thoracic duct.

The described pecularities in the circulation of lymph in the esophagus are conducive to the metastatic spread of cancer from this organ, both into the lymph nodes of the mediastinum and abdominal cavity (in the region of the stomach) and by way of the thoracic duct, receiving lymph directly from the esophagus, to more remote organs.

The sources of *innervation* of the esophagus are the vagus nerves and branches of the sympathetic trunk.

The cervical and upper third of the thoracic esophagus are innervated by branches of the recurrent laryngeal nerves and by branches originating directly from the trunk of the vagus nerve. The branches communi-

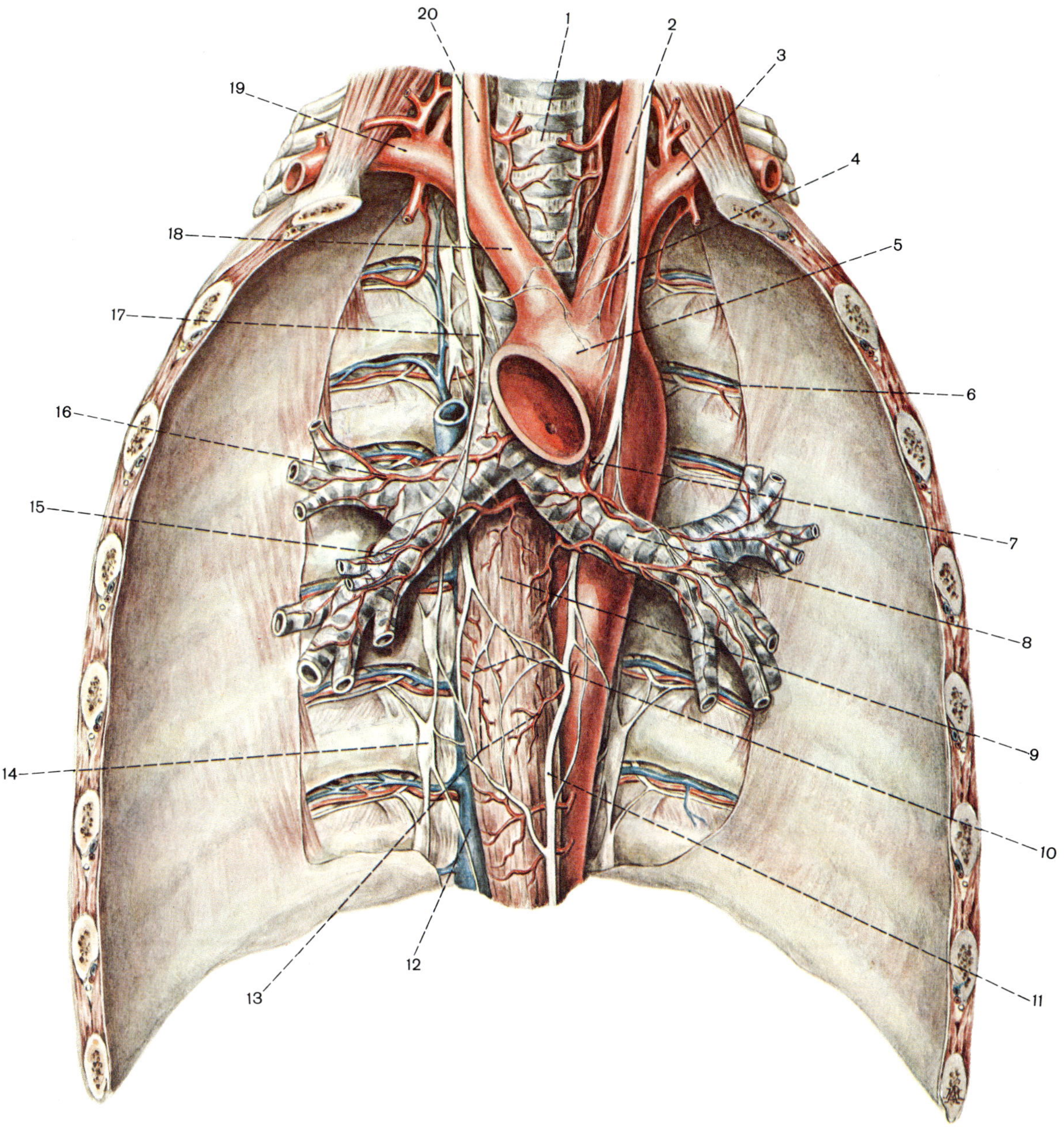

Fig. 48. Syntopy of thoracic part of esophagus. (After E. Pernkopf.)

1 Trachea
2 Left common carotid artery (a. carotis communis sinistra)
3 Left subclavian artery (a. subclavia sinistra)
4 Left vagus nerve (n. vagus sinister)
5 Arch of aorta (arcus aortae)
6 Intercostal artery and vein (a. et v. intercostales)
7 Left recurrent laryngeal nerve (n. laryngeus recurrens sinister)
8 Left primary bronchus (bronchus principalis sinister)
9 Esophagus
10 Esophageal branch of recurrent laryngeal nerve (r. esophagei n. laryngeus recurrentis)
11 Left vagus nerve (n. vagus sinister)
12 Azygos vein (v. azygos)
13 Mediastinal arteries (aa. mediastinales)
14 Sympathetic trunk (truncus sympathicus)
15 Right primary bronchus (bronchus principalis dexter)
16 Bronchial artery (a. bronchialis)
17 Right vagus nerve (n. vagus dexter)
18 Brachiocephalic trunk (truncus brachocephalicus)
19 Right subclavian artery (a. subclavia dextra)
20 Right common carotid artery (a. carotis communis dextra)

cate expansively with one another on the anterior and posterior surfaces of the esophagus. Nerves innervating the esophagus also give off branches here to the mediastinal organs (heart, trachea), forming interorgan nerve connections. The middle third of the esophagus receives branches from the vagus nerves; these branches form nerve plexuses on the posterior surface of the root of the lung (esophagopulmonary plexuses).

Numerous connections between the left and right vagus nerves form on the anterior and, to a lesser degree, on the posterior surfaces of the esophagus. Some authors define them as plexuses; they also contain sympathetic nerves originating from the thoracic portion of the sympathetic trunk.

Branches of the vagus nerves form plexuses on the anterior and posterior surfaces of the lower parts of the esophagus. In the lowest portions the plexuses again gather to form the trunks of the vagus nerves, which stretch on the left anterior (left trunk) and right posterior (right trunk) surfaces. Sometimes more than two trunks, forming the anterolateral and posterolateral plexuses of the esophagus, are found here.

In the supradiaphragmatic part the main trunks lie very closely to the esophagus; having penetrated the diaphragm they branch out, the left on the anterior and the right on the posterior surfaces of the stomach.

The syntopy of the esophagus is distinguished by considerable variability (Fig. 48).

The cervical esophagus is behind the trachea, with which it is joined by a number of connective tissue strands. The posterior surface of the esophagus adjoins the prevertebral fascia and the loose fatty tissue (retroorgan cellular space). The recurrent laryngeal nerves stretch on the right and left of the esophagus in the grooves between it and the trachea. Both common carotid arteries run along the sides of the esophagus, the left lying directly on it, while the right is separated from it by a layer of fatty cellular tissue. Over a short distance the left lobe of the thyroid gland comes in contact with the esophagus.

The upper third of the thoracic esophagus is to the back and somewhat to the left of the trachea and is separated from the vertebral column by loose cellular tissue. The left common carotid artery and the left recurrent laryngeal nerve are situated to the left and in front of the esophagus; the thoracic duct ascending obliquely from back to front and the left subclavian artery adjoin the esophagus on the lateral side. In some cases the right mediastinal pleura reaches the posterolateral surfaces of the esophagus along a short distance.

The esophagus lies close to the trachea, and there are many connective tissue strands between these organs, some of which acquire the nature of a muscle.

The topographo-anatomical relations of the midthird of the thoracic esophagus are most complex. The esophagus here is surrounded by large vessels. The arch of the aorta adjoins the esophagus in front and to the left of it at the level of the fourth thoracic vertebra; the bifurcation of the trachea and the left bronchus are slightly lower; the descending aorta is in back; the right vagus nerve is on the right, and the azygos vein is on the right and to the back. The mediastinal pleura in this part does not come into direct contact with the esophagus.

A number of connective tissue and muscular bundles are distinguished in the cellular tissue around this part of the esophagus; they serve as its ligaments. There are descriptions of ligaments stretching to the esophagus from the vertebral column, left bronchus, and pericardium, and also of muscular bundles joining the esophagus with the left bronchus and left mediastinal pleura, aorta, etc.

The lower third of the thoracic esophagus is in close contact with the aorta. There may be two extreme variants in the relationship of these organs. In the first the esophagus crosses the aorta in front, almost in the middle of its descending part, forming a clearly defined esophago-aortic intersection. In the second variant the esophagus and aorta run almost parallel to each other, and it is only in the lowest part that the esophagus makes a sharp turn to the left. Forward of the esophagus here are the pericardium and a small area of the posterior wall of the left atrium not covered by the pericardium, and at the back where the esophagus leaves the vertebral column is the thoracic aorta.

The lower third of the thoracic esophagus comes in contact with the right pleura over a considerable distance. In some cases the pleura covers its posterior surfaces here. The area of contact between the right pleura and the esophagus depends on the extent of the latter's displacement to the left.

The left pleura only comes in contact with the lowest part of the esophagus.

The lower part of the esophagus is attached to the opening in the diaphragm by means of the Morozov-Savvin connective tissue ligaments stretching to the front and to the back of the esophagus and encasing it. These ligaments are shaped like plates firmly secured to the posteroinferior corners of the pleural sacs on the sides and with the margins of the opening in the diaphragm at the bottom. When the Morozov-Savvin ligament is cut out on the right and to the back of the esophagus, a serous sac is revealed adhering to the esophageal wall in 25% of cases. If this sac is cut open during the operation, it may seem that the pleura had been accidentally injured.

The abdominal esophagus located in the opening in the diaphragm varies most in length. It is covered with the peritoneum in front and on the sides. The left lobe of the liver adjoins it on the right and in front and the upper pole of the spleen on the left.

THE VAGUS NERVES

The vagus nerves are partly situated in the anterior and mostly in the posterior mediastinum (see Figs. 47 and 48). In passing from the neck into the mediastinum the right vagus nerve lies between the subclavian artery and the right brachiocephalic vein. At the level of the interior margin of the subclavian artery it gives off the right recurrent laryngeal nerve, which curves around the inferior and posterior surfaces of the subclavian artery and runs upward. The trunk of the right vagus nerve stretches to the back and downward, at first back of the superior vena cava on the lateral wall of the trachea and then behind the right bronchus and root of the lung. On reaching the posterolateral wall of the esophagus, the right vagus nerve gives off numerous branches and, together with the esophagus, passes into the abdominal cavity.

The left vagus nerve enters the mediastinum from the neck in front of the left subclavian artery and behind the left brachiocephalic vein. Further down it is situated on the left anterior surface of the aortic arch. At the level of the lower border of the arch it gives off the left recurrent laryngeal nerve which curves around the inferior and posterior surfaces of the aortic arch and ascends on the anterior surface of the esophagus. The left recurrent laryngeal nerve closely adjoins the ligamentum arteriosum on the lateral surface or runs in close proximity and lateral to Botallo's duct, if there is one. The trunk of the left vagus nerve then descends between the aortic arch and the left pulmonary artery and extends back of the root of the left lung to the anterolateral surface of the esophagus.

The vagus nerves contribute to the innervation of the heart, lungs, esophagus, trachea, bronchi and thymus.

THE THORACIC DUCT

The thoracic part of the lymphatic duct is situated in the posterior mediastinum, emerging from the abdominal cavity through the arotic opening in the diaphragm (Fig. 49). Inferior and superior portions are distinguished. The inferior portion of the thoracic duct (pars interazygoaortalis) stretches along the midline of the vertebral column to the right of the aorta and to the left of the azygos vein. At the level of the third vertebra the duct deviates to the left and at first runs behind the arch of the aorta, and then above it. The upper part of the thoracic duct (pars supraaortalis) is behind the left common carotid artery and the left vagus nerve, in front of the long muscle of the neck, lateral of the esophagus and left recurrent laryngeal nerve and medial of the left subclavian artery and the mediastinal pleura. According to D. Zhdanov, in 60% of cases the thoracic duct is encountered as a single trunk; in 37% of cases there is, apart from the main trunk, an accessory one stretching to the left of the vertebral column; finally, in 3% of cases, along with the right main thoracic duct there are a few segments of the left trunk connected to it. No lymphatics drain directly into them from the abdominal cavity.

The thoracic part of the lymphatic duct is about 20 to 30 cm long, whereas the total length of the duct, including its abdominal and cervical portions, is 35 to 45 cm. The diameter of the thoracic duct within the mediastinum is 2 to 4 mm.

The relationship between the thoracic duct and the mediastinal pleura is of practical significance. In the lower part the thoracic duct is in direct contact with the right mediastinovertebral pleural pocket formed where the costal pleura is continuous with the mediastinal pleura behind the esophagus. In the upper supraaortic part the thoracic duct touches the left mediastinal pleura. This may explain the occurrence of right chylothorax in injury to the lower parts of the thoracic duct and the development of left chylothorax in injury to its upper parts.

There are valves in the thoracic duct, one above the diaphragm and one or two at the site where the lower portion is continuous with the upper.

Innervation of the duct is effected by branches from the aortic and paraesophageal plexuses and from the intercostal nerves and, in the lower part, by branches of the greater splanchnic nerve. Nerve plexuses and sensory and motor endings are found in the wall of the duct.

The thoracic duct is the principal lymphatic vessel through which up to three fourths of the entire amount of lymph in the body flows. It carries lymph draining from the lower extremities and the organs and walls of the abdominal and thoracic cavities: 1 to 2 ml per minute, or 1.5 to 2.0 liters per 24 hours. The lymph of the thoracic duct differs from that of the peripheral lymphatic vessels, mainly because it contains products of liver and intestinal metabolism (pH 9).

The bulk of lymphocytes entering the blood passes through the lymphatic duct. When the flow of lymph from the thoracic duct into the blood of experimental animals is fully arrested, lymphocytes and eosinophils almost completely disappear from the blood. The lymphocyte count in the lymph of the human thoracic duct ranges between 2,000 and 20,000 per 1 ml. A certain number of erythrocytes is always found in the lymph of the thoracic duct. Since well-developed collaterals, bypassing lymphatic vessels, are present in most cases, the thoracic duct may be ligated at any level within the mediastinum.

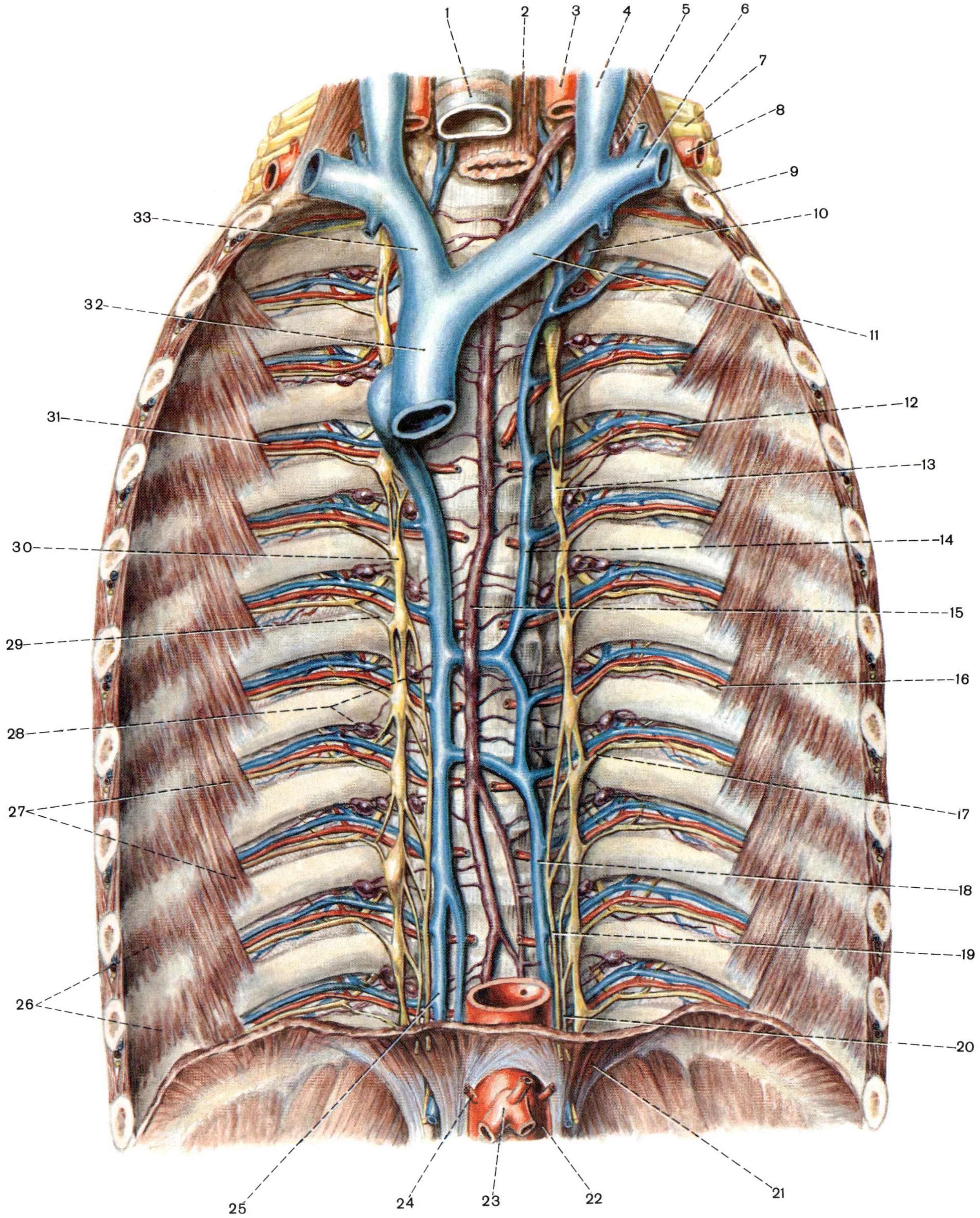

Fig. 49. Neurovascular structures of posterior mediastinum. (After E. Pernkopf.)

1 Trachea
2 Esophagus
3 Left common carotid artery (a. carotis communis sinistra)
4 Internal jugular vein (v. jugularis interna)
5 Thoracic duct, site of drainage (ductus thoracicus)
6 Left subclavian vein (v. subclavia sinistra)
7 Brachial plexus (plexus brachialis)
8 Left subclavian artery (a. subclavia sinistra)
9 First rib (costa I)
10 Left superior intercostal vein (v. intercostalis superior sinistra)
11 Left brachiocephalic vein (v. brachiocephalica sinistra)
12, 31 Intercostal artery and vein (a. et v. intercostales)
13, 30 Sympathetic trunk (truncus sympathicus)
14 Accessory hemiazygos vein (v. hemiazygos accessoria)
15 Thoracic duct (ductus thoracicus)
16 Intercostal nerve (n. intercostalis)
17, 29 Communicating branches of the sympathetic trunk (rr. communicantes trunci sympathici)
18 Hemiazygos vein (v. hemiazygos)
19 Greater splanchnic nerve (n. splanchnicus major)
20 Lesser splanchnic nerve (n. splanchnicus minor)
21 Diaphragm (diaphragma)
22 Abdominal aorta (aorta abdominalis)
23 Celiac trunk (truncus celiacus)
24 Inferior phrenic artery (a. phrenica inferior)
25 Azygos vein (v. azygos)
26 Internal intercostal muscle (m. intercostalis internus)
27 Subcostal muscle (m. subcostalis)
28 Intercostal lymph nodes
32 Superior vena cava (v. cava superior)
33 Right brachiocephalic vein (v. brachiocephalica dextra)

THE AZYGOS AND HEMIAZYGOS VEINS

The azygos and hemiazygos veins are located in the posterior mediastinum on the anterolateral surfaces of the vertebral column (see Figs. 46, 47 and 49). Arising in the retroperitoneal space, they pass into the thoracic cavity together with the greater splanchic nerves through the opening between the medial and middle crura of the diaphragm. In the thoracic cavity the azygos and hemiazygos veins receive the right and left intercostal veins. The syntopy of the azygos veins is as follows: the esophagus is in front of it, the intercostal blood vessel in the back, and the sympathetic trunk and the medial thoracic lymphatic duct lateral to it. At the level of the fourth thoracic vertebra the azygos vein runs forward, curves over the right bronchus, and drains into the superior vena cava. The hemiazygos vein consists of the upper and lower portions. The upper portion is called the superior, or accessory, hemiazygos vein. The accessory and hemiazygos veins unite at the level of the eighth or ninth thoracic vertebra and, crossing the vertebral column, drain into the azygos vein by one or more trunks.

The azygos and hemiazygos veins connect the system of the superior and inferior venae cavae, accomplishing collateral circulation when the blood flow in one of the venae cavae is impaired. Numerous connections of the azygos and hemiazygos veins with the system of the portal vein (through the veins of the lower part of the esophagus and the veins of the retroperitoneal cellular tissue) form portacaval anastomoses that play a major role when portal circulation is impaired.

THE SYMPATHETIC TRUNK

The thoracic part of the sympathetic trunk consists of 10 or 12 ganglia connected by interganglionic branches (see Figs. 46 and 49). It is located in front of the costal heads between the pleura and the endothoracic fascia. The azygos vein is medial to the right sympathetic trunk; the hemiazygos vein is medial to the left sympathetic trunk. Each sympathetic ganglion is connected with the intercostal nerve by means of white and gray communicating branches. Mediastinal branches arise from the sympathetic ganglia and great splanchnic nerve and, together with the branches of the vagus nerve, form the mediastinal nerve plexuses and also branches to the thymus.

The greater splanchnic nerve is usually derived from the branches of five to nine sympathetic ganglia. It descends obliquely to the front and medially, adjoining the bodies of the lower thoracic vertebrae. It then enters the abdominal cavity through the opening formed by the middle and medial diaphragmatic crura.

The smaller splanchnic nerve consists of bundles of fibers arising from the tenth and eleventh (sometimes also from the twelfth) ganglia of the sympathetic trunk. It penetrates the abdominal cavity through a special opening in the middle diaphragmatic crus lateral to the greater splanchnic nerve.

OPERATIONS ON THE THORACIC WALL

CLOSURE OF OPEN PNEUMOTHORAX

Surgical debridement of the wound is performed. The skin and muscles are removed by making an incision along the margins of the wound within the limits of helathy tissues. The injured rib is resected. When the defects in the rib are small, its edges are freed from the periosteum and resected with Luer's forceps; in this case the damaged areas of the intercostal muscles, pectoral fascia, and parietal pleura are excised. In more extensive injuries of the thoracic wall, excision of the injured soft tissues is followed by subperiosteal resection of the rib along the entire length of the wound. The pleural cavity is inspected, and blood clots and foreign bodies are removed. If the lungs are damaged, the wound is sutured.

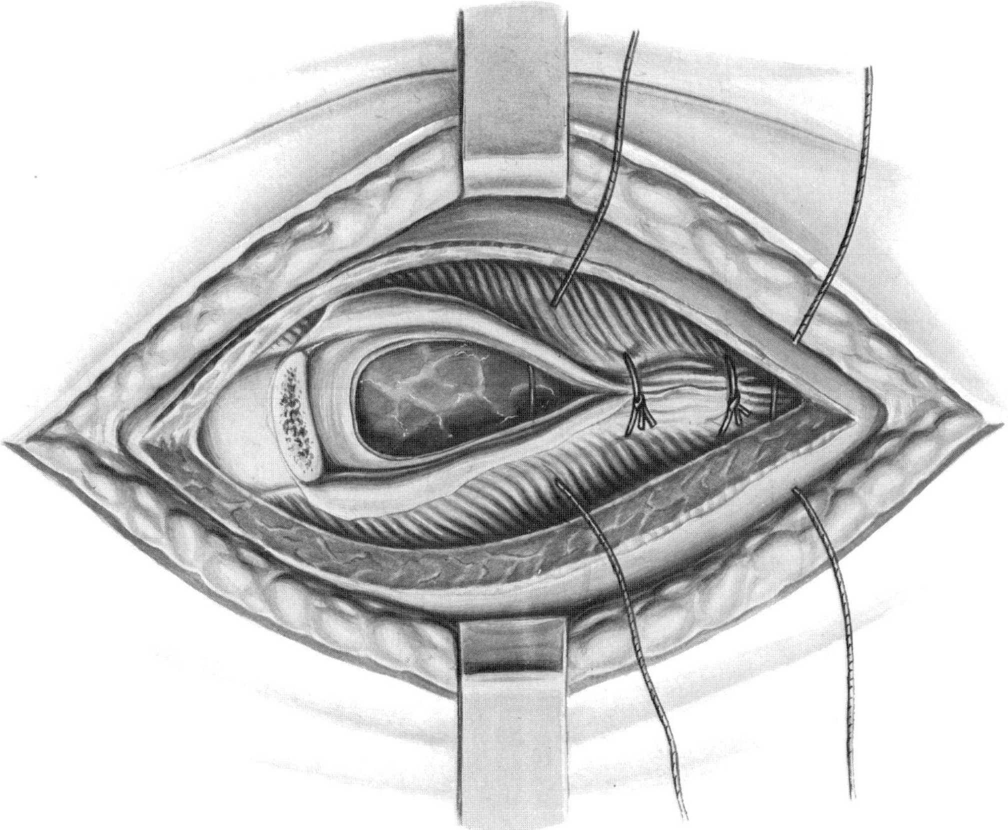

Fig. 50. Wound in thoracic wall in open pneumothorax is sutured layer-by-layer. Application of pleuromuscular sutures is shown.

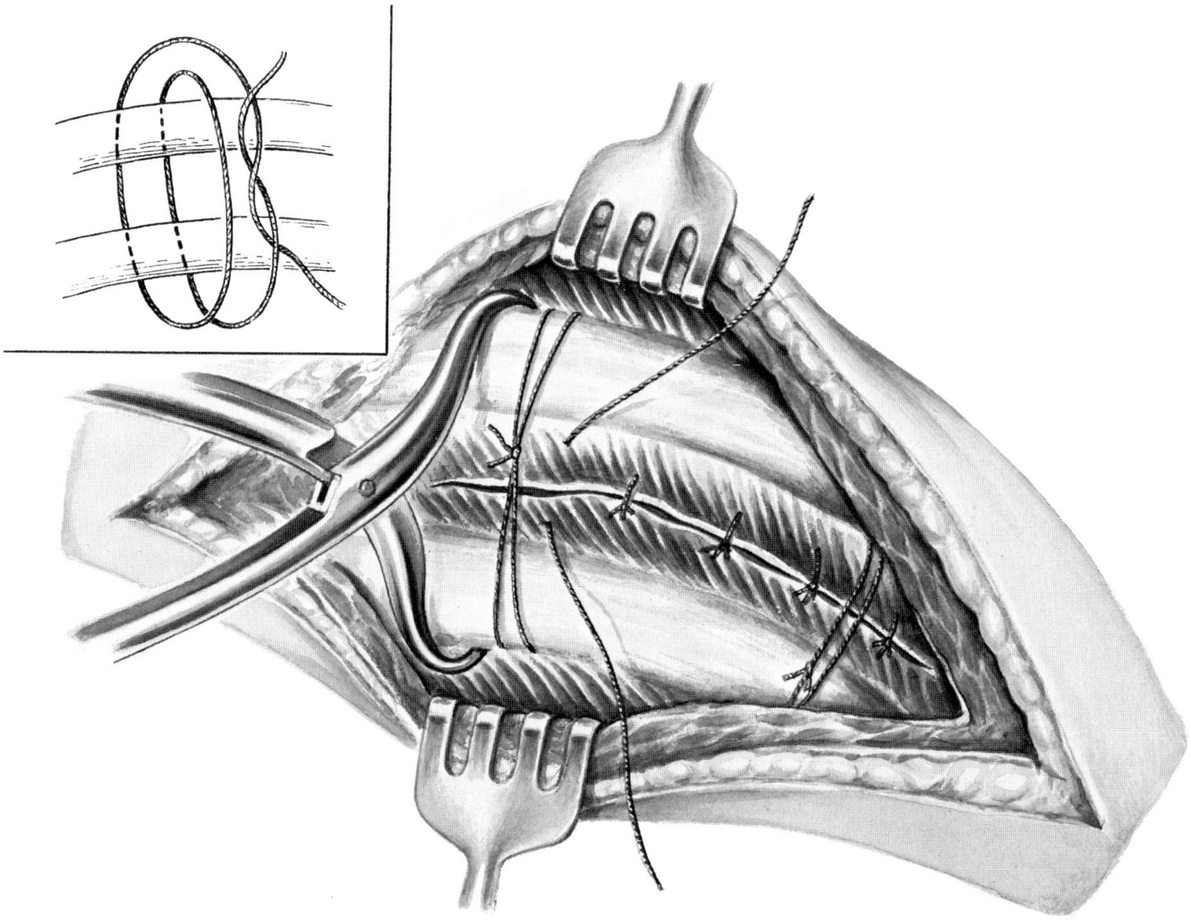

Fig. 51. Wound in thoracic wall is made airtight by means of a suture passed through all tissues grasping adjacent ribs. Course of thread is shown in left top corner.

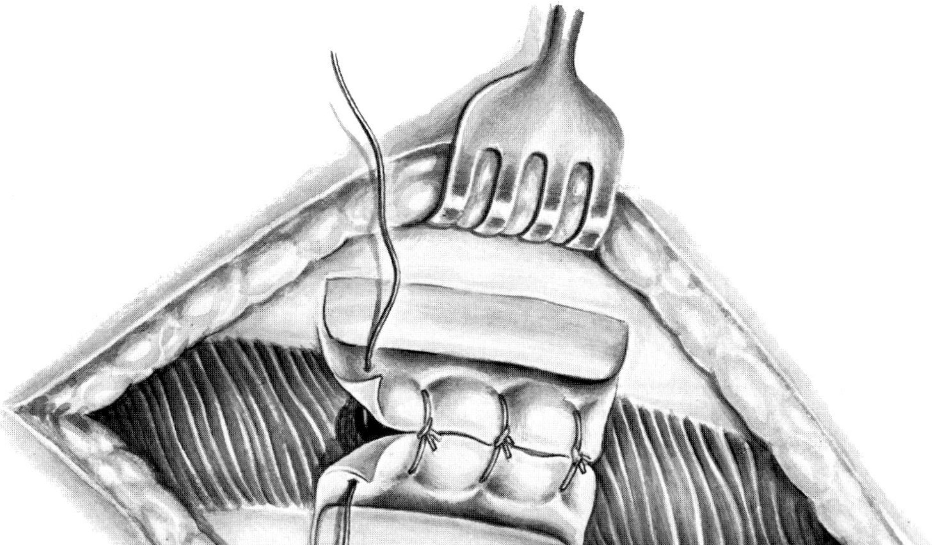

Fig. 52. Wound in thoracic wall is closed by covering it with flaps of periosteum of adjacent ribs.

The wound on the thoracic wall is closed. The pleura, endothoracic fascia, periosteum, and intercostal muscles are grasped with the first row of interrupted sutures (pleuromuscular sutures) (Fig. 50). Before the last suture is tied to make the wound airtight a catheter is introduced into the pleural cavity for aspiration of air and blood in the postoperative period. The second row of sutures is applied to the superficial muscles and skin. When there is a large defect in the tissues, it is advisable not only to apply pleuromuscular sutures, but to bring closer the two ribs adjoining the wound by means of two or three catgut sutures. With this purpose in mind, these two ribs are drawn together with forceps, and the suture is passed through the intercostal spaces (Fig. 51). Sutures are then applied to the skin. In cases with small wounds of the intercostal space the damaged areas of the muscles and pleura are excised, and flaps are then formed from the periosteum of the two adjacent ribs, and pleuromuscular periosteal sutures are applied (Fig. 52). The skin is sutured completely.

RIB RESECTION

An incision of the necessary length (depending on the indications) is made in the soft tissues along the middle of the rib's outer surface. The periosteum is cut with a scalpel, and two small transverse cuts are made at the edges of the incision on both sides. The periosteum is separated for a short distance to the level of the superior and then to that of the inferior borders of the rib with a curved raspatory (Fig. 53). After the periosteum is detached from the outer surface of the rib, it is separated from the inner surface with the raspatory. Doyen's raspatory is inserted under the rib, and by moving this instrument evenly along the length of the rib the periosteum is detached from its inner surface (Fig. 54).

Without removing the raspatory the curved blade of rib forceps is inserted under the rib, which is transected first on one and then on the other side (Fig. 55). The pleural cavity is punctured through the seat of the resected rib (Fig. 56), and the inner membrane of the periosteum and the parietal pleura are cut with a scalpel.

A drainage tube is inserted into the pleural cavity through the opening formed; the other end of it is brought out through an additional skin incision (Fig. 57).

The wound in the soft tissues is sutured layer by layer.

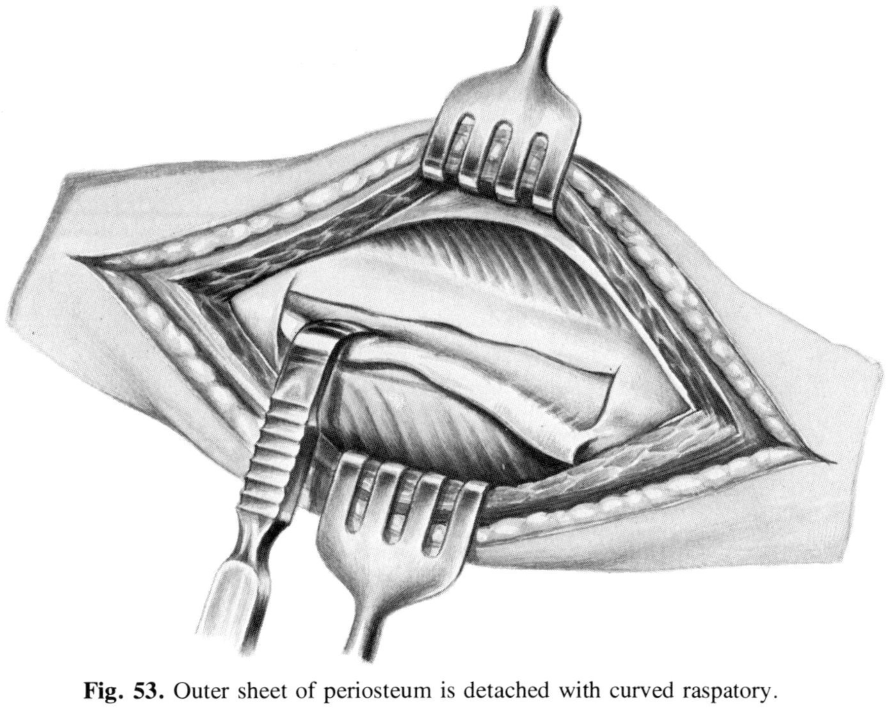

Fig. 53. Outer sheet of periosteum is detached with curved raspatory.

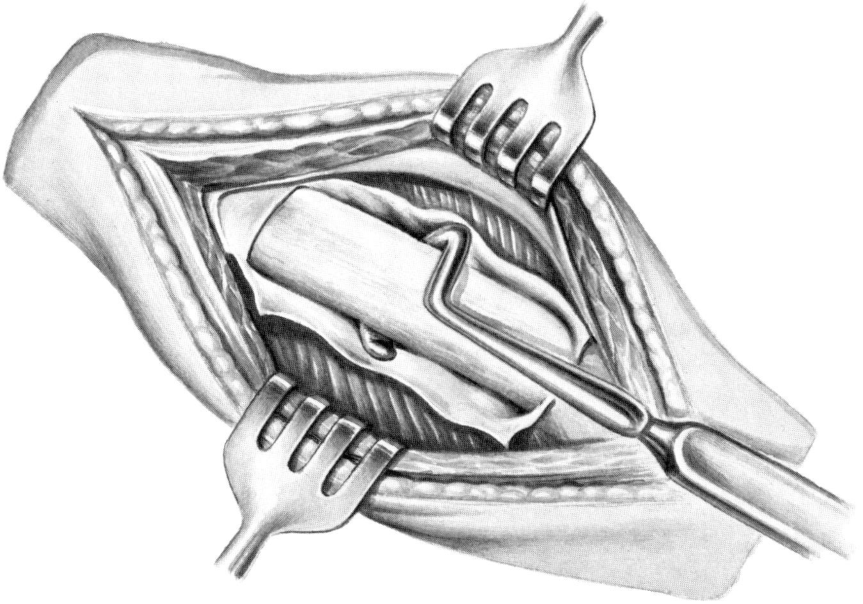

Fig. 54. Inner sheet of periosteum is detached with Doyen's raspatory.

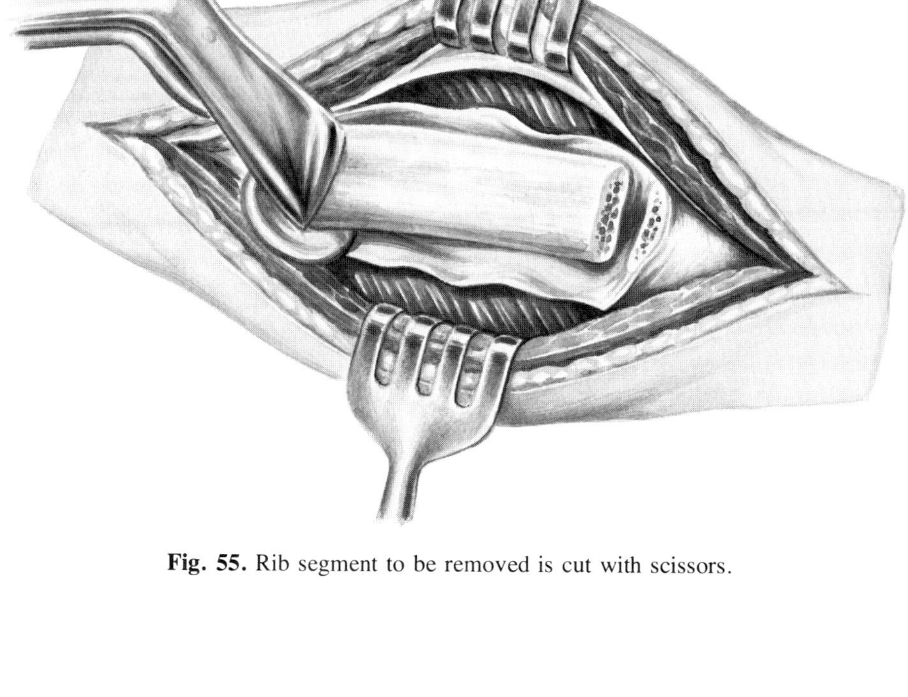

Fig. 55. Rib segment to be removed is cut with scissors.

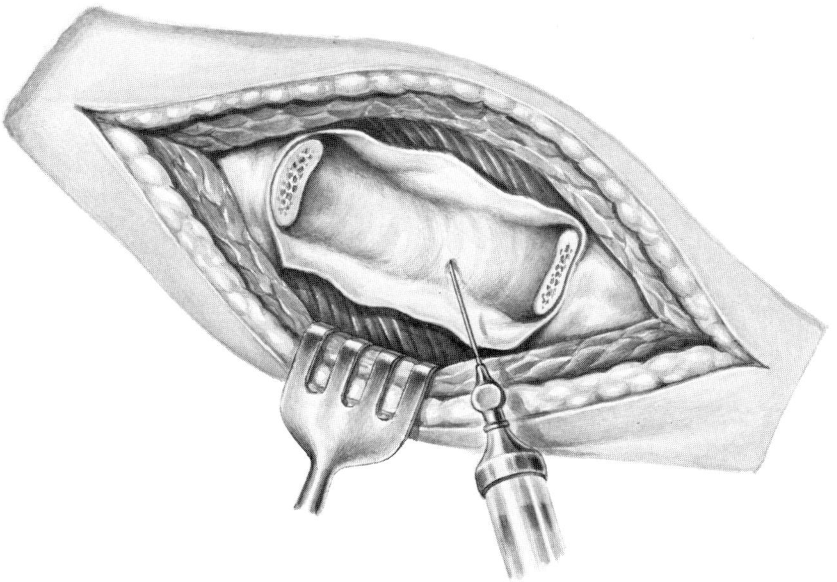

Fig. 56. Diagnostic (exploratory) puncture of pleural cavity through seat of resected rib.

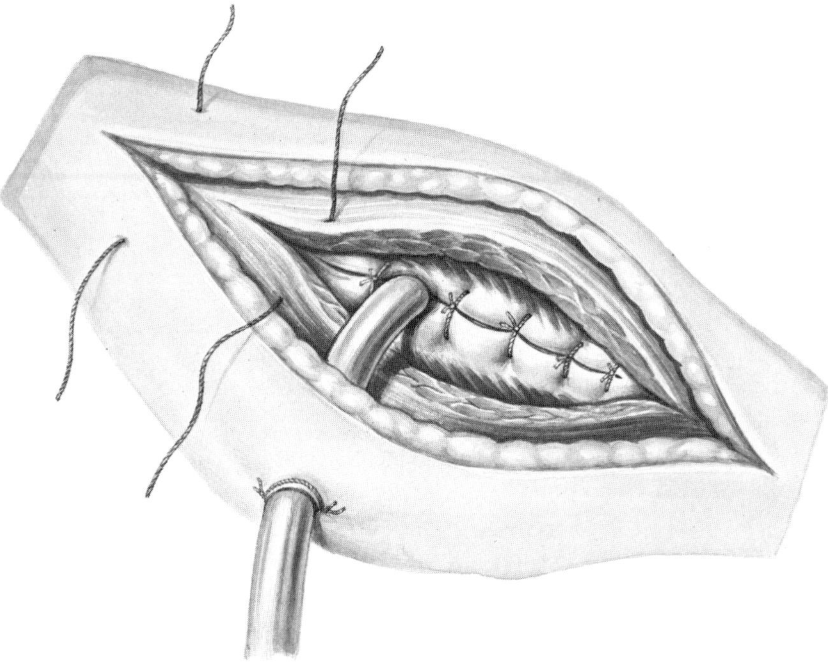

Fig. 57. After resection of rib a drain is left in pleural cavity and wound is sutured.

POSTEROSUPERIOR THORACOPLASTY

The patient is in a prone position.

The arm on the side operated on hangs down for maximum abduction of the scapula. The skin incision is begun at the level of the first thoracic vertebra, continued downward 4 to 5 cm from the line of the spinous processes and parallel to the medial border of the scapula, and then continued around its inferior angle to the posterior axillary line. The incision is made through the skin, subcutaneous cellular tissue, superficial fascia, the lower part of the trapezius muscle, the latissimus dorsi muscle, and the rhomboid muscle. It is desirable to preserve the upper part of the trapezius muscle intact. A wide hook is introduced into the subscapular space, and is used to draw the scapula away cranially and laterally. The periosteum is then cut with an electrotome beginning with the lowest rib (sixth or seventh) to be resected (Fig. 58). A raspatory is used to separate the periosteum from the rib, first from the outer surface and then from the superior and inferior borders and from the inner surface (Fig. 59).

The separation is accomplished more easily in the direction of the fibers of the intercostal muscles; that is, the raspatory should be advanced along the superior border of the rib ventrally, and along the inferior border dorsally. It is advisable first to free several ribs, including the second, from the periosteum and only after that to transect them one by one.

All the ribs are removed subperiosteally for a length of 12 to 15 cm from the transverse processes.

In patients with tuberculosis of the lungs or with a residual paravertebral cavity, where it is necessary to achieve maximum collapse, exarticulation of the paravertebral segments of the ribs serves the purpose best. This is accomplished by forcefully pressing the paravertebral segment of the rib ventrally with a bone holder, cutting the ligaments between the transverse process

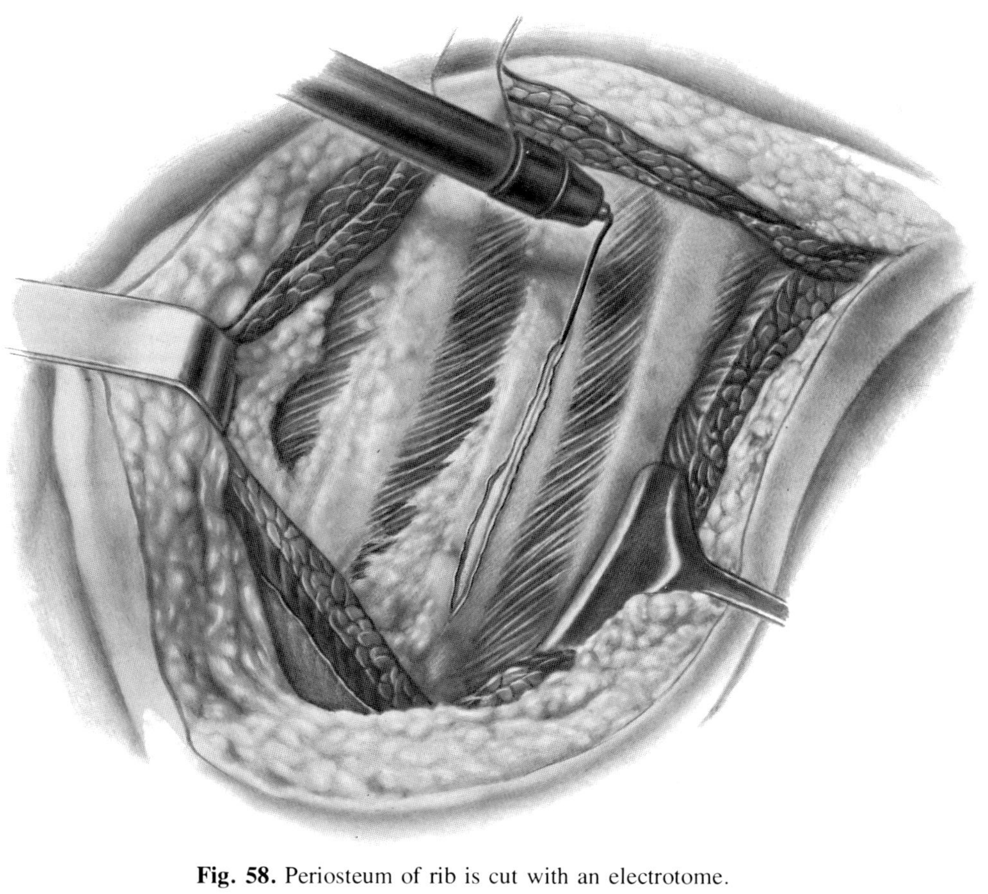

Fig. 58. Periosteum of rib is cut with an electrotome.

and the tubercle of the rib with a scalpel, and opening the joint.

The raspatory is introduced into the open joint. The head of the rib is separated from the transverse processes by light rotating movements of the raspatory and bone holder (Fig. 60). The remnants of the soft tissues are cut with scissors, and the paravertebral segment of the rib is removed.

After the heads of the ribs are removed, resection of the first rib is begun. A scalpel is used to make a small cut in the muscles overlying the paravertebral part of the rib on its posterior border. Separation of the periosteum is completed with a raspatory: first along the posterior border, then passing to the inferior surface, and finally to the superior surface of the rib. It is most convenient to use a special raspatory for the first rib to separate the periosteum from its superior surface (Fig. 61). The next step consists in cutting the vertebral part of the rib at the neck with special bone scissors, after which the rib is drawn out with a bone holder and transected in its anterior part. The removed segment of the first rib is about 5 to 7 cm long. In detaching the inner border of the rib it should be borne in mind that the subclavian artery and vein are adjacent to it here.

It is not advisable to remove the paravertebral segment of the first rib because of the risk of injuring the stellate ganglion of the sympathetic nerve.

Hemorrhage from the seat of the removed ribs is arrested by tamponade. At the end of the operation the entire surface of the wound is carefully inspected (Fig. 62). A drain is fitted along the whole length of the wound, and the muscles, subcutaneous tissue, and skin are sutured over it layer by layer. A compression bandage is applied.

The removal of six to seven ribs is typical of posterosuperior thoracoplasty.

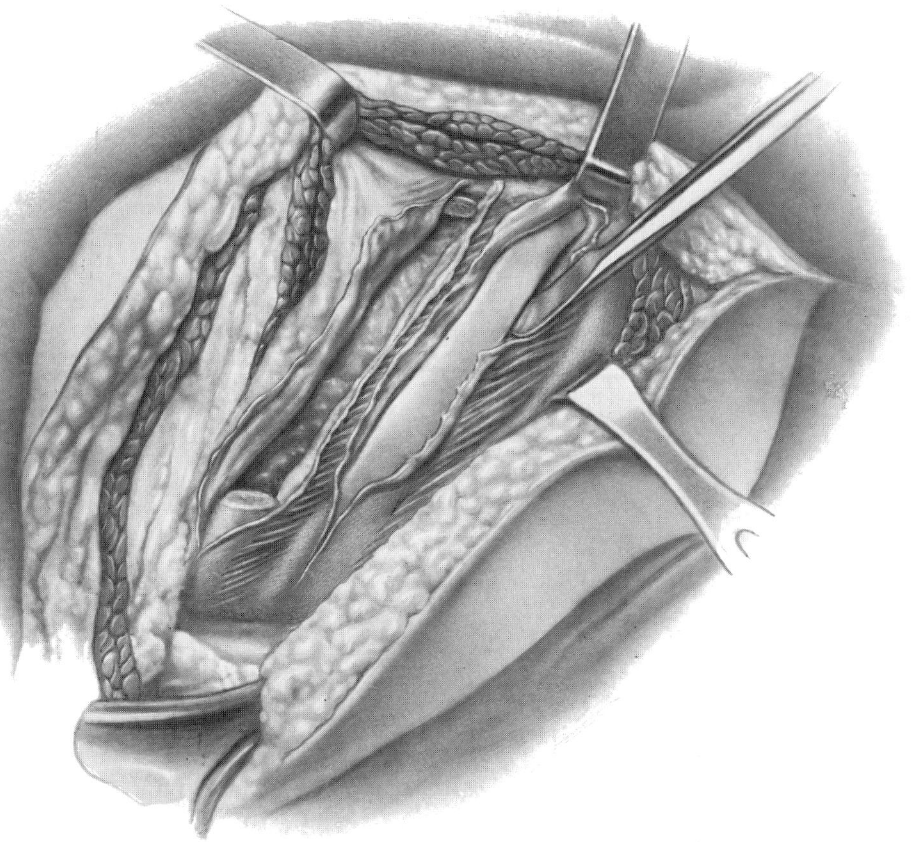

Fig. 59. Detachment of periosteum of fifth rib; sixth rib has been resected.

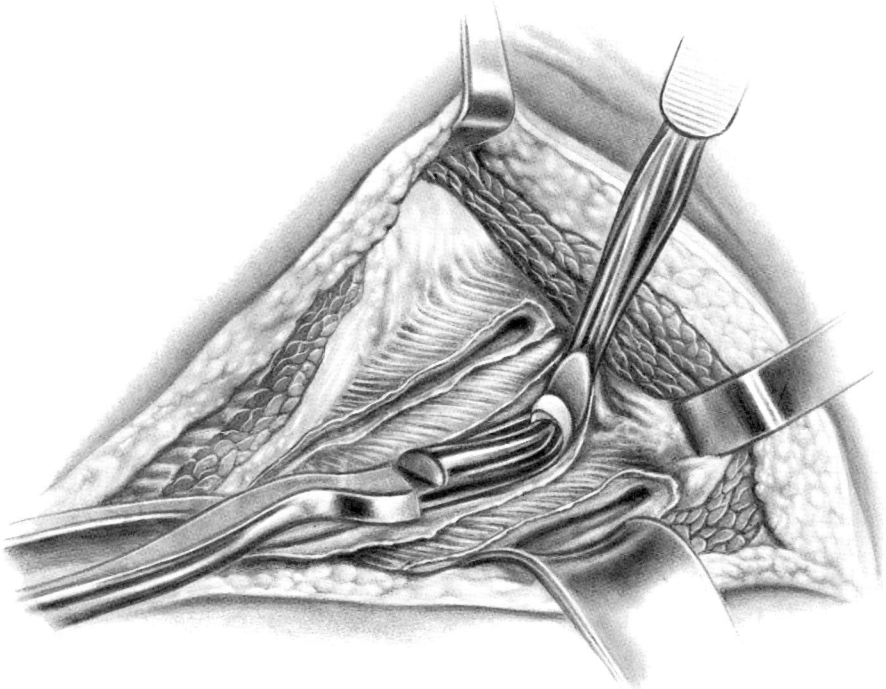

Fig. 60. Exarticulation of paravertebral rib segments. Raspatory is introduced into opened joint between rib tuberculum and transverse process. Bone holder is applied to paravertebral segment of rib.

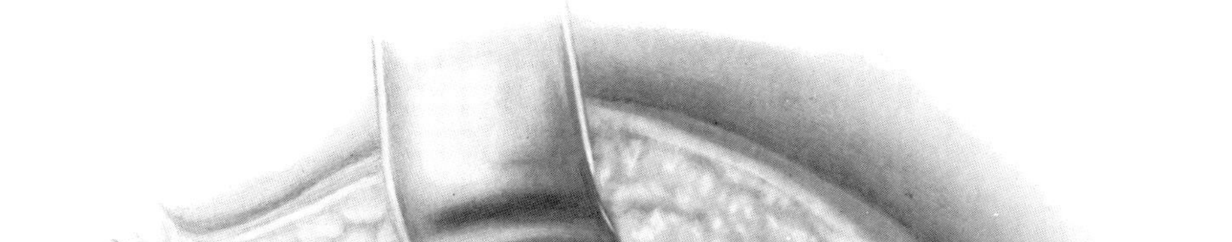

Fig. 61. Inner border of rib is freed from periosteum with special raspatory.

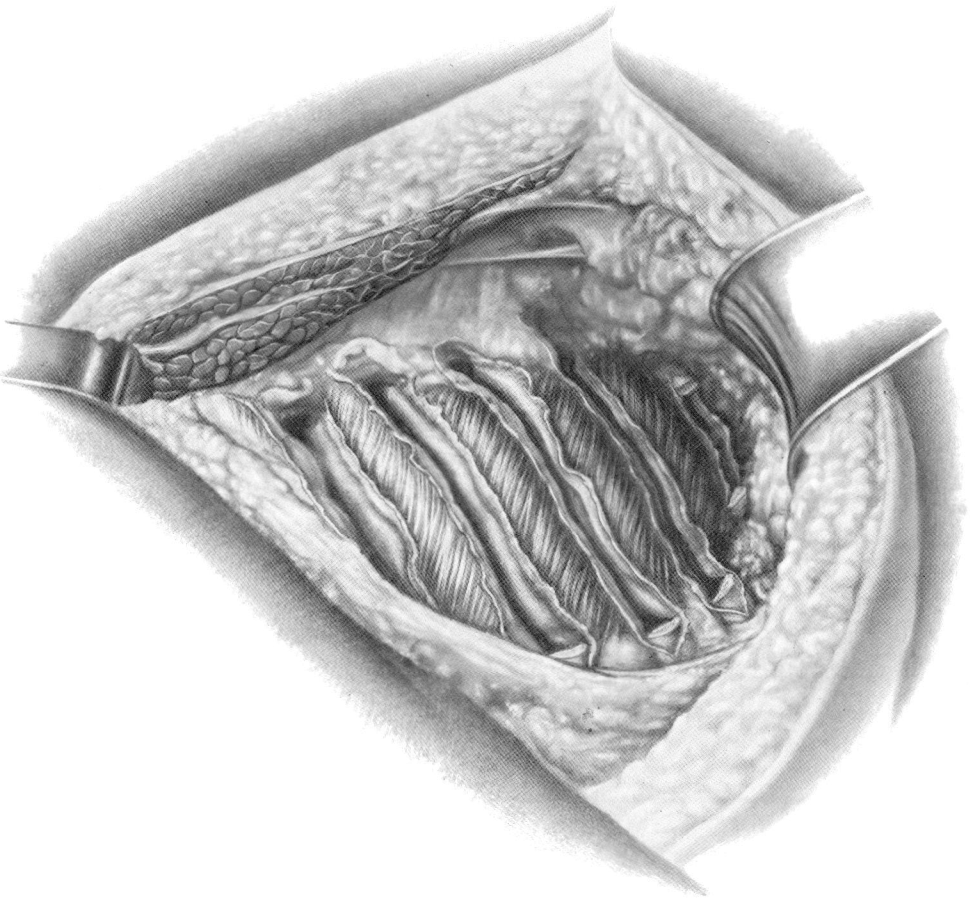

Fig. 62. Posterior segments of six upper ribs have been resected subperiosteally. Seats of resected ribs are seen.

ANTERIOR THORACOPLASTY

The patient is in a supine position.

A horizontal incision is made through the skin and subcutaneous tissue in the first intercostal space, parallel to the clavicle. The medial edge of the incision is folded down parallel to and 1.0 to 1.5 cm lateral of the sternal border.

The greater pectoral muscle is separated bluntly in the first intercostal space along the fibers. The edges of the muscle are drawn apart with blunt hooks. The border of the smaller pectoral muscle is drawn aside laterally. After this the second rib is freed from the periosteum.

The periosteum is cut with a scalpel along the middle of the external rib surface (Fig. 63) and detached with a raspatory. It is first carefully detached from the superior and inferior borders and inner surface of the rib (Fig. 64). The rib is freed for a distance of 8 to 10 cm, including the cartilaginous part, which is 2 to 3 cm long, and the freed segment is resected. A 9 to 11 cm segment of the third rib is removed in similar fashion, and, if necessary, a segment of the fourth rib too. With the second and third ribs resected the surgeon begins to free the first rib.

The periosteum on the superior surface of the first rib is cut for a distance of 0.5 cm. This incision is gradually widened with a raspatory, freeing the rib from all sides. A special raspatory for the first rib is used to move the periosteum off the inner border of the rib (Fig. 65). Resection of the first rib is the most delicate manipulation due to the close proximity of the subclavian vein. The rib is transected with bone forceps, while the sternal part in young individuals is cut with a scalpel. A segment, 3 to 5 cm long, is removed.

Bleeding from the seat of the ribs is arrested by tamponade. Several catgut sutures are applied to the greater pectoral muscle, and a drain is fitted under it. The wound is closed layer by layer. A compressing bandage is applied. Removal of the upper three or four ribs is typical of anterior thoracoplasty.

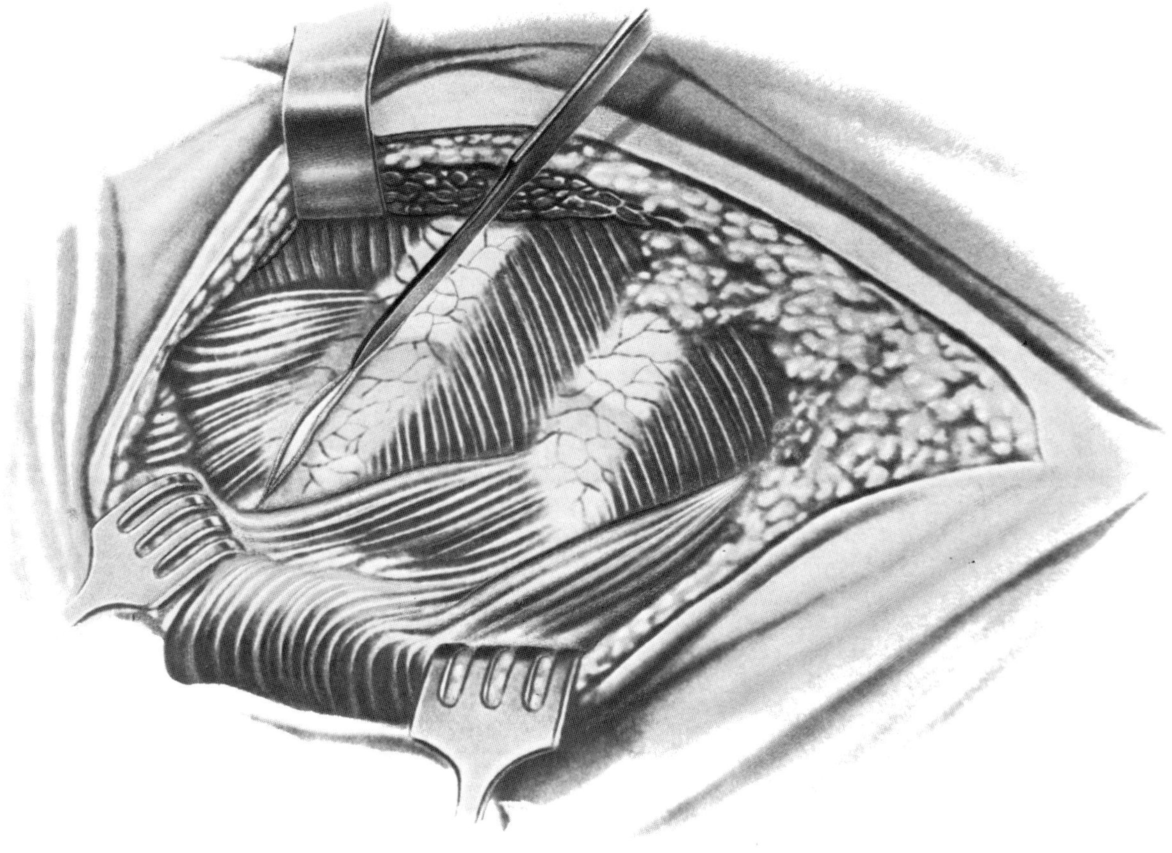

Fig. 63. External surface of periosteum is cut with scalpel.

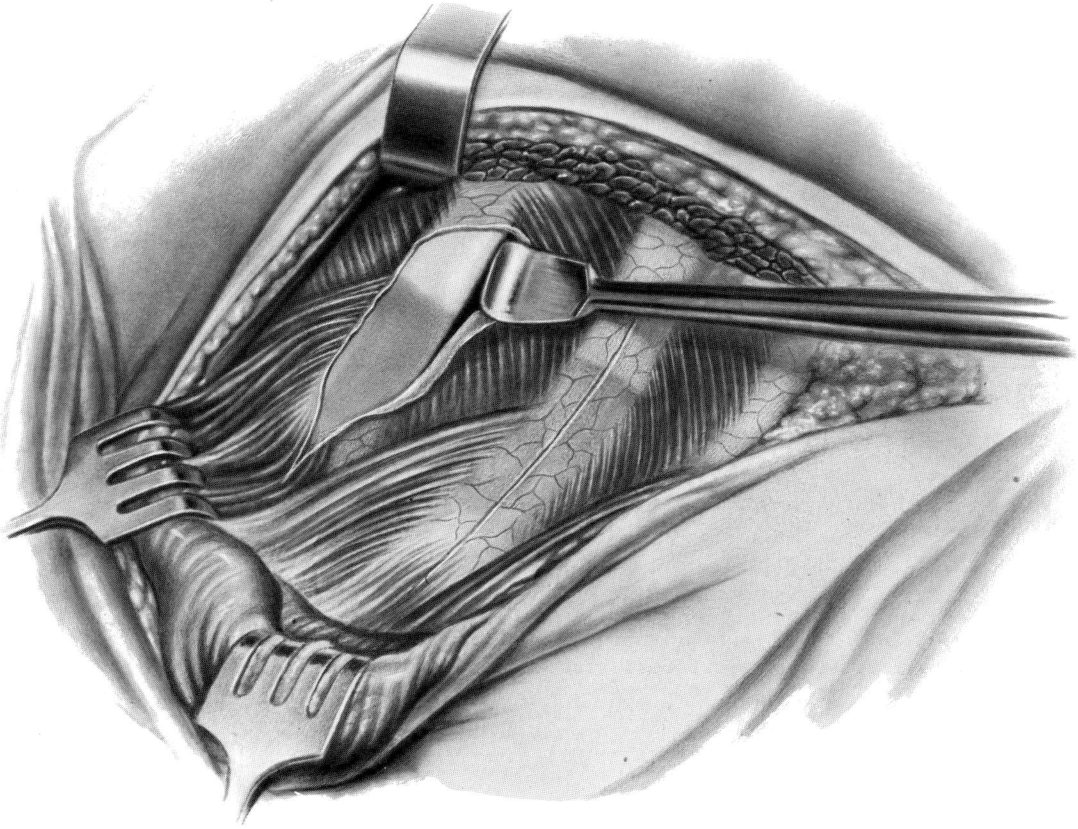

Fig. 64. Separation of periosteum and perichondrium of fourth rib; perichondrium of third rib has been cut.

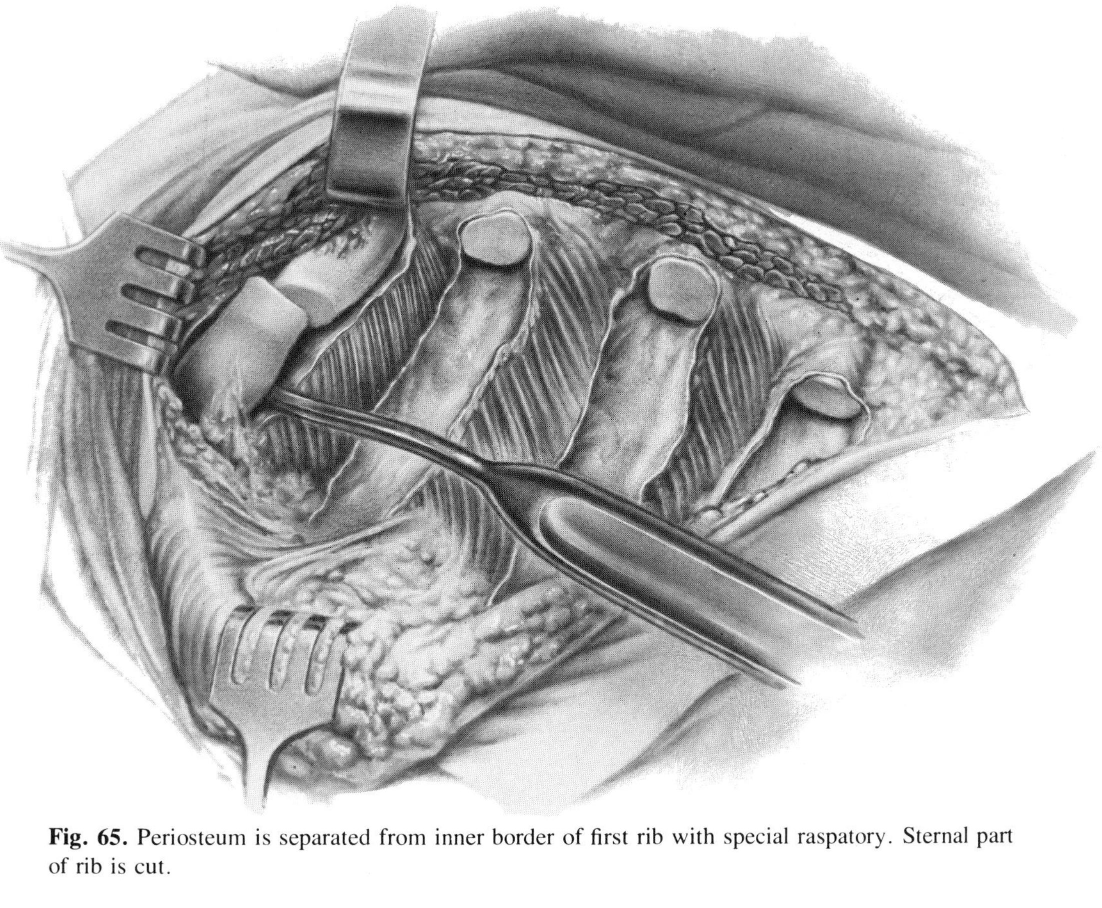

Fig. 65. Periosteum is separated from inner border of first rib with special raspatory. Sternal part of rib is cut.

LINBERG'S METHOD OF THORACOPLASTY

The patient is placed on his healthy side. The skin and muscles are cut along the medial scapular border 10 to 12 cm from the line of the spinous processes the entire length of the residual cavity. The fistulas are excised. The musculocutaneous flap is drawn upward with hooks to expose the rib in the vicinity of the fistula.

The lower rib is resected subperiosteally for a distance of 10 to 12 cm; the inner membrane of its periosteum is cut; and a finger is inserted through this opening into the pleural cavity to determine the boundary of the empyema (Fig. 66).

After that the next higher rib is resected along the length of the cavity and 2 cm beyond it on both sides, and then the seat of the rib is again cut lengthwise to open the pleural cavity.

In this way, four to five ribs are successively resected over the entire surface of the purulent cavity, cutting the seat of each rib longitudinally.

The remaining intercostal spaces, separated from each other by the incisions made in the periosteum along the lines of the resected ribs, resemble a staircase.

The intercostal muscles are cut one after the other alternatingly at the thoracic and vertebral boundaries of the cavity (Fig. 67), then freed from adhesions on the inner surface, and the cavity is cleansed and wiped with a gauze tampon moistened with alcohol.

Next, flaps shaped from the intercostal muscles are placed over the surface of the lung, which serve as plastic material for filling the cavity.

If the purulent cavity is shallow and the "cross-beams" sag unimpeded to the lung, then the intercostal muscles are not cut, but tampons are fitted loosely into the incisions in the ribs' seats (Fig. 68). The musculo-cutaneous flap is arranged in place and fastened with widely spaced sutures. The edges of the tampons are brought out to the skin surface between sutures.

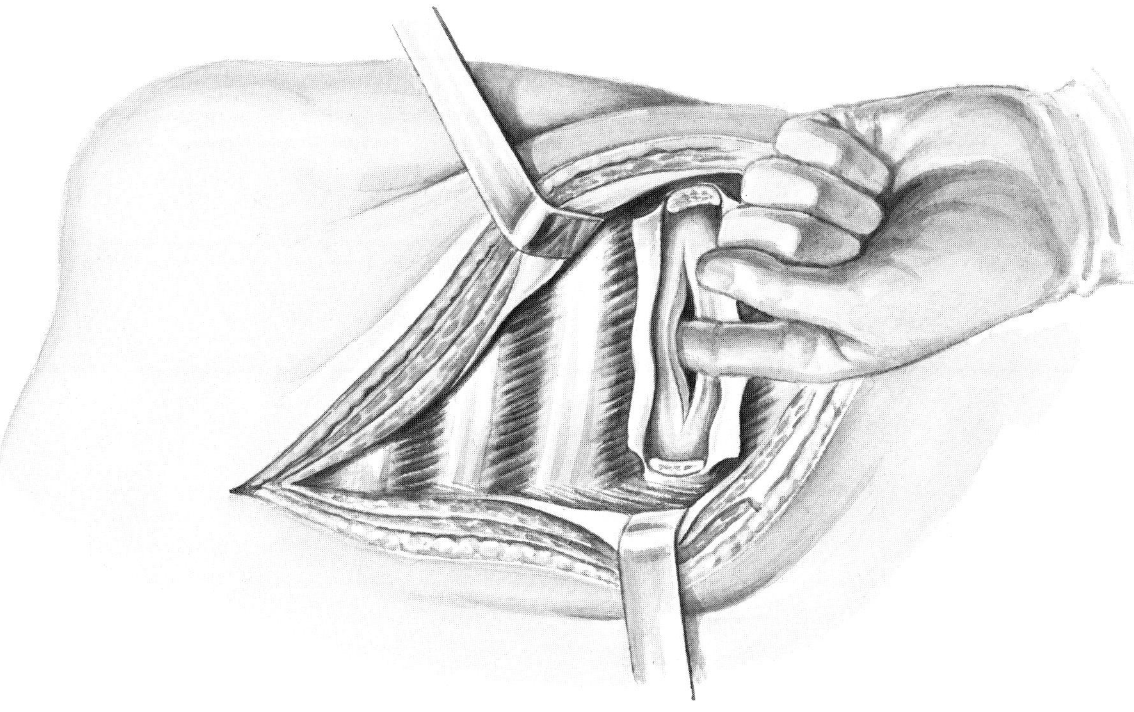

Fig. 66. Pleural cavity is opened in rib seat at level of lower border of residual cavity.

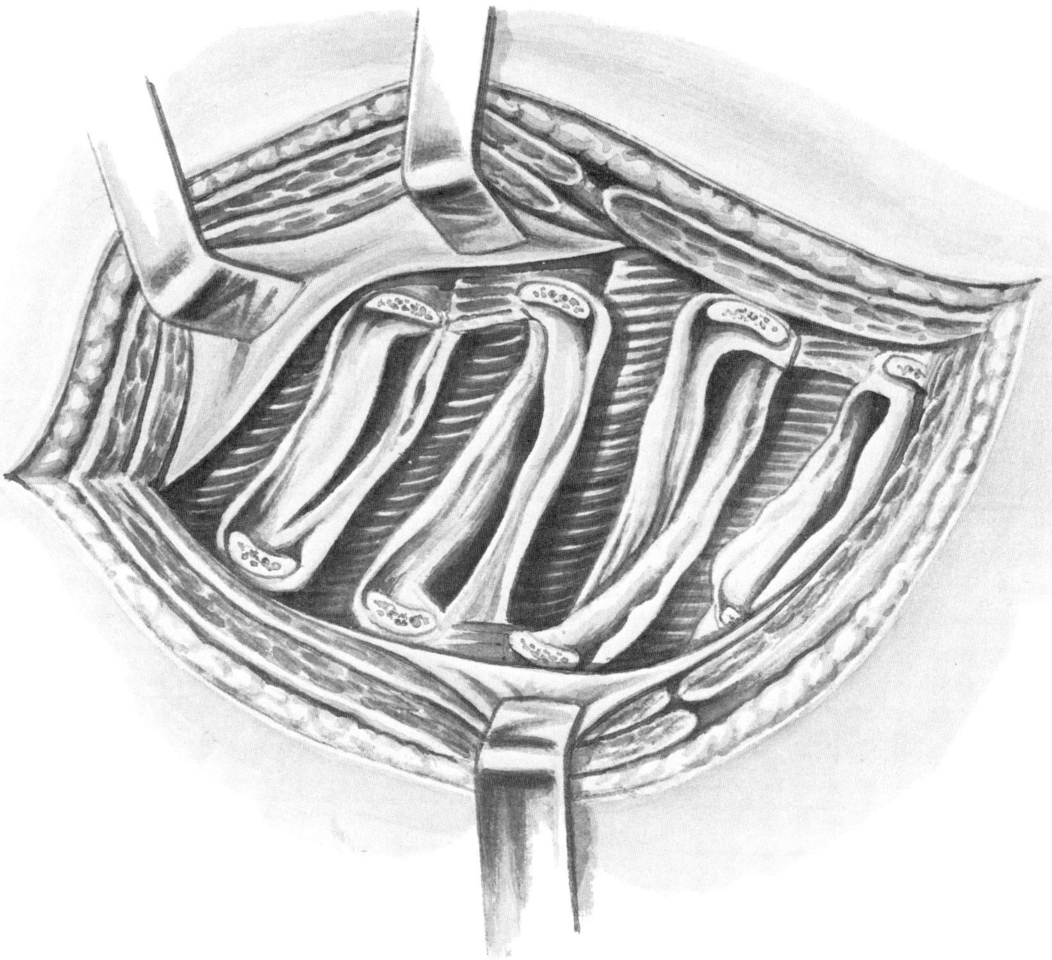

Fig. 67. Intercostal muscles that had been cut one by one are sunk into cavity of pleura (first, second, and third).

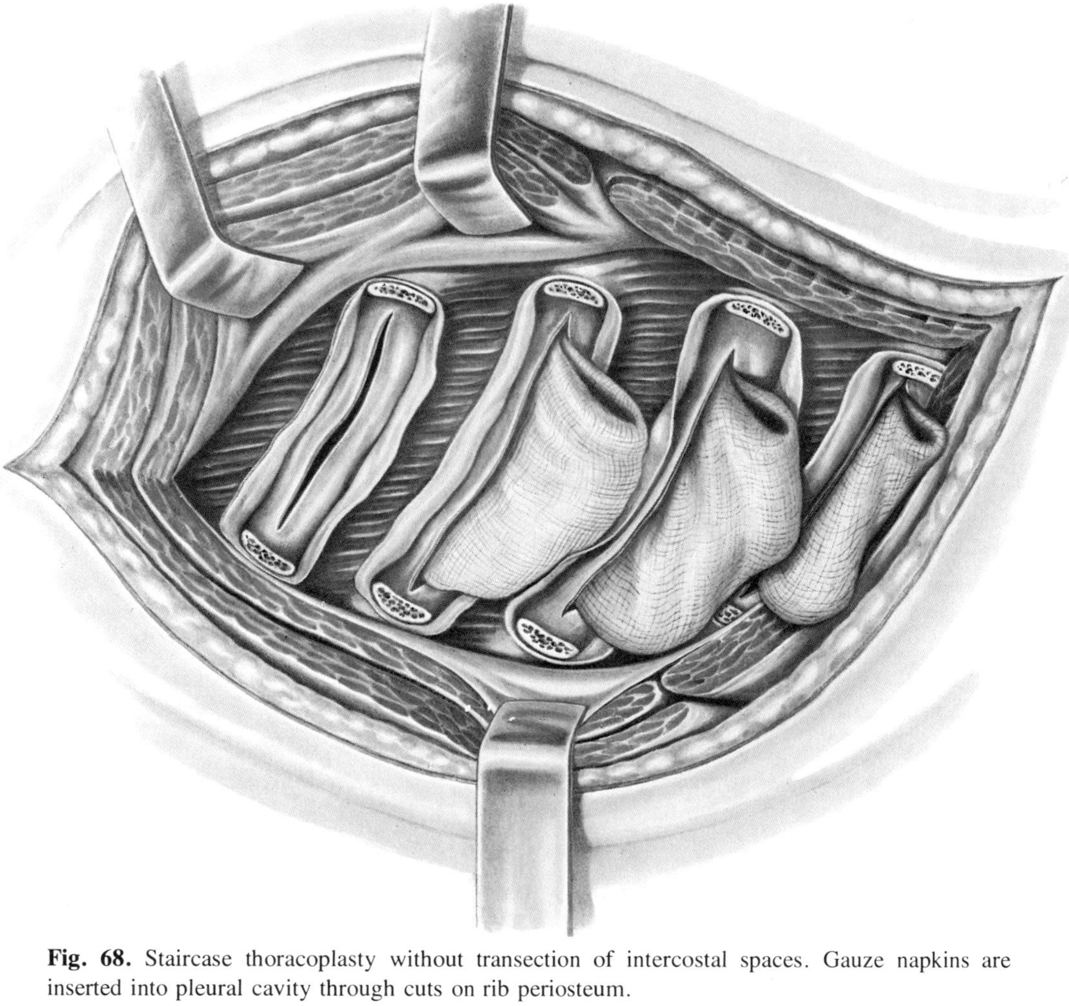

Fig. 68. Staircase thoracoplasty without transection of intercostal spaces. Gauze napkins are inserted into pleural cavity through cuts on rib periosteum.

MYOPLASTY OF RESIDUAL PLEURAL CAVITY AND BRONCHIAL FISTULAS AFTER ABRAZHANOV

The patient is placed on his healthy side with the upper limb drawn to his head.

An ellipsoid incision is made through the soft tissues on the periphery of the fistula 2 to 3 cm from its edges. The skin incision is extended in the direction of the nearest muscle chosen for grafting. The skin and muscles with the cicatricial tissues surrounding the fistula are excised in a single block (Fig. 69).

The exact size of the cavity is defined with a probe. If the cavity is large, a 5 to 8 cm rib segment is resected subperiosteally, and the periosteum is removed together with the thickened parietal pleura. The walls of the cavity are scraped with a curette. If a bronchial fistula is discovered in the depths of the wound, it is separated from the surrounding tissues and closed with a mattress suture.

The instruments and gloves are changed, and a muscular graft is shaped from the latissimus dorsi muscle (Fig. 70). The graft should be long enough to reach into the depth of the wound without being stretched. The bleeding vessels of the graft are ligated. Together with the cellular tissue, the muscular graft is sunk into the residual cavity in such a manner as to fill it entirely. It is fastened to the edges of the wound in the thoracic wall with catgut sutures (Fig. 71).

A drain is introduced into the residual cavity next to the flap, with its other end brought out through another incision (Fig. 72). The skin is sutured.

In cases with a fistula in the anterior thoracic wall the operation is carried out according to the same principle, but the graft is shaped from the greater pectoral muscle.

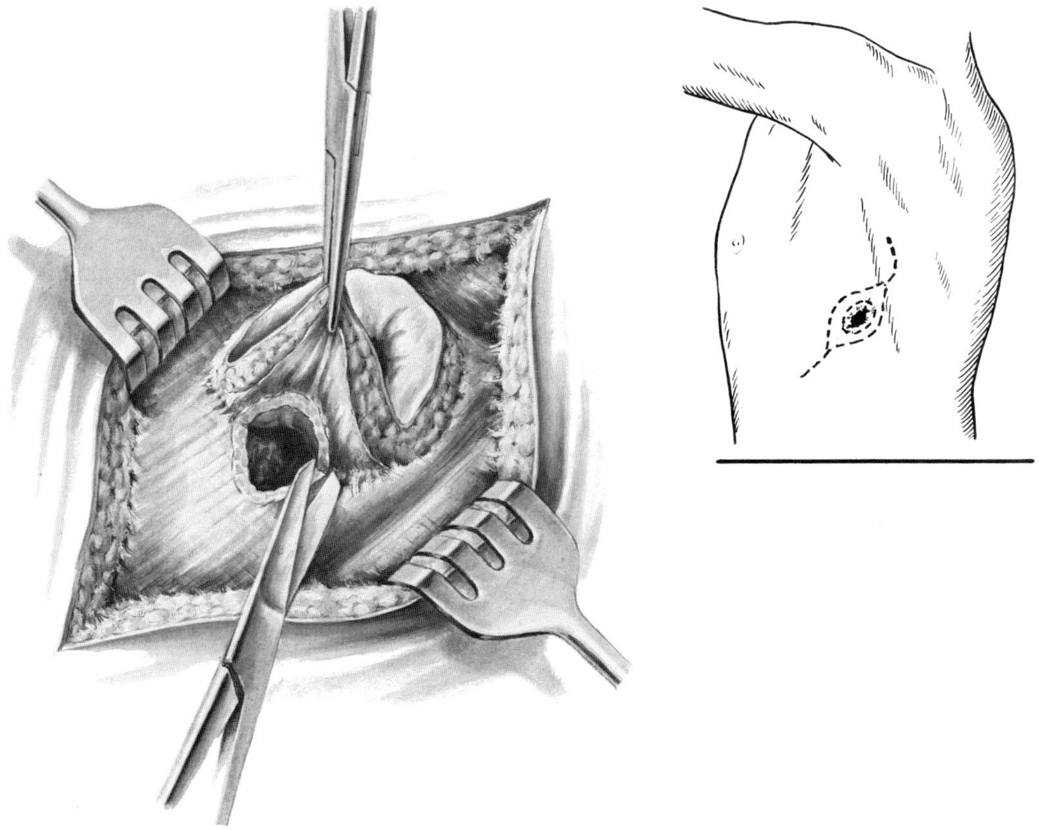

Fig. 69. Excision of cicatrized skin around fistula together with scars. Position of fistula and lines of incision are represented schematically on right.

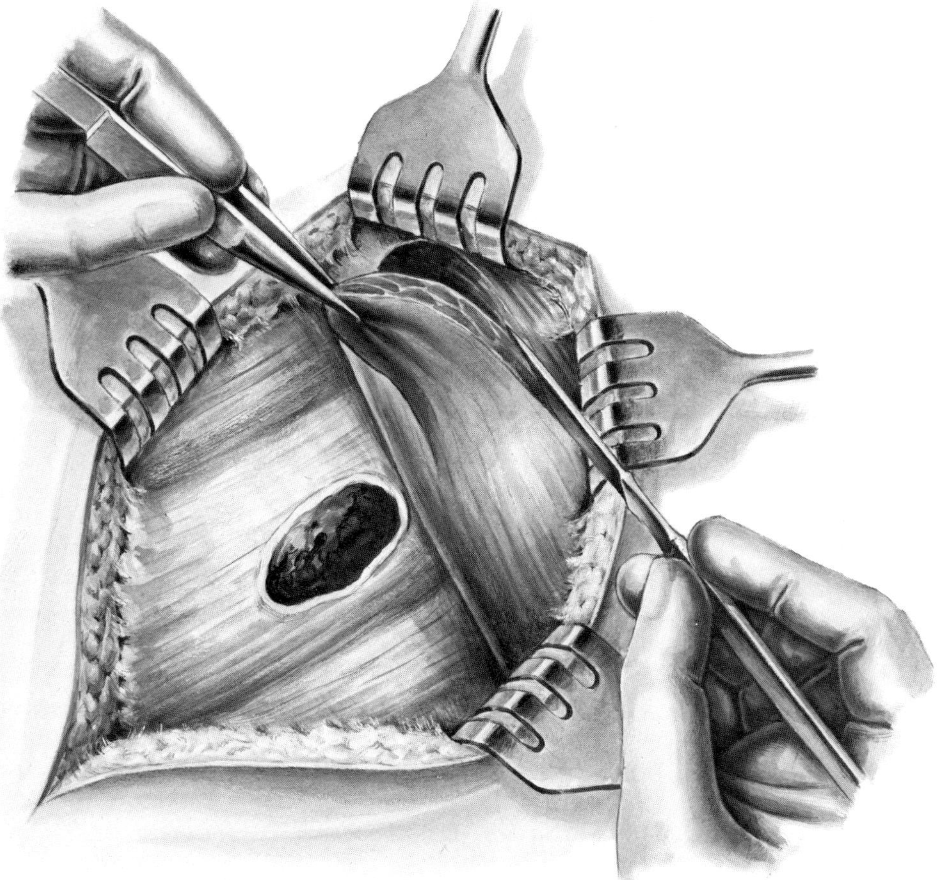

Fig. 70. Muscular graft is shaped from latissimus dorsi muscle.

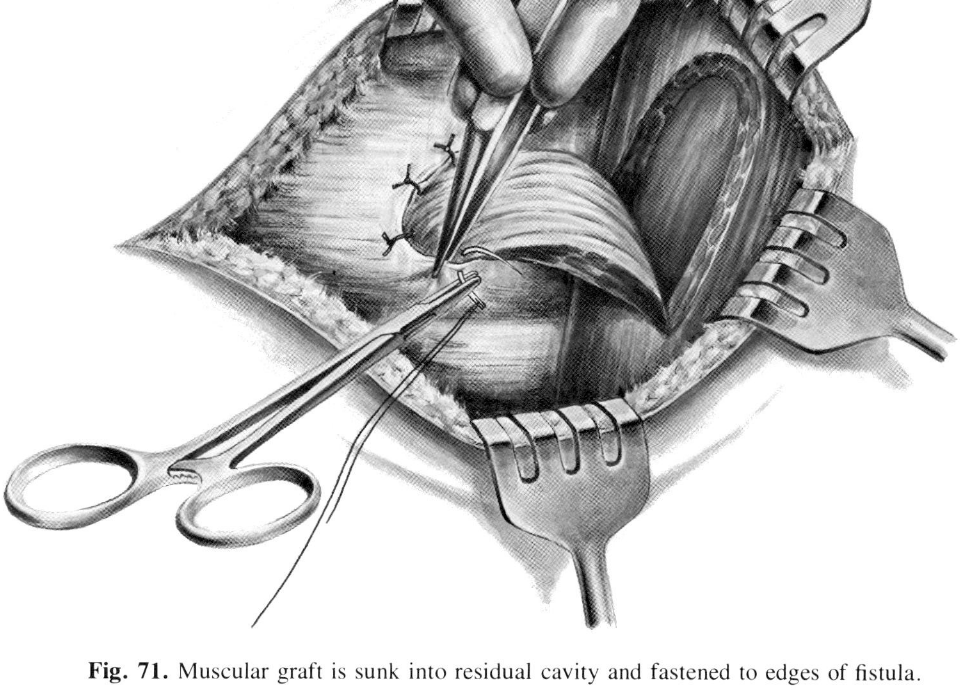

Fig. 71. Muscular graft is sunk into residual cavity and fastened to edges of fistula.

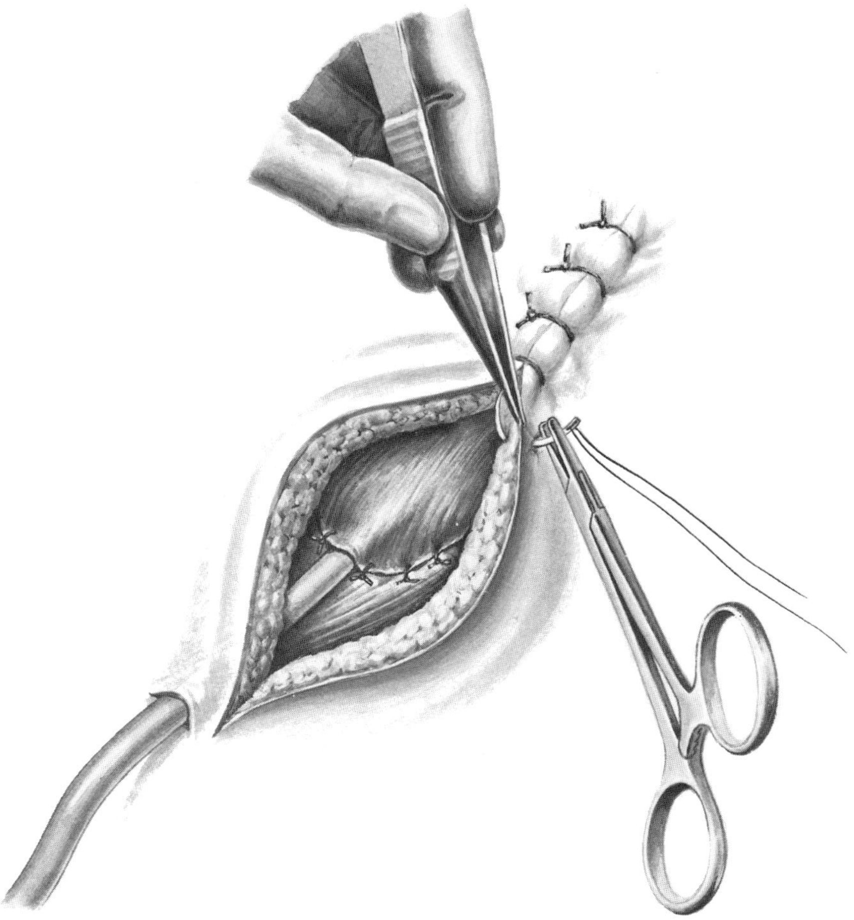

Fig. 72. Drain is inserted and wound sutured.

EXTRAPLEURAL PNEUMONOLYSIS

With the patient lying on his side the fourth rib is resected for a distance of 5 to 7 cm through a horizontal or vertical axillary incision 10 cm long (Fig. 73). The inner layer of the costal periosteum with the adjacent endothoracic fascia are cut. The finger or a small tampon is inserted into the cut, and the endothoracic fascia is separated from the parietal pleura with careful movements in different directions (Fig. 74). In doing so, it is advisable to maniuplate closer to the inner surface of the thoracic wall so as not to rupture the parietal pleura or even a cavern. When a small cavity has been formed, a gauze tampon held with curved dressing forceps is used to detach the parietal pleura. During pneumonolysis the cavity is illuminated with a special lamp for deep cavities or with the lamp of a straight thoracoscope (Fig. 75). Pneumonolysis is usually carried out from the back to the level of the sixth rib, from the front to the level of the third rib, and medially to the root of the lung. The guiding point on the right is the arch of the azygos vein and on the left the aortic arch.

The cavity formed as the result of extrapleural pneumonitis is tamponed with gauze to arrest bleeding. The tampons are then removed, and sutures are applied successively to the periosteum, muscles, and skin to make the wound airtight.

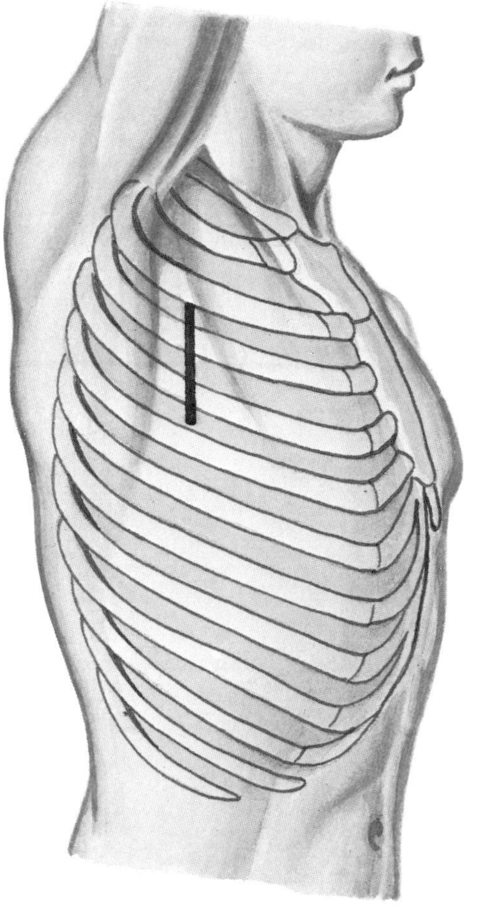

Fig. 73. Vertical axillary approach. Line of incision is shown.

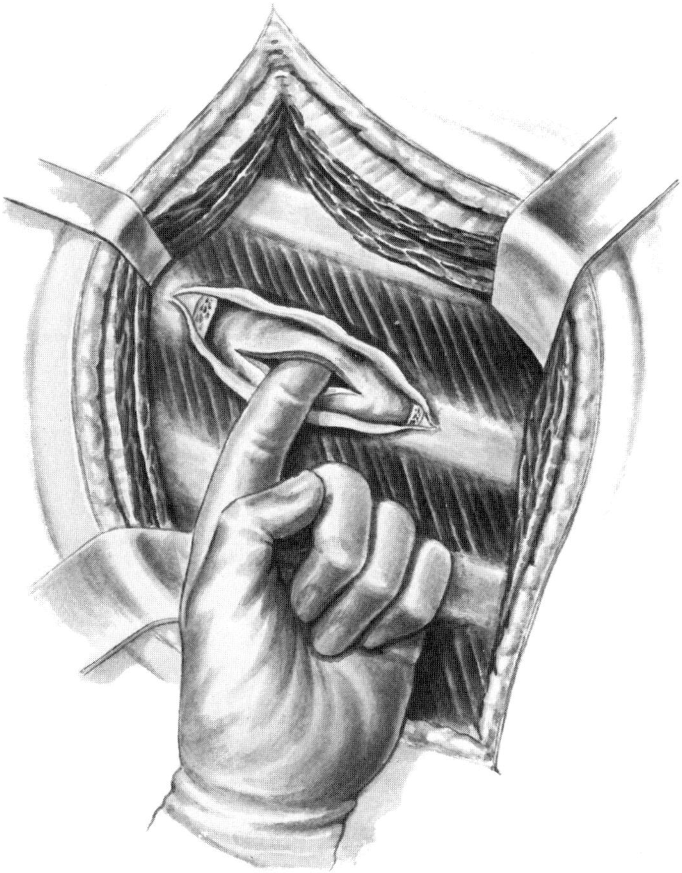

Fig. 74. Segment of fourth rib has been resected subperiosteally; periosteum is cut and the finger inserted to separate parietal pleura.

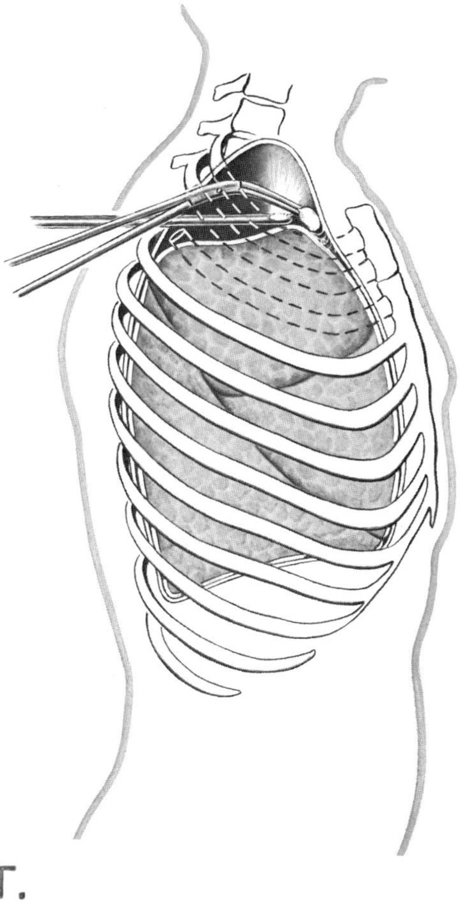

Fig. 75. Parietal pleura is detached with gauze tampon under control with a thorascope. Separated cervical pleura can be seen.

RADICAL MASTECTOMY

An incision is chosen depending on the localization of the tumor, for it must ensure extensive excision of the skin bordering upon the tumor, a wide approach for removing the regional lymph nodes and pectoral muscles, and conditions for closure of the skin defect without supplementary plastics. A skin incision in the shape of two semiovals is usually planned to encompass the mammary gland 6 to 8 cm from the tumor both on the right and left.

The incision is begun at the lateral third of the clavicle, continued in the direction of the sternum and then downward on the parasternal line, and completed at the costal arch, thus encompassing the mammary gland from the medial side (medial semioval).

The second incision (the lateral semioval) is also begun at the clavicle and continued downward obliquely along the anterior margin of the axilla; then it is directed medially to join the first incision at the costal arch (Fig. 76).

The edges of the wound are temporarily stitched through with thick threads (traction sutures) for raising them. The skin is separated with a scalpel, leaving a minimum layer (no more than 0.5 cm) of subcutaneous fat on them. The subcutaneous fat in the axilla is removed completely so that lymph nodes situated near the skin will not remain.

The skin flaps are separated from the thoracic wall cranially up to the clavicle, medially to the middle of the sternum, laterally up to the anterior border of the latissimus dorsi muscle, and caudally down to the border of the costal arch. The subcutaneous cellular tissue and the superficial fascia are cut along the entire perimeter of the wound within the limits of the folded back skin edges.

The greater pectoral muscle is freed of the subcutaneous cellular tissue in the upper corner of the wound and cut at the site of its insertion to the humerus. It is easier to divide the muscle by inserting the index finger under it, so that the fingertip protrudes between the separated muscle fibers. After that the index and middle

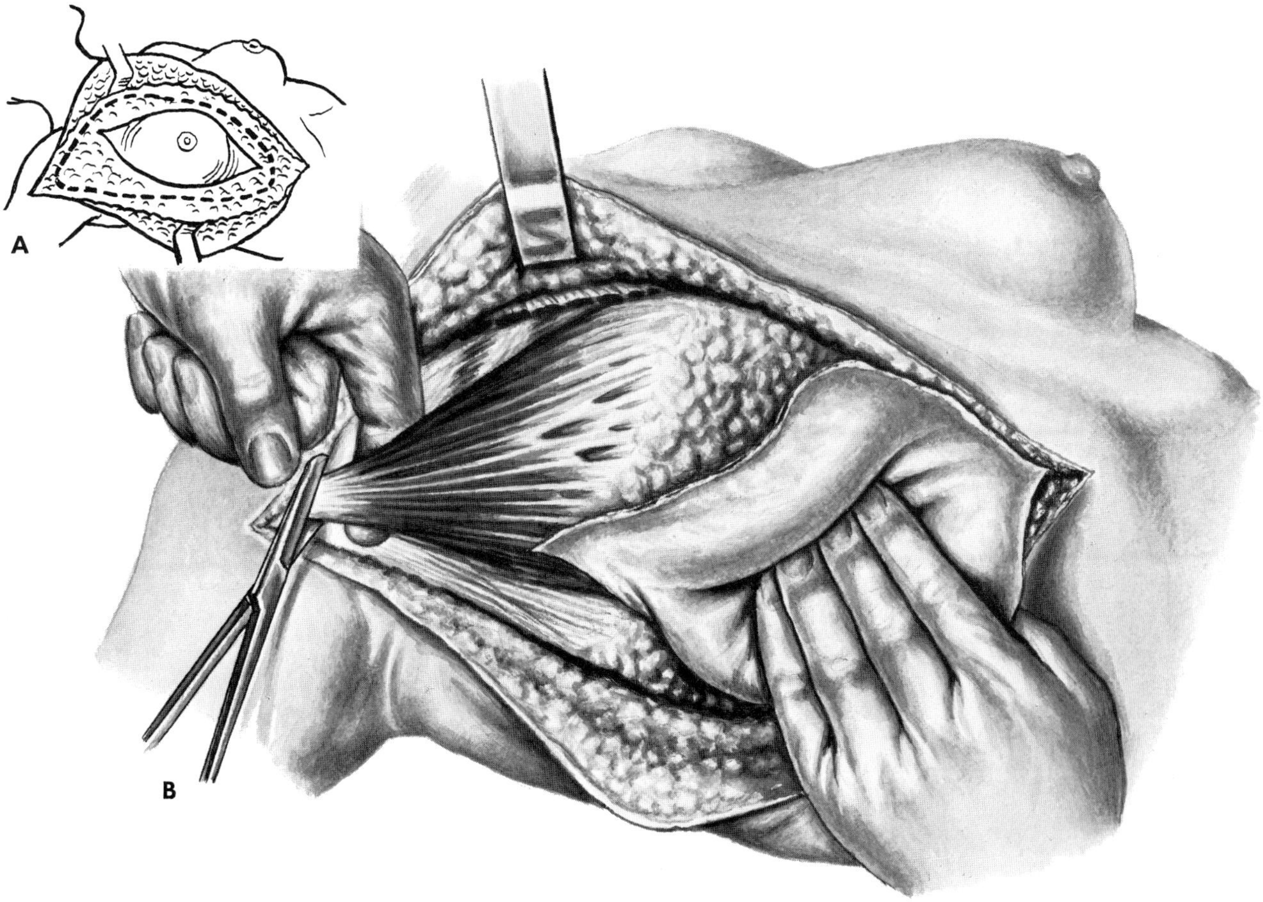

Fig. 76. A, Ellipsoid skin incision with separation of subcutaneous fat; dashed line represents line of incision of superficial thoracic fascia. **B,** Brachial part of the greater pectoral muscle is cut.

finger are placed under the clavicular part of the muscle, which is detached along the clavicle. With the muscle stretched caudally and ventrally, its fibers are cut at the clavicle.

The costal part of the greater pectoral muscle is then cut with a scalpel along the sternal border until the costal cartilages are exposed (no farther than the third rib), and the muscle and mammary gland are drawn away caudally (see Fig. 76). The coracobrachial muscle is exposed; the deep sheet of the pectoral fascia is cut along the medial border of this muscle; and the index finger is placed under the smaller pectoral muscle, which is then transected (Fig. 77).

With the greater and smaller pectoral muscles cut, the entire complex is drawn away caudally and the lymph nodes and fatty tissue are removed along the subclavian vein. The fatty cellular tissue is removed completely so that the vein and the stripped part of the thoracic wall resemble an anatomical preparation (Fig. 78).

The fatty cellular tissue and the lymph nodes are removed from the deep parts of the axilla and prescapular space with care taken not to damage the long thoracic nerve. The fascia of the anterior serratus muscle is cut; the greater pectoral muscle is separated from the thoracic wall; the smaller pectoral muscle is cut at its origin from the ribs; and the greater pectoral muscle, at the sternum. The complex comprising the mammary gland, the cellular tissue with the lymphatic nodes, and the pectoral muscles is removed as a whole. Careful hemostasis employing electrocoagulation is accomplished. The large branches of the arteries and veins are ligated separately.

A drain is introduced into the operative wound through a contra-aperture on the anterior border of the latissimus dorsi muscle (Fig. 79). To avoid the formation of decubitus ulcer, the tube should not be placed on the vessels. Sutures are applied to the skin. When the skin is stretched tightly and it is difficult to approximate the edges of the wound, the skin flaps are correspondingly rearranged in the needed direction.

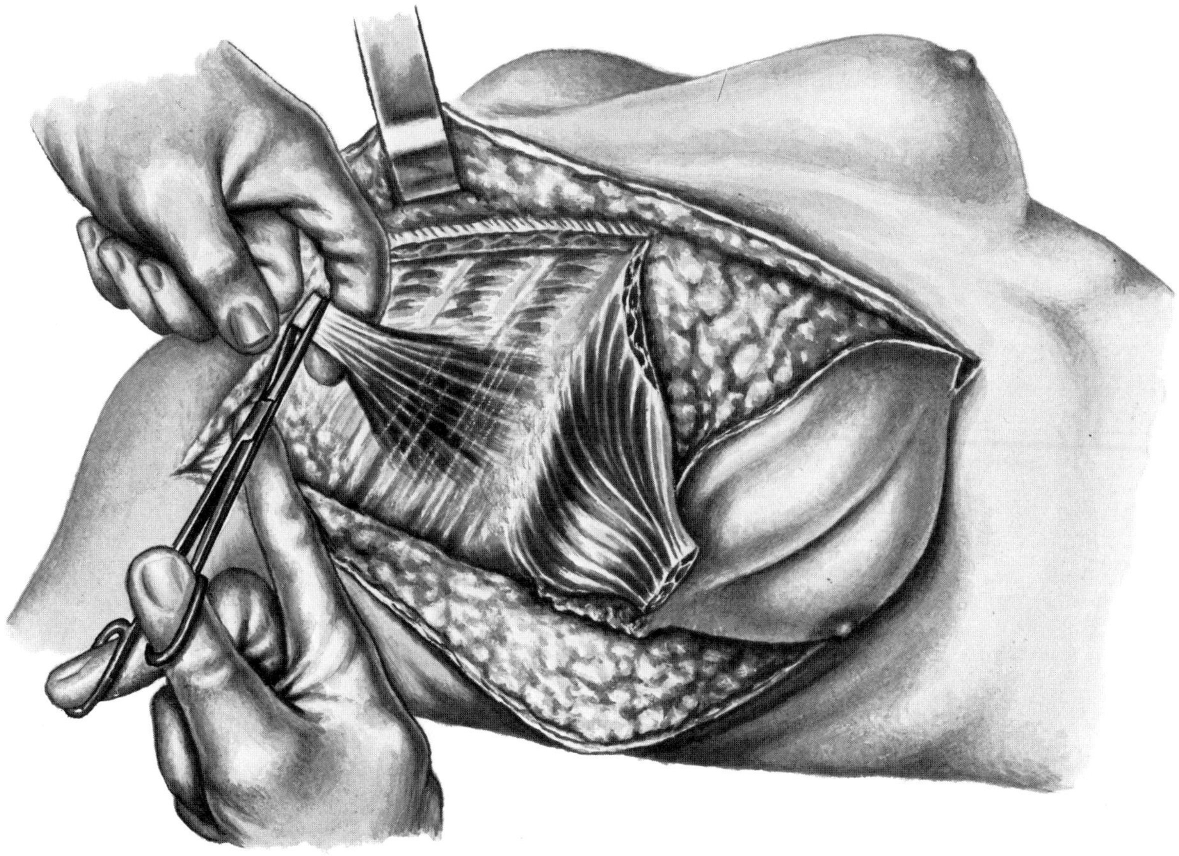

Fig. 77. Greater pectoral muscle is drawn downward, and tendon of smaller pectoral muscle is cut with scissors.

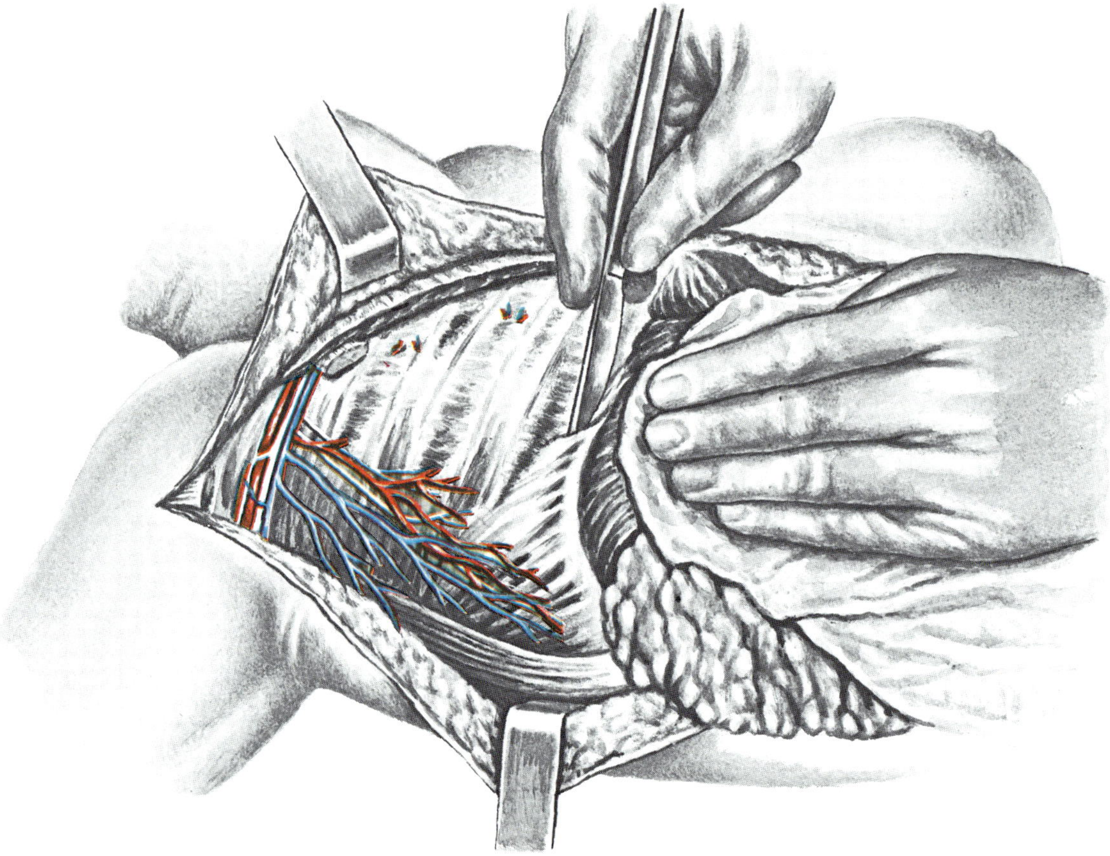

Fig. 78. Subcutaneous fat and lymph nodes are removed along subclavian vessels, and in region of fossa axillaris, muscles and mammary gland are separated from thoracic wall.

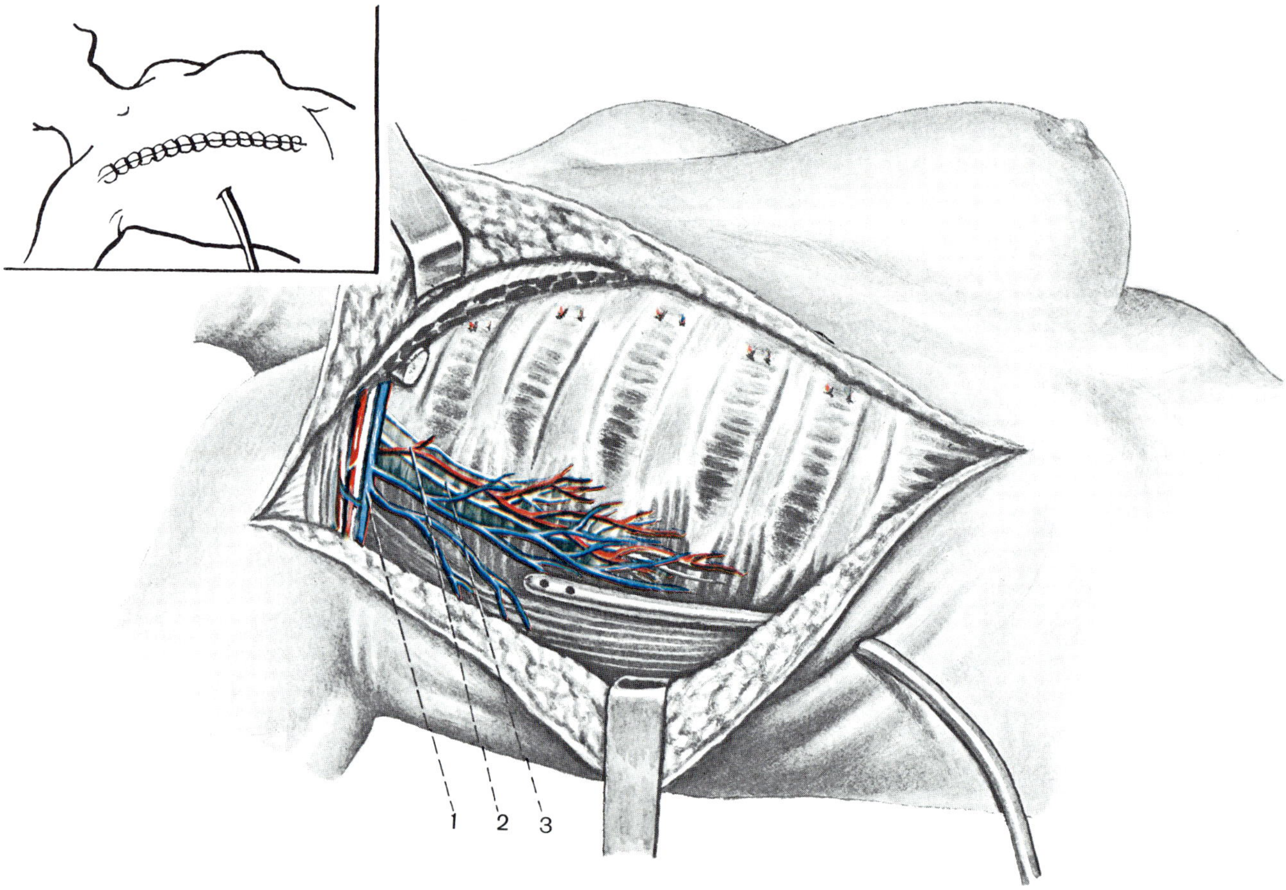

Fig. 79. Appearance of wound after removal of mammary gland. Closed postoperative wound and position of drain are represented schematically in inset. **1,** a. et v. subclavia. **2,** a. thoracalis lateralis. **3.** n. thoracicus longus.

OPERATIVE APPROACHES TO THE THORACIC ORGANS

The principal requirements adhered to in the choice of the operative approach are anatomical accessibility and practical possibility for carrying out all the stages of the operation by this approach. Besides the technical conveniences for performing the surgical intervention, one must also take into account the position of the patient on the operating table most desirable in each case. This is of vital importance in disorders of the respiratory and cardiovascular systems and in copious production of purulent sputum. In operations for purulent lesions of the lung (bronchiectases, abscess, etc.), for instance, it is expedient to use a posterior approach in which the patient is placed in a prone position. In severe disorders of the cardiovascular system an anterolateral approach is preferable.

Anterolateral approach. The patient lies on his healthy side or on his back. The skin incision is begun on a level with the third costal cartilage at a small distance from the parasternal line, continued caudally to the inferior border of the fourth rib, curved round the nipple, and extended along the fourth intercostal space to the posterior axillary line (Fig. 80).

With the skin, cellular tissue, superficial fascia, and the presternal part of the greater pectoral muscle cut, the fibers of the anterior serratus muscle are transected in the dorsal part of the wound. The border of the latissimus dorsi muscle protruding into the dorsal part of the incision is drawn laterally with a hook, or some of the fibers of this muscle are cut. After that the intercostal muscle, endothoracic fascia, and parietal pleura are cut with a scalpel. Through the opening thus made the intercostal space is cut the entire length of the skin wound with scissors. Care should be taken not to injure the internal thoracic vessels in the medial corner of the wound. When it is necessary to provide a wider access into the pleural cavity or the mediastinum, the third or fourth costal cartilage is cut, or, in some cases, the rib is resected.

The choice of the intercostal space for opening the pleural cavity is determined by the character of the forthcoming surgical intervention (Fig. 81).

Posterolateral approach. The patient lies face downward or in a semiprone position, inclined to the side opposite the one to be operated on. The incision of the soft tissues is begun at the level of the spinous process of the third or fourth thoracic vertebra and continued on the paravertebral line to the level of the scapular angle. It is then passed around and below the angle of the scapula and extended along the sixth rib to the anterior axillary line (Fig. 82).

All the tissues are cut successively down to the ribs: the inferior fibers of the trapezius muscles and the underlying inferior fibers of the greater rhomboid muscle in the vertical part; the latissimus dorsi muscle and part of the serratus muscle in the horizontal part. The pleural cavity is opened in the intercostal space or through the seat of the resected rib. To gain a wider operative approach, the necks of two adjacent ribs are resected and the intercostal ridges in which blood vessels are located are transected and ligated.

The posterior approach is rather damaging because a thick layer of muscles has to be cut and the ribs transected.

Lateral intercostal approach. In the lateral approach the thoracic cavity is opened along the fifth or sixth ribs from the paravertebral to the midclavicular line (Fig. 83). The lateral intercostal approach creates good conditions for manipulating in all parts of the thoracic cavity, from the cervical pleura to the diaphragm, and from the vertebral column to the sternum. The disadvantages of this approach are connected with the necessity for keeping the patient on his healthy side, due to which the purulent contents from the bronchi of the side operated on may seep into the bronchi of the healthy side.

Inferior anterolateral approach. The patient lies on his healthy side with a bolster placed under him. The skin incision is begun 3 cm below the xiphoid process and extended slightly caudally; then, at the level of the seventh intercostal space, it crosses the costal arch and extends in the seventh intercostal space to the angle of the scapula (Fig. 84). The skin, subcutaneous cellular tissue, and muscles are cut. A cut is made in the rectus abdominis muscle at the costal arch. The pleural cavity is opened in the seventh intercostal space, after which the costal arch is transected. The lower half of the pleural cavity may be opened widely with a wound retractor. The diaphragm is also incised in interventions on the cardia and esophagus.

Superior anterolateral approach. The patient lies on his side. The skin is cut in the second or third intercostal space between the parasternal line and the anterior axillary line. The pleural cavity is opened by cutting the skin and muscles successively, one after the other, and transecting the cartilages of the second and third ribs close to the sternal border.

Longitudinal sternotomy. The patient lies on his back. The midsternal skin incision is begun 2 to 3 cm above the manubrium and extended 3 to 4 cm below the xiphoid process (Figs. 85 and 86). The fascia and the sternal periosteum are cut, and the latter is slightly separated along the wound with a raspatory. In the lower part of the wound the linea alba is cut over a distance of a few centimeters. A tunnel is made between the posterior surface of the sternum and the sternal part of the diaphragm with a blunt instrument or the index

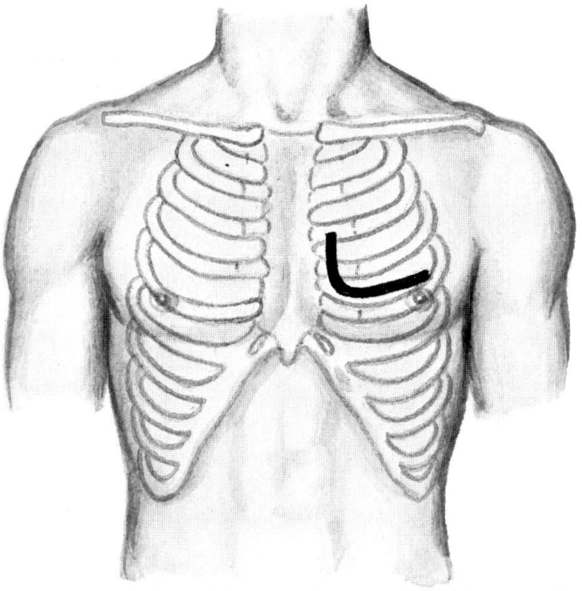

Fig. 80. Anterolateral intercostal approach with transection of costal cartilages. Line of incision is shown.

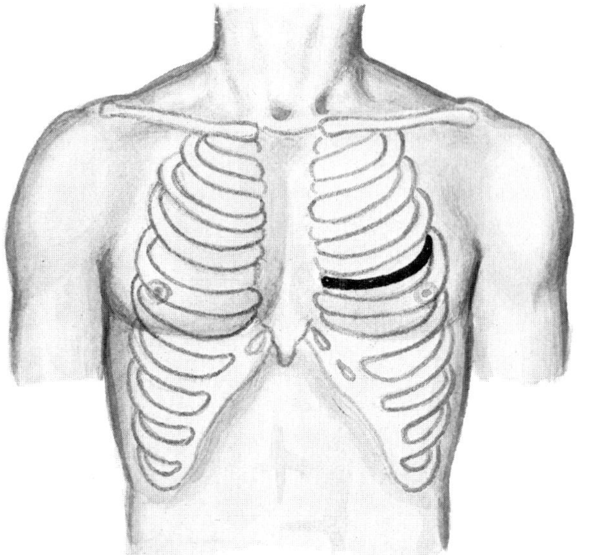

Fig. 81. Anterolateral intercostal approach without transection of costal cartilages. Line of incision is shown.

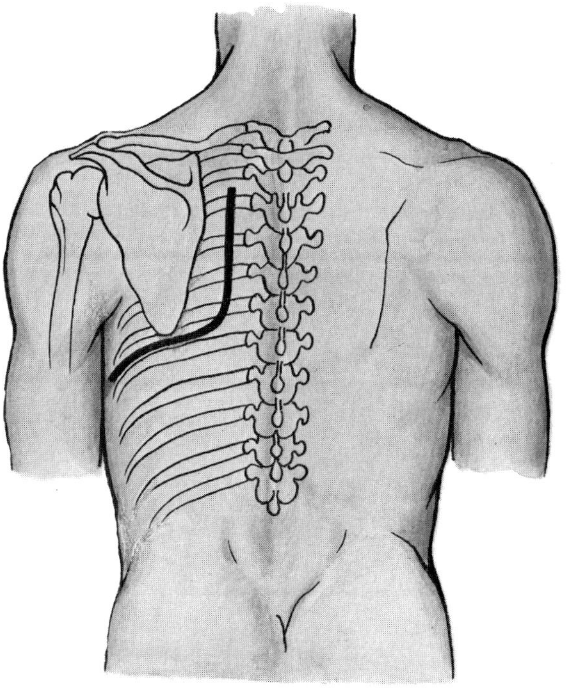

Fig. 82. Superior posterolateral operative approach to lung. Line of incision is shown.

finger, gaining entrance into the cellular space of the mediastinum. The sternum is raised with a hook; a sternotome is inserted into the wound; part of the sternum is then cut through on the midline; sternotomy is then continued step by step along the entire length of the bone (Fig. 87).

Careful hemostasis is essential after the sternum has been cut. Bleeding from the edges of the bone is arrested by rubbing sterile wax into them.

Longitudinal sternotomy ensures wide access to the organs of the anterior mediastinum (Fig. 88).

In children under 5 years of age the sternum may be cut with straight scissors. Longitudinal sternotomy may also be accomplished with Gigli's saw inserted behind the sternum directly along its posterior surface with long straight dressing forceps.

At the end of the operation the edges of the sternum are approximated and fastened with special clamps or strong sutures. With this purpose in view, five or six strong Lavsan sutures are stitched through the intercostal spaces or through the bone. To correct displacement of the sternal edges in the frontal plane, they may be

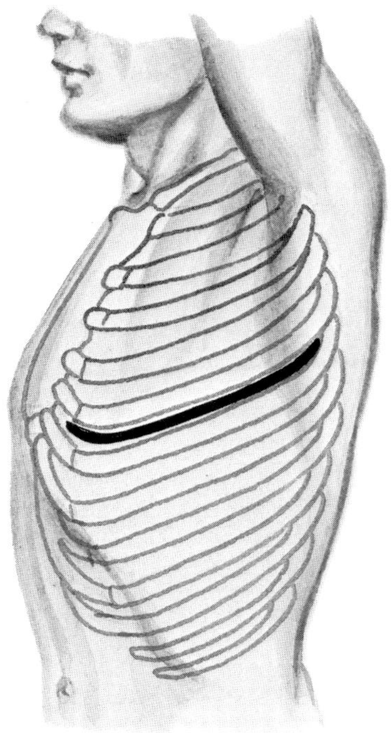

Fig. 83. Lateral intercostal approach. Line of incision is shown.

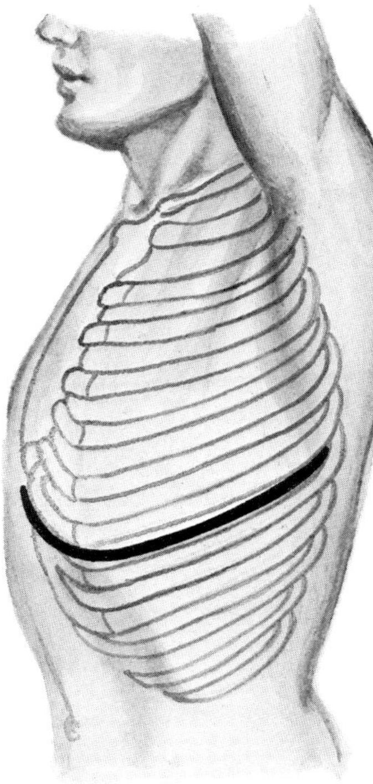

Fig. 84. Inferior anterolateral approach. Line of incision is shown.

fastened with two or four tantalum pins (Fig. 88).

Transverse transbipleural approach. The skin incision is made in the right fourth intercostal space from the midaxillary line across the sternum and extended in the corresponding intercostal space on the opposite side (Fig. 89). The internal thoracic vessels on each side are ligated and cut between the ligatures.

The periosteum of the sternum is cut, and the bone is then cut through across on this line with a sternotome or bone scissors (Fig. 90).

Bleeding from the edges of the sternum is arrested by rubbing sterile wax into them. The ends of the transected sternum are drawn apart together with the ribs by means of a wound retractor, exposing the heart and the roots of the lungs.

At the end of the operation the thoracic wall is closed with catgut blanket sutures passed through the intercostal spaces on both sides. The sternal perioseum is repaired with fine sutures (Fig. 91).

The transbipleural approach provides access to all parts of the heart and large vessels, but its use is restricted because it causes damage.

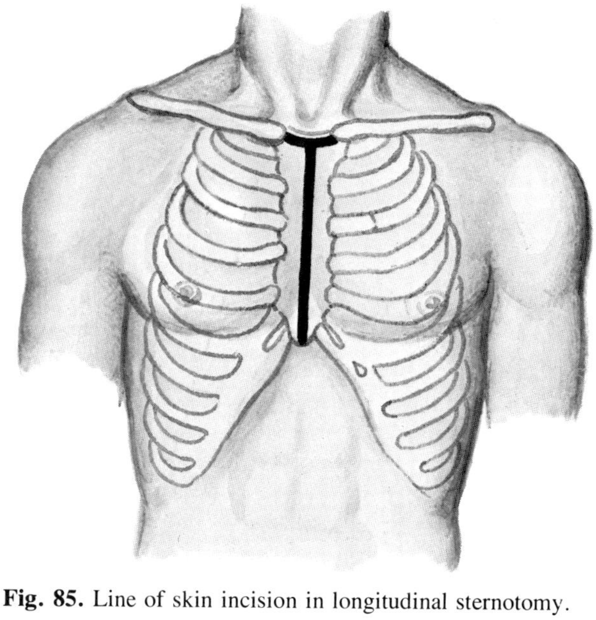

Fig. 85. Line of skin incision in longitudinal sternotomy.

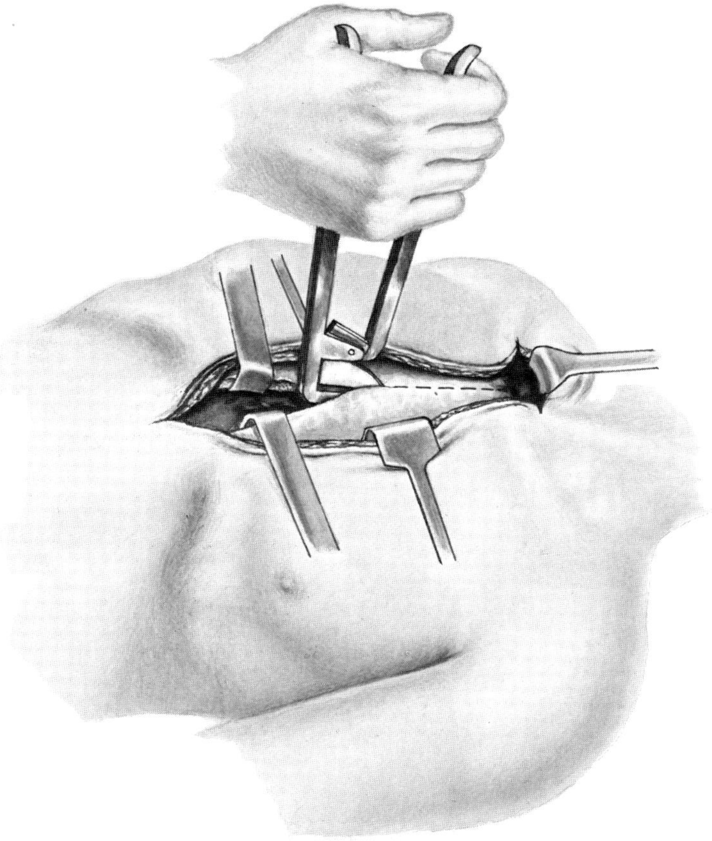

Fig. 86. Cutting the sternum with a sternotome.

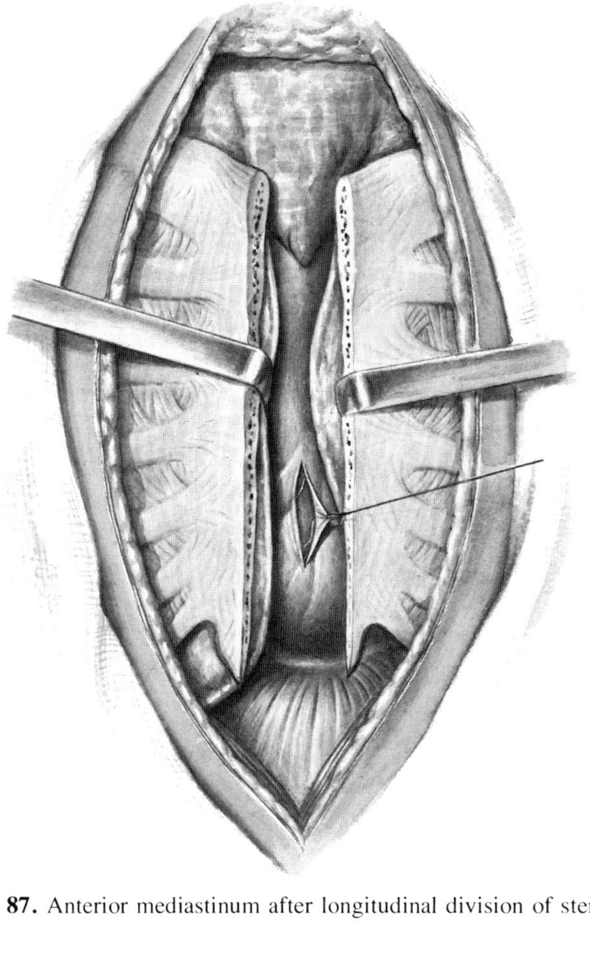

Fig. 87. Anterior mediastinum after longitudinal division of sternum.

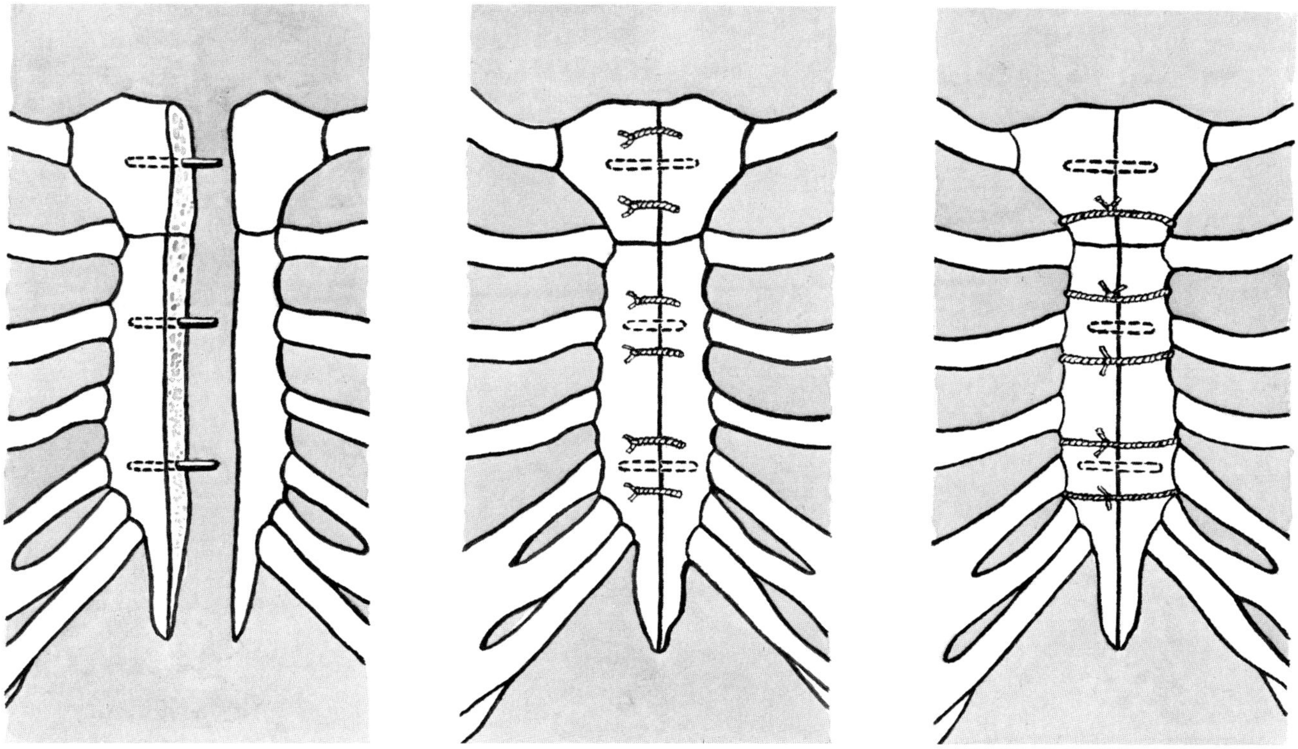

Fig. 88. Joining the edges of sternum after longitudinal sternotomy.

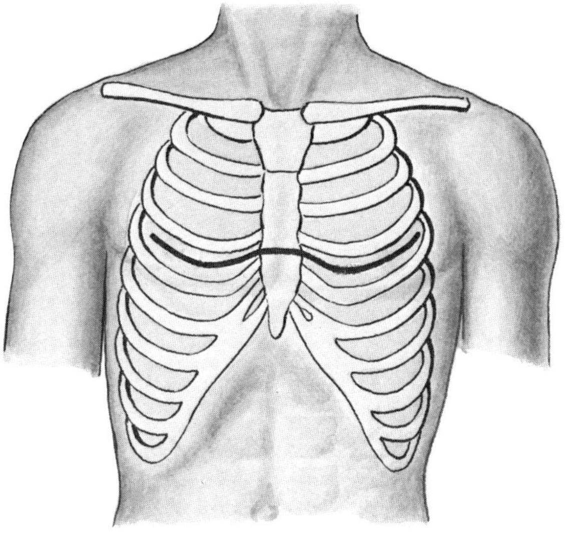

Fig. 89. Transbipleural approach. Line of incision is shown.

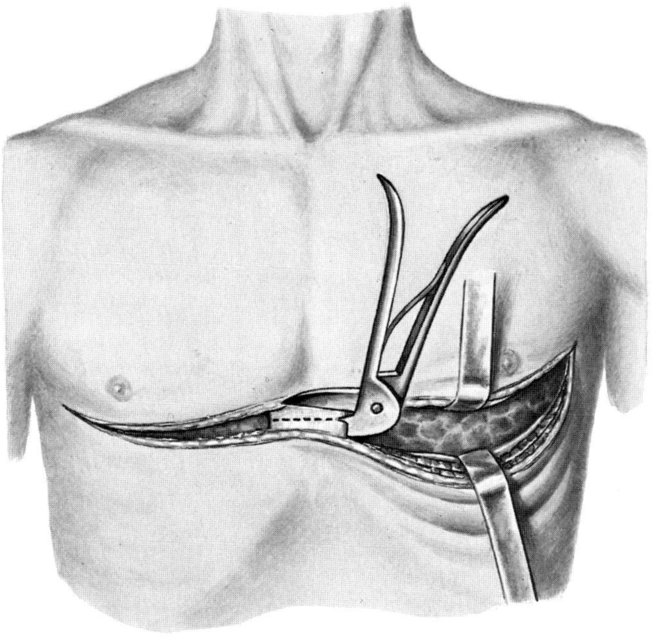

Fig. 90. Transbipleural approach with transection of sternum and intercostal spaces.

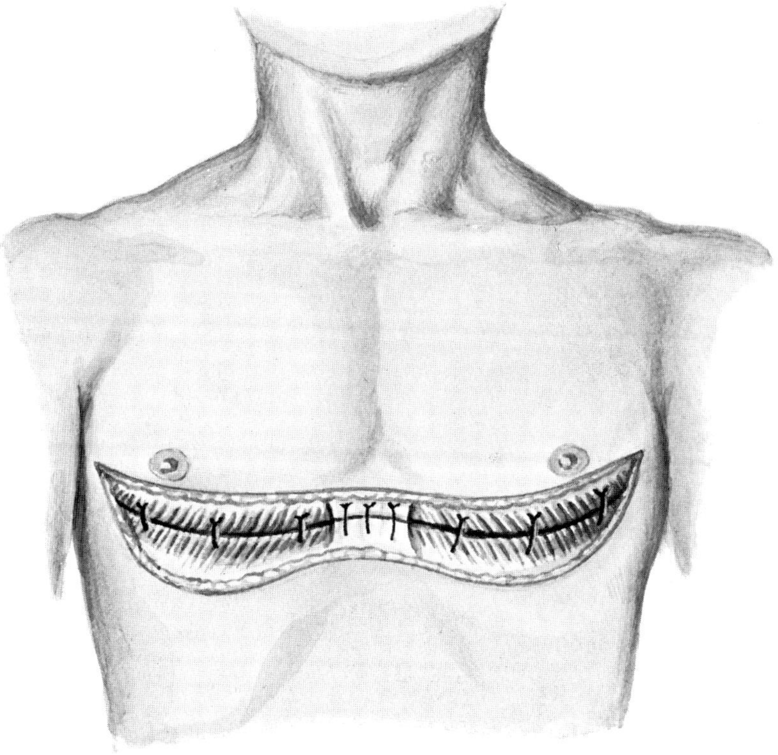

Fig. 91. Closure of wound after thoracotomy with transection of sternum.

OPERATIONS ON THE LUNGS

General problems of operative methods and techniques

PNEUMONOLYSIS

Pneumonolysis, a manipulation in which the lung is freed from adhesions, is usually the first and compulsory stage of any operation on the lungs. Depending on the degree to which these adhesions have developed and the intended volume of the resection, the method of pneumonolysis may vary.

In removal of a lung fused firmly with the parietal pleura over its entire surface, pleuropneumonectomy is preferable. Extrapleuropneumonolysis is attended with less bleeding; it prevents the rupture of subpleural caverns, caseous foci, and superficially located abcesses; and it makes it possible to remove the lung together with the sac of the empyema without opening the latter. If the adhesions are very thick and their division is accompanied by considerable bleeding, all the components of the pulmonary root should first be treated, and the root may then be removed after the major vessels and bronchus have been cut.

Similar tactics should be followed in partial resection of the lung. Middle and inferior lobectomy need not always be followed by total pneumonolysis on condition that the remaining superior lobe inflates well.

Pneumonolysis may be carried out by blunt or sharp techniques in accordance with the anatomical situation and the operative techniques called for. It is quite permissible to alternate extrapleural and intrapleural freeing of the lung. Adhesions are particularly strong and thick in the region of the diaphragm.

Partial resection of the diaphragm with its subsequent closure is admissible in a few such cases. Special caution is required during separation of the lung from the mediastinum. It is always desirable to separate the root of the lung intrapleurally.

INTRAOPERATIVE DIAGNOSIS

Intraoperative diagnosis is a compulsory component of any surgical intervention. It allows the extent, character, and topography of the pathological changes in the lung, pleura, and regional lymph nodes to be determined more precisely. When the pleural cavity is opened, the ability of different parts of the lung to inflate may be appraised with sufficient objectivity, and certain physiological tests may be carried out. In neoplasms of the lung, macroscopic diagnosis provides a complete picture of the dimensions of the tumorous node and its relationships with the surrounding tissues, bronchi, and large vessels; the state of the lymph nodes may be determined visually; in doubtful cases emergency biopsy is carried out. The great possibilities of bronchotomy should also be emphasized; in patients with benign endobronchial new growths it helps to determine the place where the tumor originated and to carry out economical resection.

Patients suffering from chronic, nonspecific suppurative diseases practically always have concordant inflammation of the bronchi of those segments that adjoin the irreparably diseased areas of the lung. Such bronchitic and bronchiectatic processes cannot always be recognized prior to operation.

To avoid the removal of normally functioning segments, it is necessary to make a close study of the macroscopic picture, which is appraised according to several indices. The vessels of the root of the diseased parts have a small diameter and are surrounded by scars and hyperplastic lymph nodes; the test for elasticity is drastically impaired (the parenchyma does not collapse on expiration and in aspiration of air through the intubation tube); the abnormal tissues are paler, and anthracosis is less marked than in the healthy parenchyma; a field of compact or nodular fibrosis and crepitation are easily determined by palpation. In tuberculosis of the lung, palpation of all the segments is of utmost importance; it helps to determine the boundaries of the tuberculoma, cavern, or infiltrate and also to detect focal changes unrecognized prior to the operation.

As a result of intraoperative diagnosis the planned volume of the resection may be either increased or reduced. Sometimes it is found that the operation cannot be performed.

It is unnecessary to inspect the lung during the operation if it is entirely involved in the pathological process and there is no room for doubt that it must be removed (bronchiectases, cysts, caverns, etc.). Of all the methods of intraoperative functional diagnosis, of utmost importance is the recording of pressure in the pulmonary artery prior to and after its clamping in order to decide whether or not pulmonectomy is permissible.

PREPARATION OF THE PULMONARY VESSELS AND BRONCHI

The basic principle consists in separate preparation of each component of the root of the lung. The succession in which the vessels and bronchi are exposed depends on a number of circumstances: the operative approach, anatomical conditions, peculiarities of the pathological process, the character of the operation to be performed, the amount of sputum expectorated, and the operative techniques.

In typical cases the arteries are prepared first so as to prevent the deposition of blood, after ligation of the pulmonary veins, in the part of the lung to be removed. In pulmonary cancer, however, it is preferable, contrary to this rule, to prepare the pulmonary veins first. According to some reports this may prevent the discharge into the blood of cancer cells during manipulations on the lung.

In purulent processes with the patient expectorating much sputum the bronchus may be given priority treatment. The bronchus, however, may be prepared later if reliable methods to block it are applied or separate intubation is carried out.

Preparation of the pulmonary vessels. In approach to the vessels from the ventral surface of the root of the lung, an incision is made in the mediastinal pleura overlying the artery or vein to be treated. The mediastinal cellular tissue is pushed off the vessel with a tampon. The adventitia is grasped with forceps and cut along the length of the vessel (Fig. 92). The flaps formed make it simple to separate the lateral and posterior walls of the vessel and to advance the dissector under it (Fig. 93). The vessel is tied with two ligatures, one of which is stitched through it or a suturing instrument, the vascular stump stitcher (УС), is used (Figs. 94 and 95).

When there are gross perivasal adhesions, it is necessary to resect some of the hyperplastic lymph nodes and cut the cicatricial sheath around the vessel. The further separation of the vessel meets with no difficulty. Preparation of the vessel together with the adhesions surrounding it is more difficult and hazardous, and less reliable, because the ligature may slip off the central stump.

Vessels with no signs of severe sclerosis may be sutured with an instrument of the УС type. The instrumental method is also convenient when the vessel is short or when it is in the depth of the wound.

When the strength of the sutures central to the tantalum staples causes doubt, a circular ligature may be applied.

Preparation of the bronchus. The bronchus is separated by means of scissors, dissector, and gauze tampons (Fig. 96). The peripheral part of the bronchus separated from the surrounding tissues is clamped. The central segment of the bronchus is stitched through at the edges on both sides with sutures that will serve first to hold the bronchus and then to close its stump (Fig. 97).

The bronchus is transected in such a way as to leave a stump no longer than 5 to 7 mm. The contents of the stump and the bronchi above are thoroughly aspirated with a soft catheter connected to an aspirator. The stump is closed by passing a fine round needle through all its layers. The sutures are applied so as to pull the membranous part evenly to the cartilaginous part of the bronchus. In doing so, it is convenient to place the central suture first, thus dividing the stump into two halves (Fig. 98). There should be as few as possible subsequent sutures, though sufficient in number for

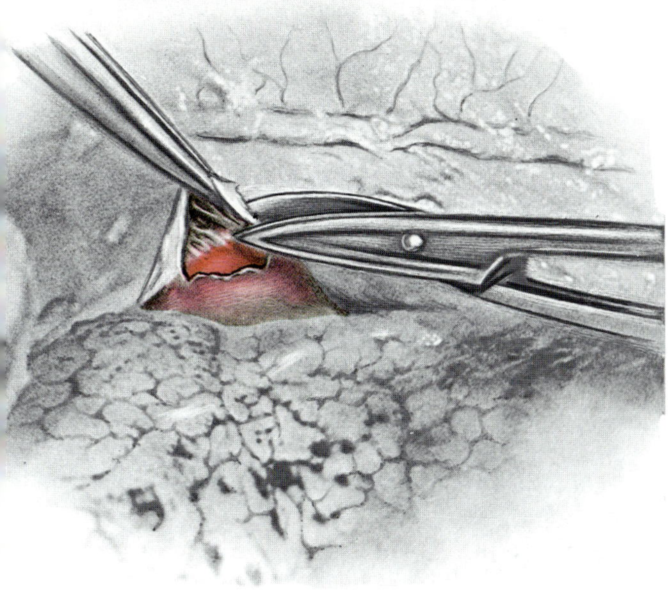

Fig. 92. Adventitia is cut and vessel exposed.

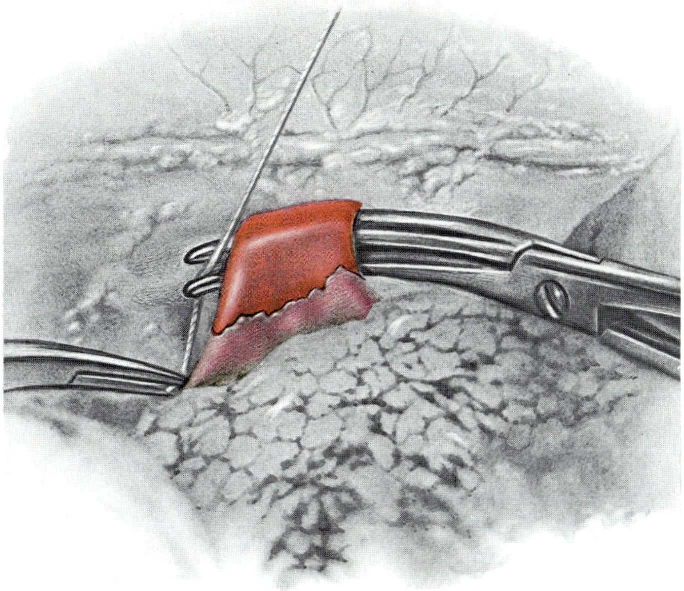

Fig. 93. Ligature is drawn under the vessel.

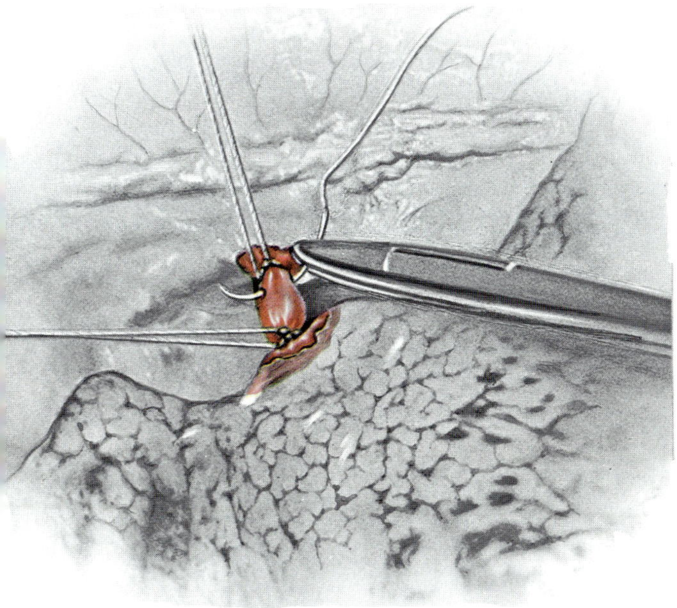

Fig. 94. Vessel is tied. Ligature for tying it is stitched through central end of vessel.

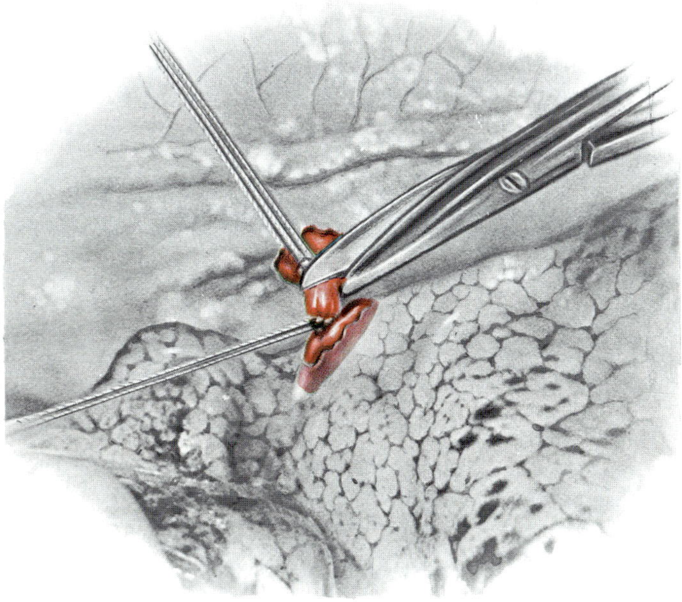

Fig. 95. Ligated vessel is transected.

making the stump airtight. The closure of the main bronchus, for instance, requires five to seven sutures. A properly closed stump has a crescent shape (Fig. 99).

Any fine threads that do not untwist may be used for suturing. The sutures are tied to draw the walls of the bronchus close together, but without applying force. The stump is covered with mediastinal pleura or the surrounding pulmonary tissue (see Fig. 99). In the preparation of a segmental bronchus, in children in particular, it is sufficient to stitch it through and tie it with a circular ligature.

When the wall of the resected bronchus is neither sclerosed nor inflamed, the stump may be closed by means of the УО stitching instrument; in children the vessel-stitching (УС) instrument suits the purpose.

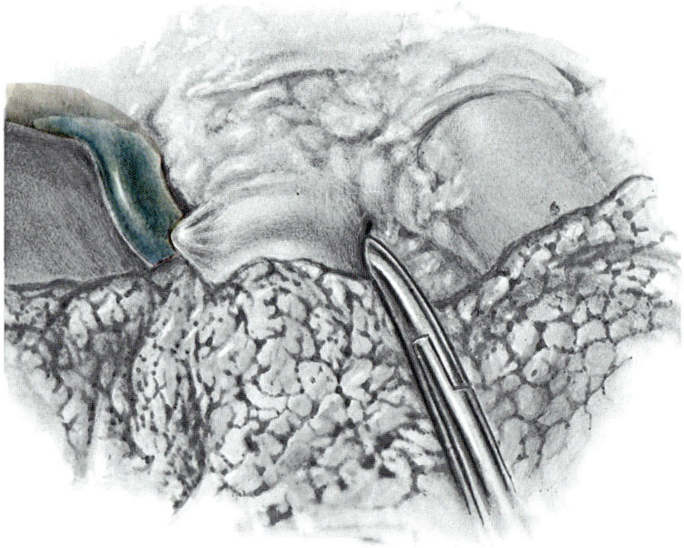

Fig. 96. Bronchus is separated.

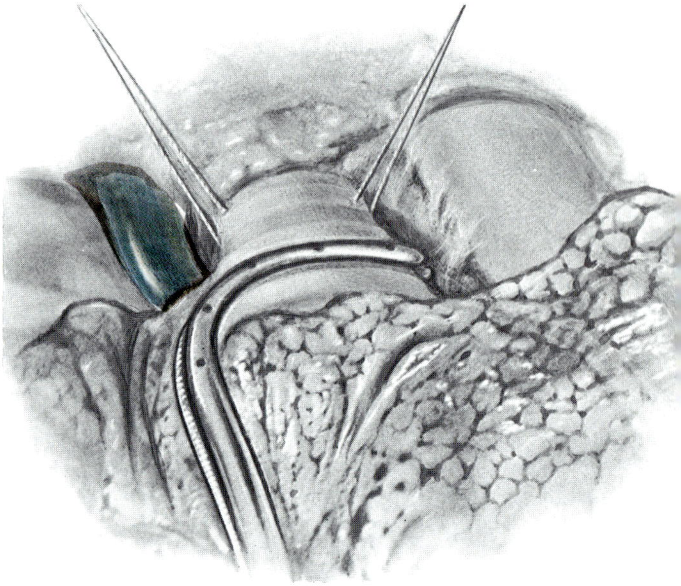

Fig. 97. Traction sutures are applied to bronchus.

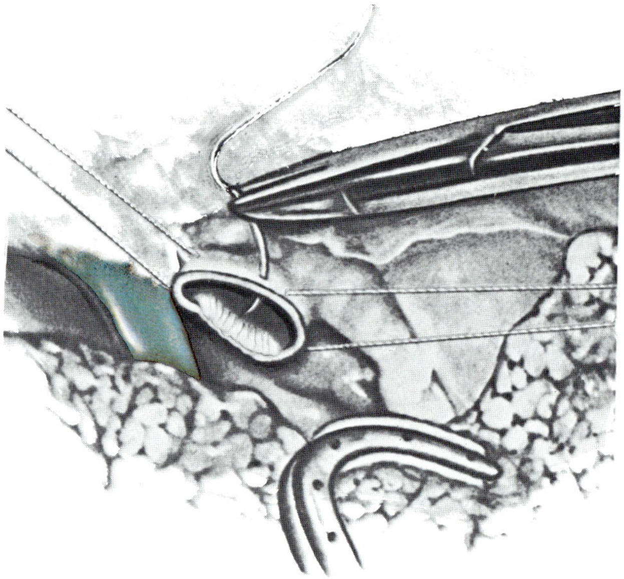

Fig. 98. Stump of transected bronchus is sutured.

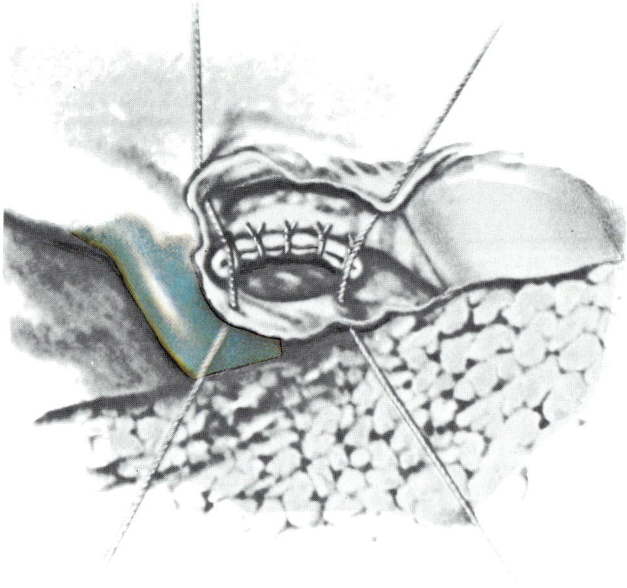

Fig. 99. Bronchial stump has been sutured. Mediastinal pleura is being stitched to it.

SEPARATION OF THE LOBES AND SEGMENTS

In lobectomy the lobes are usually separated along the interlobar fissures by means of scissors and gauze tampons. If the fissures are not clearly defined or if they are grown over, this method of separation is practically impossible without causing damage to the parenchyma. One of the following three manipulations is resorted to in such cases.

1. The pulmonary parenchyma is divided between clamps applied to the edge of the lobe that is to be resected and is atelectatic after transection of the bronchus; the tissue of the remaining parenchyma is stitched through with interrupted or figure-of-eight sutures.

2. A tunnel is made under the grown-over or poorly discernible interlobar fissure; the blade of a large stitching instrument is advanced into the tunnel. One or two cartridges of tantalum staples are stitched through the remaining tissue, and the part to be removed is cut off.

3. The lobe to be removed is drawn up by the clamp placed on the peripheral end of the transected bronchus, and the adhesions with the remaining lobe are separated by the sharp and blunt techniques.

Segments should always be removed strictly according to anatomical boundaries from the root to the periphery, drawing the end of the transected segmental bronchus upward. There are two methods for separating the segments from each other.

In the first ("the two-finger technique") the lung is raised on the index finger of the left hand in such a way that the part to be removed is on the palm surface, and the segments to be preserved are on the back surface. In other words, the parenchyma of the lung is doubled over the intended boundary of the resection. This makes it a simple matter to palpate and clamp the intersegmental vascular connections. After these vessels have been prepared separately, the segments intended for removal are freed from the surrounding parenchyma.

In the second method ("the tapping technique") the bronchial stump of the segments to be resected is pulled with the left hand while the line dividing the remaining segments from the part to be removed is tapped with a tight gauze tampon held with the right hand.

Both methods are actually used in practice. If segmental resection is carried out properly, bleeding is scarce and air does not escape from the wound in the lung. Parenchymal hemorrhage is arrested with tampons moistened in hot physiological saline solution. All small bleeding vessels should be ligated. A small escape of air, the intensity of which is assessed under a layer of fluid poured into the pleural cavity, is no reason for suturing the lung. Small ruptured bronchial branches should also be ligated.

It is a matter of strict individual approach whether or not to suture the wound in the lung. Suturation of the wound always reduces the volume of the lung and aggravates its aeration. At the same time, if the parenchyma is not sufficiently airtight, serious complications may develop after segmental resections. This is why to make the wound reliably airtight after the removal of one or two segments the tissue of the remaining segments may be stitched through with the YO stitching instrument. When there is a considerable escape of air, the edges of the pulmonary wound are sutured. If this causes gross deformity of the parenchyma and reduces its volume, it would be inexpedient to preserve it. In these circumstances lobectomy is preferable to segmentectomy.

It is essential to test whether or not the bronchial stump and parenchyma are airtight after any type of pulmonary resection. Warm physiological saline solution is poured into the pleural cavity, and the remaining segments are inflated by means of the sac of an anesthetic machine and held in a state of inspiration for 10 to 15 seconds. This makes it possible to define exactly the places where much air escapes and eliminate such leaks. In small ruptures of the pulmonary tissue occurring after pneumonolysis it is best not to suture them but to grasp their edges with Luer's fenestrated forceps and then tie them with a circular ligature.

DRAINAGE OF THE PLEURAL CAVITY

After removal of a lung it is always advisable to drain the pleural cavity with one tube introduced into the supradiaphragmatic space. The end of the drain fitted with a valve by Petrov's technique is lowered into a flask containing an antiseptic solution (Fig. 100). This drain provides for the timely detection of intrapleural hemorrhage and prevents hemothorax clotting and displacement of the mediastinum toward the healthy lung.

After partial lung resection the pleural cavity is drained with two tubes. The upper drain is introduced into the second intercostal space in front or in the axillary region. Inside, the end of the drain is fastened to the dome of the thoracic cavity with a thin catgut suture. The lower drain is introduced on the posterior axillary line in the eighth or ninth intercostal space and fitted along the spine to the level of the root of the lung (see Fig. 100). The drain may also reach the cervical pleura.

Following segmental resections, one of the drains may be brought up directly to the postresection surface of the lung, due to which the air escaping from it will not spread to the cervical pleura. The upper and lower drains are joined by means of a T-tube with the source of a constant vacuum. When the lung is sealed off properly, continuous aspiration at a negative pressure of 30 to 40 mm Hg is carried on. If there is noticeable leakage of air or interpleural hemorrhage persists, aspiration is either temporarily stopped or conducted at a pressure of 5 to 10 mm Hg. With the postoperative period following an uneventful course, the drains are removed on the second or third day.

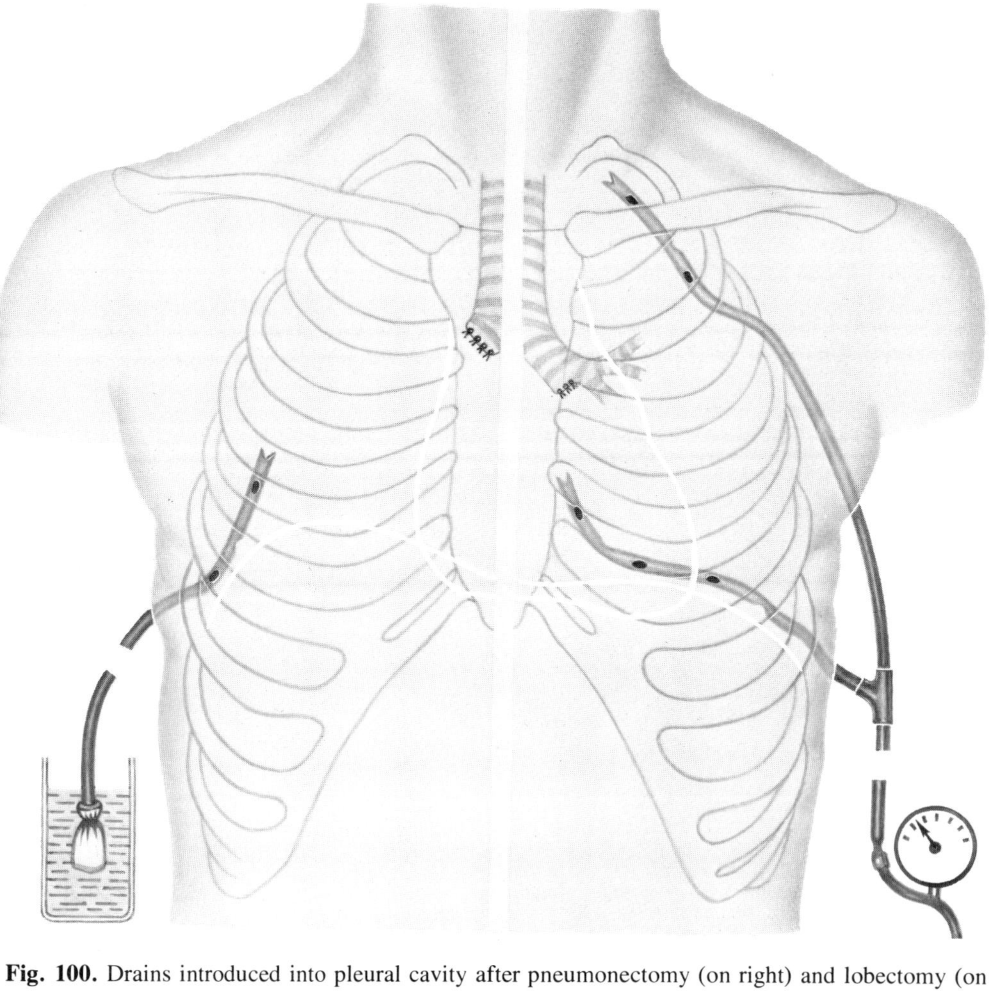

Fig. 100. Drains introduced into pleural cavity after pneumonectomy (on right) and lobectomy (on left).

Resection of the lungs

OPERATIONS ON THE RIGHT LUNG

PNEUMONECTOMY

The pleural cavity is opened through a lateral approach in the fifth or through a posterior approach in the sixth intercostal space. The lung is freed from adhesions along the entire length, and the pulmonary ligament is dissected. In total adhesions, particularly in the region of the diaphragm, pneumonolysis is conducted at the end of the operation. In case of a sudden hemorrhage, however, the root of the lung should be freed on all sides before its components are separated.

The mediastinal pleura is cut in the region of the

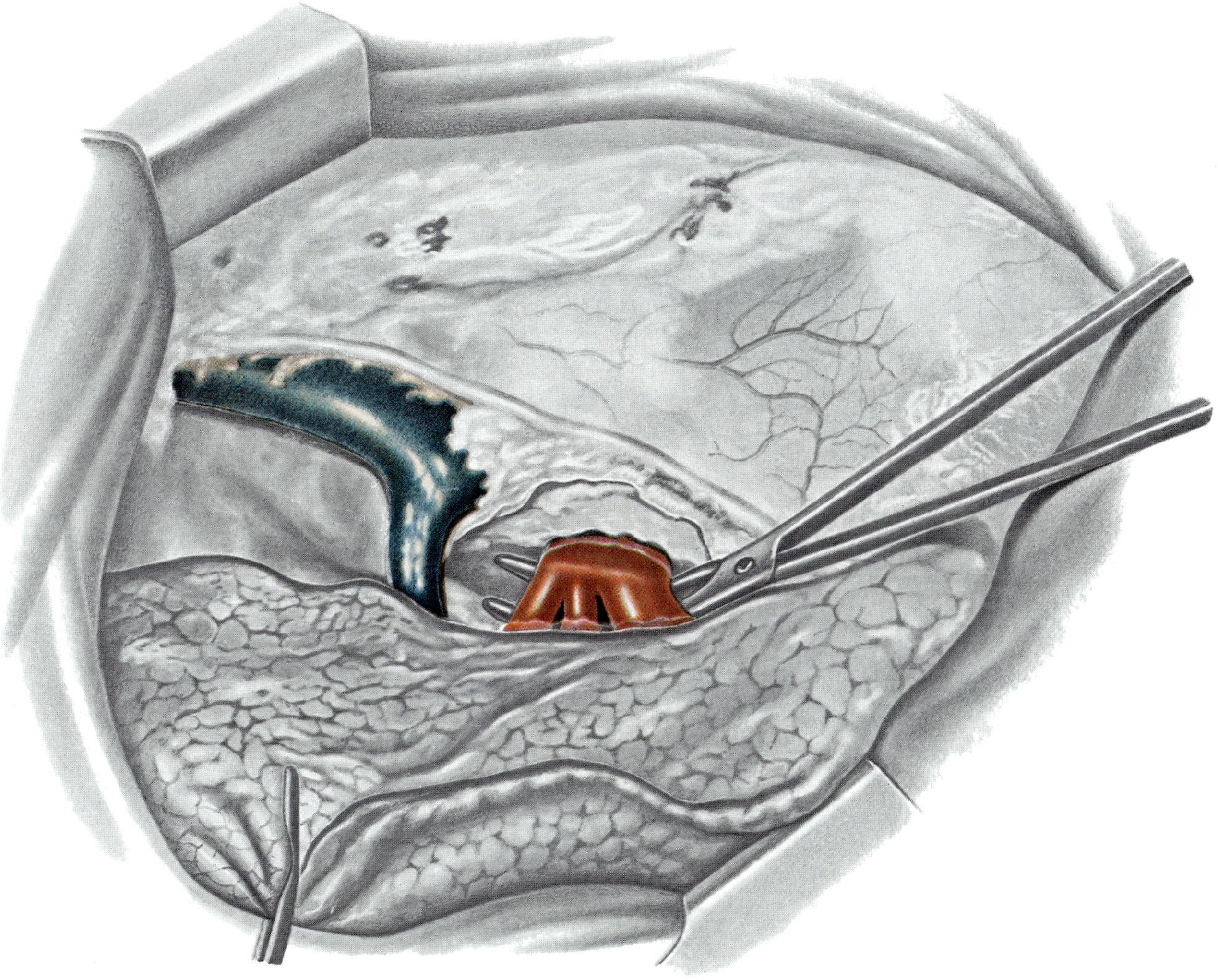

Fig. 101. Dissector is advanced under right pulmonary artery.

pulmonary artery dorsal and parallel to the phrenic nerve. The anterior trunk of the pulmonary artery is found, and with it as a landmark, the right pulmonary artery is freed from the mediastinal cellular tissue by the acute and blunt techniques. To make the manipulations easier, the superior vena cava is moved medially with a tampon and the superior pulmonary vein caudally. A dissector (Fig. 101) or Fedorov's clamp is brought under the pulmonary artery, which is then treated by the ligature method or by means of the УС instrument.

Then the superior pulmonary vein is separated and prepared for the greatest possible distance (Fig. 102).

To gain access to the inferior pulmonary vein, the inferior lobe is drawn aside laterally. If there are no gross adhesions, the vein is separated with a finger or dissector, treated by the ligature or instrumental method, and divided (Fig. 103). The right main bronchus is separated to the level of the trachea. Its peripheral segment is grasped with Fedorov's clamp; traction sutures are applied to the central segment, and the bronchus is cut. Its stump is closed with interrupted sutures or by means of the УО instrument (Fig. 104).

The mechanical suture is used only if the bronchial walls are soft, yielding, and not inflamed. The stump is

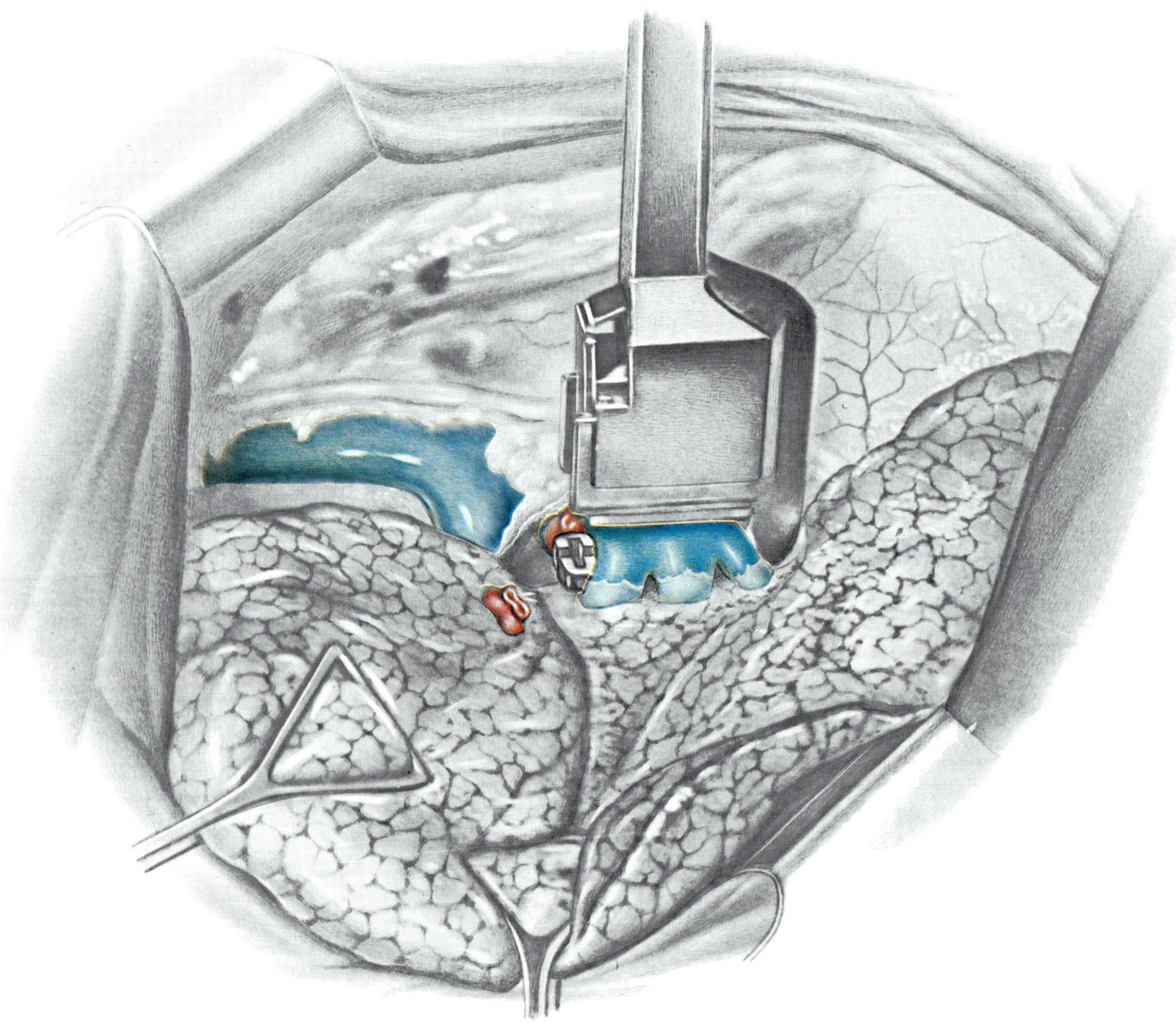

Fig. 102. Superior pulmonary vein is stitched through with УС instrument.

covered with mediastinal pleura or the arch of the azygos vein (Fig. 105).

Intrapericardial ligation of vessels in extended pneumonectomy. In some patients the inflammatory infiltration, scars, tumor, or the pathologically altered lymph nodes block access to the vessels of the root of the lung completely. The bronchus in such cases may be intact. Intrapericardial ligation of the vessels is thus made expedient. It should be noted, however, that the indications for this intervention must be well grounded. The pericardium is opened for a distance of 6 to 8 cm dorsal and parallel to the phrenic nerve. The pericardial flaps are drawn aside by the traction ligatures. The inferior pulmonary vein is found on the dorsal wall of the pericardium where the superior vena cava drains into the right atrium. Just like the superior pulmonary vein and pulmonary artery, the inferior pulmonary vein is situated mesopericardially. The pericardium covering it is transected (Fig. 106). The vein is carefully separated with scissors and a dissector, its dorsal wall protected from injury, and then treated by the ligature method (Fig. 107).

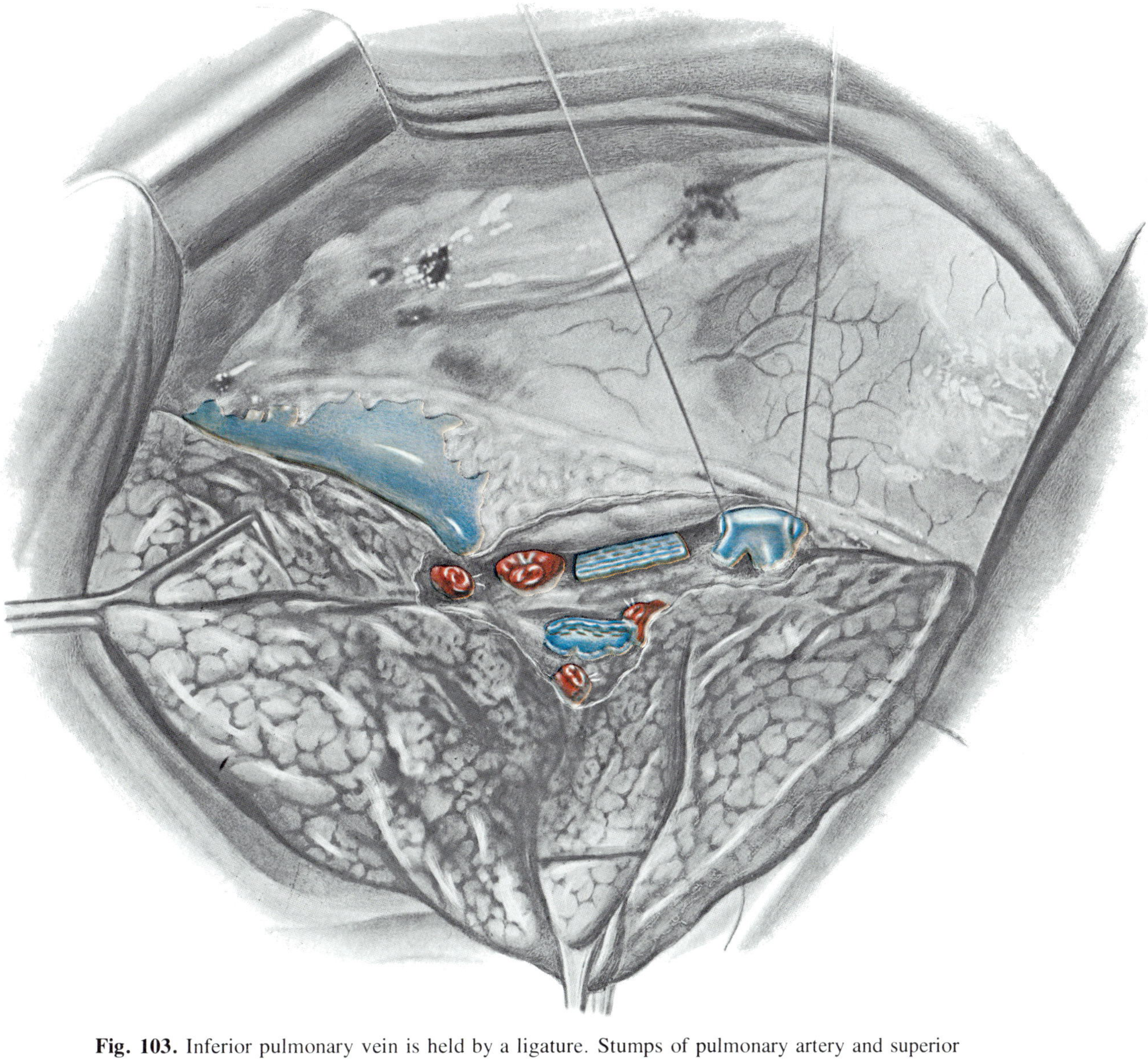

Fig. 103. Inferior pulmonary vein is held by a ligature. Stumps of pulmonary artery and superior pulmonary vein are visible.

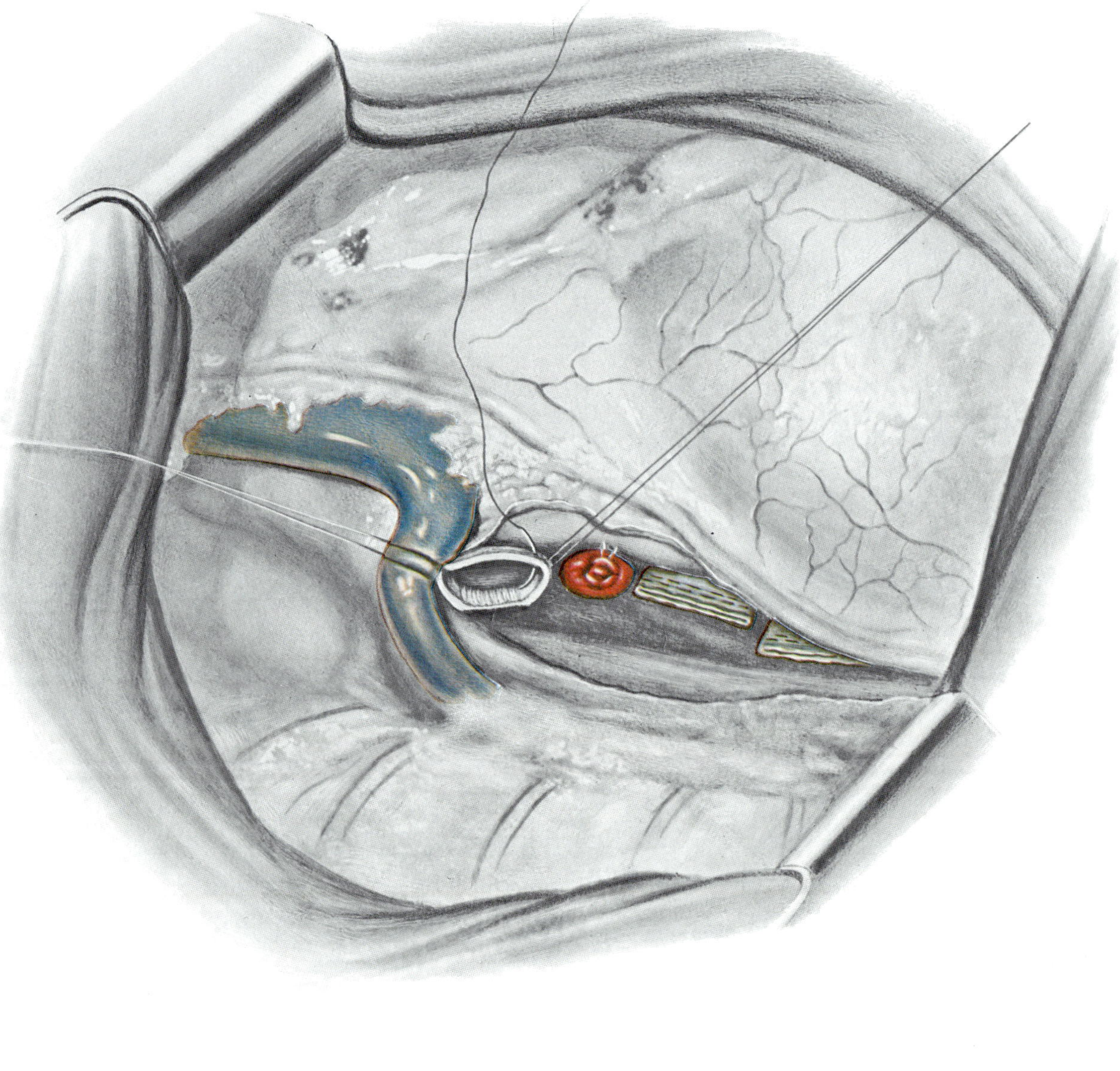

Fig. 104. Stump of main bronchus is sutured. Left lung has been removed. Stumps of vessels are seen.

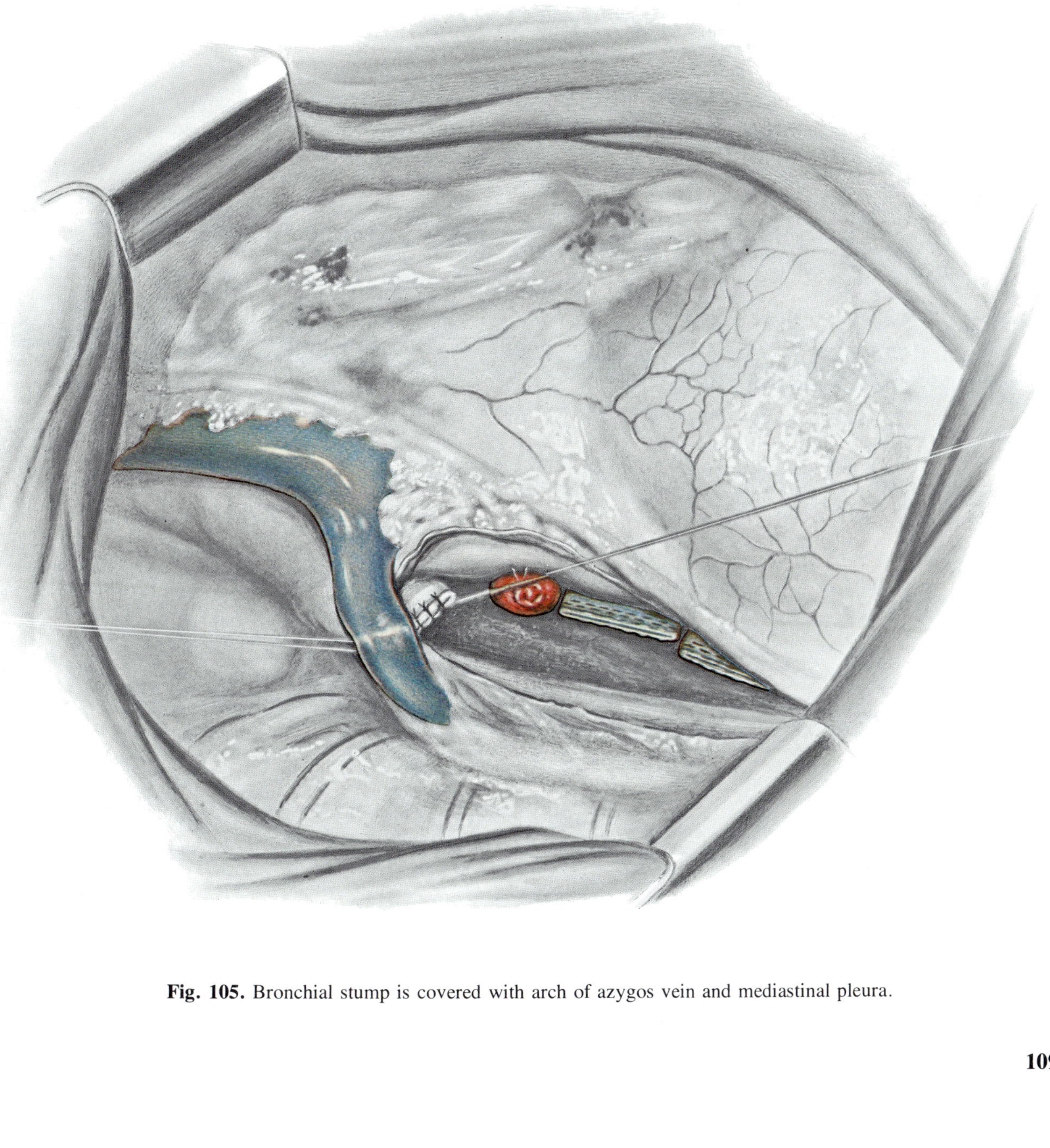

Fig. 105. Bronchial stump is covered with arch of azygos vein and mediastinal pleura.

The superior pulmonary vein located slightly more cranially is prepared in a similar manner (Fig. 108). With both pulmonary veins cut, a convenient approach is obtained to the right pulmonary artery, which is often fused with the superior vena cava and covered by it. The latter is displaced medially, but care must be taken not to occlude its lumen. After the pericardial fold is cut, the pulmonary artery is treated by the ligature method (Fig. 109).

This sequence in the preparation of the vessels is dictated in the first place by considerations pertaining to oncology and secondly by the fact that it is difficult to

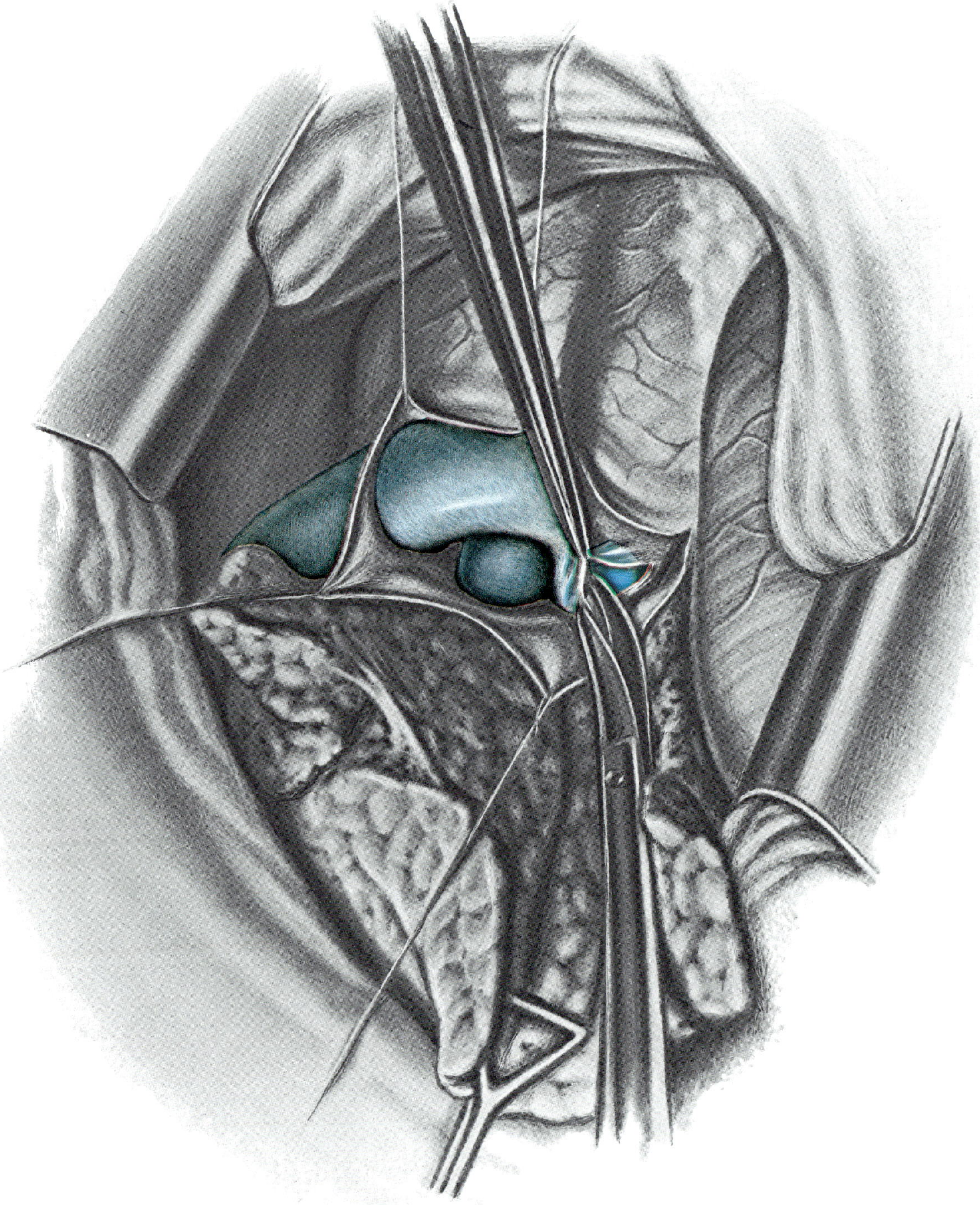

Fig. 106. Dorsal sheet of pericardium covering inferior pulmonary vein is cut.

gain access to the pulmonary artery before cutting the pulmonary veins. In some cases the intrapericardial vascular segments are very short. To make their treatment easier, an instrument for applying a linear vascular suture, the УС, may be employed.

When preparation of the vessels has been completed, the bronchus is divided and sutured. The lung is removed with part of the pericardium. The defect formed is closed with several sutures so as to prevent the heart from prolapsing into the pleural cavity. Openings are left between the sutures on the pericardium.

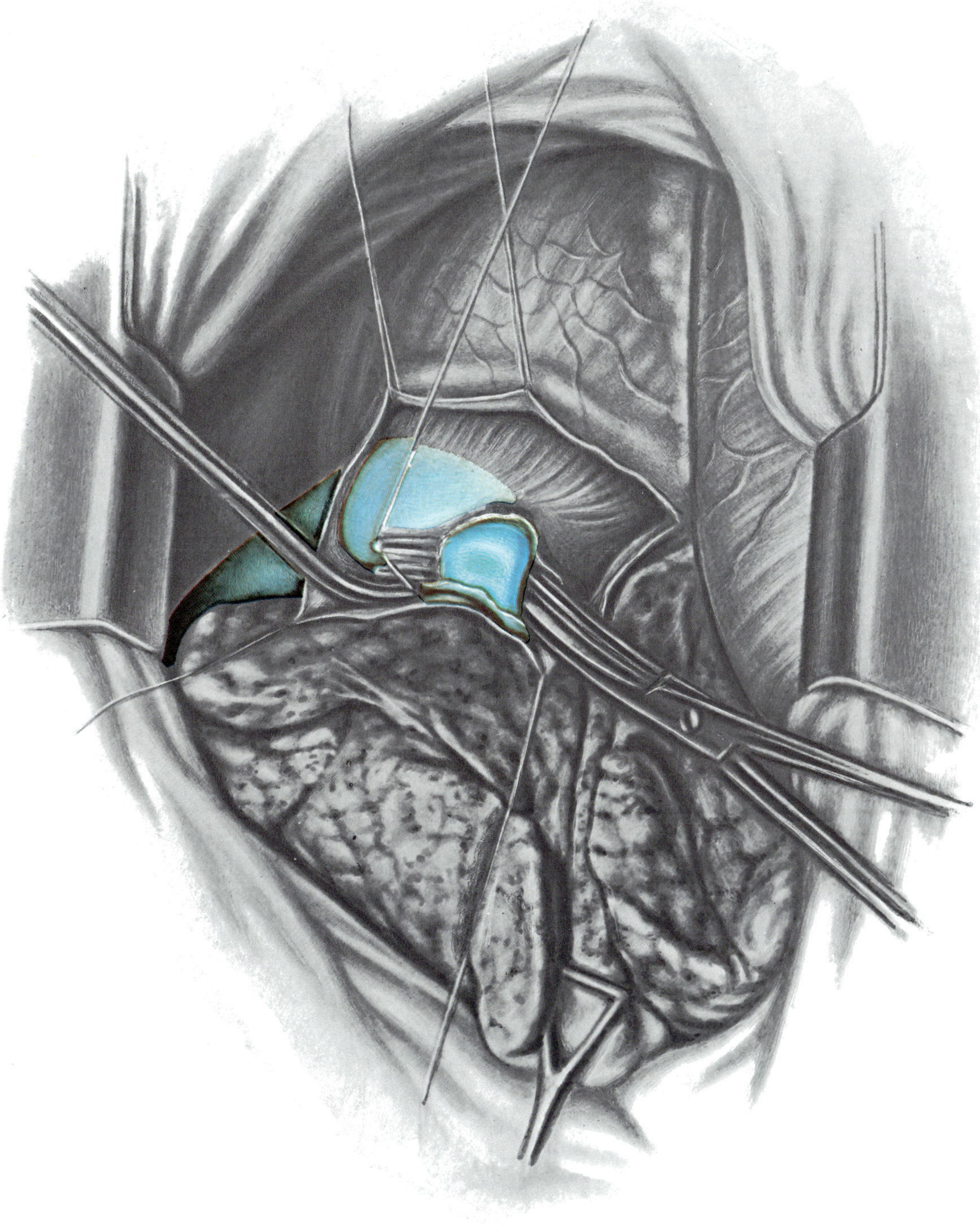

Fig. 107. Ligatures are brought under inferior pulmonary vein.

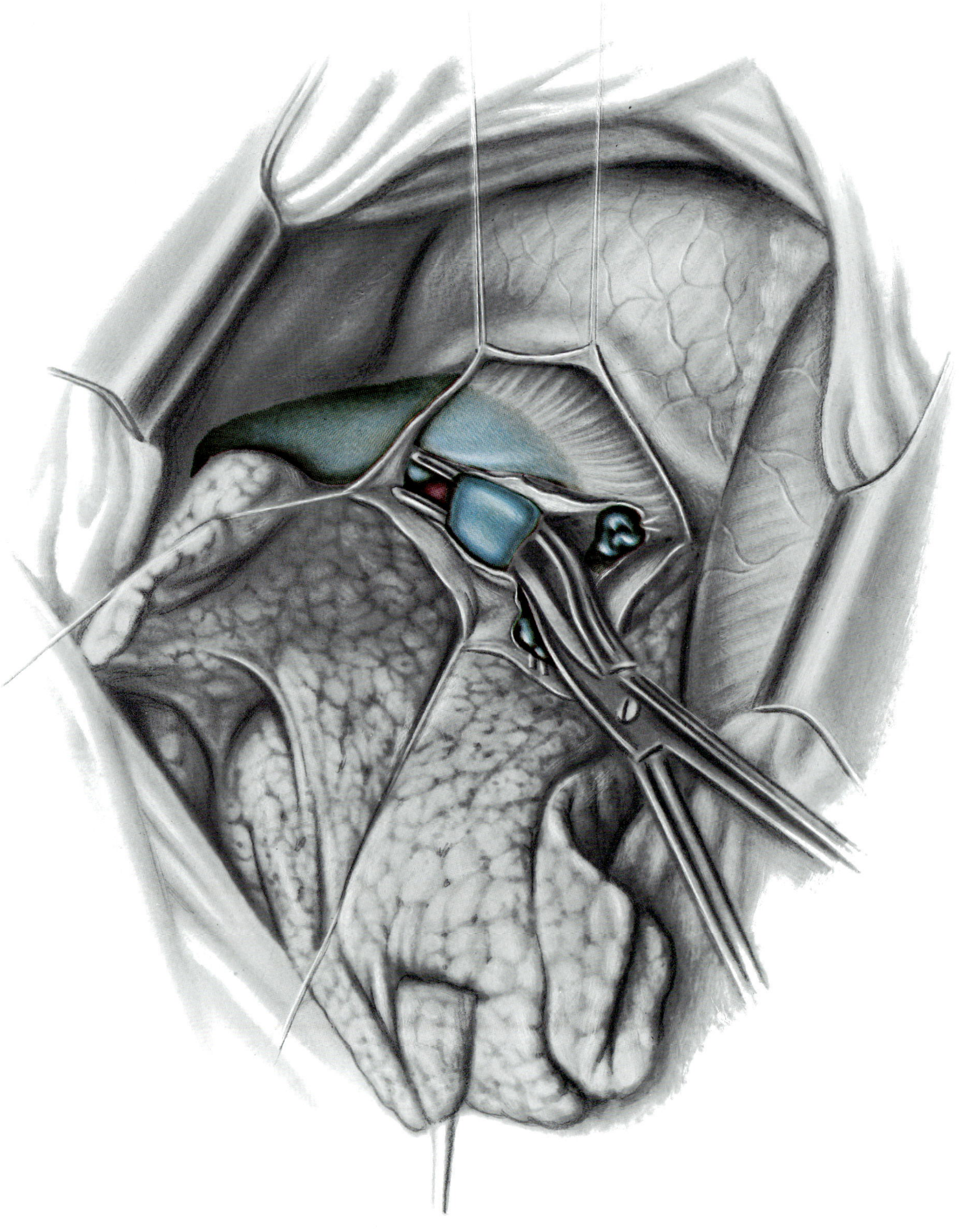

Fig. 108. A dissector is brought under superior pulmonary vein.

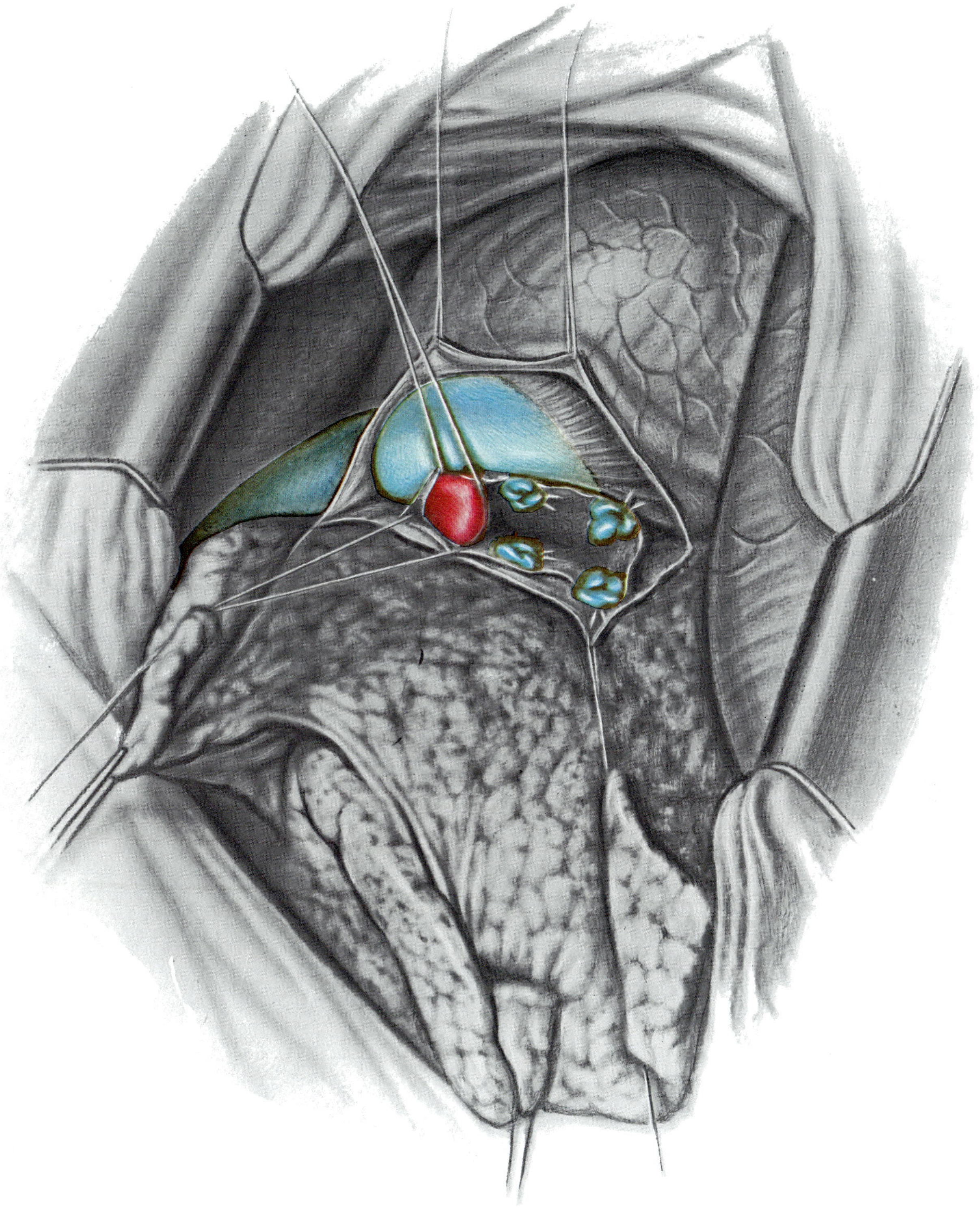

Fig. 109. Right pulmonary artery is ligated. Both pulmonary veins have been transected.

The pleural cavity is opened by a lateral approach in the fifth intercostal space.

The superior lobe is freed from the adhesions. The mediastinal pleura is cut dorsal and parallel to the phrenic nerve over the root of the lung. In cases with cancer, $V_{1,2,3}$ are prepared first, while in all other cases it is advisable to separate the anterior trunk of the pulmonary artery in the first place.

A_{1+2}, forming the anterior trunk of the pulmonary artery, is situated in the cranial part of the root of the lung between the arch of the azygos vein and the superior pulmonary vein. It is easier to prepare this artery (Fig. 110) when the superior lobe is drawn aside laterally. A_{1+2} is treated by the ligature method or with the УC instrument.

The superior pulmonary vein is exposed by the blunt and sharp techniques. The branch related to the middle lobe is scrupulously identified and protected from damage. The common $V_{1,2,3}$ trunk is prepared and treated by the ligature method or is stitched through with the УC instrument (Fig. 111).

After A_{1+2} and $V_{1,2,3}$ have been cut, access to the superior lobar bronchus is free. Since the bronchus is very short, it is separated toward the periphery to the site of its division into segmental branches. The bronchial arteries are ligated separately whenever possible. The dorsal wall of the bronchus is prepared, exercising caution in regard to the adjacent A_2. Traction sutures are applied to the bronchus, and a clamp to its caudal segment. The bronchus is divided (Fig. 112). Its stump

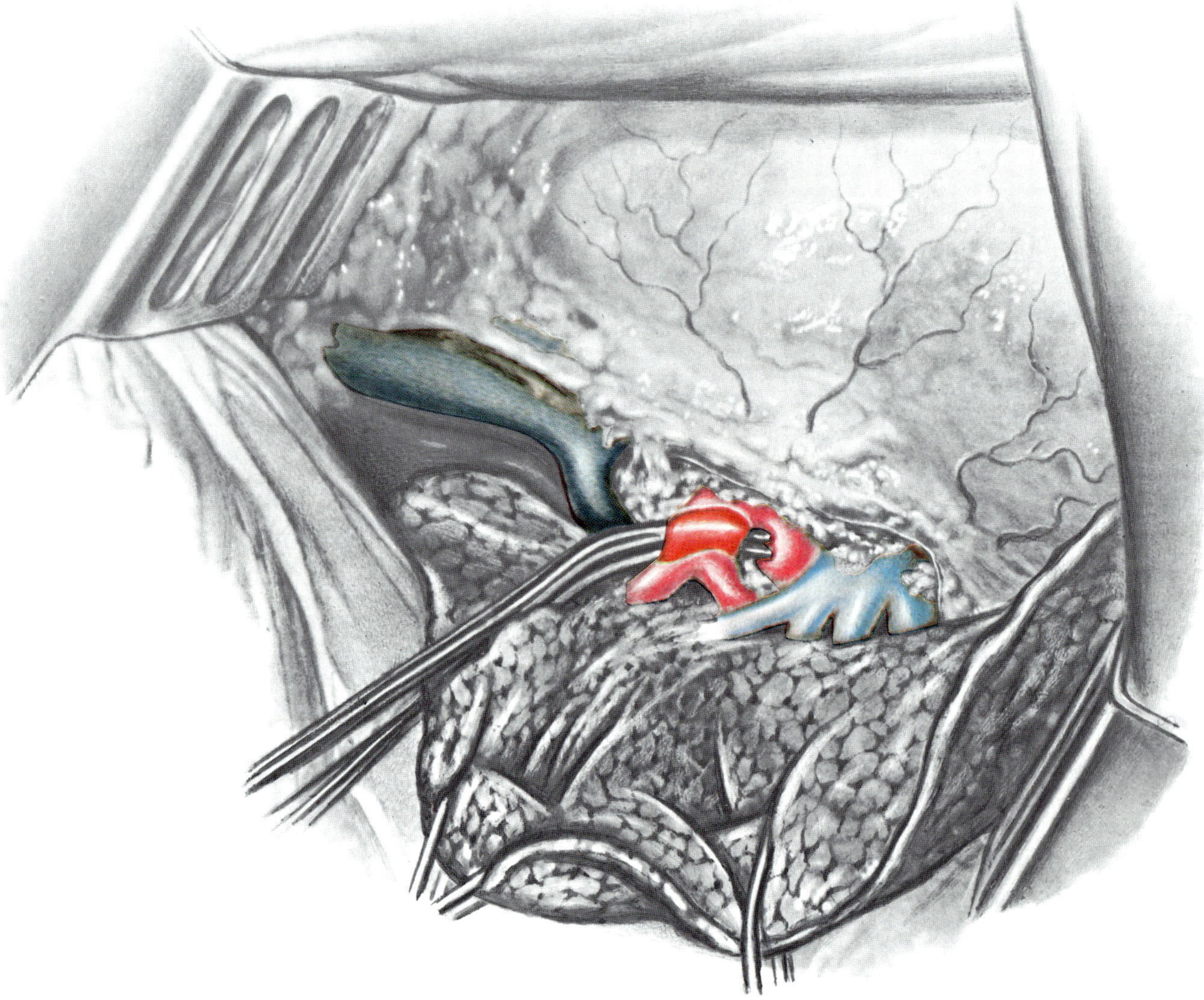

Fig. 110. Separation of anterior trunk of pulmonary artery.

is sutured by hand and covered with a graft of mediastinal pleura or by the neighboring tissues.

The superior lobe is moved in the lateral caudal direction, and A_2 is found and treated by the ligature method (Fig. 113). In some cases it is possible to ligate this artery immediately after the veins have been prepared, but sometimes it is easier to separate it after cutting the bridges between S_2 and S_6. The tactics are determined by the concrete circumstances of the operation.

As a rule, the superior and inferior lobes are connected by a small parenchymal bridge between S_2 and S_6; after clamps are applied, this bridge is dissected or stitched through with the УО instrument. When the superior lobe is intimately connected with the middle one, they are separated by means of the УО instrument. After trial inflation of the middle lobe the border of its resection is marked out, and the blades of the УО are advanced from the side of the main interlobar fissure in the direction of the root of the middle lobe (Fig. 114). To prevent the middle lobe from shrinking, it is necessary to avoid crimping its parenchyma during stapling. When the bridge is large, it is best to employ two cartridges of УО staples. If the superior and middle lobes are sufficiently demarcated by the smaller interlobar fissure, division may be achieved with clamps or by manipulations of the type of segmentectomy. The places where air escapes from the wound in the lungs are closed with interrupted Halsted sutures.

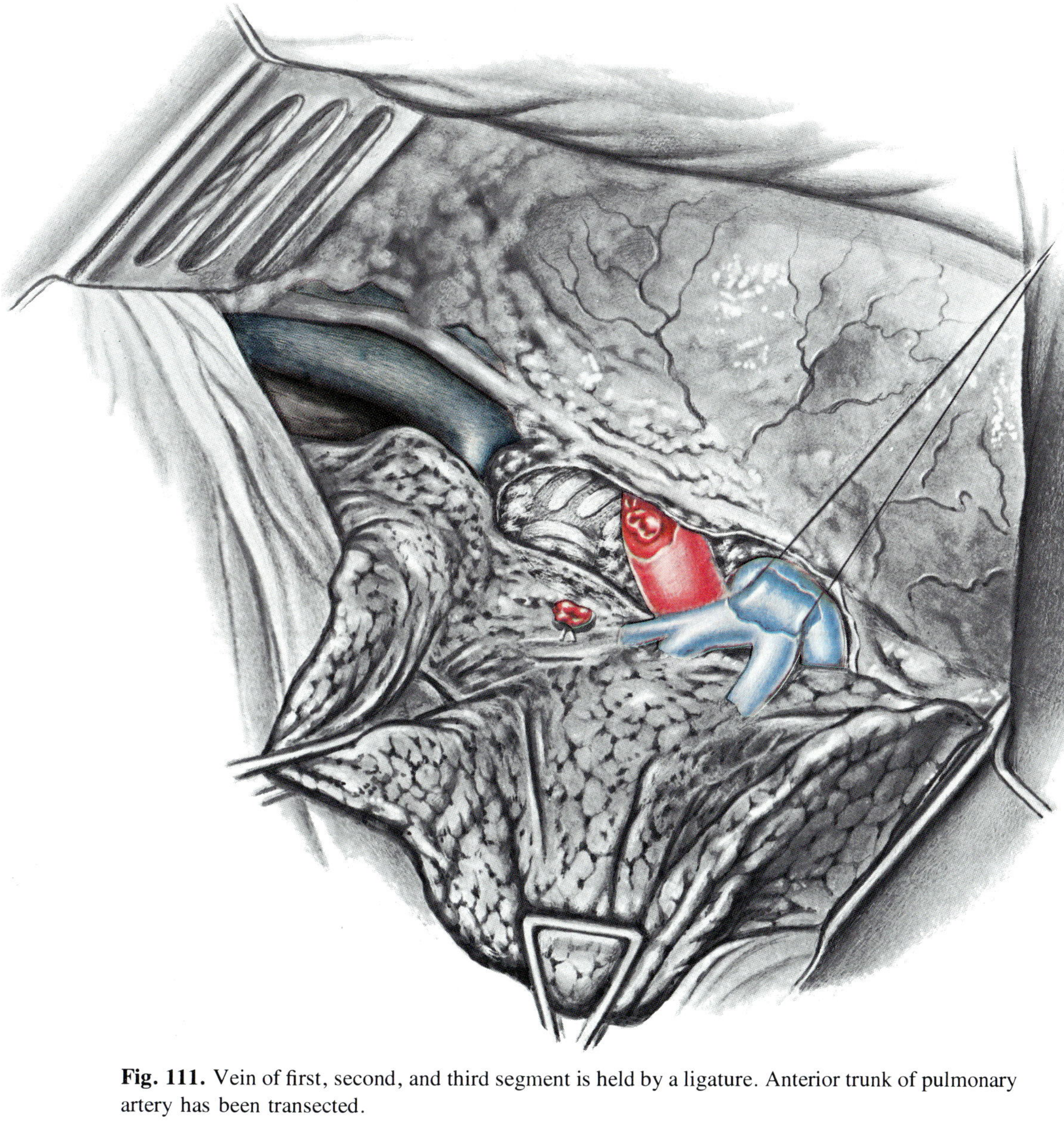

Fig. 111. Vein of first, second, and third segment is held by a ligature. Anterior trunk of pulmonary artery has been transected.

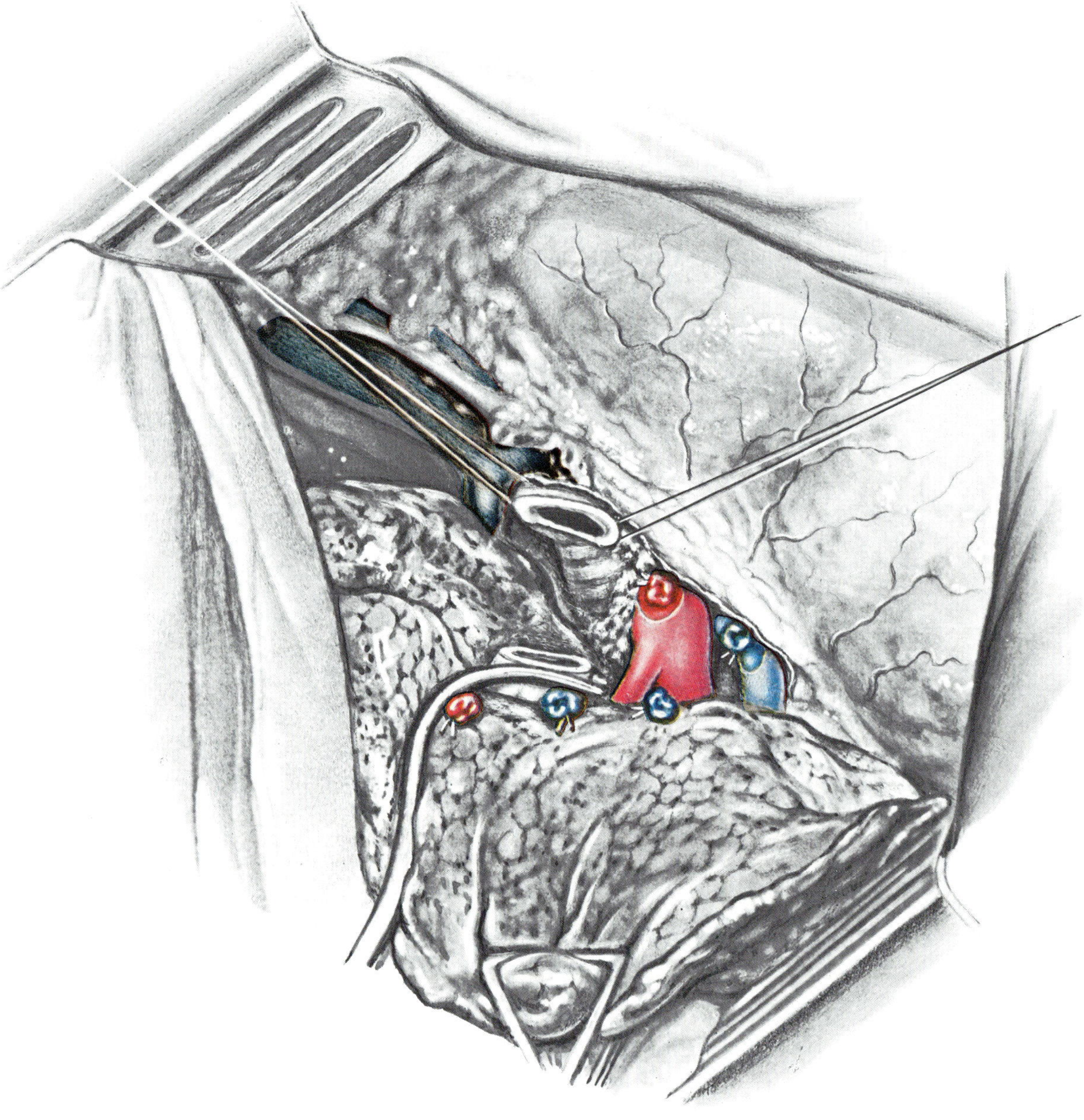

Fig. 112. Bronchus has been transected and traction sutures applied to its stump.

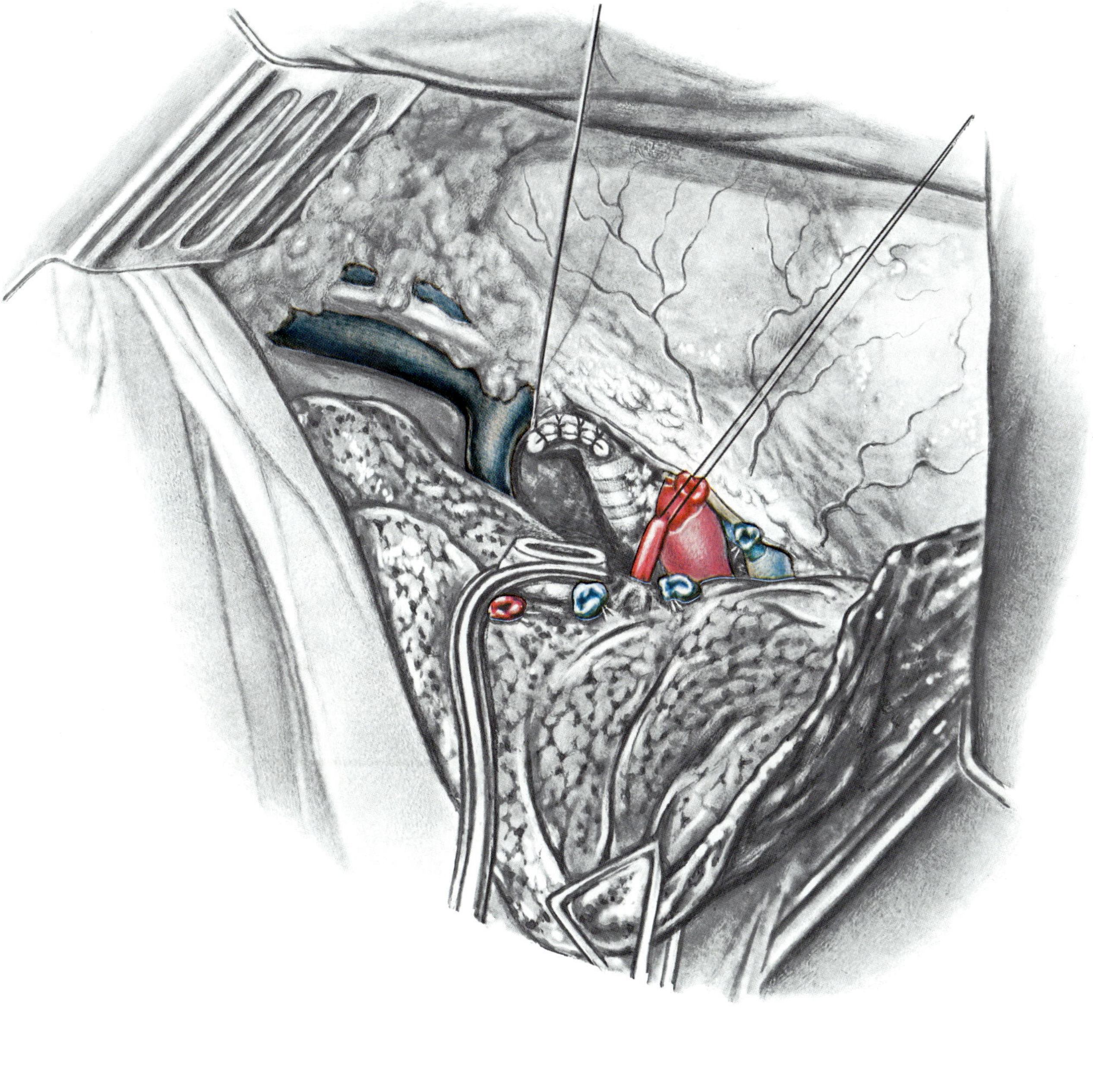

Fig. 113. Preparation of A_2. Bronchial stump has been closed with sutures.

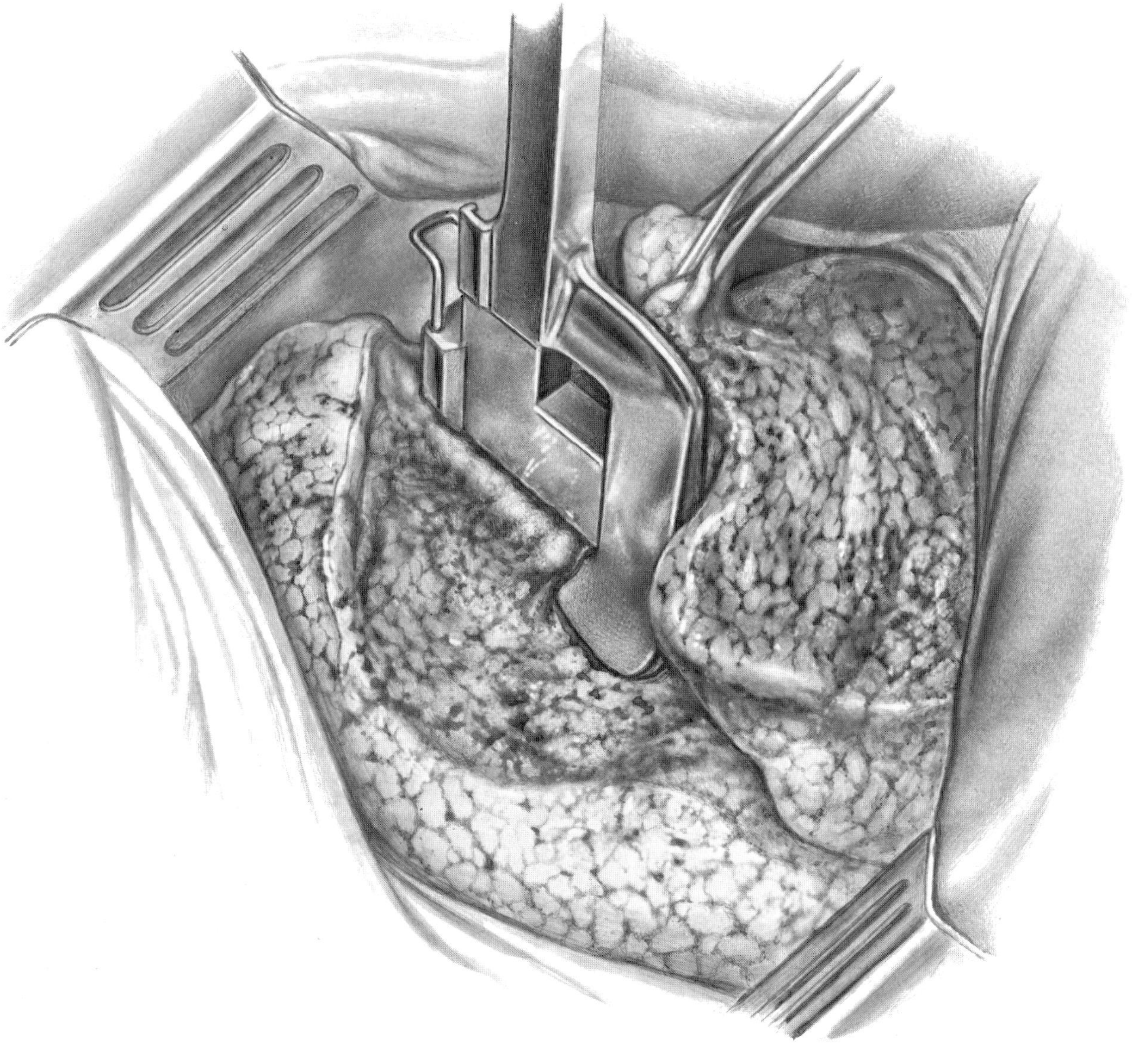

Fig. 114. Bridges between superior and middle lobes are stitched through with УО instrument.

INFERIOR LOBECTOMY

The pleural cavity is opened by a lateral approach in the sixth intercostal space.

The inferior lobe is completely freed from the adhesions. It is best to begin the manipulation from the side of the mediastinum, where the adhesions are usually weaker. The greatest difficulties often arise in the separation of the inferior lobe from the diaphragm. This stage of the operation may be accomplished after all the components of the root of the lobe have been prepared.

The pulmonary ligament is divided and ligated. The main interlobar fissure is opened widely. The inferior lobar artery is found in the dorsal third of this fissure; the artery is often wrapped in a pack of hyperplastic lymph nodes. These nodes are removed and the arterial branches separated. It is convenient to separate the artery of the basal segment first; ascending along it in the direction of the root of the lung, it is a simple matter to find A_6. Since the site where $A_{4,5}$ branches off is very near, it is necessary to protect this artery from being constructed when the ligatures are applied. The arteries are treated by the ligature method and divided (Fig. 115).

The inferior lobe is drawn away laterally. The inferior pulmonary vein is found and prepared and then treated by the ligature method or stitched through with the УС instrument (Fig. 116).

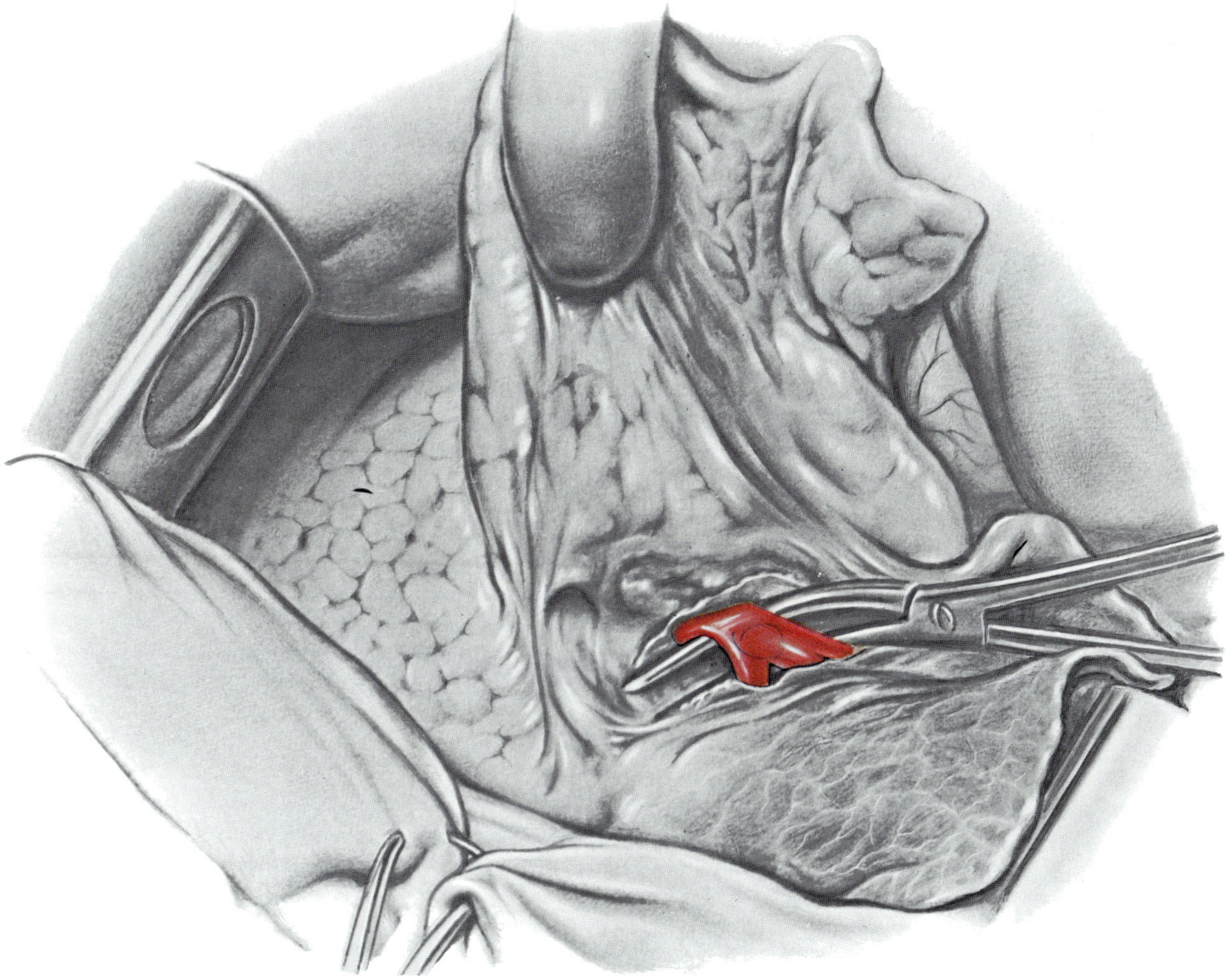

Fig. 115. Preparation of inferior lobar artery from side of interlobar fissure.

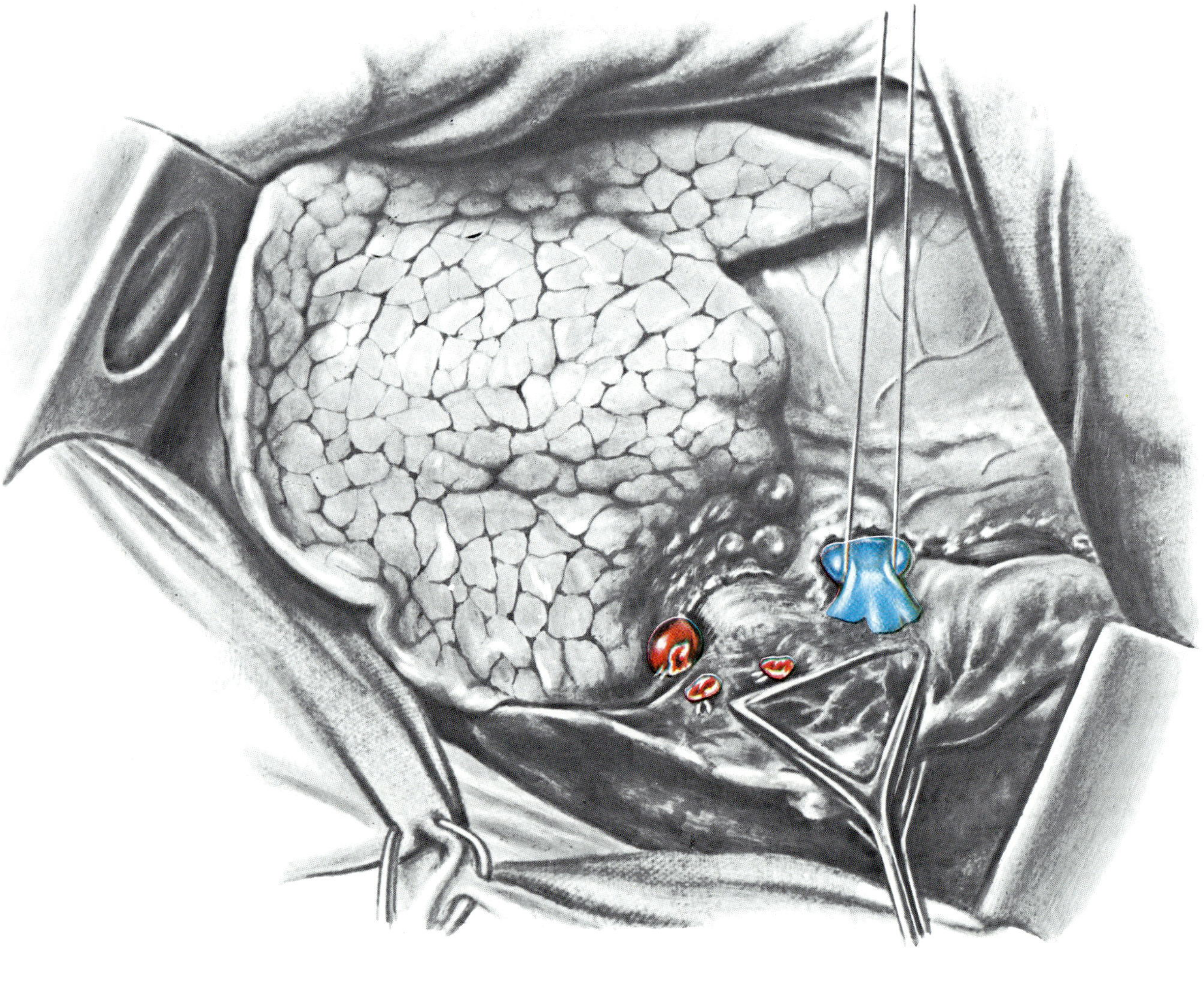

Fig. 116. A ligature has been drawn under inferior pulmonary vein.

The main interlobar fissure is again opened, and the inferior lobar bronchus located deep inside it close to the arterial stump is prepared. B_6 usually originates at the level of $B_{4,5}$. To avoid narrowing the latter, B_6 and the bronchus of the basal segment are prepared separately; in a favorable anatomical situation, one bronchial stump is formed. Bearing this in mind, it is always preferable to close the bronchial stump with manual sutures (Fig. 117).

After the components of the root have been transected, the bridge between S_6 and S_2 is stitched through with the УО instrument or cut between clamps. The inferior lobe is removed. The stump of the bronchus is covered with pleura whenever possible.

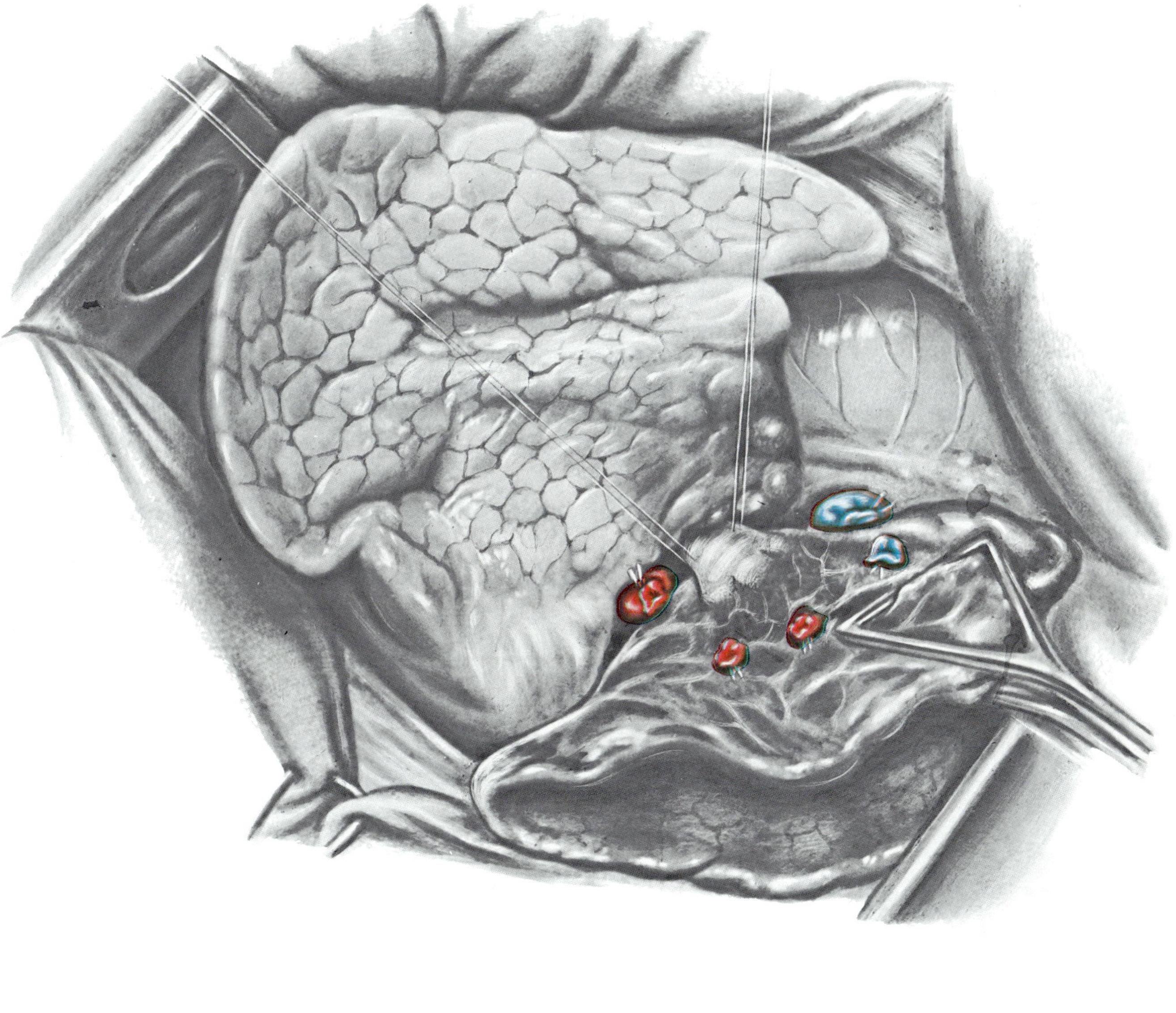

Fig. 117. Inferior lobar bronchus is prepared and held by traction sutures. Vessels have been transected; their stumps are visible.

MIDDLE LOBECTOMY

The pleural cavity is opened by an anterolateral or lateral approach in the fifth intercostal space. The middle lobe is drawn out laterally, as a result of which the branches of the superior pulmonary vein become clearly outlined. The overlying mediastinal pleura is cut. The middle lobar vein is prepared and treated by the ligature method (Fig. 118).

The middle lobar bronchus is immediately under the vein and is usually surrounded by scars and hyperplastic lymph nodes. These nodes are removed or displaced toward the lung. The ventral wall of the bronchus is exposed by blunt and sharp techniques. The middle lobar artery, stretching along the dorsocranial border of the bronchus, is carefully separated from the bronchial wall and treated by the ligature method (Fig. 119). Under definite conditions the middle lobar artery may be

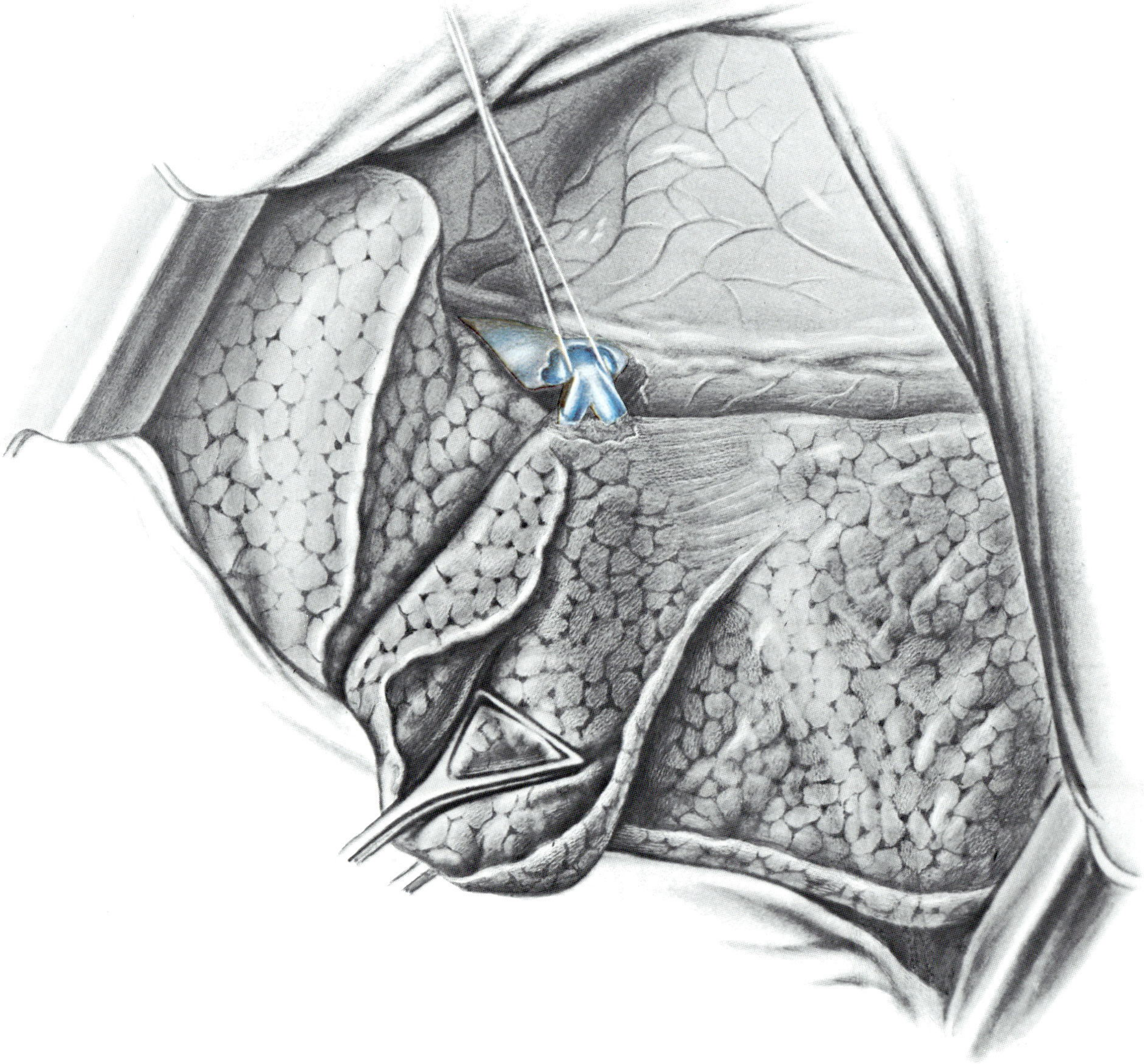

Fig. 118. Treatment of middle lobar vein.

ligated after the bronchus is transected or from the side of the main interlobar fissure.

With the vessels prepared, the middle lobar bronchus is separated. Preparation of its dorsal wall requires tremendous caution, because the inferior lobar artery lies in close contact with it. To avoid injuring the artery, it is advisable to pass the dissector around the bronchus as close as possible to the lung. The peripheral segment of the bronchus is clamped, traction sutures are applied to the central segment, and the bronchus is divided (Fig. 120). The bronchial stump is closed with interrupted sutures; in children it is stitched through and tied.

The middle lobe is removed by the method of segmentectomy. The intersegmental venous anastomoses are clamped together with S_3 and ligated. In extensive adhesions between the middle and superior lobe the УО instrument is used to separate them.

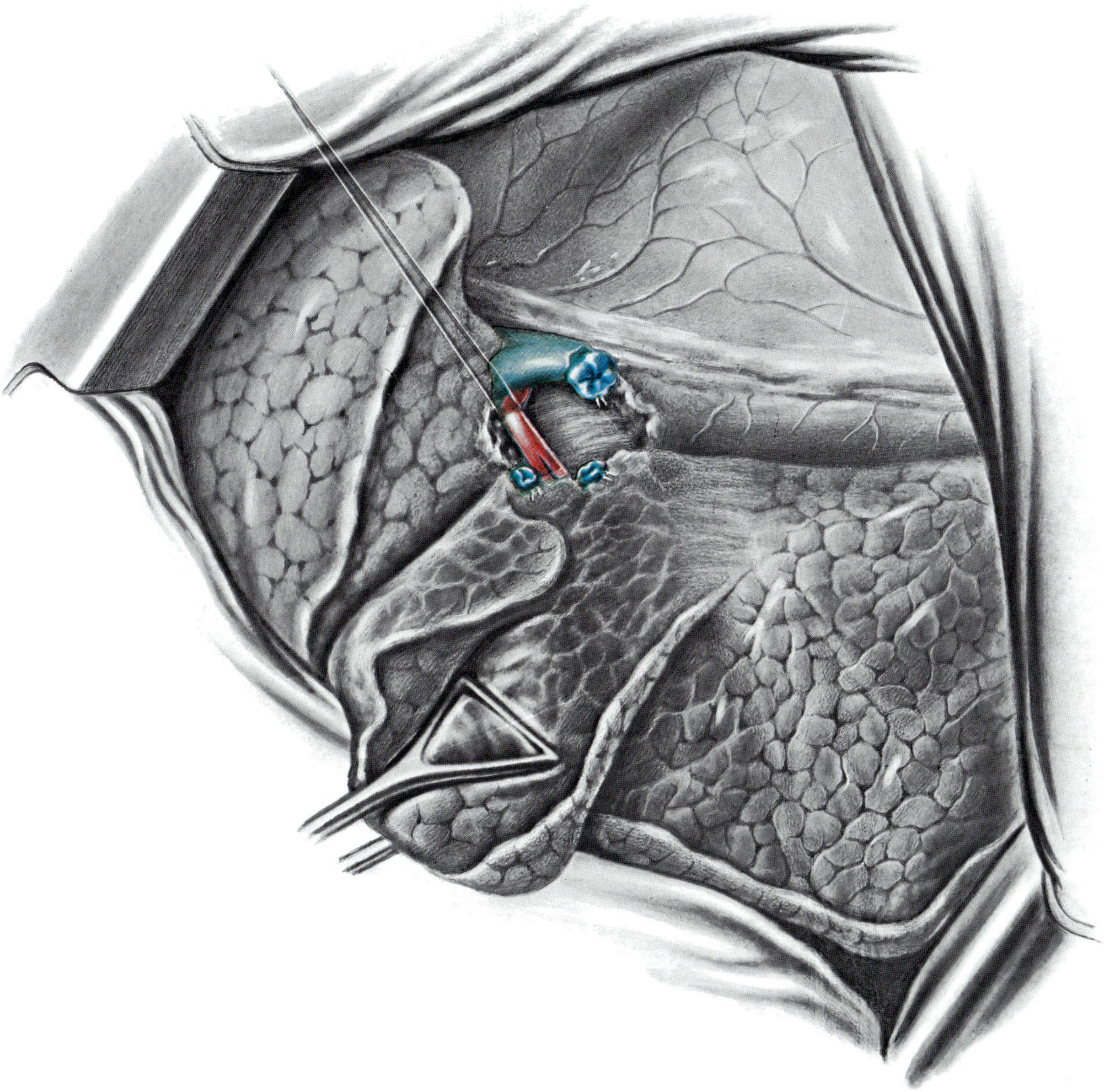

Fig. 119. Middle lobar artery has been prepared and is held by a ligature. Middle lobar vein has been transected.

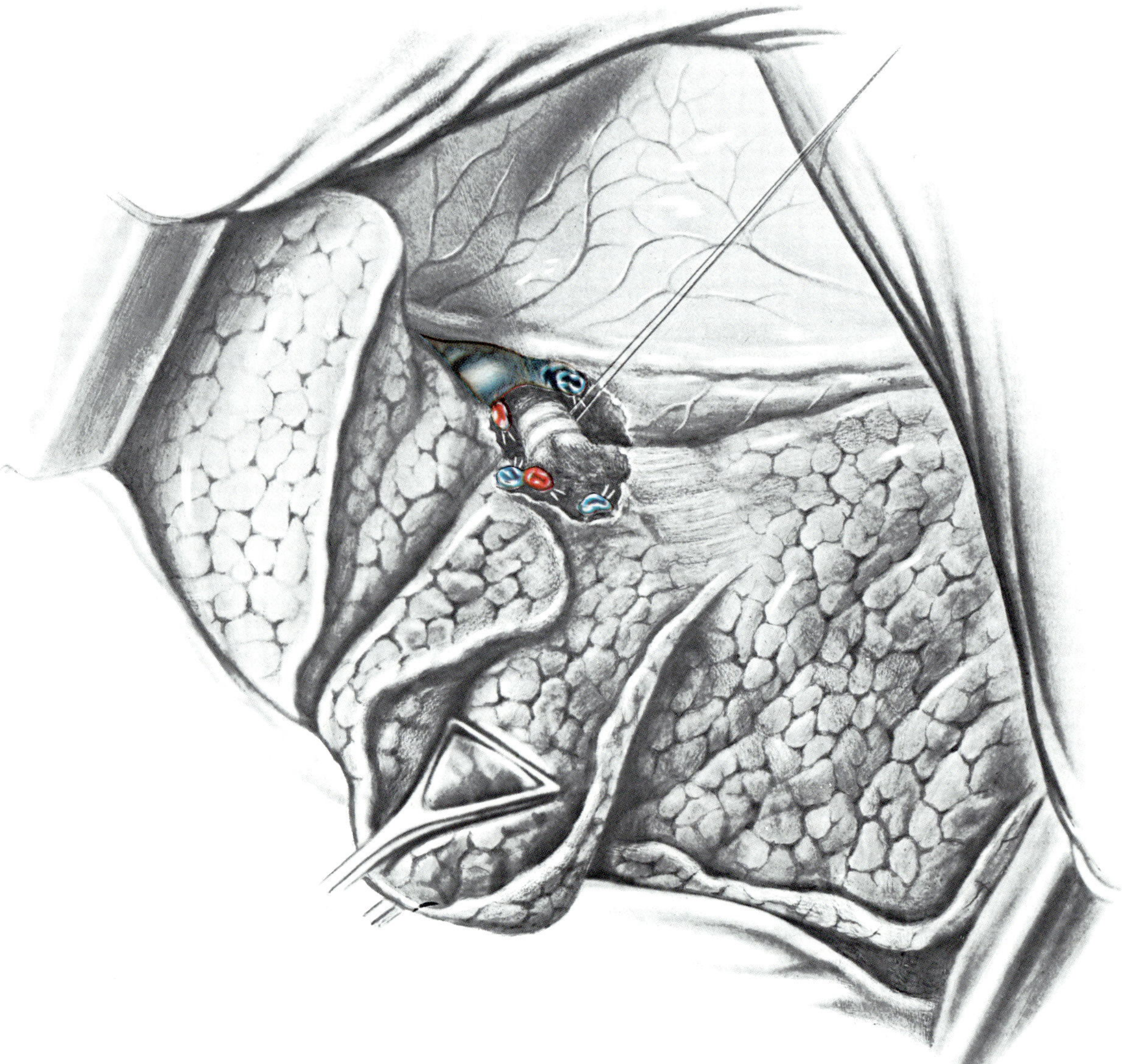

Fig. 120. Traction sutures are applied to middle lobar bronchus. Stumps of artery and vein are visible.

INFERIOR BILOBECTOMY

The pleural cavity is opened by a lateral approach in the fifth or sixth intercostal space.

The inferior and middle lobe are freed from the adhesions, and the pulmonary ligament is cut.

The main interlobar fissure is drawn widely apart, and the arteries of the inferior and middle lobe are found on its floor on the boundary between the dorsal and middle thirds. The arterial branches are scrupulously identified and treated by the ligature method (Fig. 121).

The lung is drawn aside laterally. $V_{4,5}$ is separated in the root of the middle lobe and prepared (Fig. 122). The inferior pulmonary vein is then prepared (Fig. 123).

Separation of the intermediate bronchus is the most complicated stage of the operation; it can be accomplished by either of two methods. In the first variant the bronchus is prepared in the interlobar fissure and separated to the site of the origin of the superior lobar bronchus (Fig. 124). In the second variant the bronchus is approached from the ventral surface, cranial to the middle lobar bronchus. In both cases it is expedient to separate the inferior and middle lobes from the superior lobe prior to cutting the intermediate bronchus; stitching instruments are used for this purpose.

The intermediate bronchus is transected 3 to 5 mm from the superior lobar bronchus. The inferior and middle lobes are removed as one. The stump of the bronchus

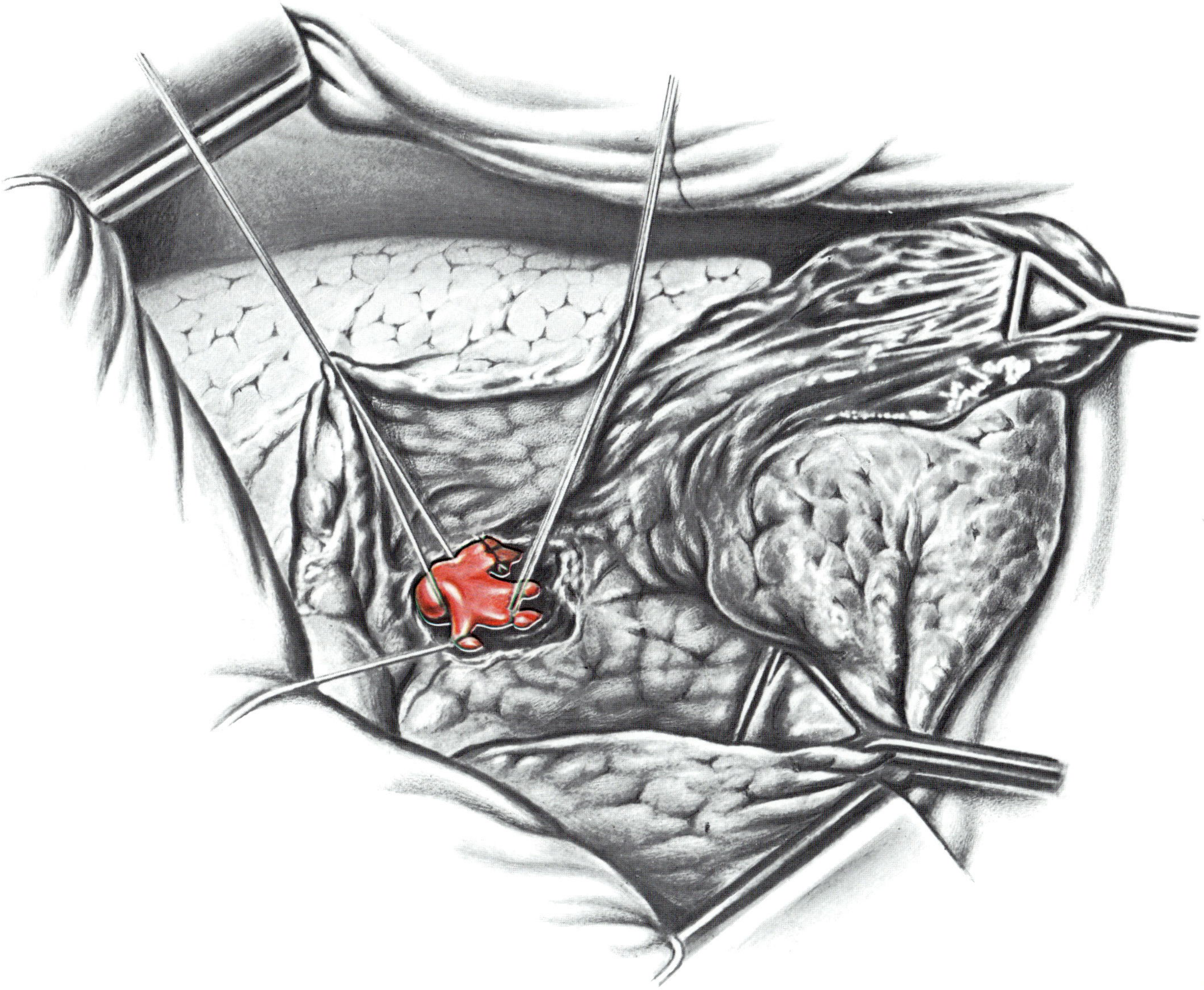

Fig. 121. Exposure and preparation of arteries of inferior and middle lobes from side of main interlobar fissure.

is sutured by hand and covered with mediastinal pleura (Fig. 125). Under appropriate circumstances (a soft bronchial wall with no inflammatory changes in it) the bronchus may be closed with the YO instrument.

In cases where the root of the lung is infiltrated and the separation of its components is very difficult technically, it is advisable to operate in two stages, removing first the middle and then the inferior lobes. Since in this case the middle and inferior bronchi have to be cut separately, reamputation of the bronchus is performed after the lobes have been removed and a common stump of the intermediate bronchus is created.

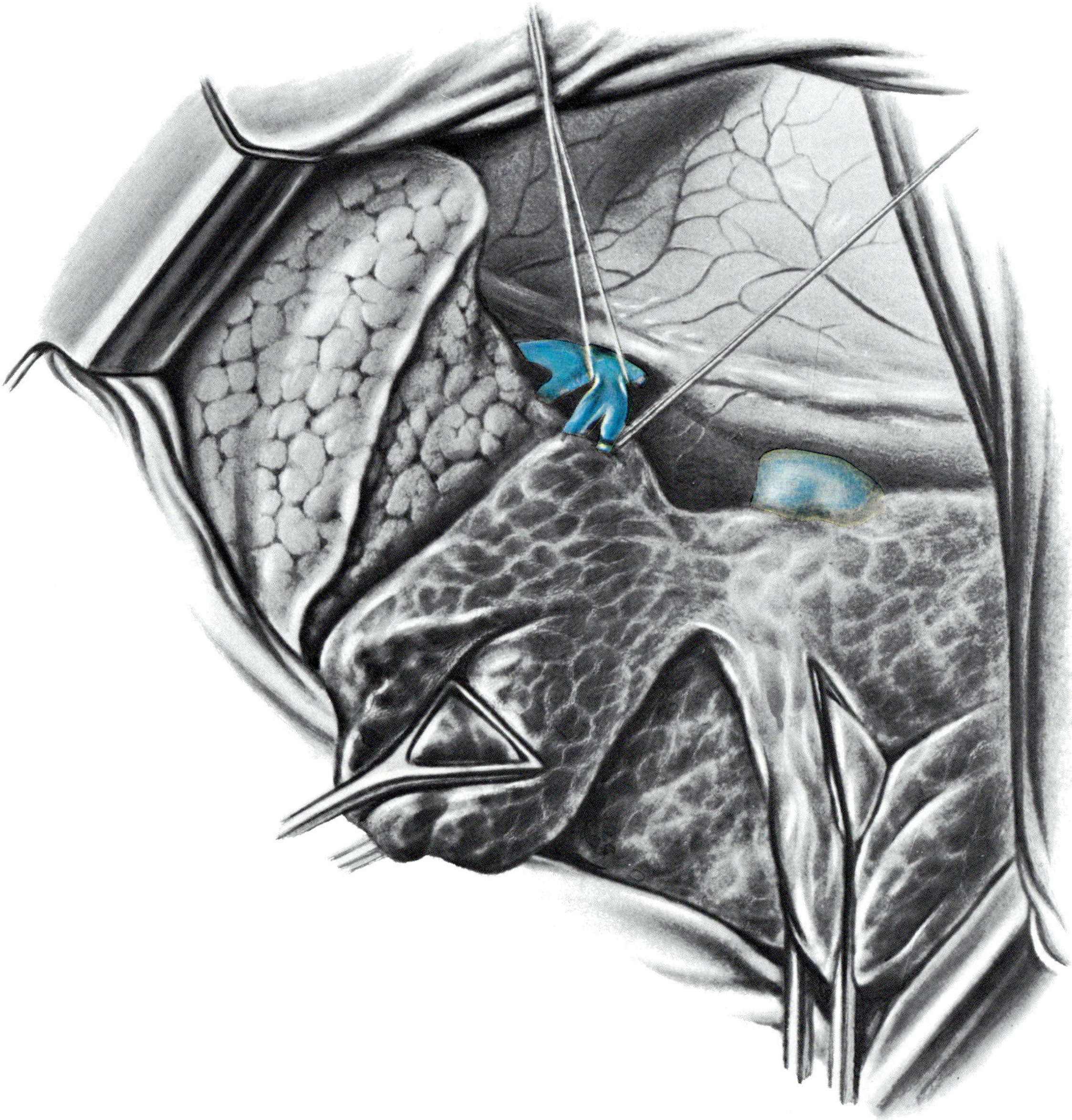

Fig. 122. Separation and ligation of middle lobar vein.

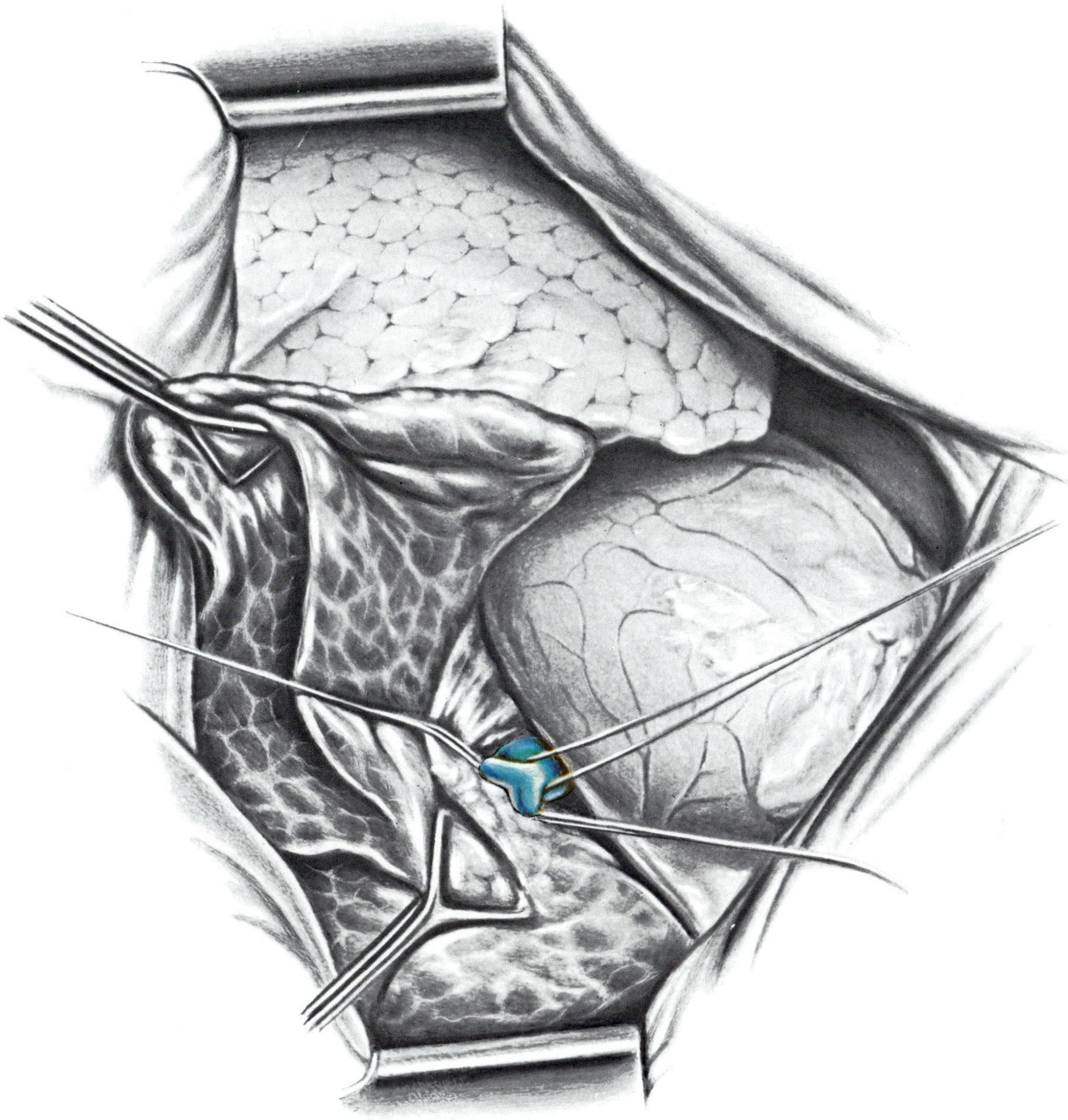

Fig. 123. A ligature is drawn under inferior pulmonary vein.

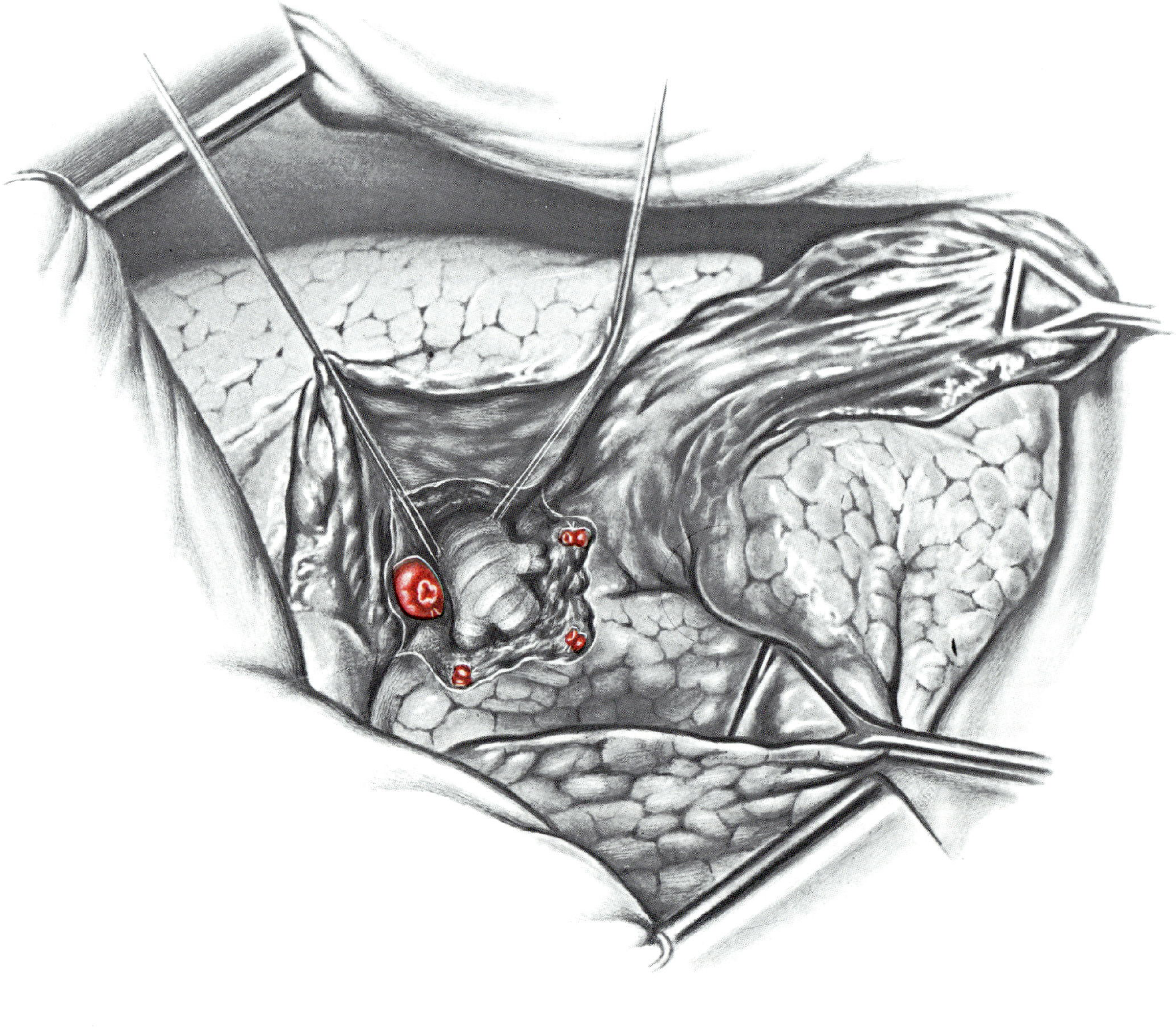

Fig. 124. Separation of intermediate bronchus by manipulating from side of interlobar fissure. Traction sutures have been applied to bronchus.

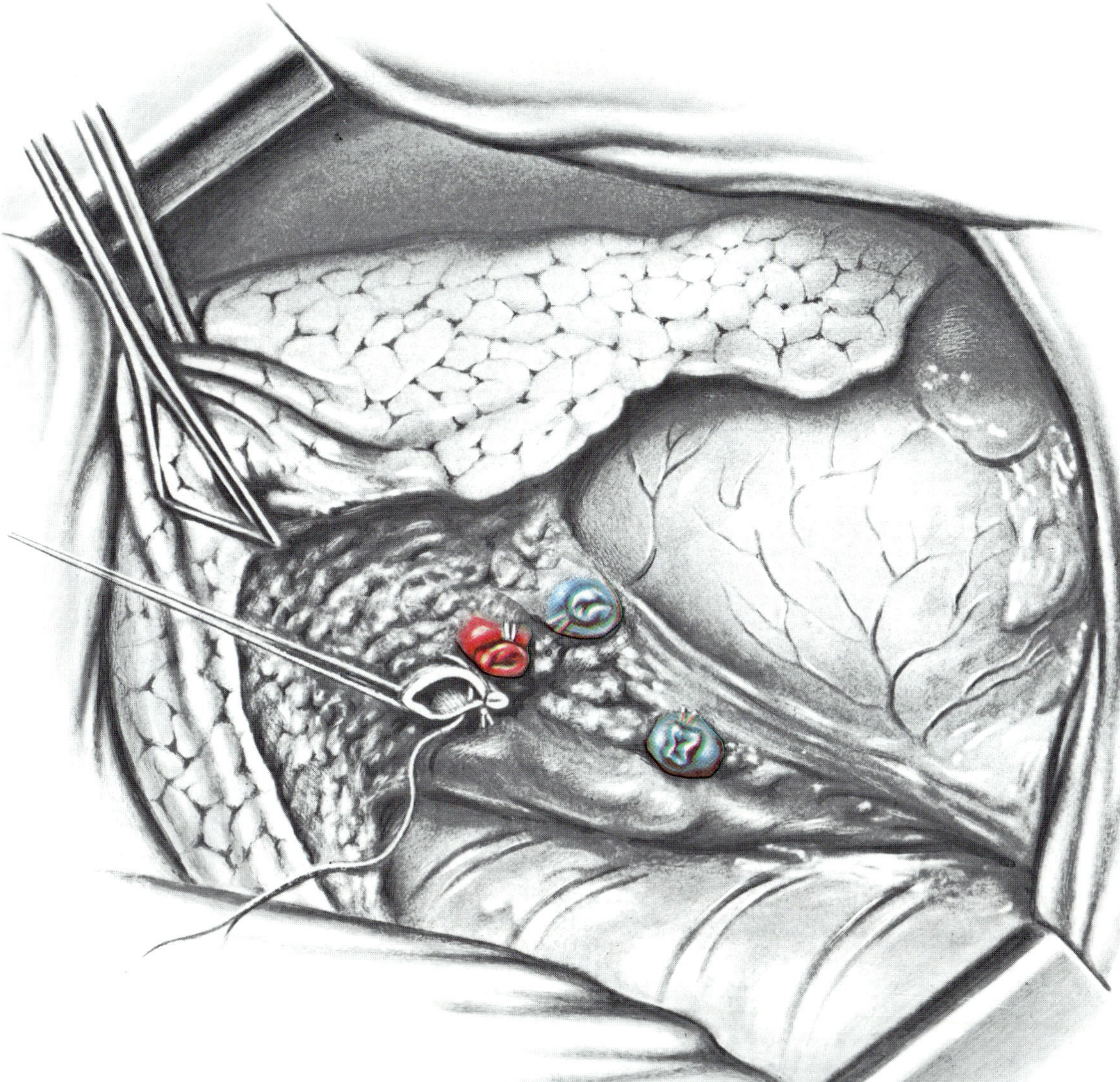

Fig. 125. Closure of stump of intermediate bronchus with sutures.

S_1 RESECTION

The pleural cavity is opened by a lateral approach to the fourth intercostal space.

The superior lobe is freed from the adhesions. The mediastinal pleura is cut on the ventral surface of the cranial part of the root of the lung. A_1 is found and prepared (Fig. 126). In about half the cases the anterior trunk of the right pulmonary artery gives off a branch to S_2; this branch should be left intact. V_1, which is a cranial branch of the superior pulmonary vein, is separated and ligated.

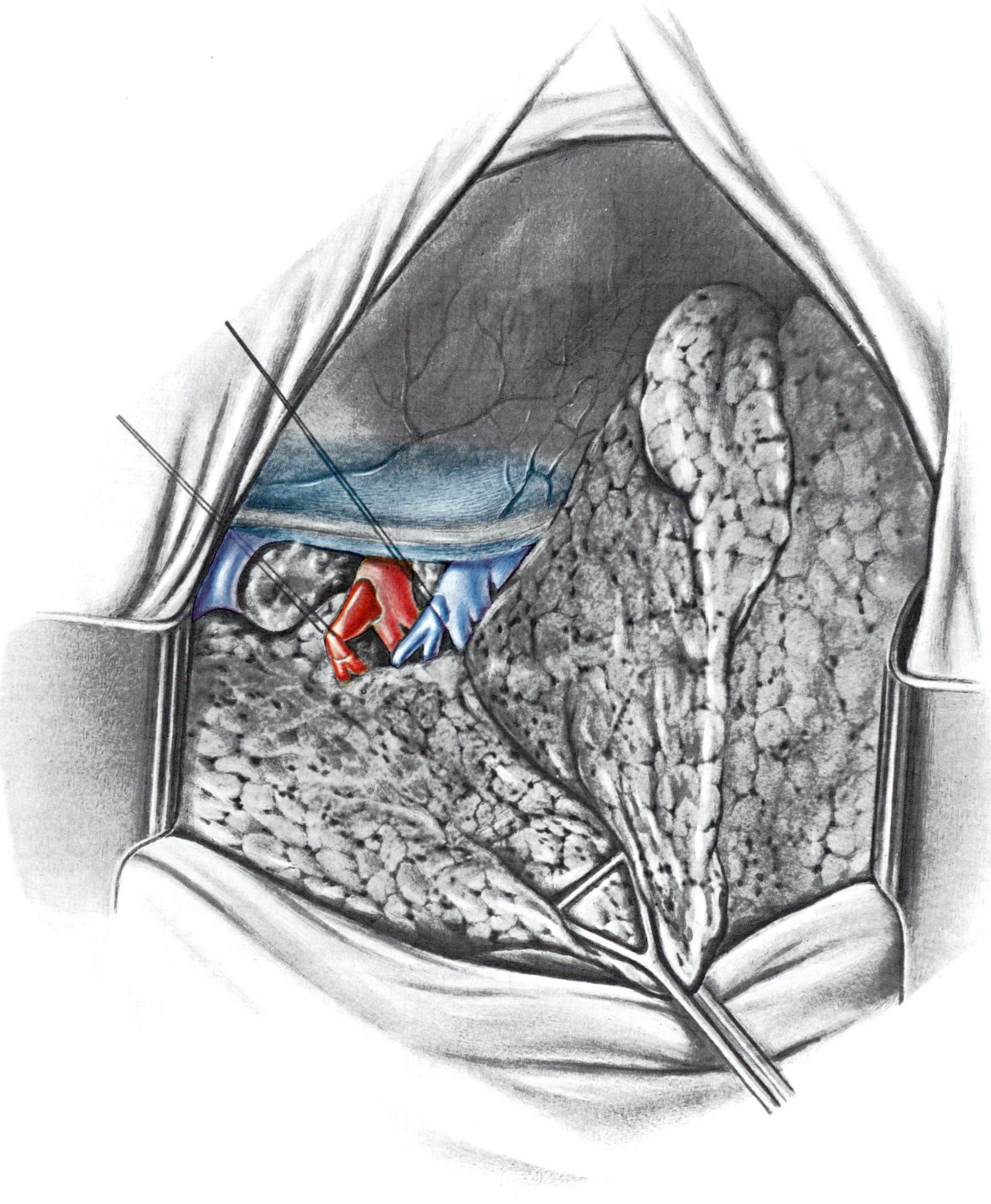

Fig. 126. Ligatures are drawn under artery and vein of first segment.

B_1 is found immediately under the artery of the first segment and separated. The bronchus is clamped and then transected, and its stump is sutured (Fig. 127). With the peripheral bronchial stump being pulled on, the intersegmental veins are found, grasped, and cut. The segment is resected (Fig. 128). The defect formed in the parenchyma of the superior lobe may be repaired by suturing together the edges of S_3 and S_2 with interrupted sutures.

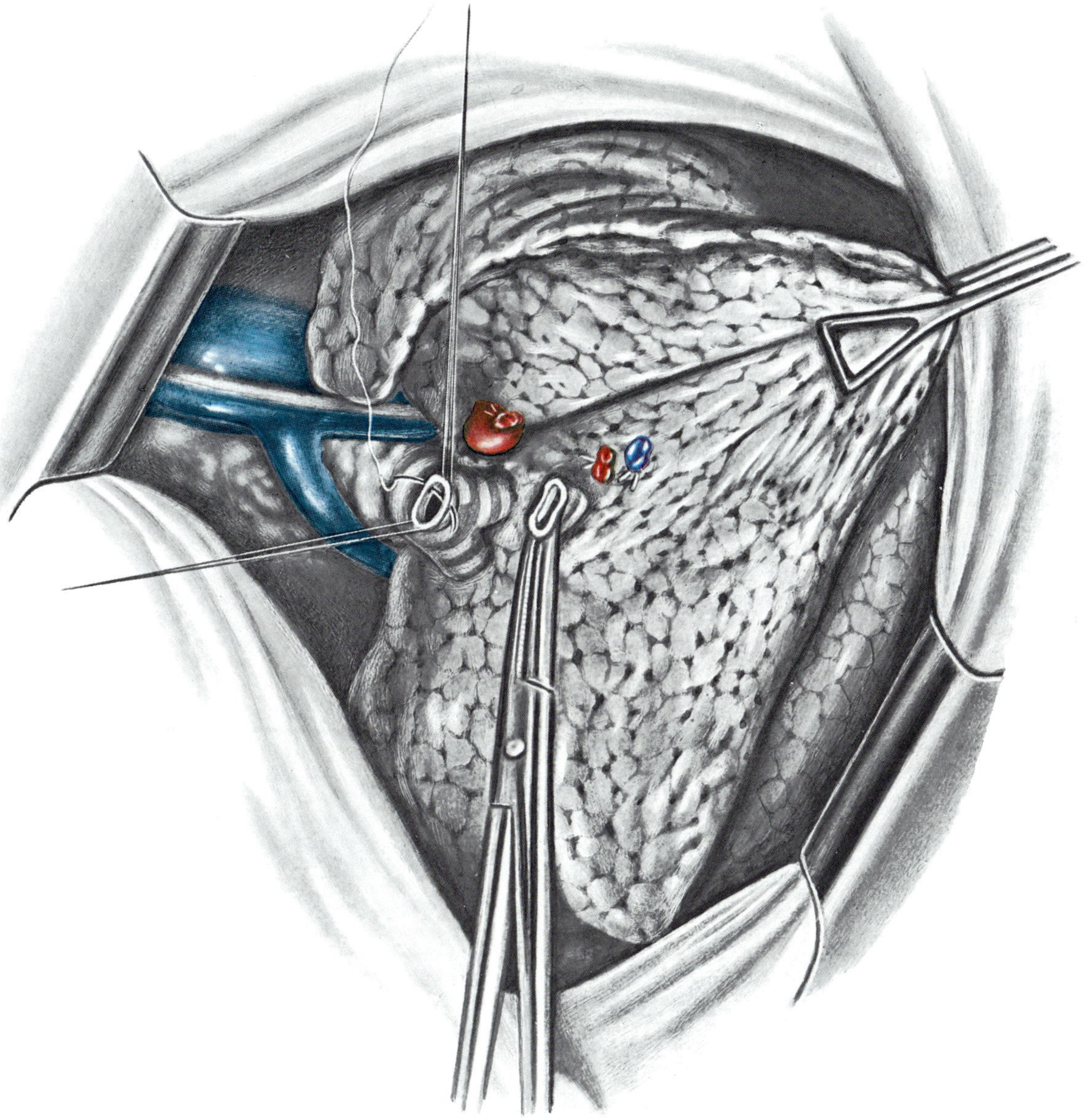

Fig. 127. Transection of B_1 and closure of its stump with sutures.

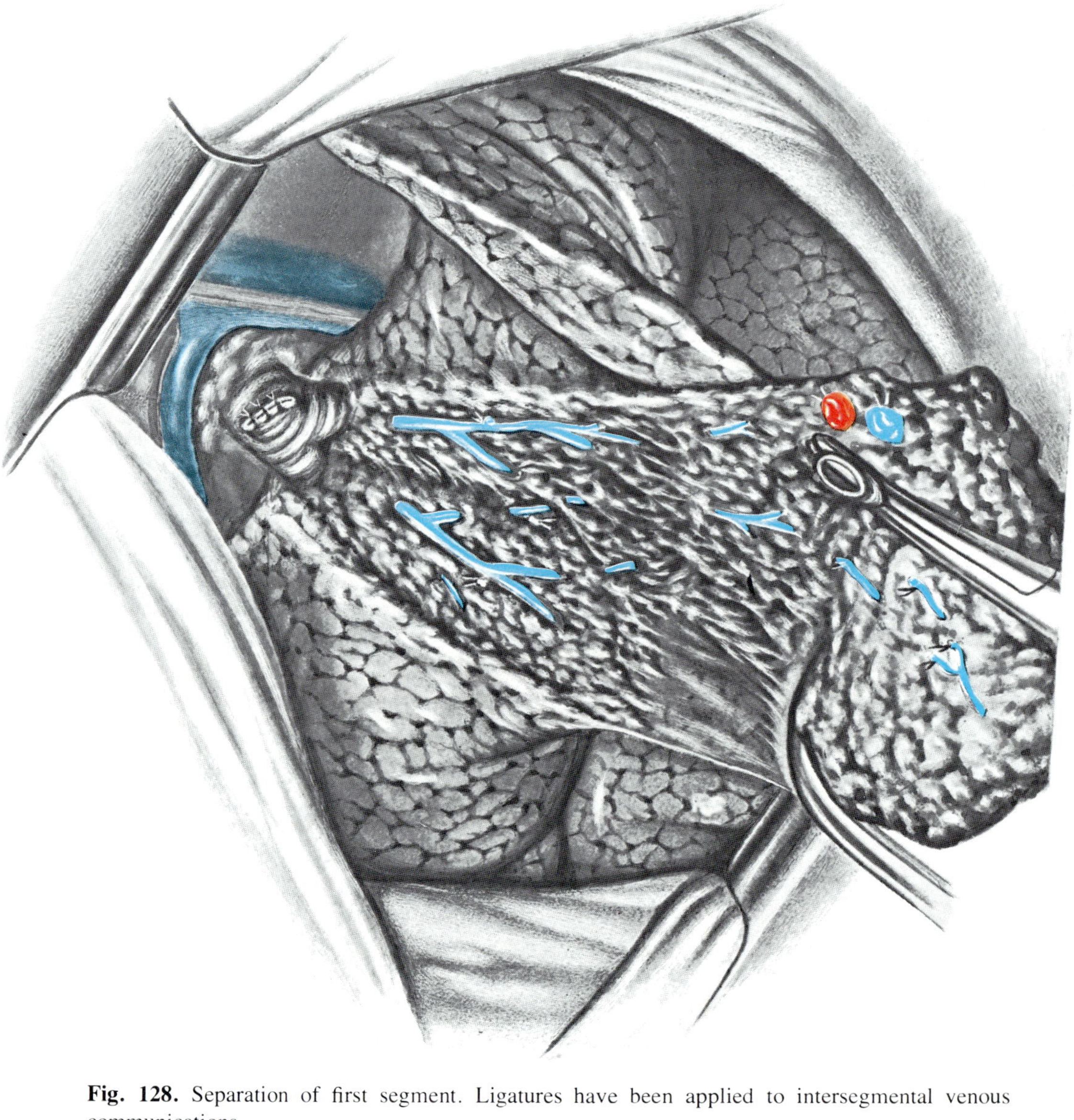

Fig. 128. Separation of first segment. Ligatures have been applied to intersegmental venous communications.

S_{1+2} RESECTION

The pleural cavity is opened by a lateral approach in the fourth intercostal space.

The pleura is cut on the ventral surface of the cranial part of the root of the lung. A_1 is separated and treated by the ligature method (Fig. 129).

The superior lobe is drawn aside laterally and caudally. The pulmonary tissue is pushed off the superior lobar bronchus with tampons, and V_1 and V_2 are prepared (Fig. 130). The segmental bronchi are cut, and their stumps sutured separately.

With the bronchi cut, access is opened to A_2, which is ligated and cut (Fig. 131).

Since S_1 and S_2 communicate closely through the system of venous drainage, at first only the clearly outlined V_1 is ligated. It is located on the ventral surface of the root of the superior lobe, and its preparation is not difficult. In contrast, V_2 passes deep in the pulmonary tissue and is only found after the segmental bronchus has been cut. This vein also receives blood from S_3; that is why it is advisable to leave its trunk on the surface of

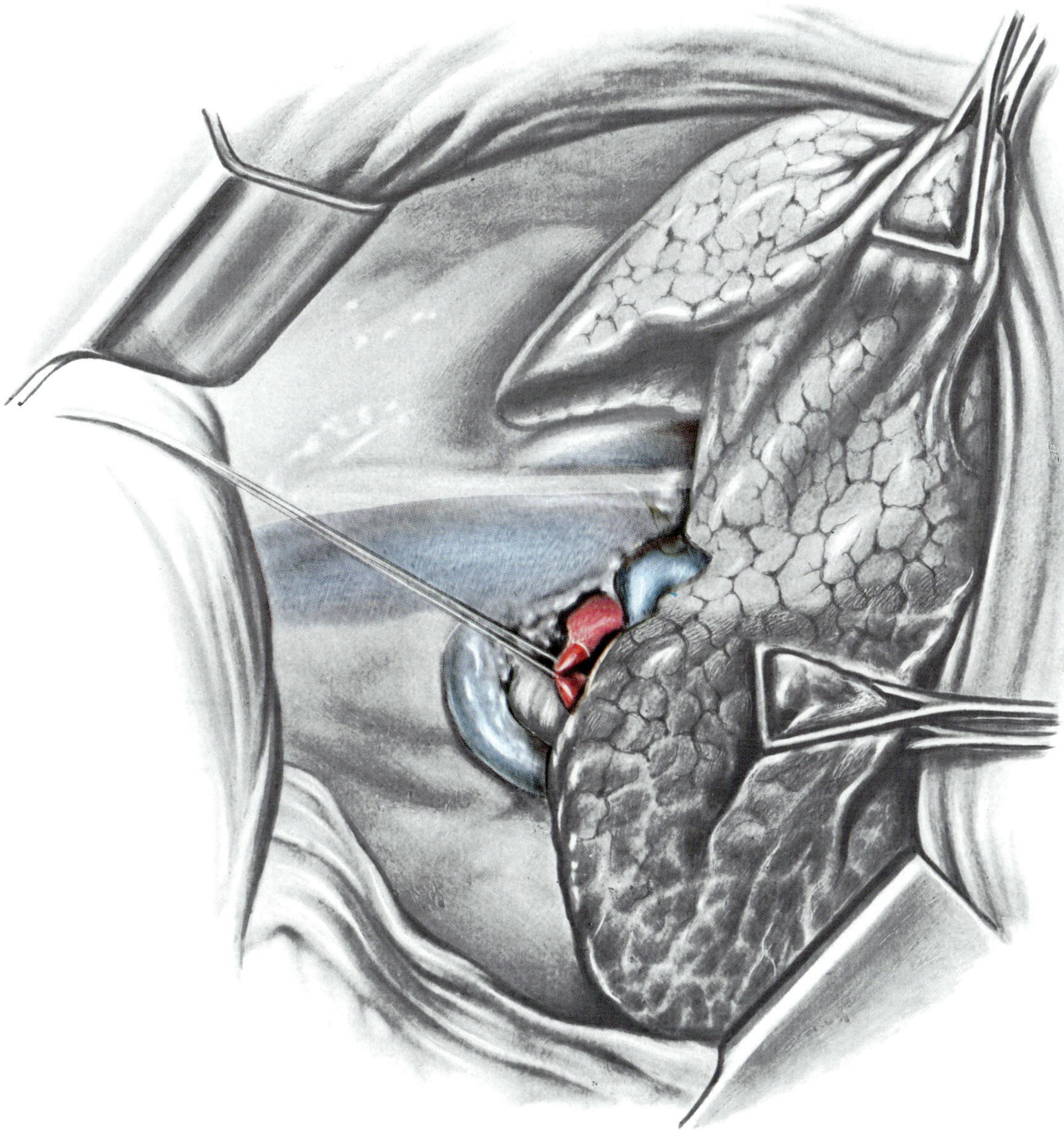

Fig. 129. Separation and ligation of A_1.

S_3 intact. For this purpose the segments to be removed are pulled by the peripheral bronchial stump, and the small veins draining into V_2 are cut. It is safe to ligate V_2 only when its main part is in the parenchyma of the segments being removed and an accessory branch of S_3 remains on the intersegmental surface.

After preparation of the veins, the segments are removed (Fig. 132). The surface of S_3 after resection is not sutured. The stumps of B_1 and B_2 are covered with the neighboring tissues.

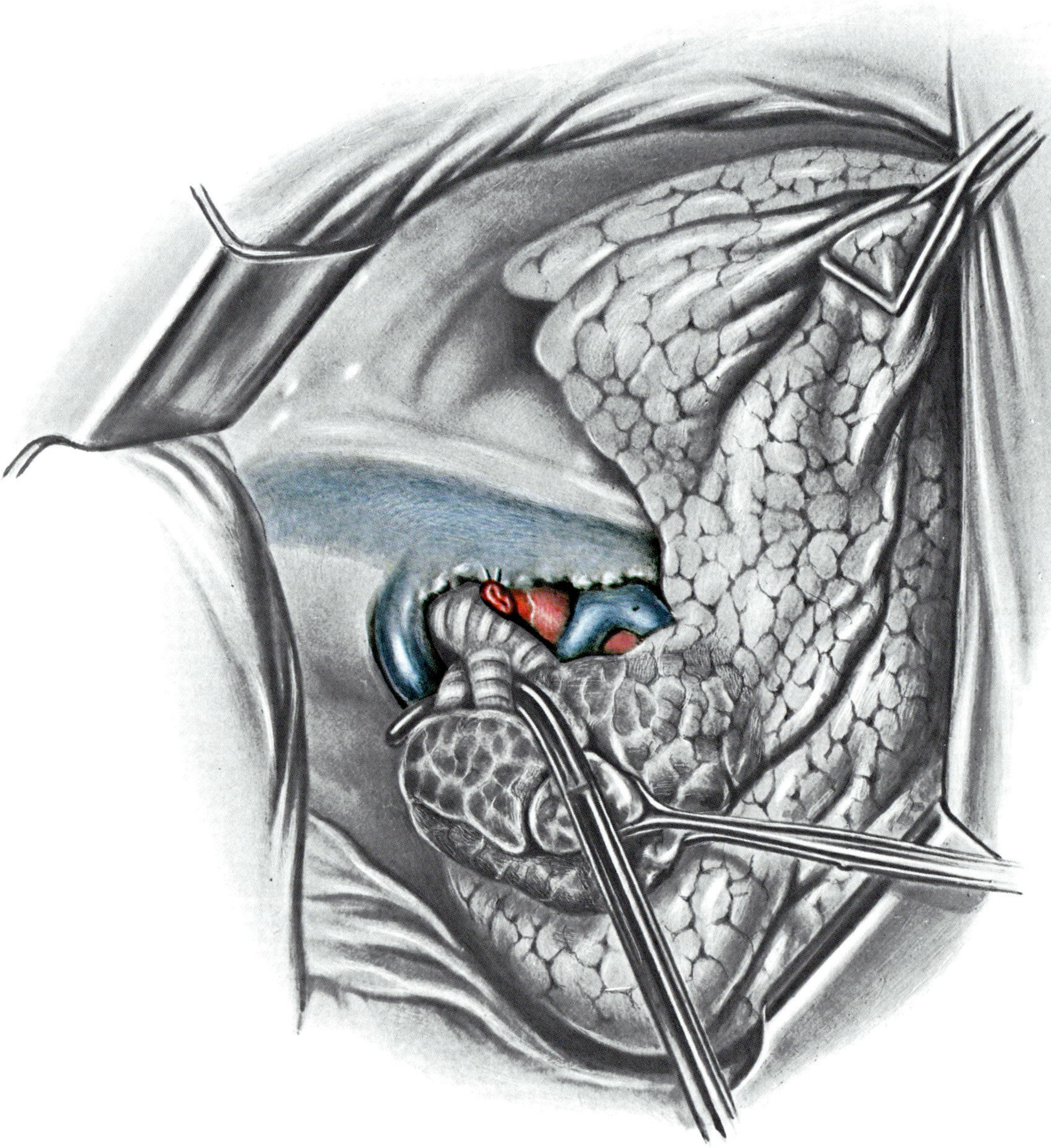

Fig. 130. A dissector is brought under B_1 and B_2. Stump of A_1 is visible.

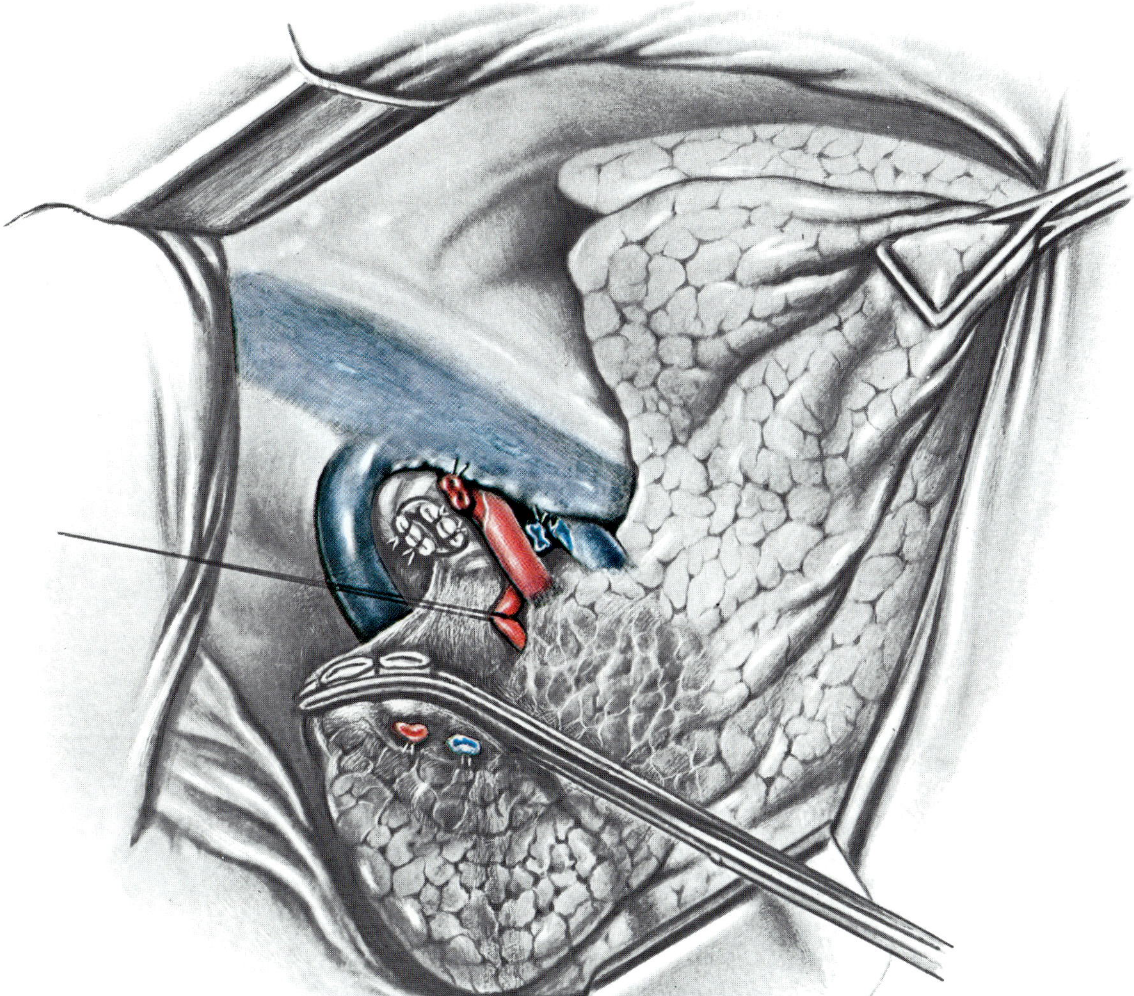

Fig. 131. A_2 is separated and ligated. Bronchial stumps are sutured.

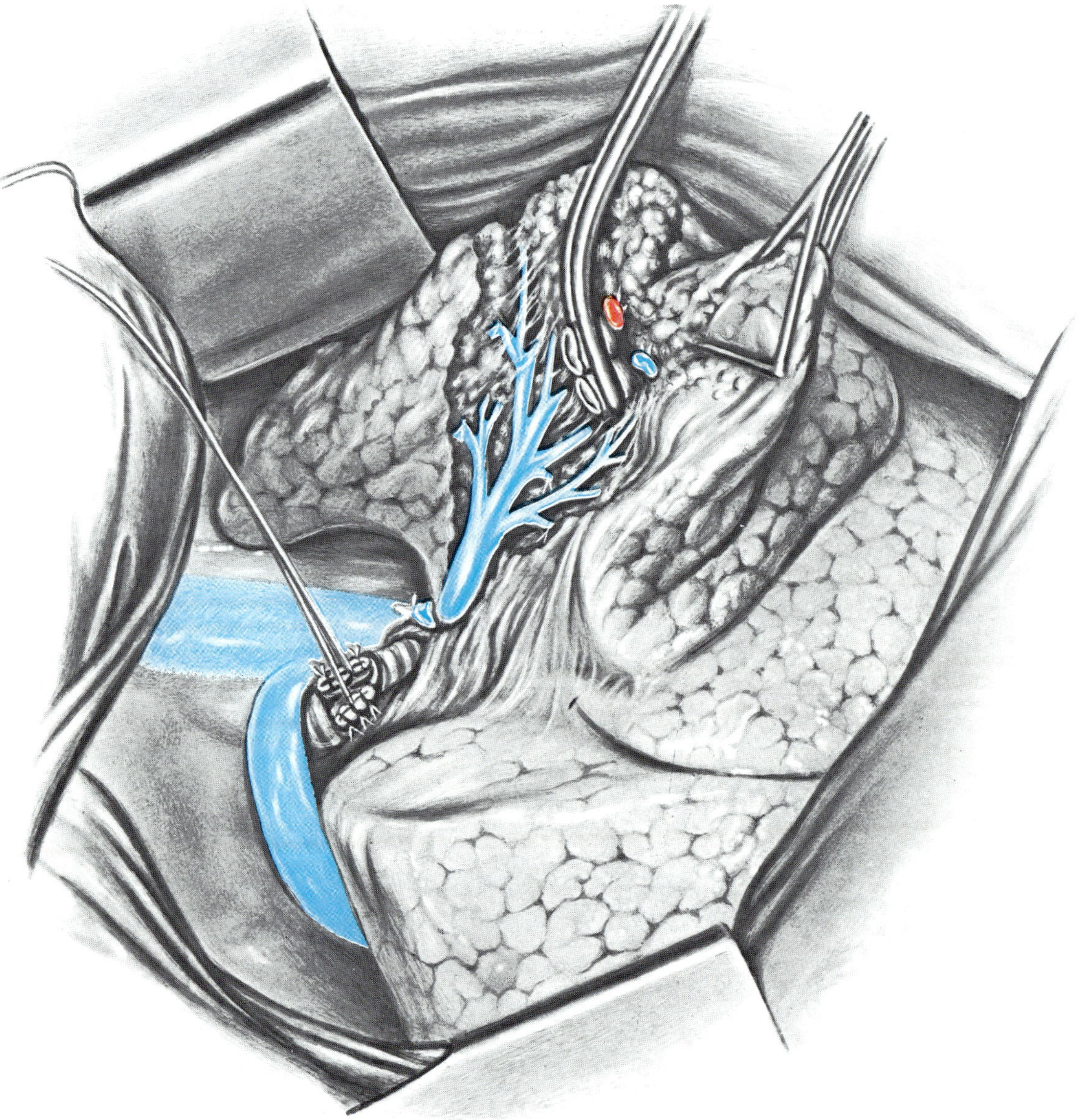

Fig. 132. Separation of segments with preparation of intersegmental venous communications.

S_3 RESECTION

The pleural cavity is opened by a lateral or antero-lateral approach in the fourth intercostal space.

The peculiarities of this operation consist in the root of the segment being located under the branches of the superior pulmonary vein and in the very close contact between the segments and the middle lobe.

The mediastinal pleura is cut over the ventral surface of the superior lobar root. The anterior trunk of the right pulmonary artery is exposed, and A_3 is prepared. A_3 is often covered with the vein of the first segment, which is moved aside with a tampon.

To identify V_3 one should inspect all the branches of the superior pulmonary vein, the vein of the middle lobe among others. The venous branch located immediately cranial to $V_{4,5}$ usually receives blood from S_3 and may be ligated (Fig. 133).

Treatment of the bronchus covered with the branches of the superior pulmonary vein is the most difficult stage.

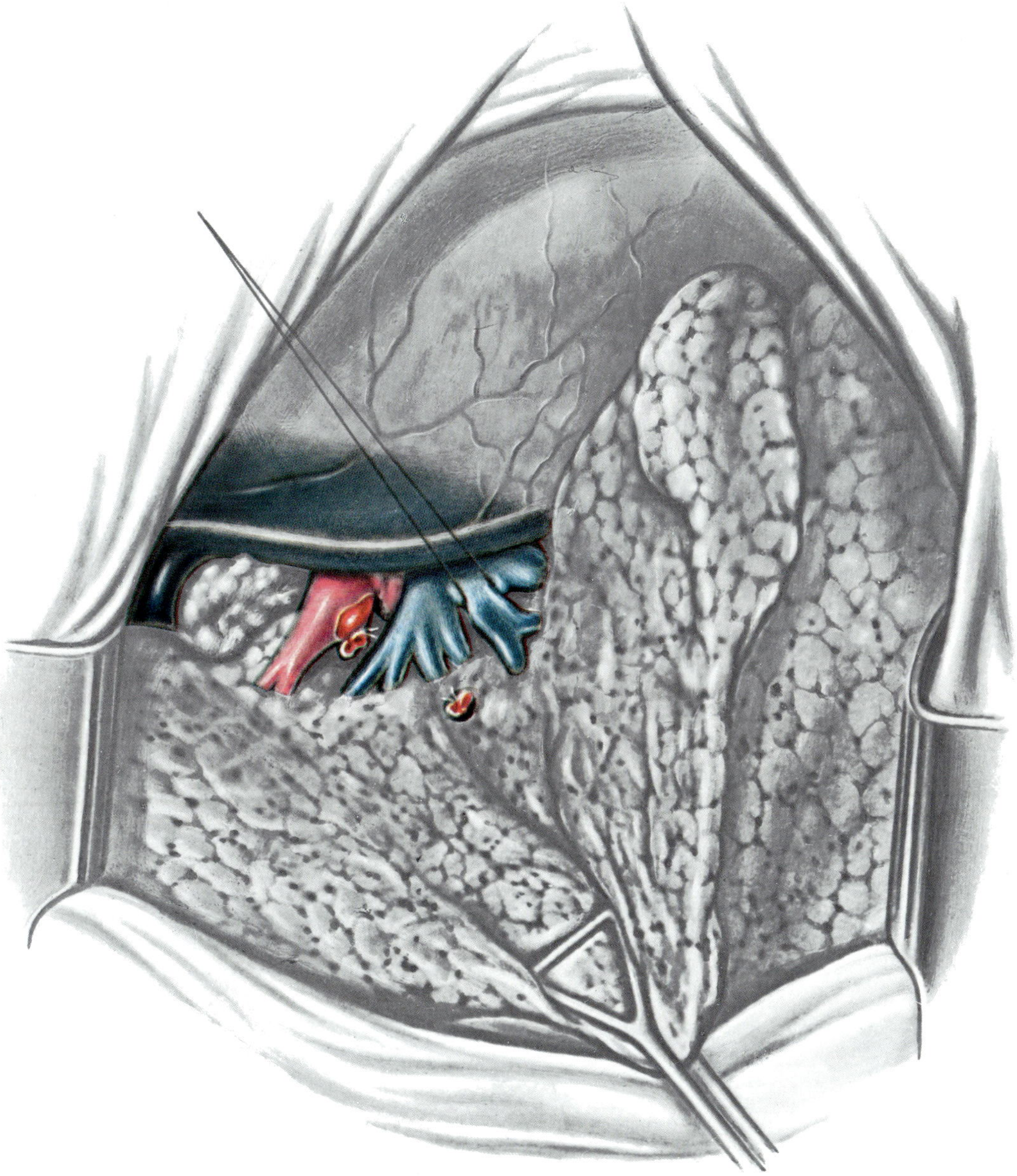

Fig. 133. Separation of veins of third segment. A_2 has been transected.

V_1 is held on a thick thread and moved cranially. The bronchus of the third segment is found and separated (Fig. 134). It is cut, and its stumps are drawn out from under V_1, which is fitted back in place. The stump of B_3 is closed with interrupted sutures. After a trial inflation of the lung the boundaries of S_3 are defined and cuts are made in the pleura according to them. With the peripheral stump of the bronchus being pulled on, the segment is removed, carefully ligating the intersegmental veins. The wound surface of the superior and middle lobe may be closed with several interrupted sutures.

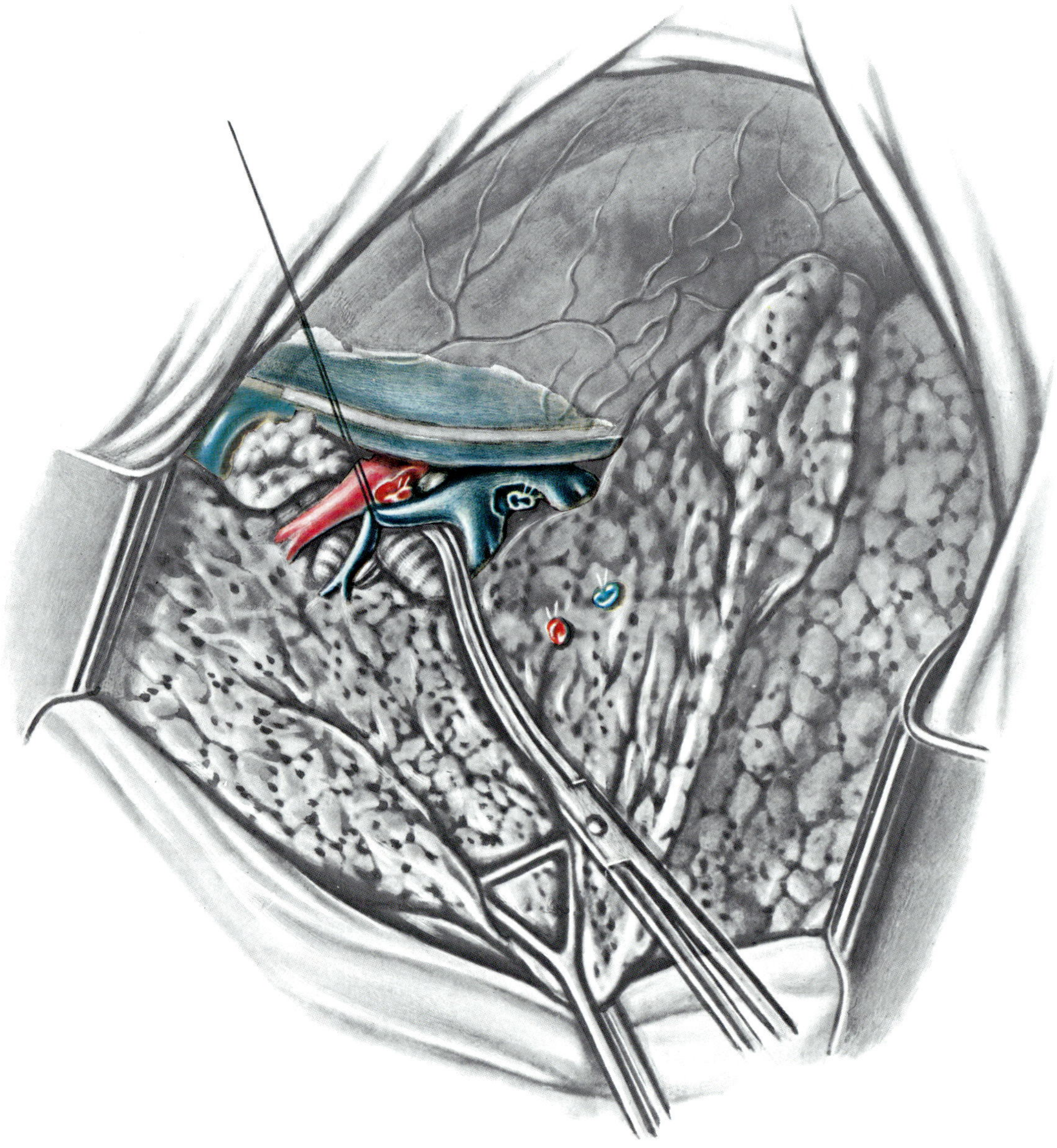

Fig. 134. B_3 separation. V_1 is drawn aside on a relaxation ligature.

S_6 RESECTION

The pleural cavity is opened by a lateral approach in the fifth intercostal space.

The inferior lobe is freed from the adhesions, and the main interlobar fissure is opened. The inferior lobar artery is found on its floor in the dorsal third. The first branch extending in the dorsolateral direction belongs to the sixth segment. A_6 is treated by the ligature method (Fig. 135). In rare cases the artery of the basal segments gives off a branch to S_6. This is also ligated and divided. Further, depending on the concrete topographoanatomical conditions, either the bronchus or the vein of the sixth segment is prepared.

B_6 is found immediately under A_6. The bronchus is transected, and its stump sutured by hand and pulled

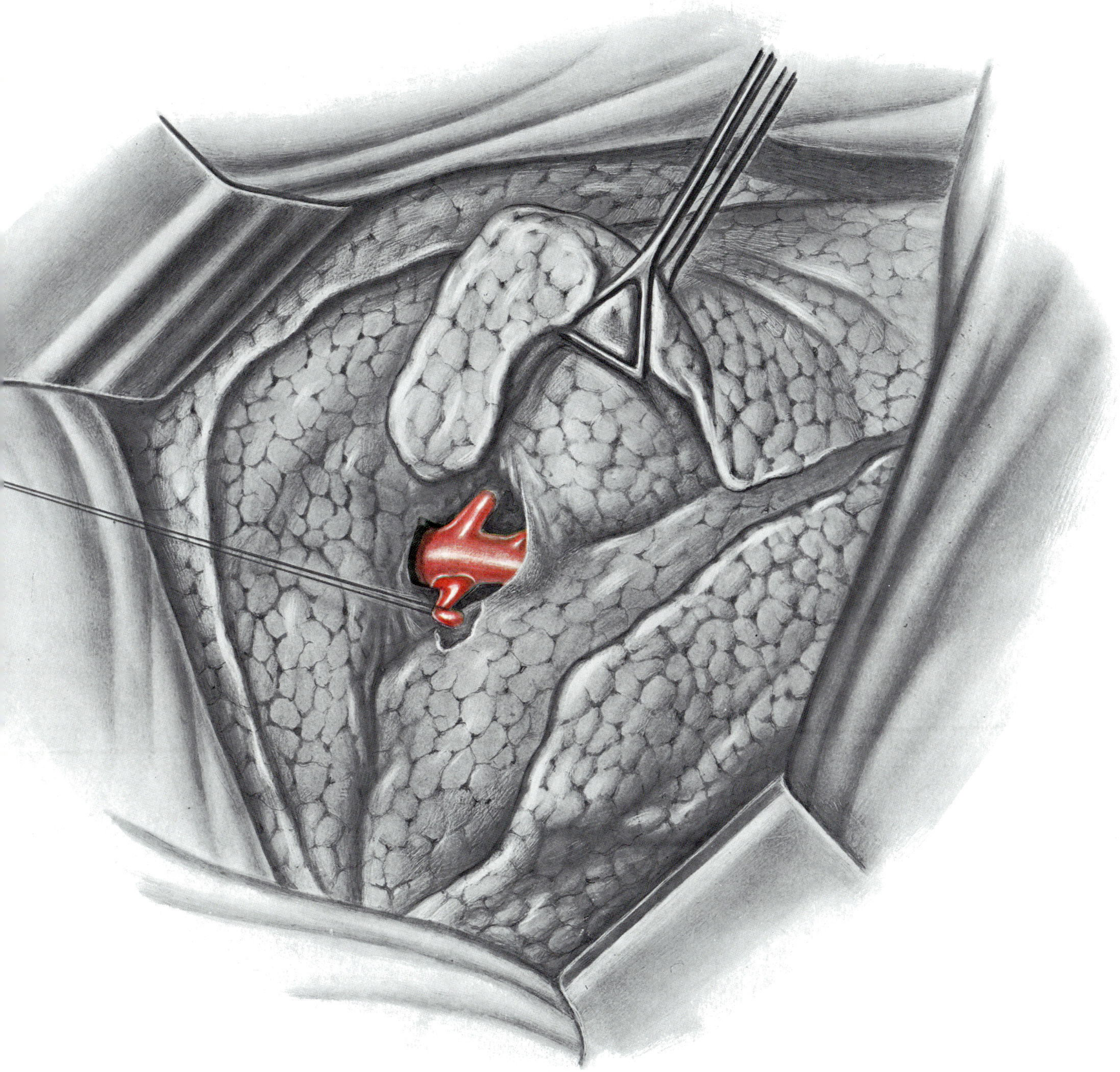

Fig. 135. Separation of A_6 from side of interlobar fissure.

ventrally by traction sutures (Fig. 136). V_6 is found in its immediate locality somewhat caudally and is prepared.

The vein of the sixth segment may be exposed from the dorsal surface of the lung, as shown in the resection of S_6 on the left.

The bridge between S_2 and S_6 is disconnected. The segment is removed by the peripheral bronchial stump with the small intersegmental veins carefully treated. The wound surface of the basal segments is not sutured.

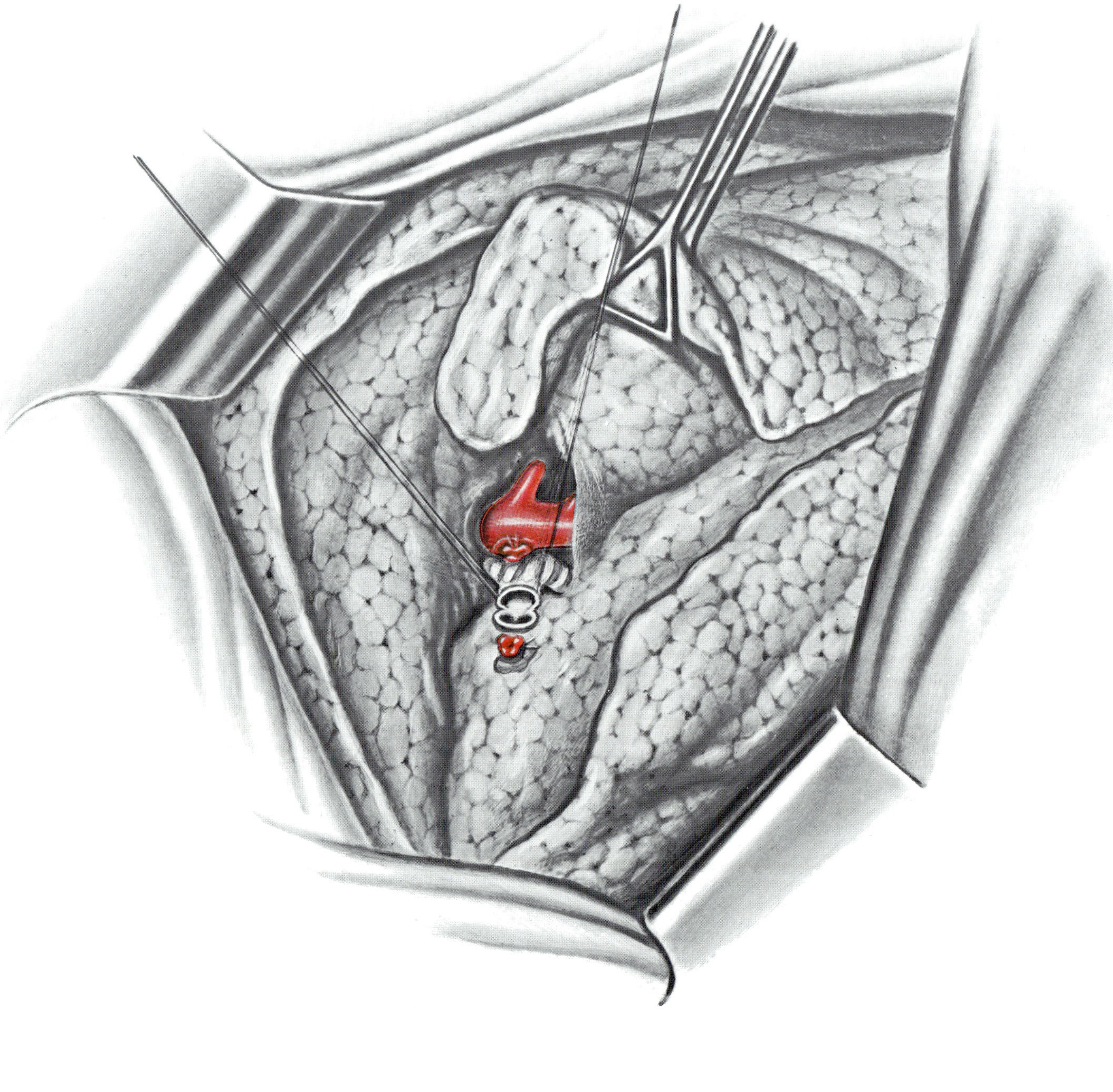

Fig. 136. B_6 has been transected, and traction sutures are applied to stump.

S_7 RESECTION

The pleural cavity is opened by a lateral or anterolateral approach in the fourth intercostal space.

The main interlobar fissure is opened. A_7, which is the extreme medial branch of the artery of the basal segment, is found in the middle third of the fissure. A_7 is ligated and transected (Fig. 137).

B_7 is palpated immediately under A_7 and prepared. The bronchus is transected, and its stump is closed with interrupted sutures or with a circular ligature passed through it (Fig. 138).

With the peripheral bronchial stump being pulled on, the segment is removed while the branches of the intersegmental vein are carefully ligated.

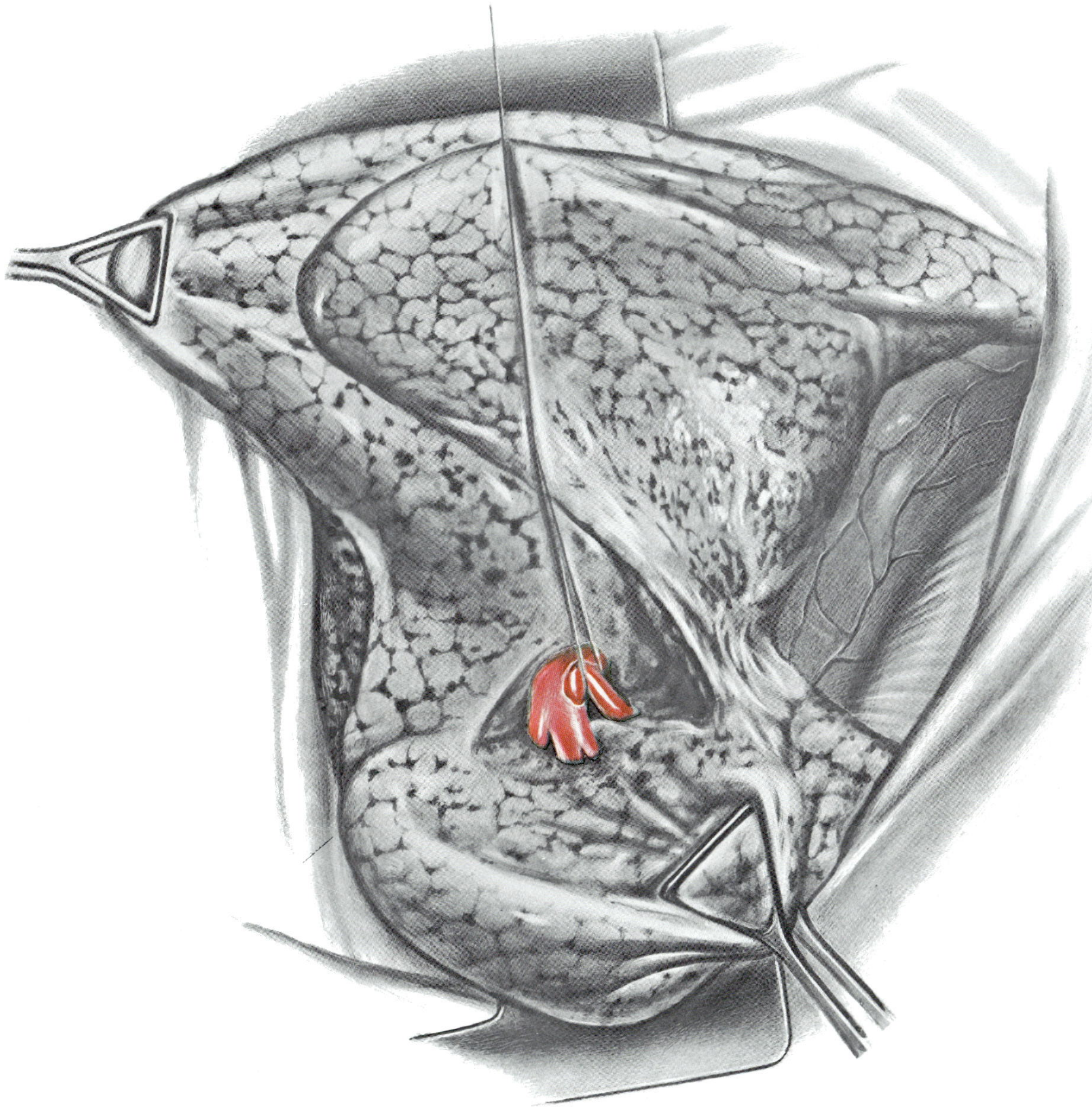

Fig. 137. Separation and ligation of A_7 from side of interlobar fissure.

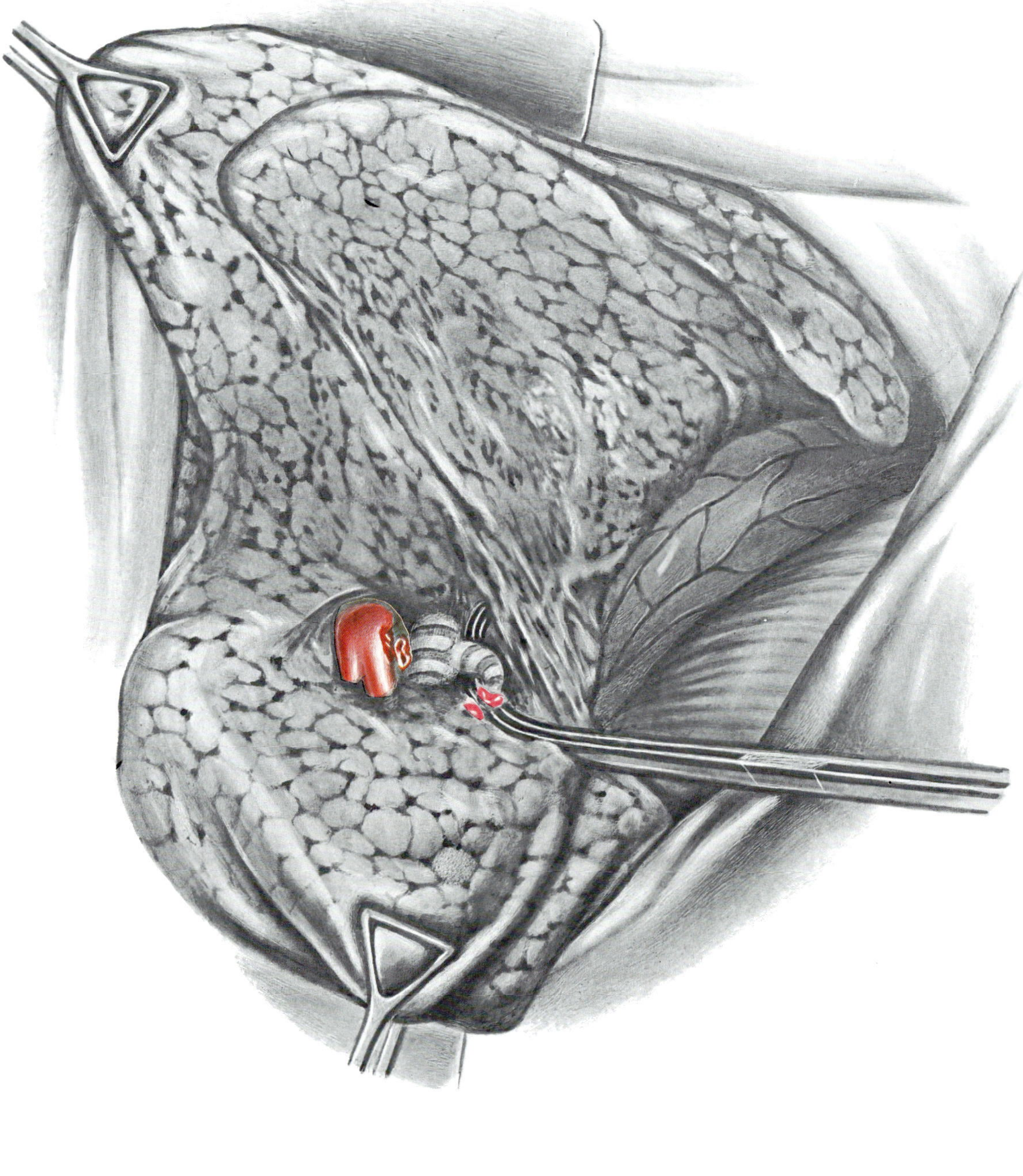

Fig. 138. A dissector is brought under B_7. Stumps of A_7 are visible.

$S_{9,10}$ RESECTION

The pleural cavity is opened by a lateral approach in the sixth intercostal space.

The main interlobar fissure is widely opened. The artery of the basal segment is exposed in the middle third of the fissure. $A_{9,10}$ is found on the dorsolateral wall of this artery below the orifice of A_6 and is prepared (Fig. 139). In rare cases two arterial branches extend to $S_{9,10}$. These are ligated separately.

$B_{9,10}$ is found under the artery in the space between A_6 and A_8 and is prepared. The bronchus is clamped, and after trial inflation of the inferior lobe it is transected. The bronchial stump is sutured by hand (Fig. 140).

It is very difficult to remove the segments because they are closely connected with S_6 and S_8.

S_6 is first disconnected. Pulling on the peripheral stumps of the bronchi, S_6 and $S_{9,10}$ are folded over the line of the intended resection. The intersegmental venous communications are ligated and transected. After that, $S_{9,10}$ are disconnected from S_8 in a similar way (Fig. 141). The defect thus formed in the parenchyma of the inferior lobe is repaired by stitching together the edges of S_6 and S_8 (Fig. 142).

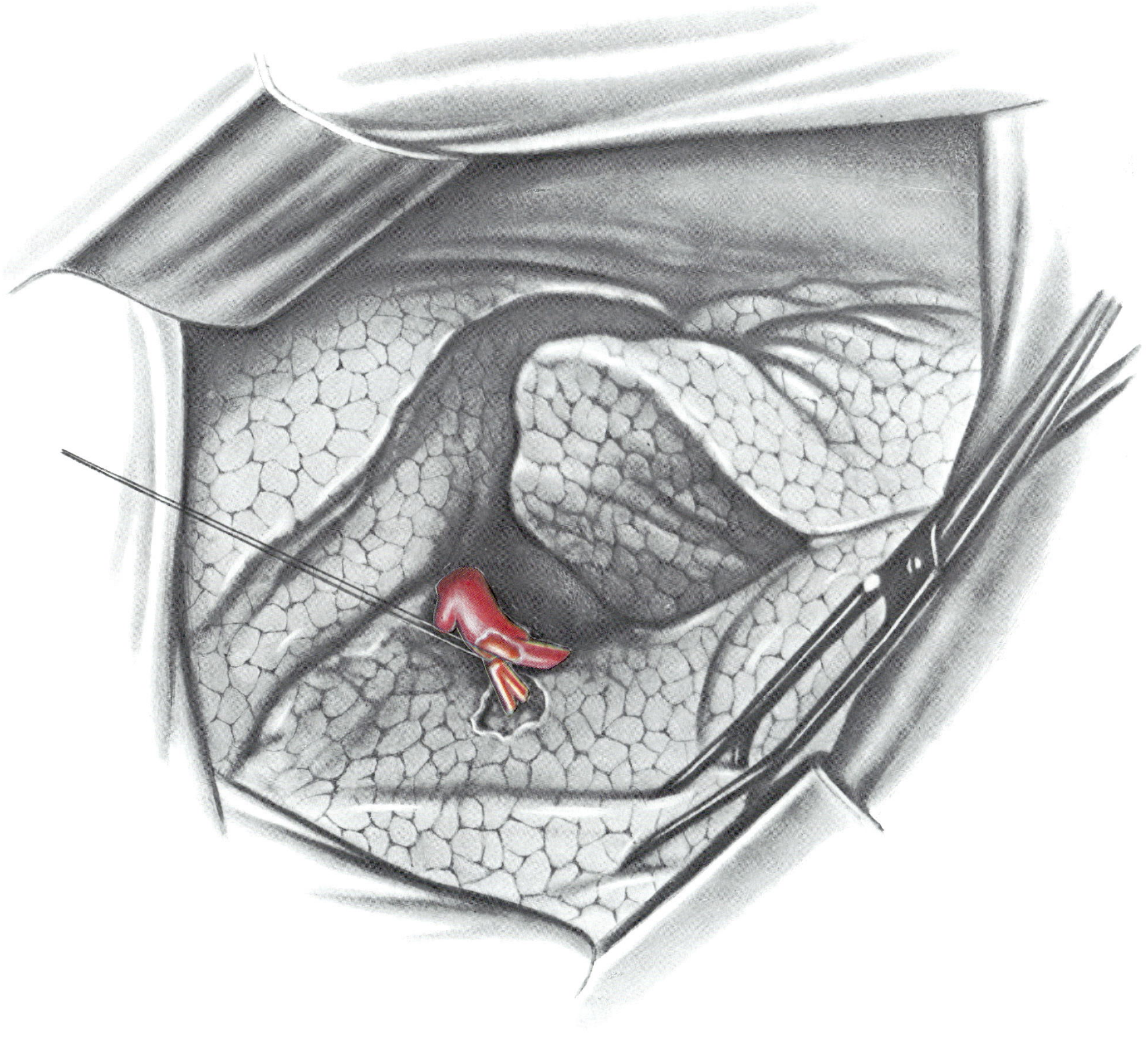

Fig. 139. A ligature has been brought under $A_{9,10}$.

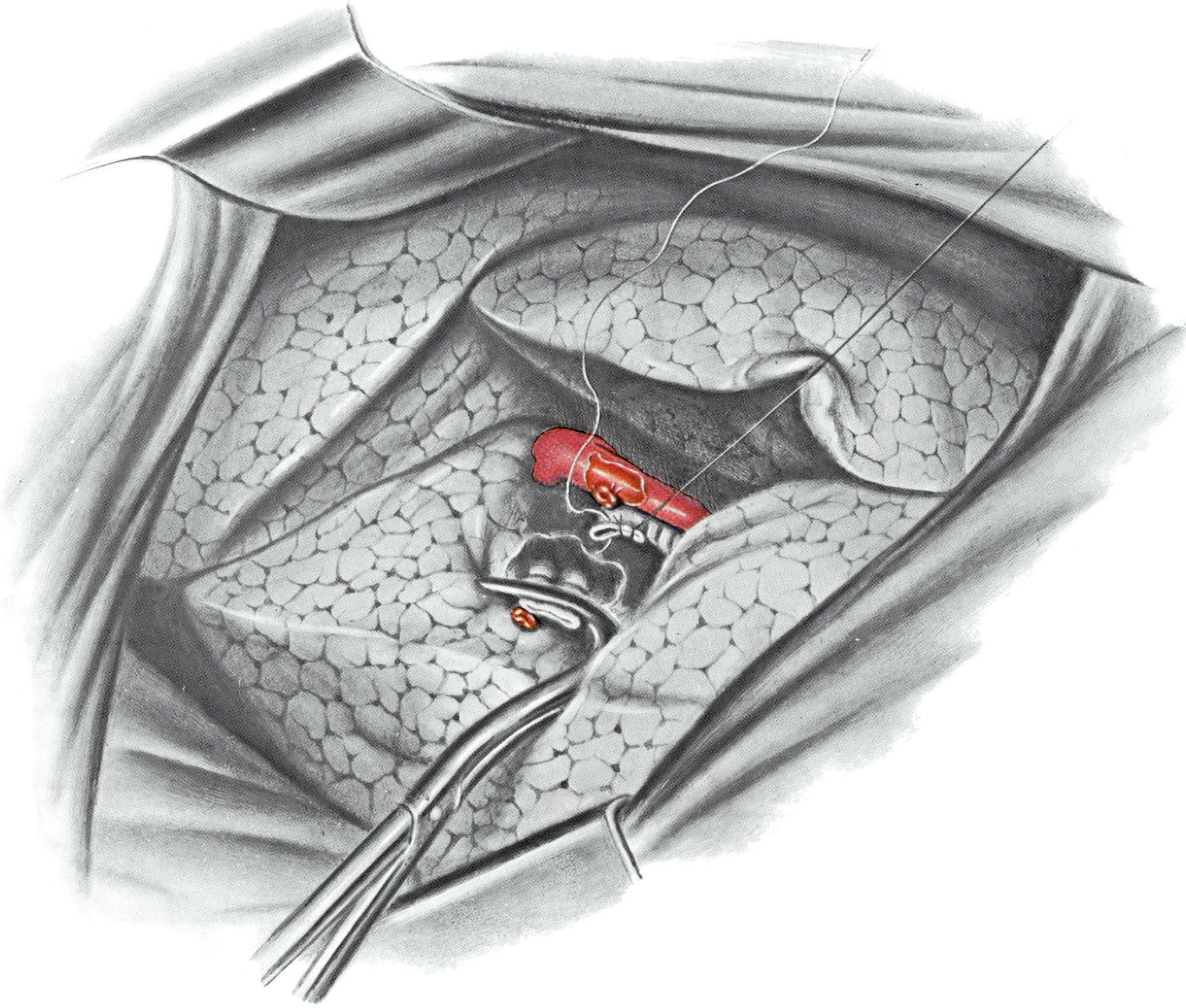

Fig. 140. Stump of $B_{9,10}$, which has been separated by manipulating from side of main interlobar fissure, is closed with sutures.

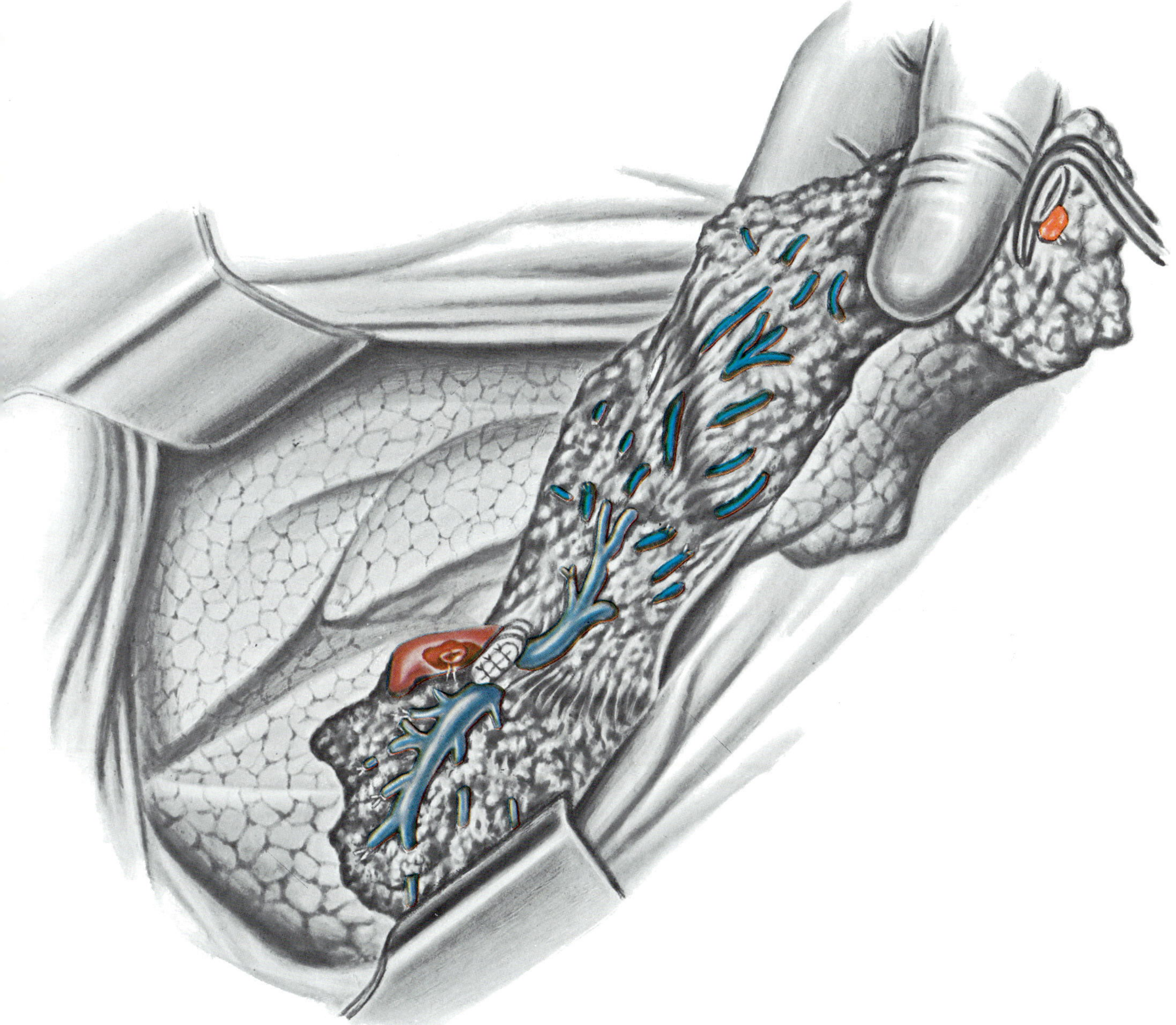

Fig. 141. $S_{9,10}$ is separated from S_8. Bronchial stump is closed with sutures. V_6 and V_8 intersegmental branches are visible.

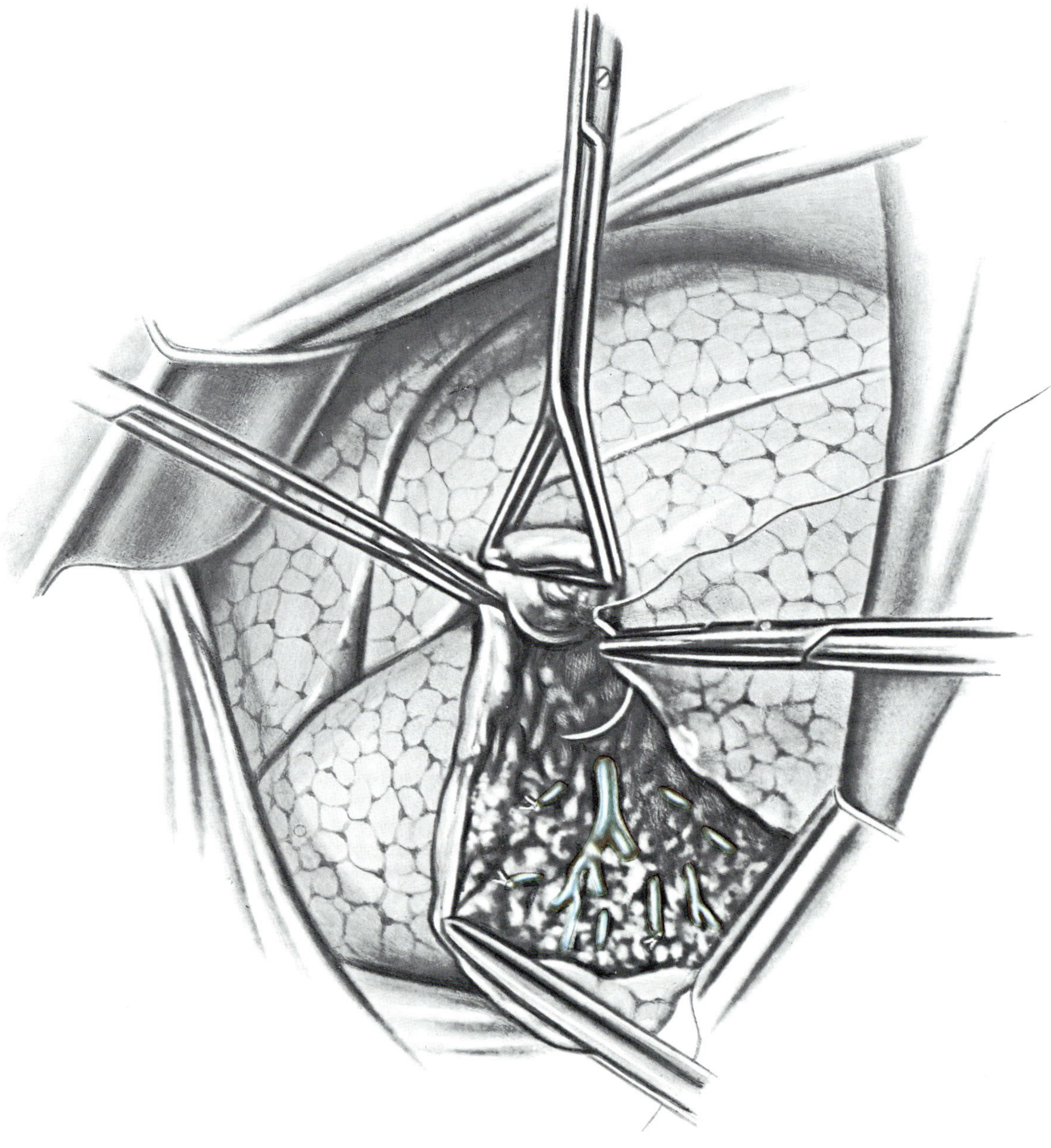

Fig. 142. S_6 and S_8 are stitched together.

RESECTION OF $S_{7,8,9,10}$ (BASAL SEGMENTS)

The pleural cavity is opened by a lateral approach in the fifth or sixth intercostal space.

The inferior lobe is freed from the adhesions, and the pulmonary ligament is cut. The main interlobar fissure is opened, and the artery of the basal segment is found on the floor of its dorsal third and treated by the ligature method (Fig. 143). The inferior lobe is pulled laterally, and the mediastinal pleura is cut above the inferior pulmonary vein. The basal vein is ligated and transected (Fig. 144). V_6 is separated from the dorsal wall of the basal bronchus with tampons.

The main interlobar fissure is again opened, and the bronchus of the basal segments is found somewhat medially to the arterial stump, cut, and sutured by hand (Fig. 145).

With the peripheral bronchial stump and the vascular stumps being pulled on, the basal segments are removed while stripping a flap of the pulmonary pleura from them (Fig. 146). This flap is placed on the wound surface of S_6 and stitched to its edges. If the pleural flap cannot be obtained, the wound surface is not sutured. The apex of S_6 is fastened to S_2 with a single suture.

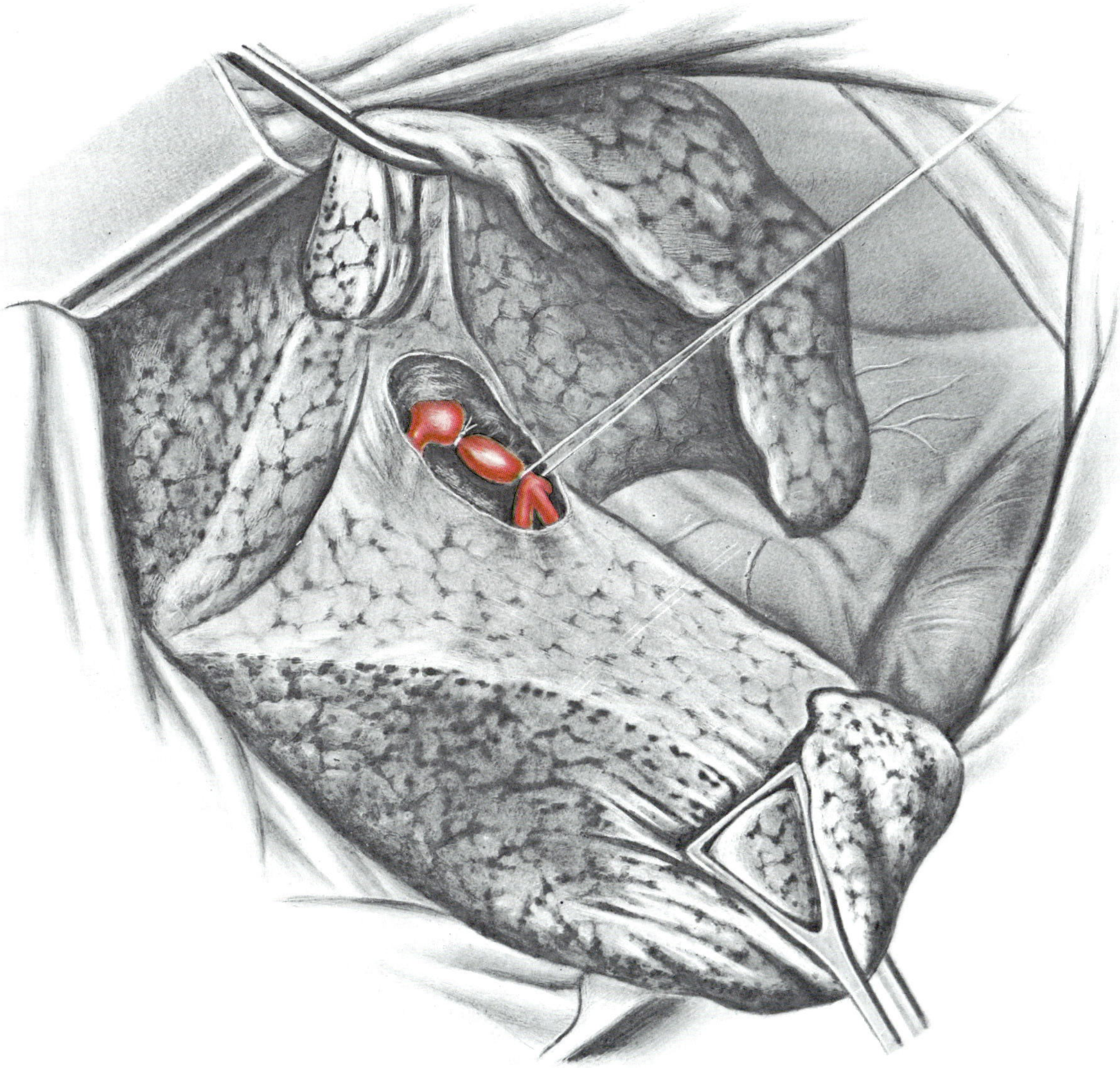

Fig. 143. Separation and ligation of arteries of basal segments from side of main interlobular fissure.

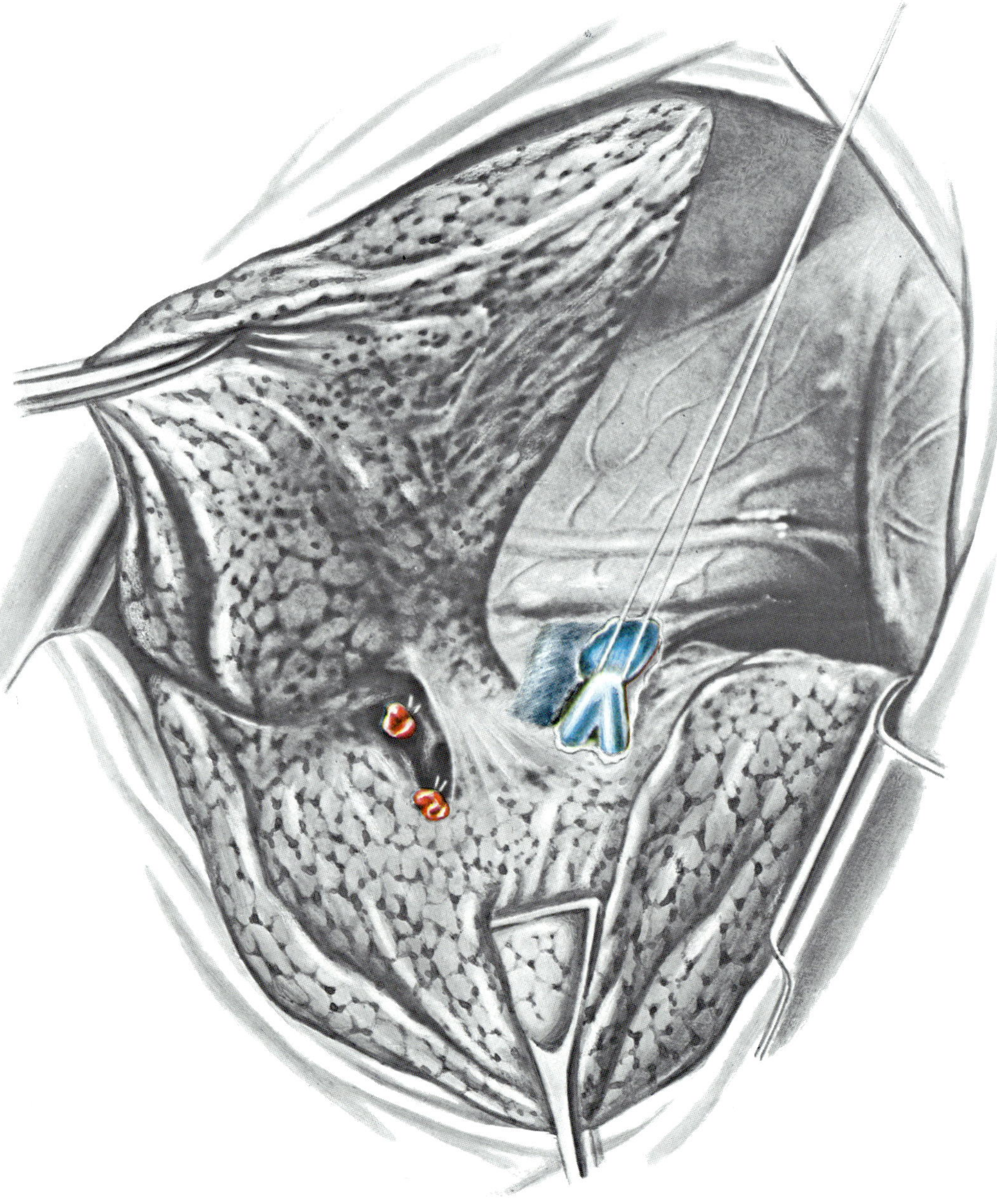

Fig. 144. Vein of basal segment is held by a ligature; artery has been transected.

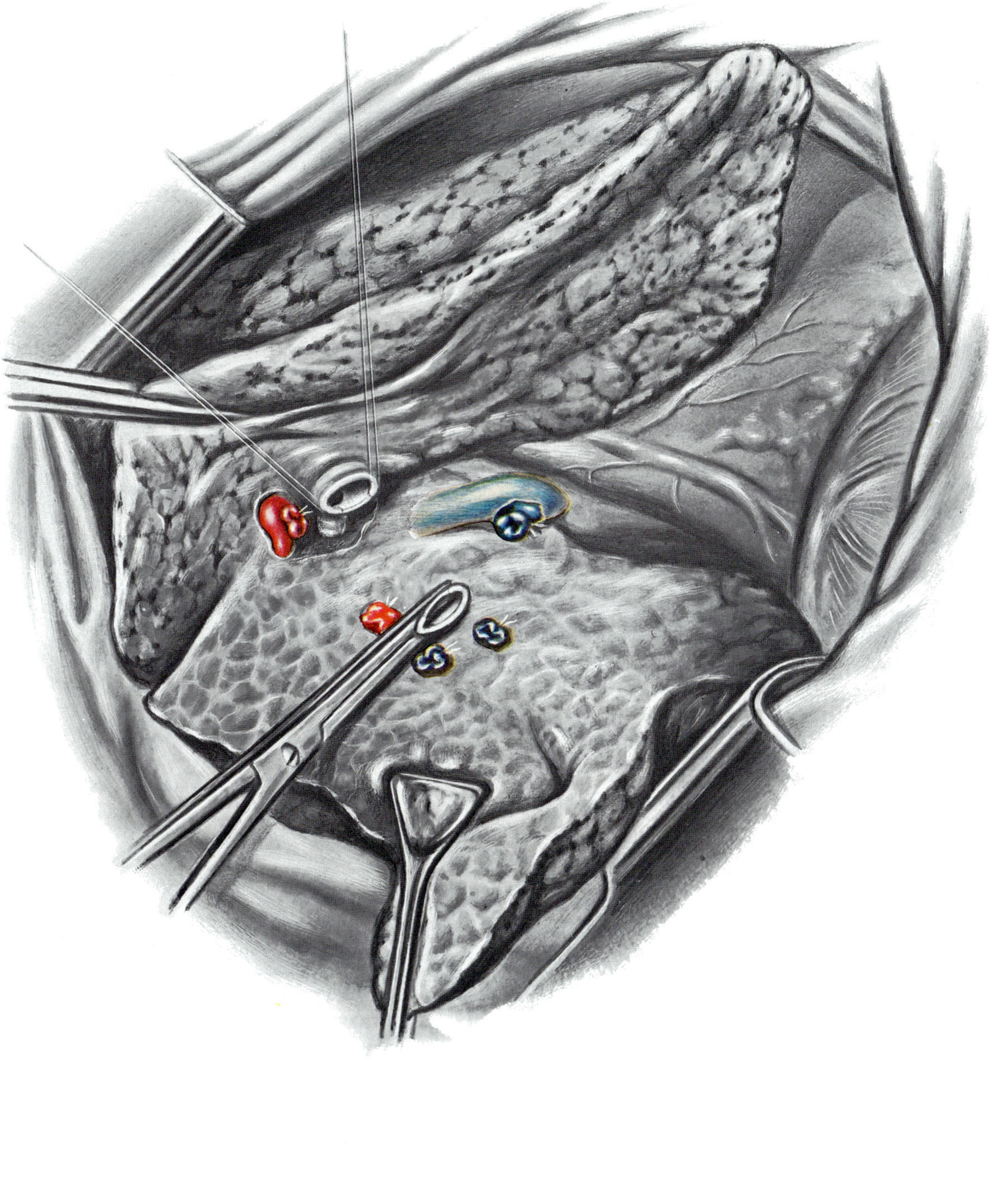

Fig. 145. Bronchus of basal segment has been transected, and traction sutures have been applied to its stump.

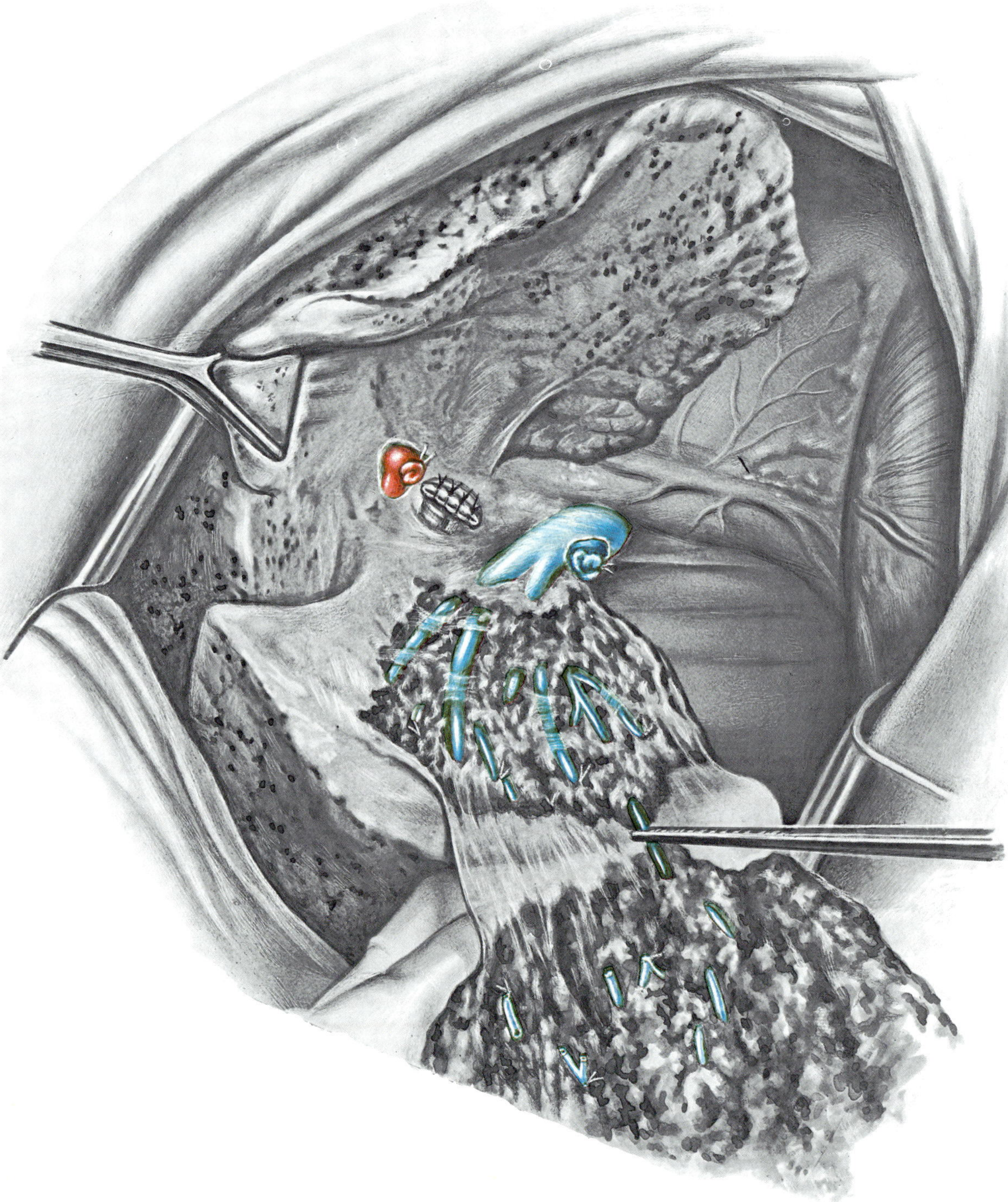

Fig. 146. Separation of basal segments from S_6. Each intersegmental vein is tied separately. Bronchial stump is closed with sutures.

OPERATIONS ON THE LEFT LUNG

PNEUMONECTOMY

The pleural cavity is opened by a lateral approach in the fifth intercostal space.

The lung is freed from the adhesions, and the pulmonary ligament is cut. In total adhesions, particularly in the region of the diaphragm, it is best to carry out pneumonolysis at the end of the operation. In case of unforeseen complications, however, the root of the lung should be exposed on all sides prior to the preparation of its components.

The mediastinal pleura is cut dorsally and along the phrenic nerve under the root of the lung. In the cranial part of the root the left pulmonary artery is prepared

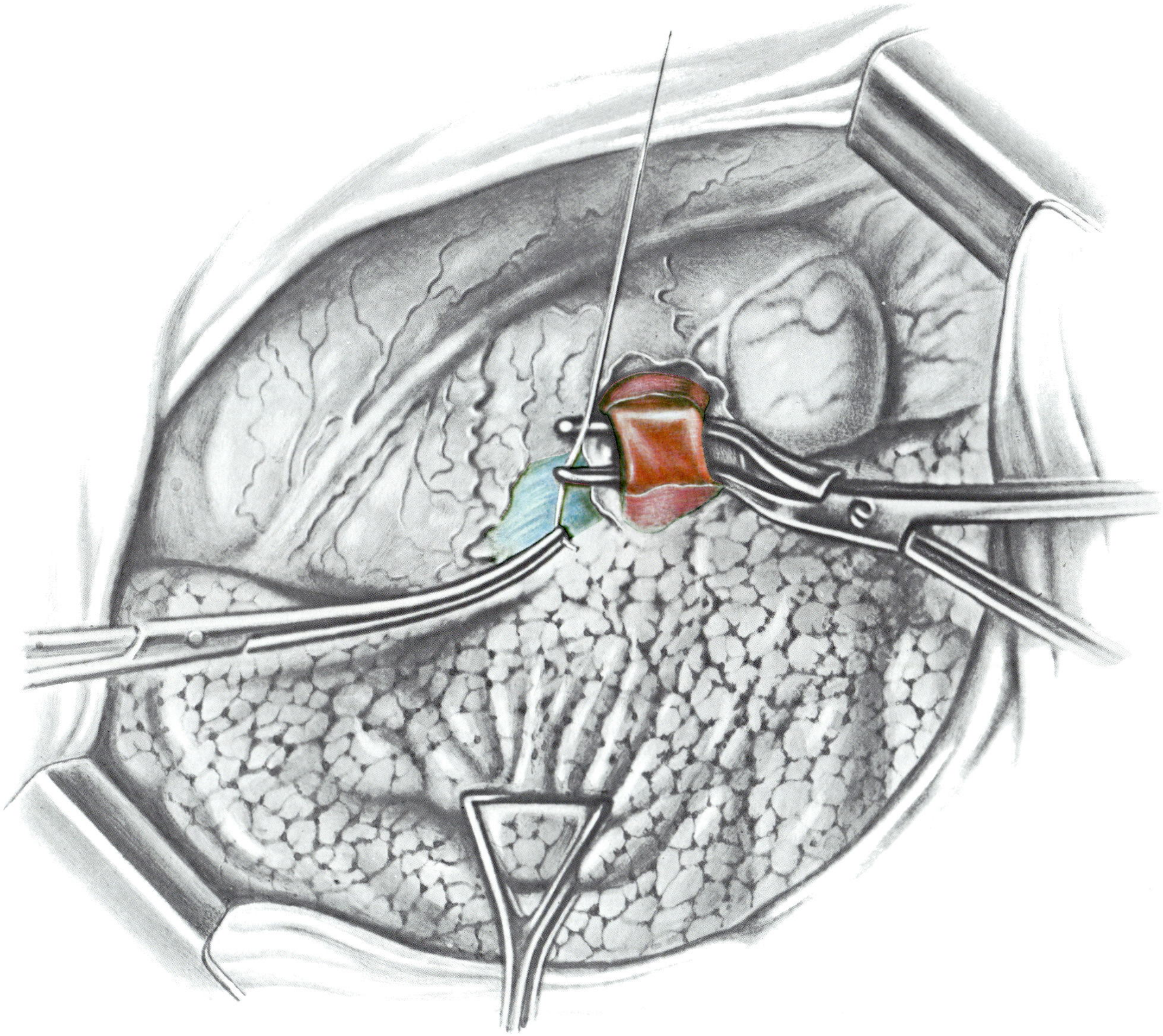

Fig. 147. A ligature is brought under left pulmonary artery.

for a distance of no less than 3 cm. It is treated by the ligature method or stitched through with the УС instrument (Fig. 147).

The superior pulmonary vein situated on the ventral surface of the root of the lung is then exposed. It is prepared up to the pericardium, treated by the ligature method, and transected (Fig. 148).

The inferior lobe is grasped with pulmonary forceps and drawn far away to the lateral side. Due to this, the inferior pulmonary vein is clearly outlined, and the overlying mediastinal pleura is cut. The vein is separated with the finger or a dissector, treated by the ligature method or stitched through with the УС instrument, and transected (Fig. 149).

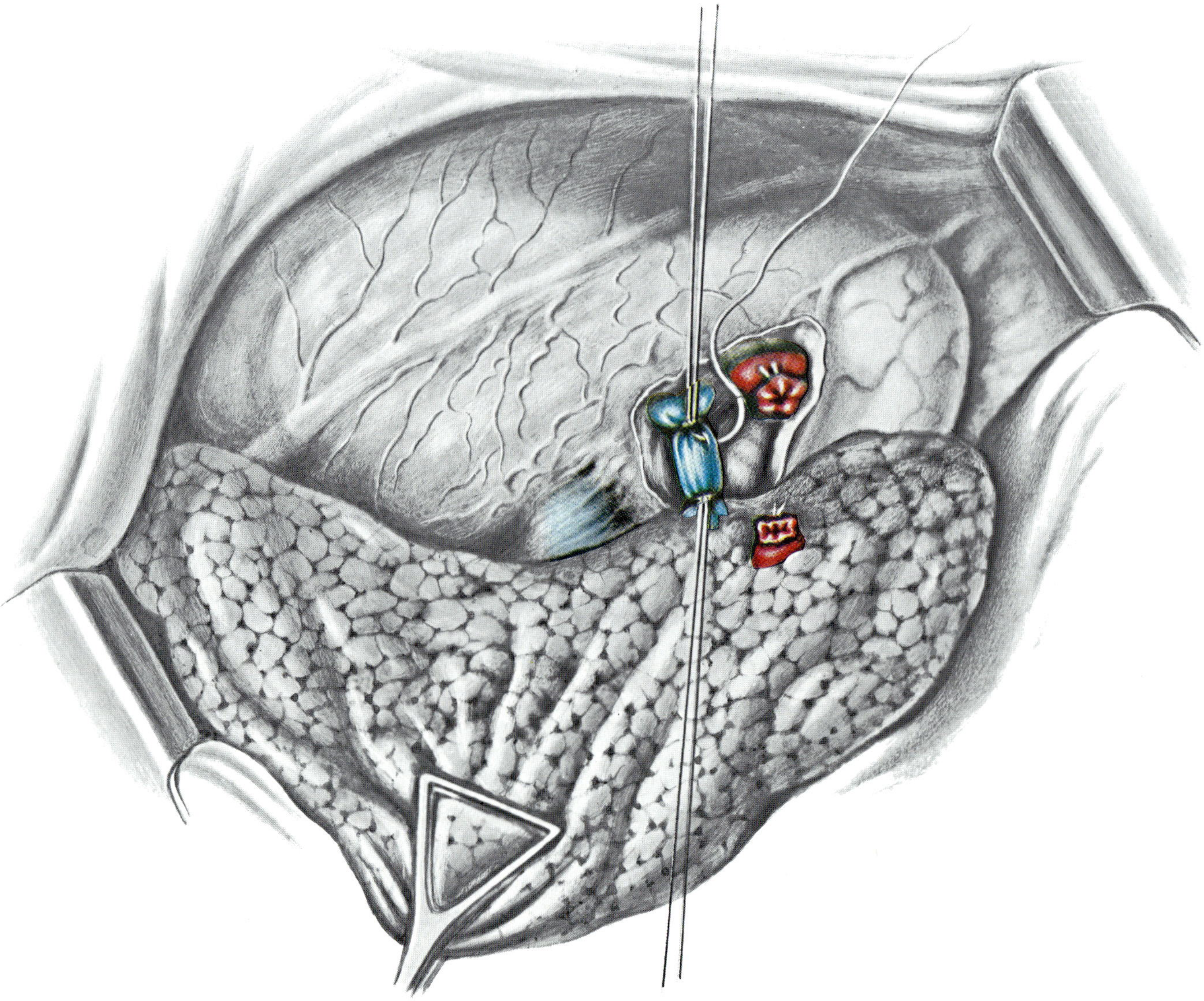

Fig. 148. Superior pulmonary vein is ligated with threads that had been passed through it. Pulmonary artery has been transected.

The ventral wall of the left main bronchus is exposed by the blunt and sharp techniques. If possible the bronchial artery should be clamped right there and ligated. A finger or a dissector is passed around the dorsal surface of the bronchus, and Fedorov's clamp is applied to its cranial part. The bronchus is pulled out as much as possible from the mediastinum and separated from the surrounding tissues up to the tracheobronchial angle. Traction sutures are applied (Fig. 150). The bronchus is treated by hand or stitched through with the УО instrument and transected. The lung is removed. Since the bronchial stump will be deep under the aortic arch, there is no need to cover it with the pleura.

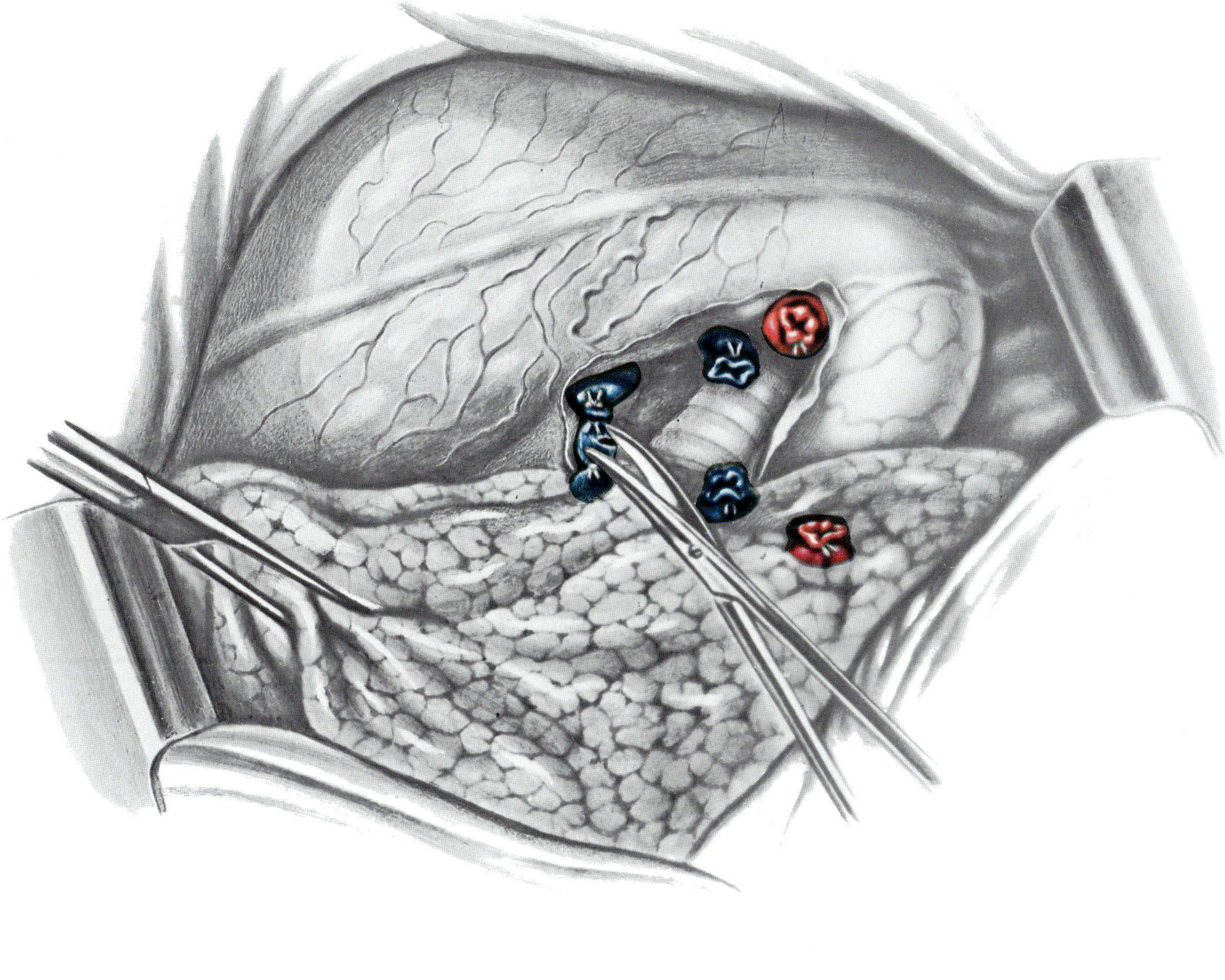

Fig. 149. Ligated inferior pulmonary vein is transected.

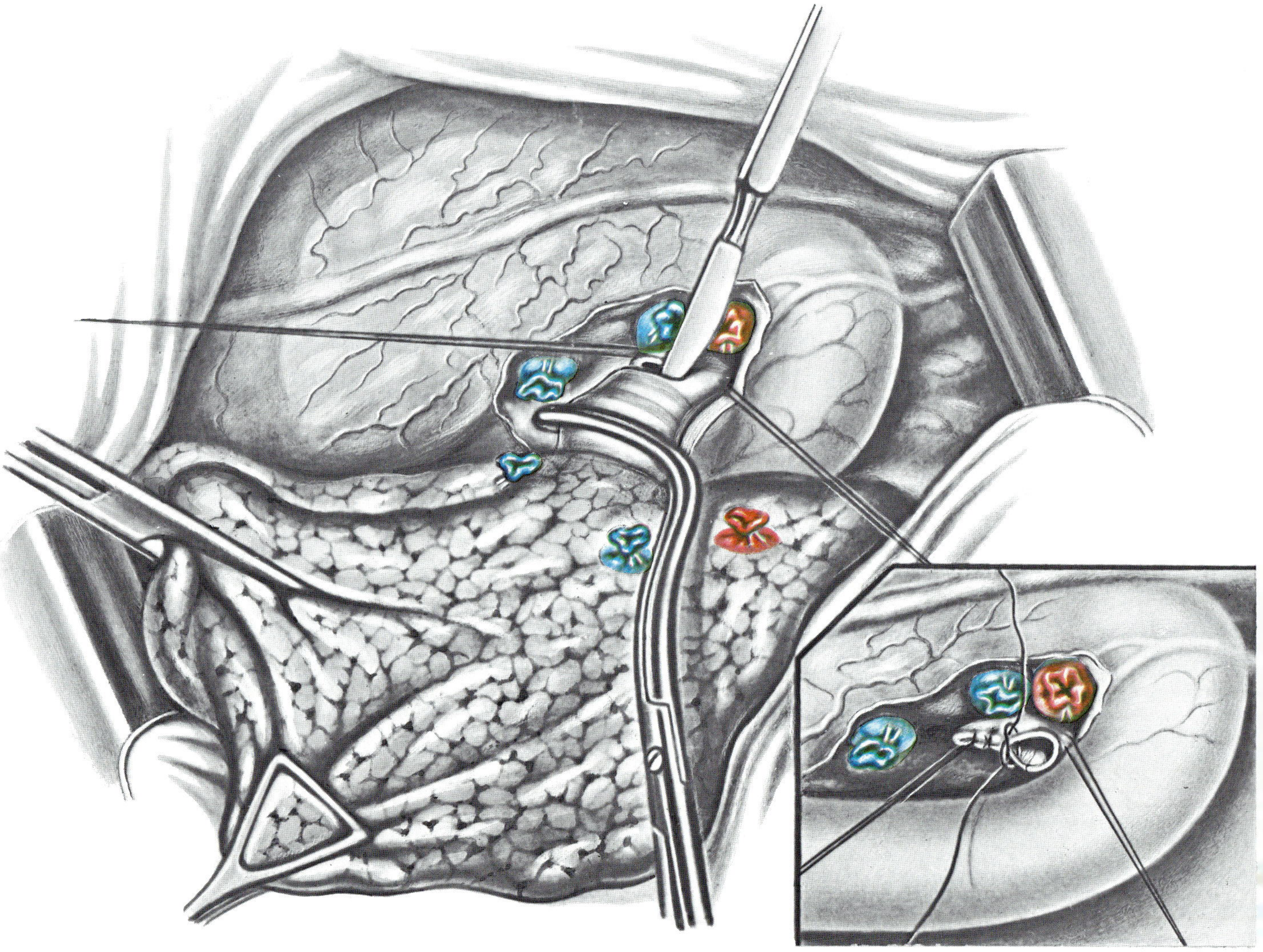

Fig. 150. Left main bronchus is transected and its stump sutured.

Intrapericardial ligation of vessels in extensive pneumonectomy. Just as in the case of pathological processes on the right side, indications for this intervention are relatively rare.

The pericardium is opened dorsally and along the phrenic nerve for 6 to 8 cm. The pericardial flaps are drawn aside by traction sutures. The vessels of the lung are located on the dorsal surface of the pericardial cavity and are covered with the pericardium on three sides. This is why the preparation of each one of them is begun by cutting the pericardial covering.

An inflammatory or cancerous process often makes it difficult to approach the pulmonary artery, which is very short in the pericardial cavity, no longer than 2 cm. That is why it is prepared last.

The inferior pulmonary vein, which is found immediately caudally and dorsally to the left atrial auricle, is prepared first. It is treated by the ligature method and

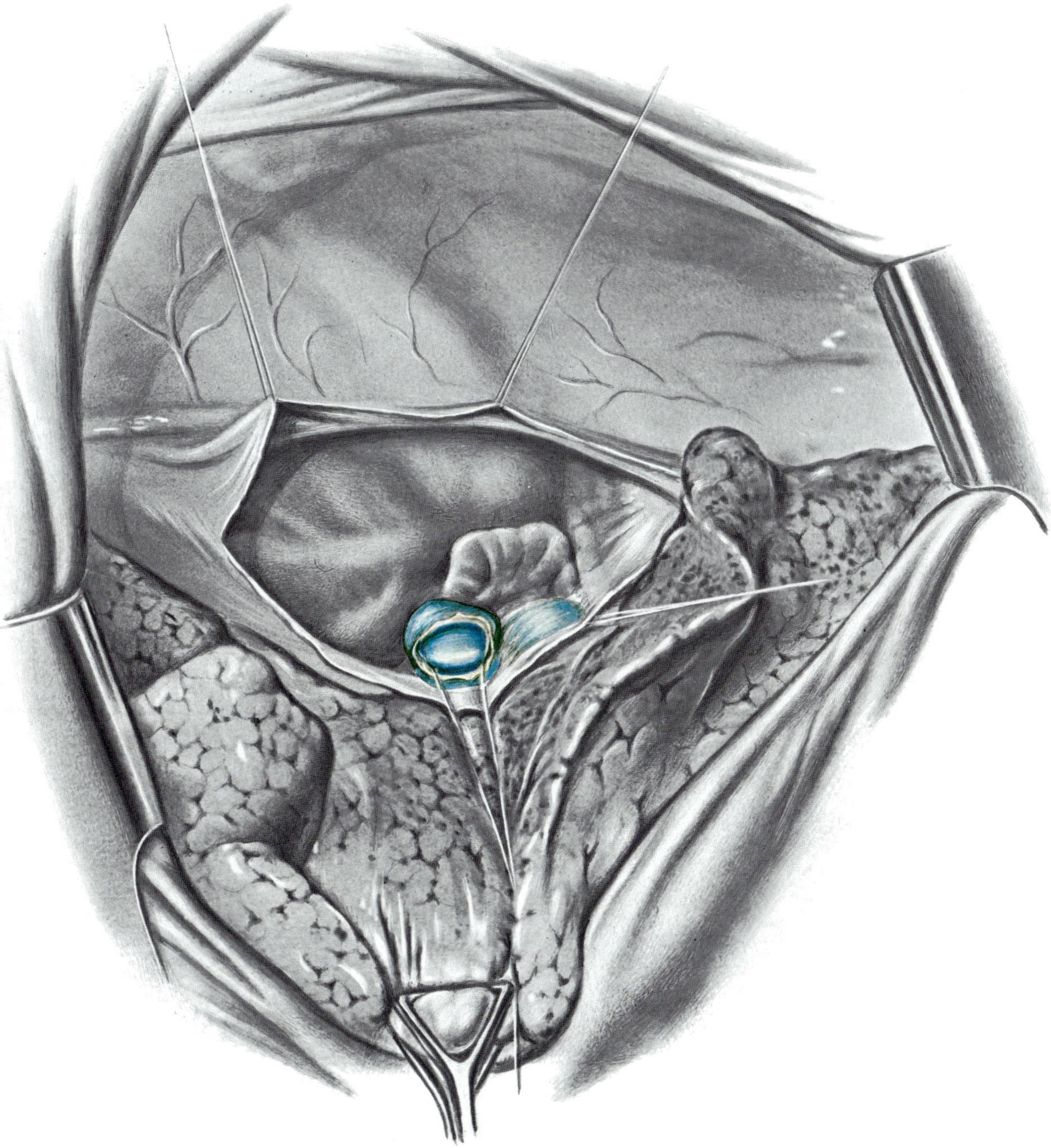

Fig. 151. Inferior pulmonary vein is separated and held with a ligature.

transected (Fig. 151). The superior pulmonary vein is at the level of the atrial auricle or its cranial border. It is also treated by the ligature method (Fig. 152).

With both pulmonary veins transected, access to the pulmonary artery improves, but its preparation is still difficult, not only because it is short, but because the pulmonary trunk lies close and if injured may cause dangerous hemorrhage. Besides, the walls of the artery are often sclerosed and involved in the infiltration. This is why the posterior wall of the vessel is separated with great caution and a ligature is drawn under it (Fig. 153). It is most convenient to carry out final ligation and transection of the artery after the main bronchus has been cut away.

The lung is removed together with part of the pericardium. The defect thus formed is corrected, if possible, but not sutured tightly.

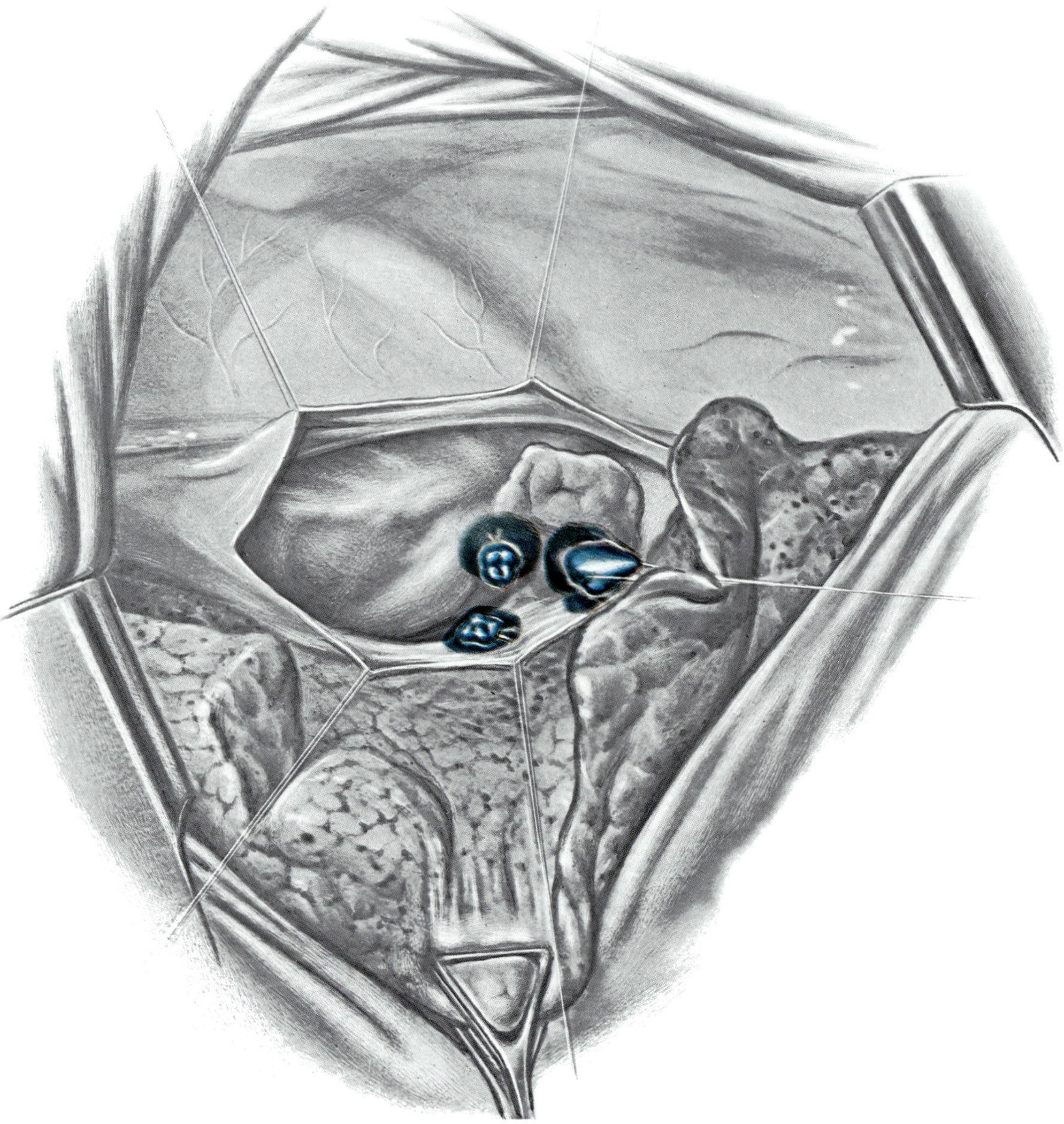

Fig. 152. Treatment of superior pulmonary vein. Inferior pulmonary vein has been transected.

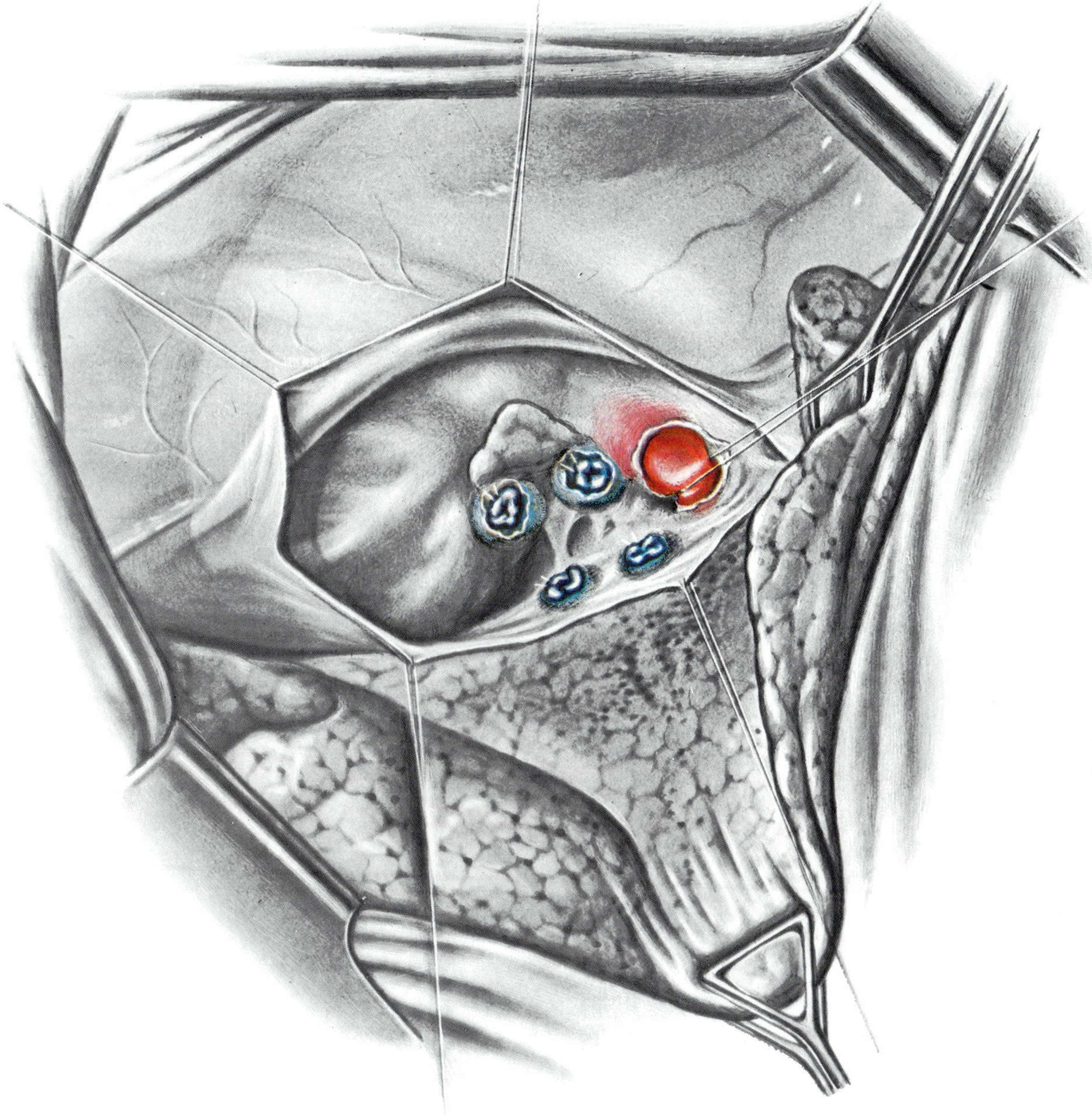

Fig. 153. Ligation of left pulmonary artery. Pulmonary veins have been transected.

SUPERIOR LOBECTOMY

The pleural cavity is opened by a lateral approach in the fifth intercostal space.

The superior lobe is freed from the adhesions. The mediastinal pleura is cut over the root of the lung dorsal to the phrenic nerve. The left pulmonary artery is found in the cranial part of the root, and the branches given off to the superior lobe are ligated one by one and transected (Fig. 154). In some cases it is more convenient to treat the artery of the lingular segment from the side of the main interlobar fissure, particularly when this artery arises at the level of or below A_6 (Fig. 155). If the fissure is obliterated, the lingular artery may be ligated after the bronchus has been transected. The superior pulmonary vein is prepared on the ventral surface of the root of the lung. It is advisable to separate its central part up to the pericardium. The vein is tied by the ligature method or stitched through with the УС instrument and transected (Fig. 156).

The superior lobar bronchus is located immediately deep below the superior pulmonary vein. In separating its dorsal wall caution should be exercised so as not to injure the artery of the inferior lobe. Since the superior lobar bronchus is short, it is always preferable to treat it by hand. Federov's clamp is applied to the peripheral

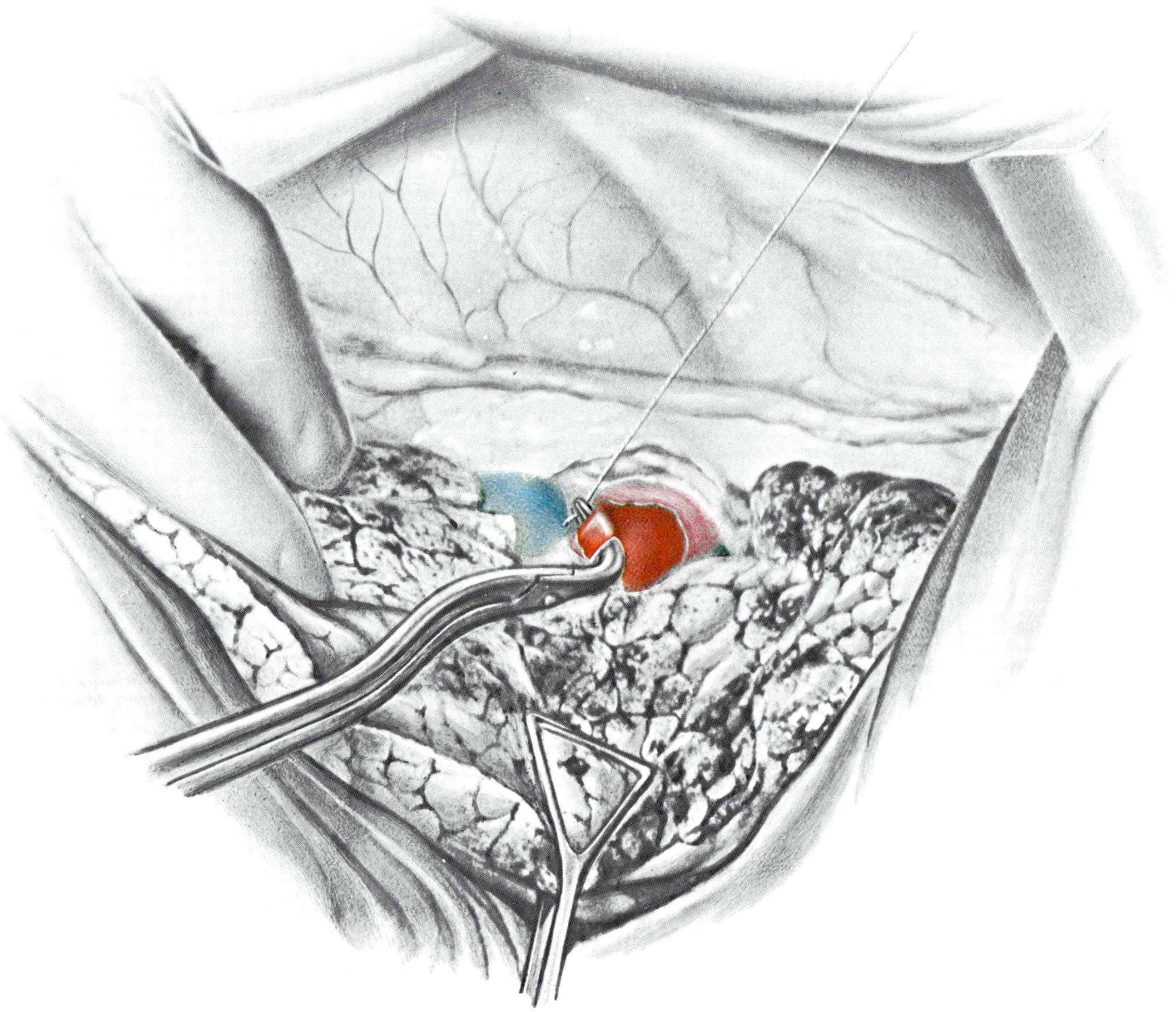

Fig. 154. Successive ligation and transection of arteries of superior lobe. A dissector is brought under A_1.

part of the bronchus, and traction sutures to the central part (Fig. 157). The bronchus is transected where it divides into the segmental branches, and the stump is closed with interrupted sutures and covered with the mediastinal pleura.

The superior lobe is drawn away cranially and ventrally and separated from the inferior lobe from the side of the interlobar fissure by means of the УО stitching instrument. The pulmonary ligament is cut to lend more mobility to the inferior lobe.

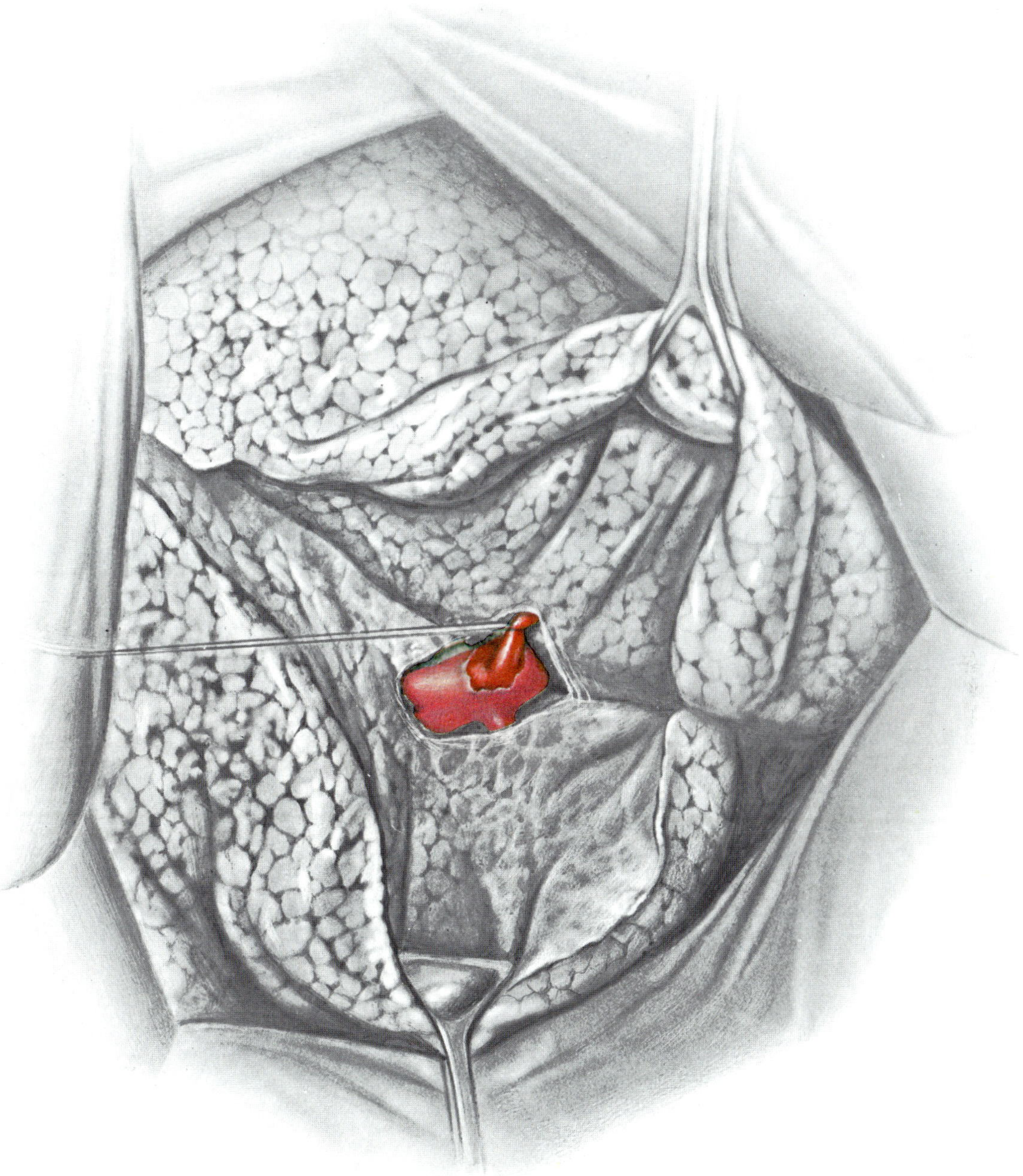

Fig. 155. Preparation of lingular artery from side of main interlobar fissure.

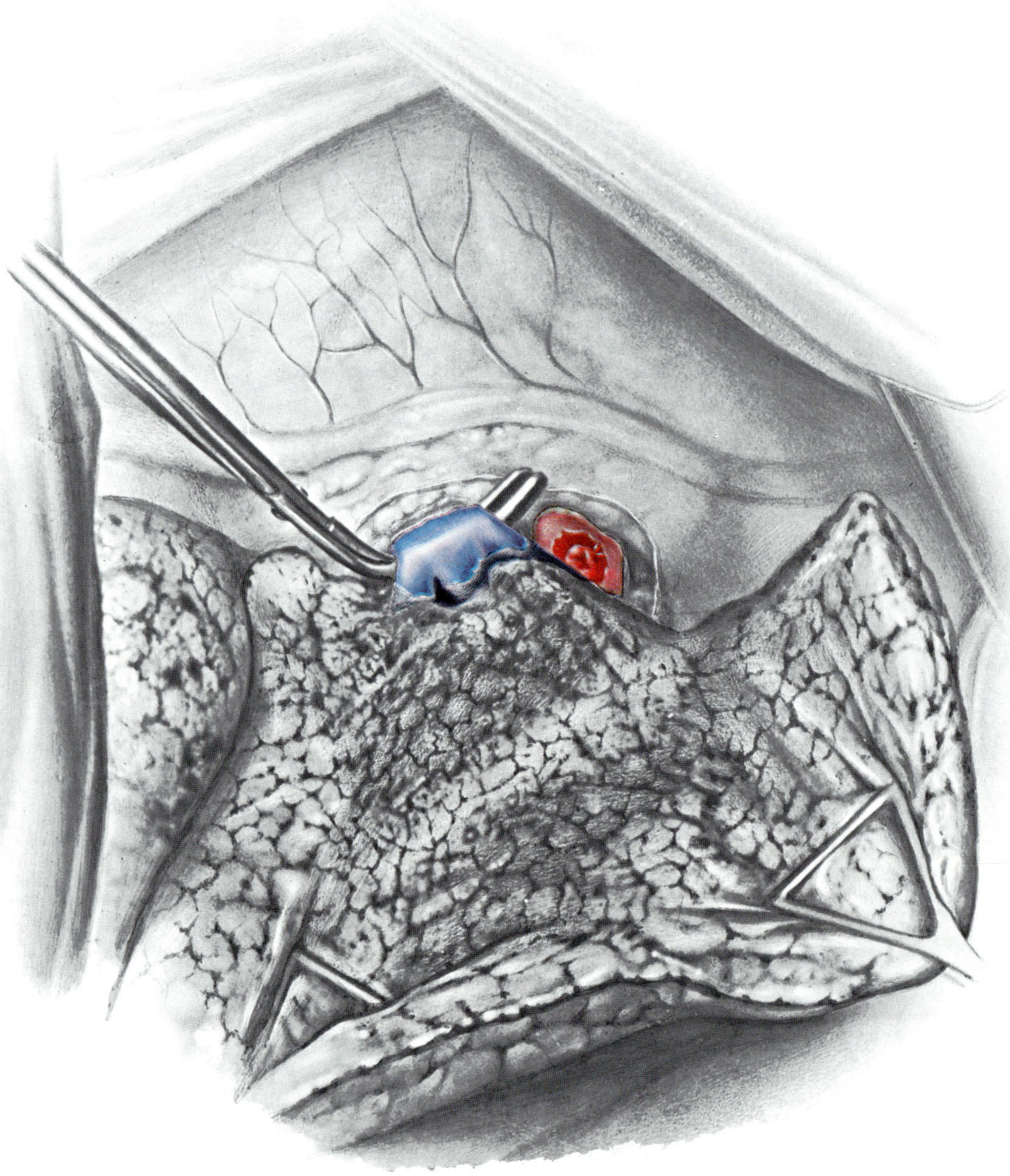

Fig. 156. Superior pulmonary vein has been exposed and a dissector brought under it. Left pulmonary artery with stump of A_3 is visible.

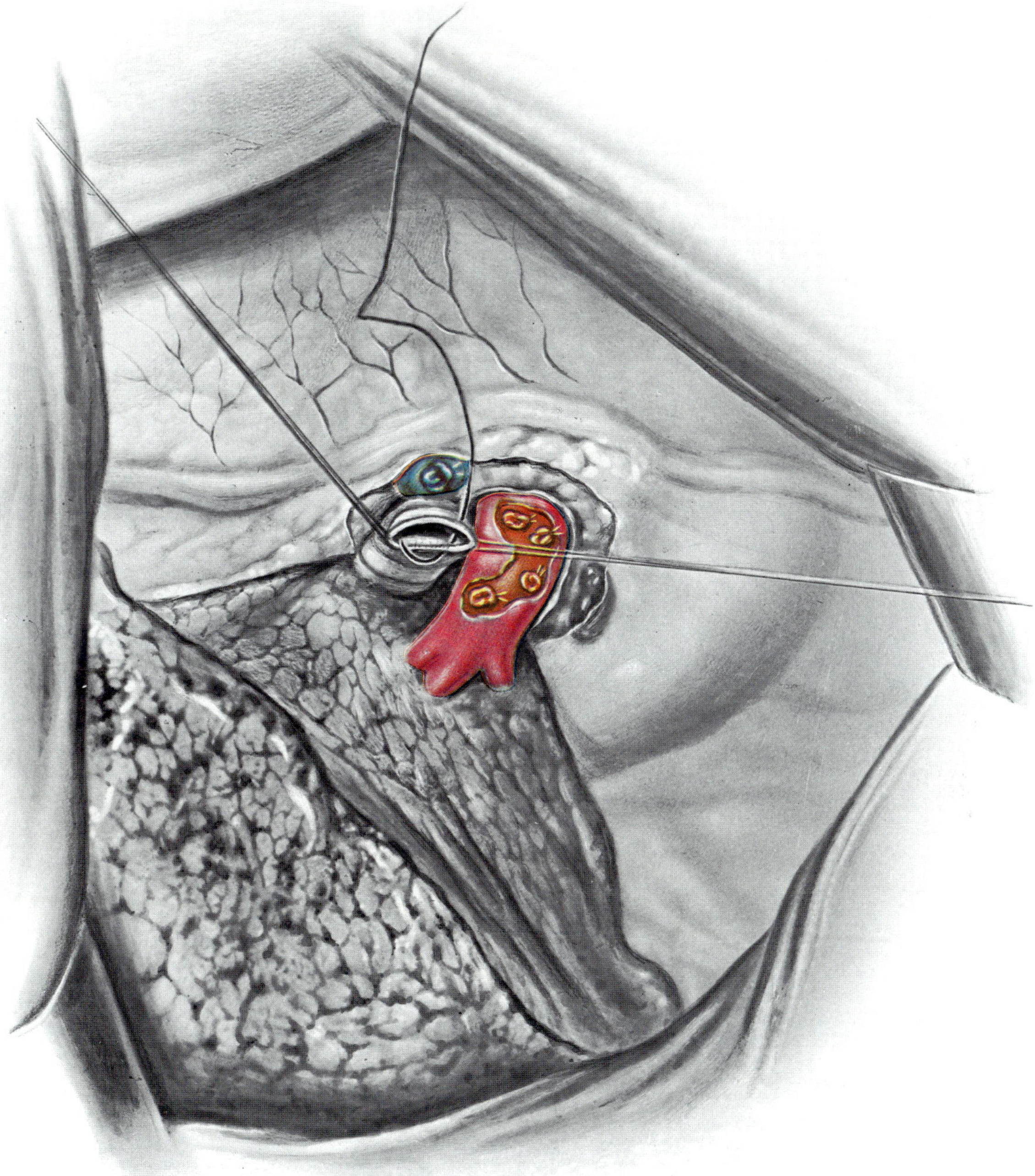

Fig. 157. Stump of superior lobar bronchus is sutured.

The pleural cavity is opened by a lateral approach in the fifth or sixth intercostal space.

The inferior lobe is freed from the adhesions, and the pulmonary ligament is cut. The interlobar fissure is opened widely, and the artery of the inferior lobe is found on its floor under the pulmonary pleura approximately on the boundary between the middle and dorsal thirds. A_6 is the first cranial branch; $A_{4,5}$ branches off on the opposite side (Fig. 158). In some cases the artery of the lingular segments arises below the level of A_6. That is why the branches of the artery of the basal segments must be precisely identified when it is exposed and prepared. To prevent the narrowing of $A_{4,5}$ it is preferable to ligate the artery of the basal segments and A_6 separately.

The inferior lobe is then pulled away laterally from the pericardium. The mediastinal pleura is cut over the inferior pulmonary vein, which is exposed by the blunt

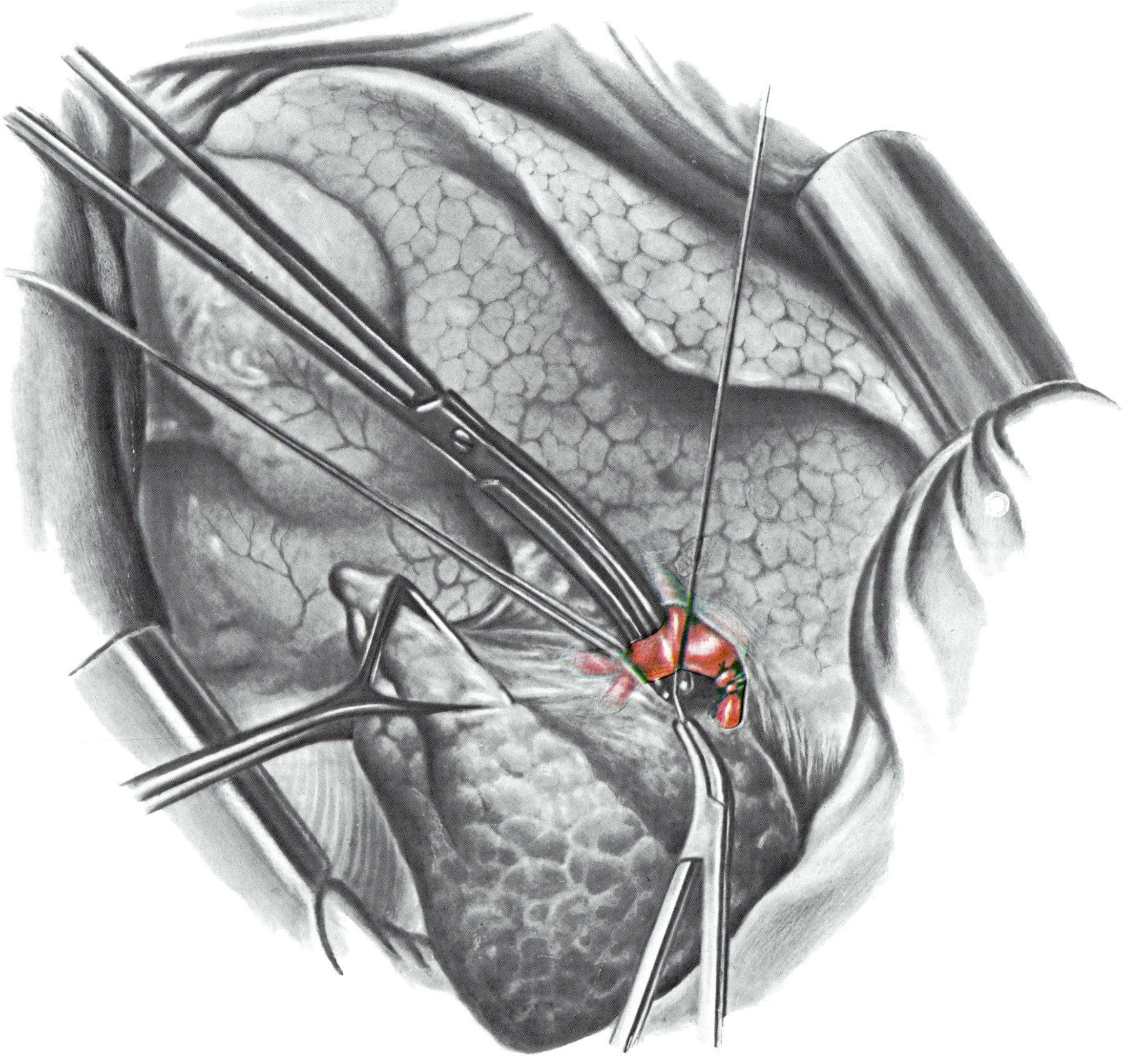

Fig. 158. Arteries of inferior lobe are prepared from side of interlobar fissure. Ligature is brought under artery of basal segments. A_6 has been ligated.

and sharp techniques (Fig. 159). The vein is treated by the ligature method or stitched through with the УС instrument and is transected.

The interlobar fissure is again opened, and the inferior lobar bronchus is found on its floor medial to the arterial stump and is separated. Since it is very short, it is preferable to treat it by hand. Fedorov's clamp is applied to the peripheral end of the bronchus, and traction sutures to the central segment (Fig. 160). The inferior lobar bronchus is transected where it divides into the bronchus of the basal segment and B_6. The stump is closed with interrupted sutures and is covered with mediastinal pleura.

The parenchymatous communications between the inferior and superior lobes are divided by means of clamps or the УО instrument.

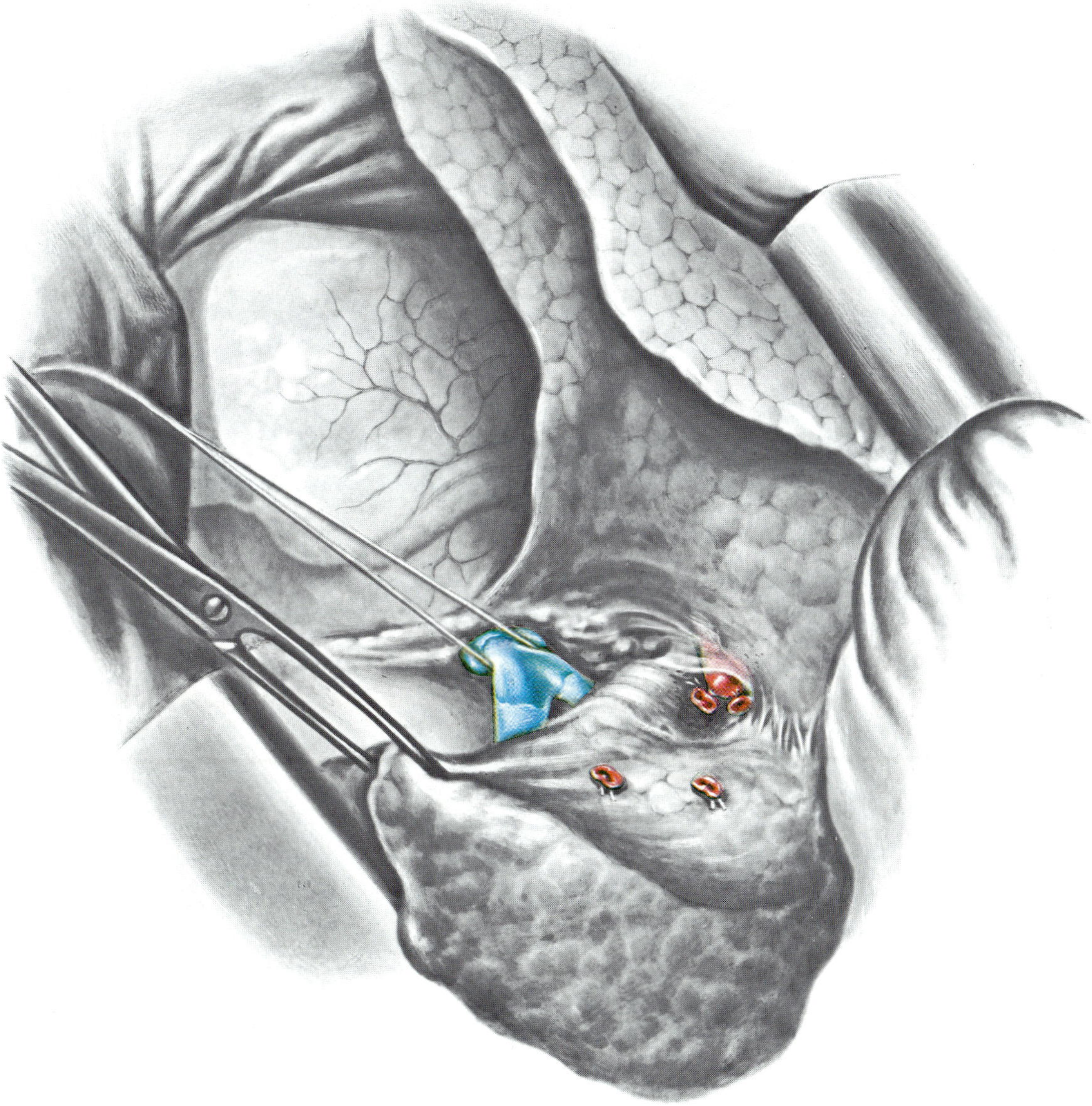

Fig. 159. Ligature has been brought under inferior pulmonary vein. Arteries of inferior lobe have been transected.

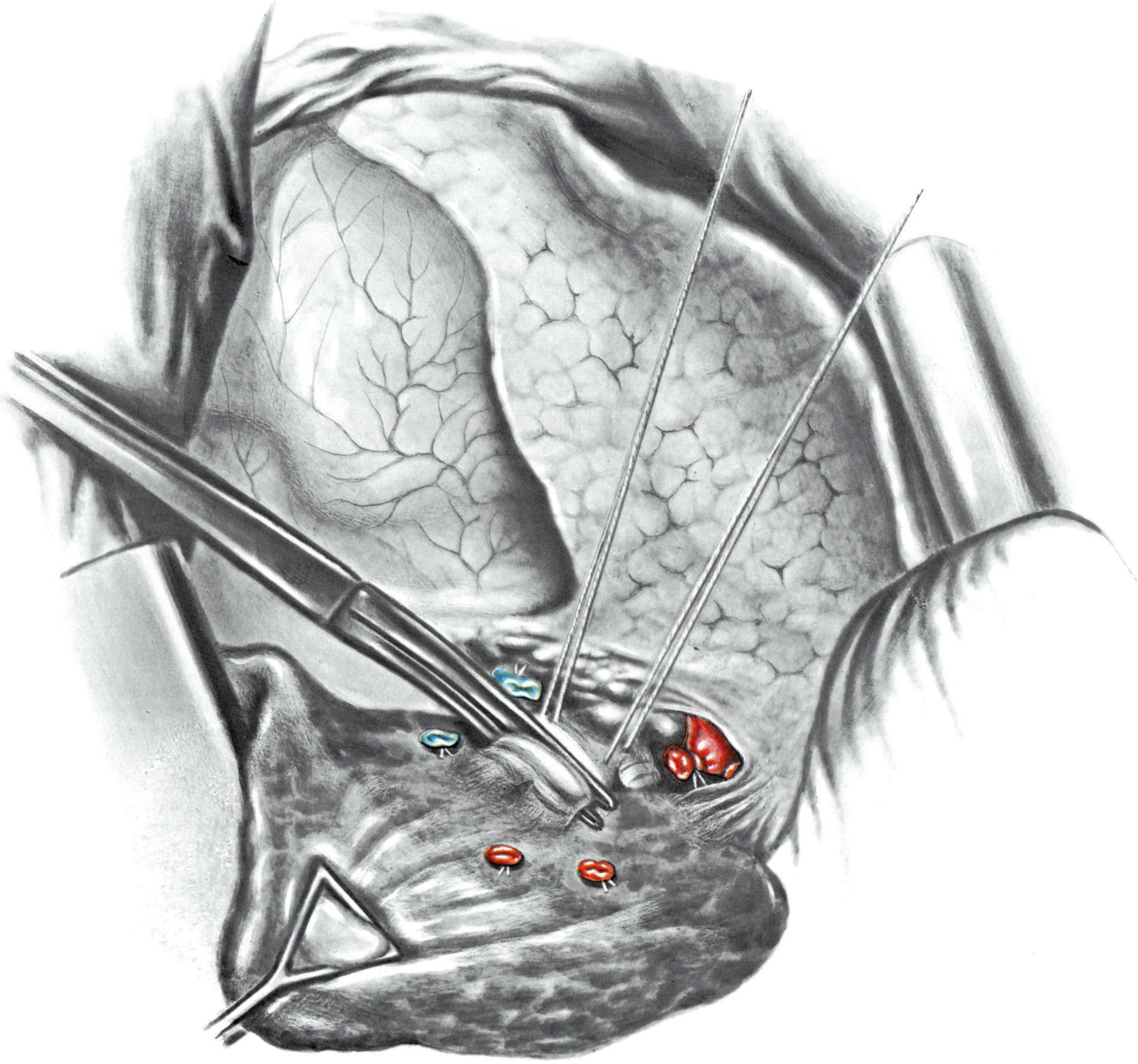

Fig. 160. Inferior lobar bronchus has been exposed, and traction sutures have been applied to it.

INFERIOR LOBECTOMY WITH RESECTION OF THE LINGULAR SEGMENTS

The pleural cavity is opened by a lateral approach in the fifth intercostal space.

The whole lung is freed from the adhesions, and the pulmonary ligament is transected. The main interlobar fissure is opened wide. The arteries of the inferior lobe and lingular segments are found in its floor on the boundary between the middle and dorsal thirds after cutting the pleura. Since these arteries are marked by considerable variability, each branch should be clearly identified before preparation. In most cases it has proven possible to apply one ligature immediately cranially to $A_{4,5}$ (Fig. 161). But if A_2 arises near to the artery of the lingular segments or if they originate as a common trunk, then the artery of the basal segments, $A_{4,5}$, and A_6 are treated separately.

The inferior lobe is pulled away laterally from the pericardium. The mediastinal pleura is cut over the inferior pulmonary vein, which is then separated and treated by the ligature method or by means of the C instrument (Fig. 162).

The operation may be continued in two ways: the lingular segments are resected first, and the inferior lobe after them, or vice versa. The decision is based entirely on the concrete topographoanatomical conditions.

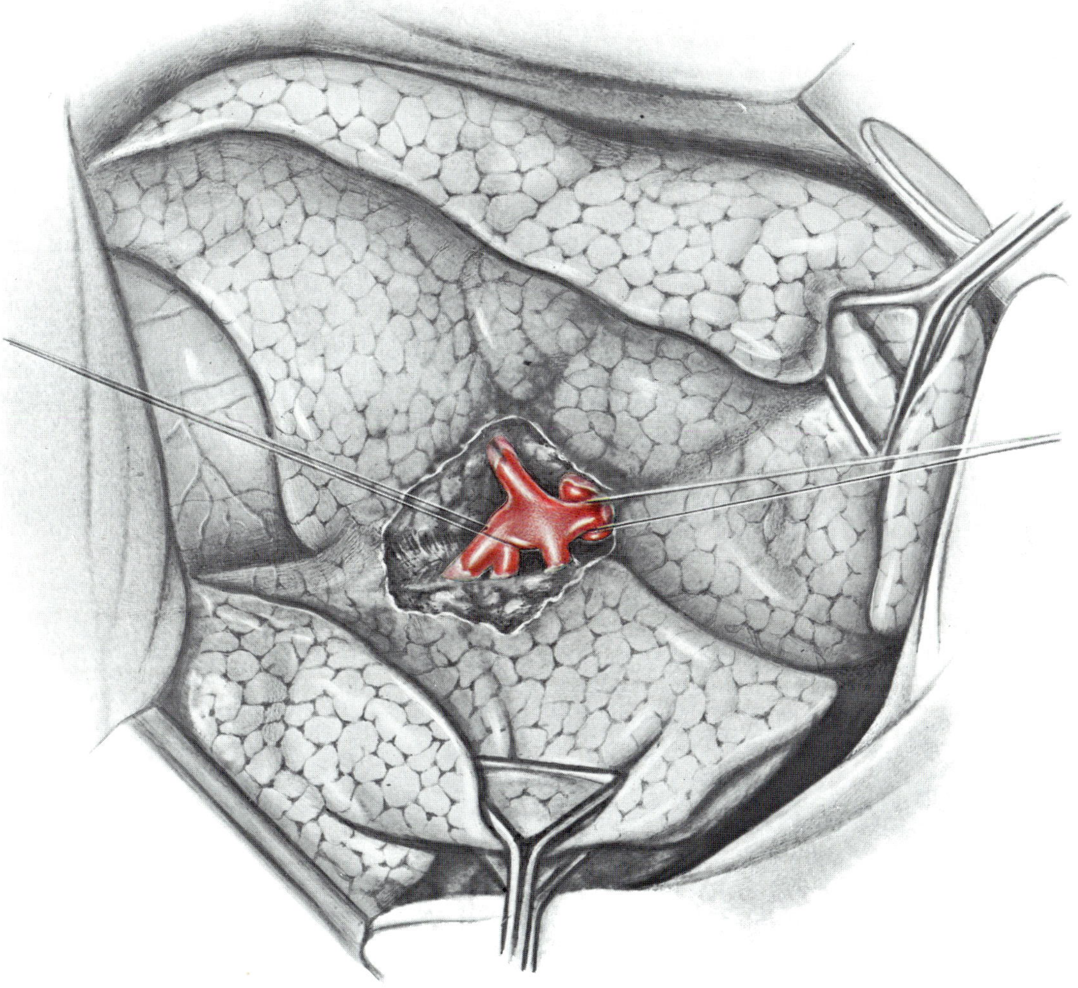

Fig. 161. Preparation of arteries from side of main interlobar fissure. Common trunk of artery of inferior lobe and arteries of lingular segments and artery of basal segments are held with ligatures.

The lingular segments are drawn away in the laterocaudal direction, and $V_{4,5}$ is treated (Fig. 163).

The bronchus of the lingular segments is found immediately under $V_{4,5}$ and separated. It is transected, and its stump closed with interrupted sutures or ligated.

The inferior lobe is pulled in the laterocaudal direction, and its bronchus is exposed, treated by hand or stitched through with the YO instrument, and transected (Fig. 164). The stumps of the inferior lobar and lingular bronchi are covered with mediastinal pleura. The wound surface of the remaining segments is not sutured, as a rule. Interrupted or Halsted sutures are only necessary when hemostasis is insufficiently reliable and there is no assurance that air stasis is perfect.

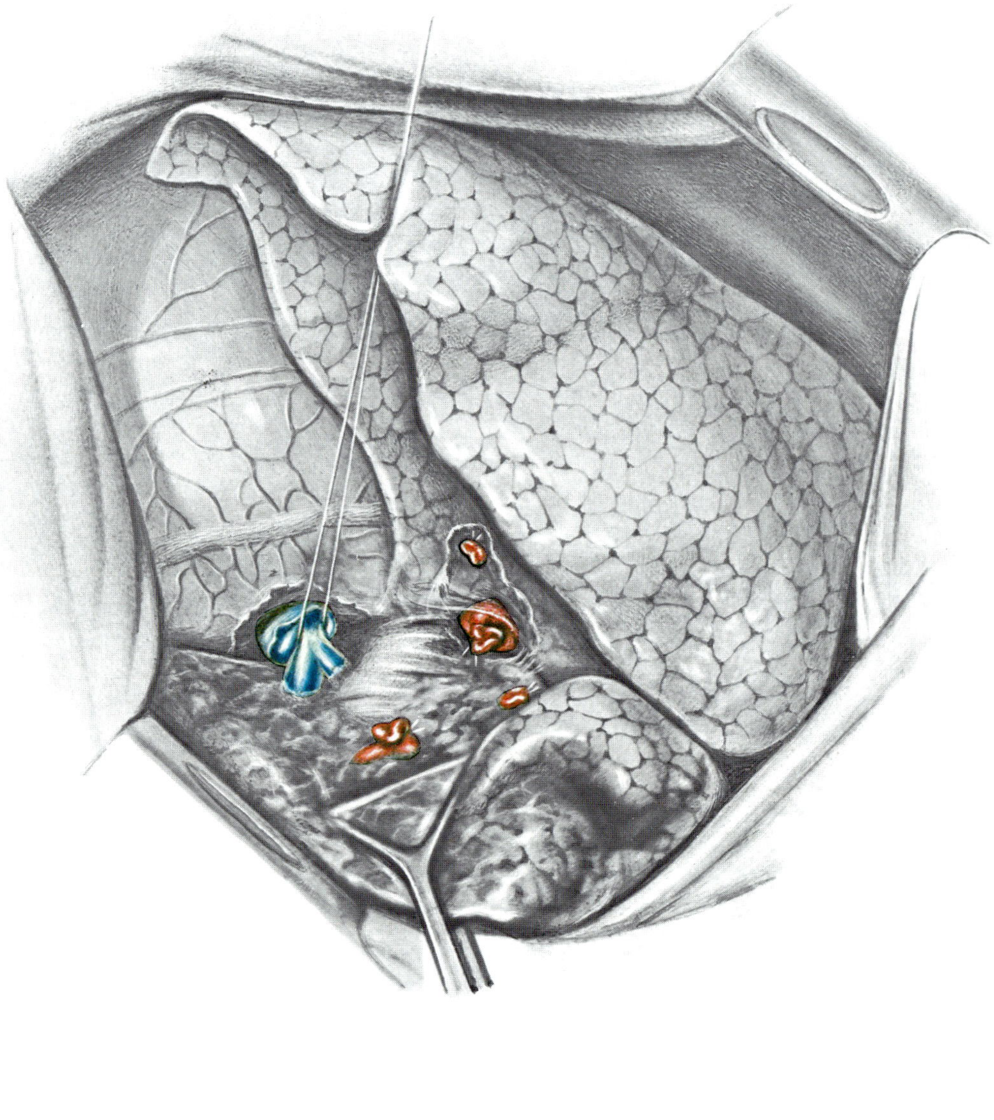

Fig. 162. Ligature is brought under inferior pulmonary vein.

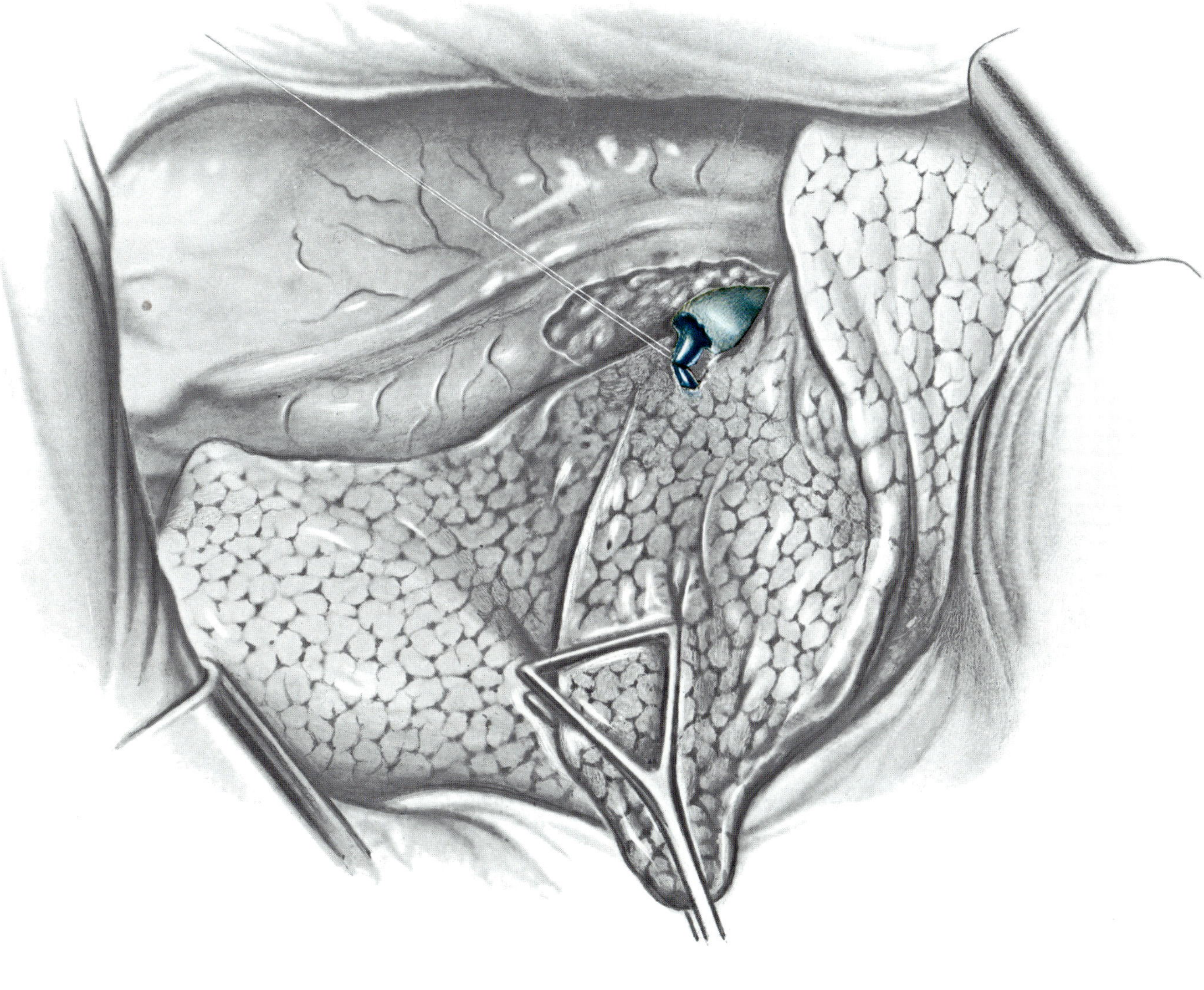

Fig. 163. Treatment of vein of lingular segments.

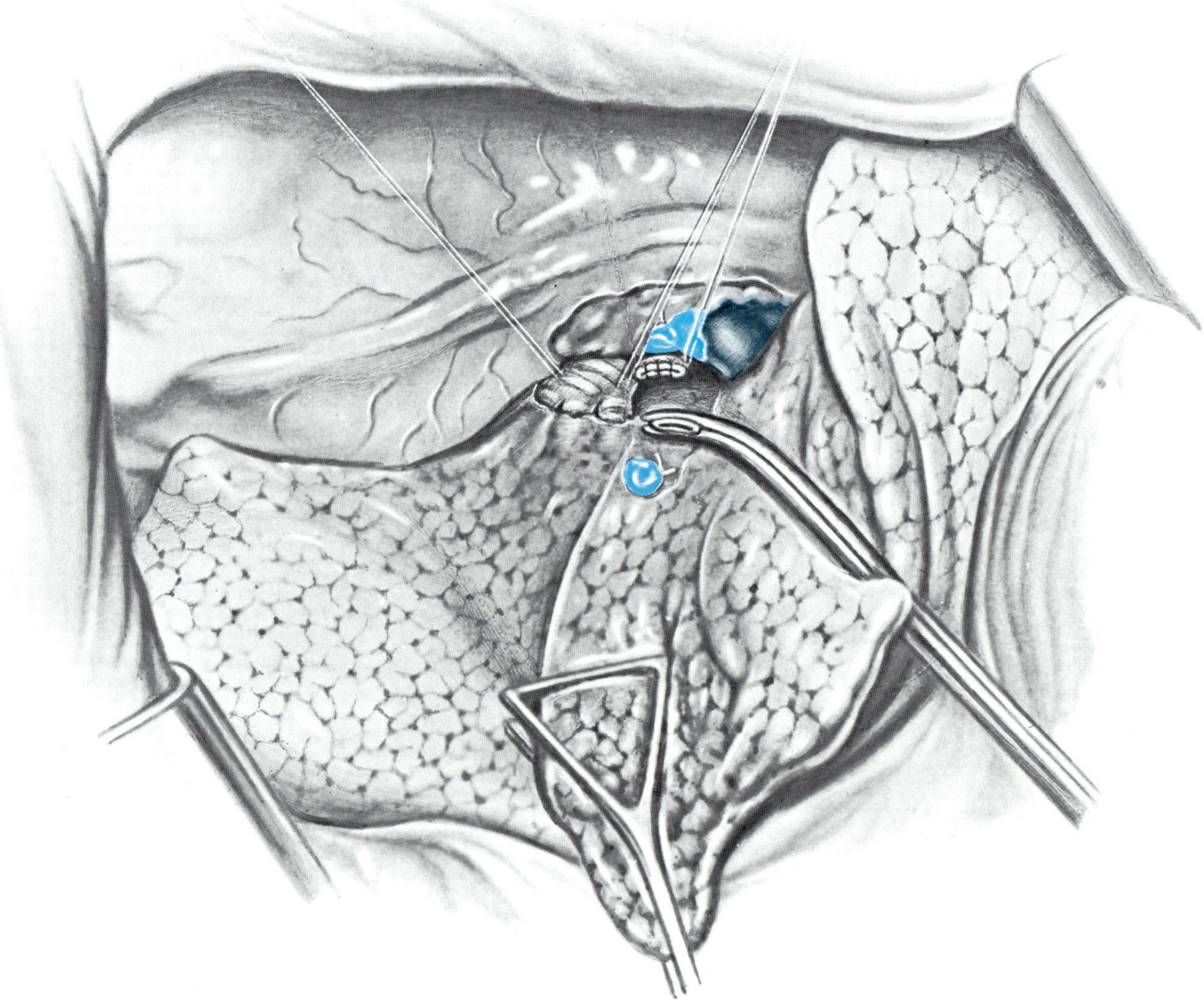

Fig. 164. Inferior lobar bronchus is separated and held by traction sutures. Bronchus of lingular segments has been transected and its stump sutured.

$S_{1,2}$ RESECTION

The pleural cavity is opened by the lateral approach in the fourth intercostal space.

The apex of the lung is freed from the adhesions, and the cranial part of the root of the superior lobe is exposed. The mediastinal pleura is cut over the left pulmonary artery and superior pulmonary vein.

The vascular network of the superior lobe of the left lung is extremely variable. In view of this, each arterial and venous branch is cut only with the full assurance that it belongs to the segments being removed.

The segmental branches of the pulmonary artery are carefully separated and identified. A_1 arises from the most cranial point of its arch; it is ligated and transected (Fig. 165). Due to the great variability of A_2 it is treated either from the side of the dorsal surface of the lung or from the main interlobar fissure. $A_{4,5}$ and A_6 serve as orientation points. When doubt arises, the final treatment of the arterial branches extending to S_2 is carried out after the bronchus has been transected.

V_1, the most cranial branch of the superior pulmonary

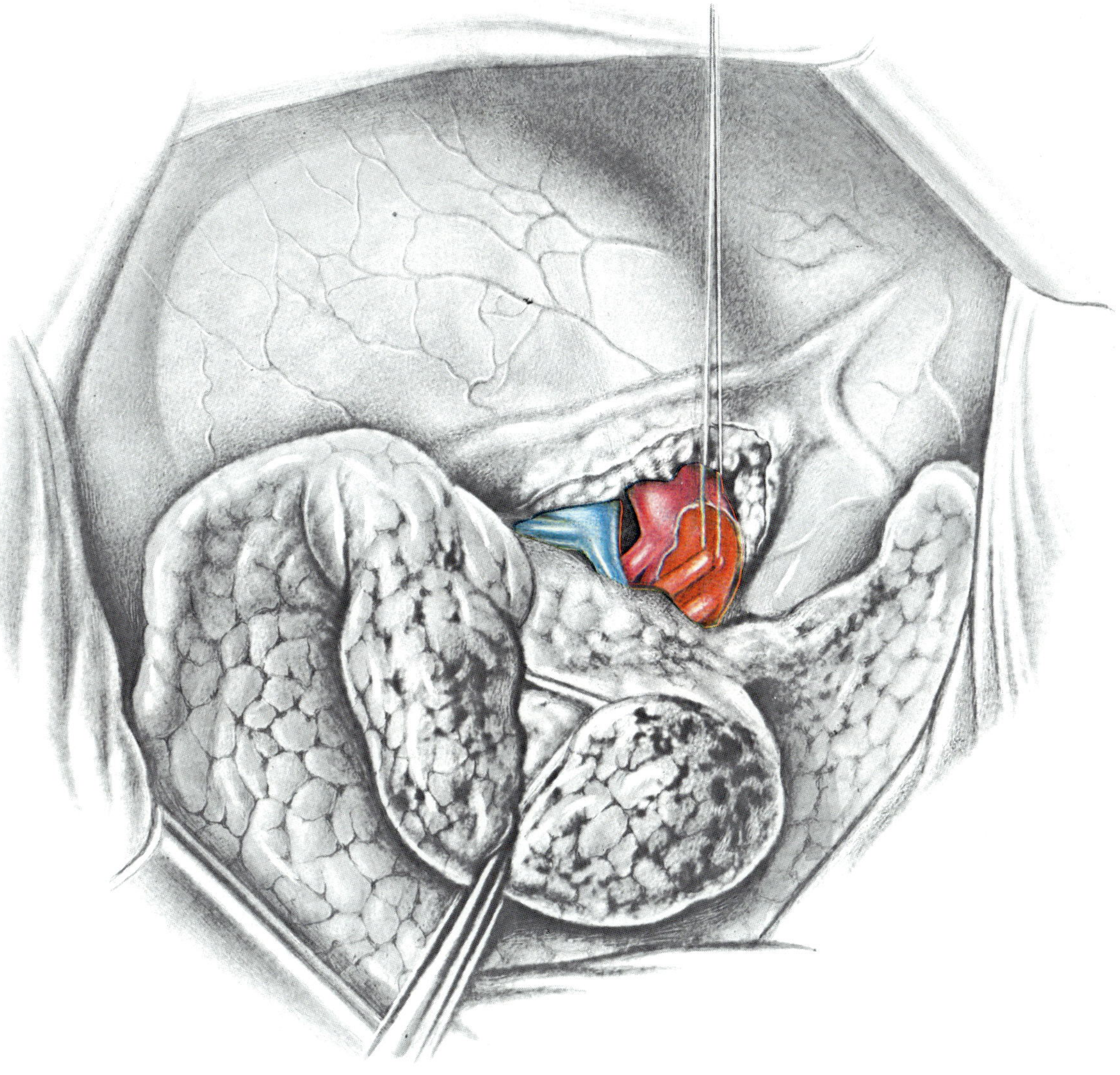

Fig. 165. Treatment of A_1 held with a ligature.

vein, is ligated on the ventral surface of the root of the superior lobe and transected (Fig. 166). V_2 is usually an intersegmental vessel for $S_{1,2}$ and S_3; it is situated deep in the pulmonary parenchyma, and therefore it is preferable to treat it during the separation of the segments.

$B_{1,2}$ is found immediately under V_1 and medial to A_3 and is exposed (Fig. 167). After trial inflation of the superior lobe, $B_{1,2}$ is transected, and the stump sutured by hand.

With the peripheral stump of the bronchi being pulled on, branches of V_2 are found and prepared. The bridge between S_2 and S_6 is separated. The segments are removed, the segmental venous communications, as a rule, being locally ligated and cut. The wound surface of S_3 is not sutured.

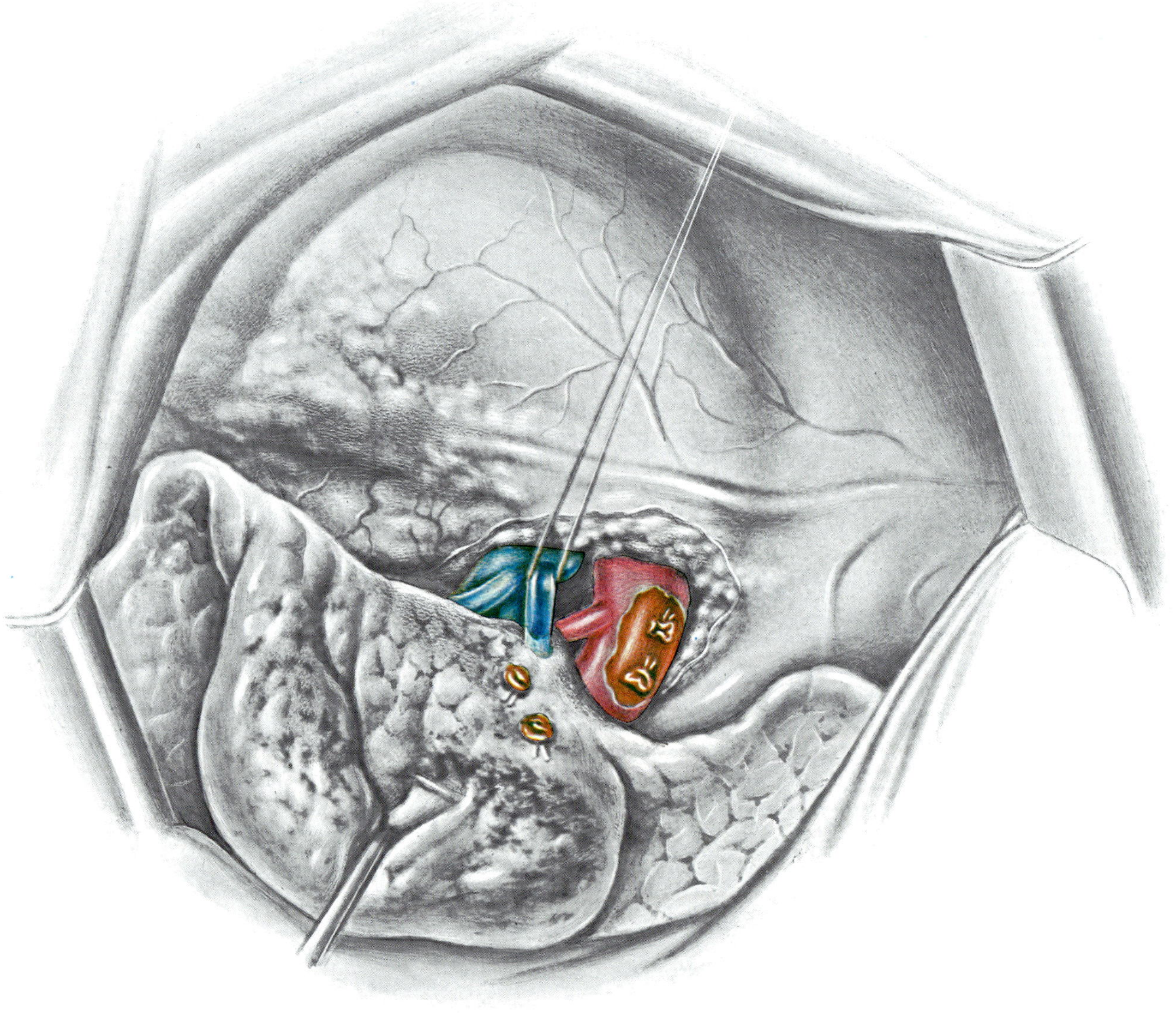

Fig. 166. Separation and ligation of V_1. A_1 and A_2 have been transected.

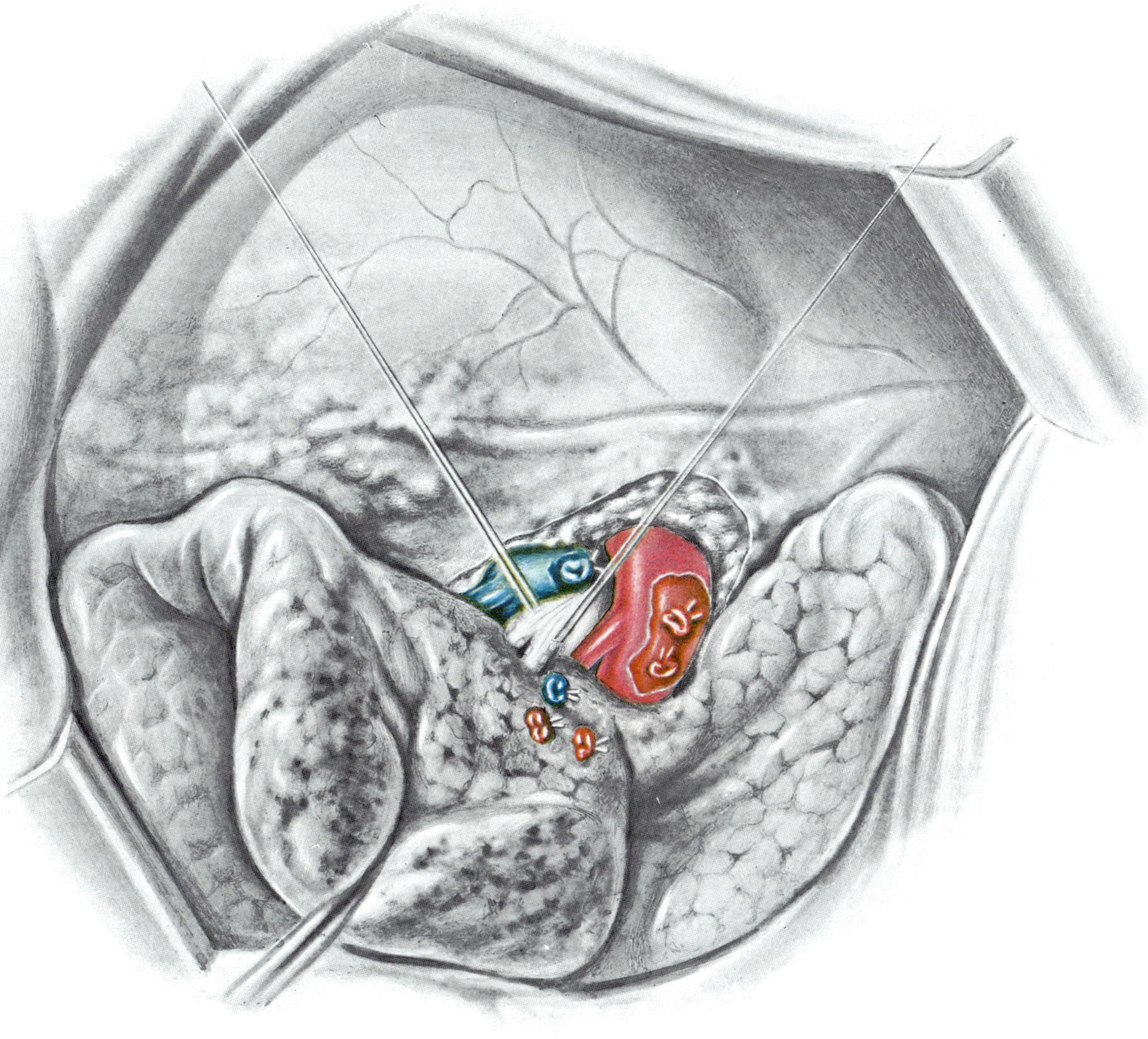

Fig. 167. $B_{1,2}$ has been separated and held by traction sutures from side of membranous part. A_1, A_2, and V_1 have been transected.

$S_{1,2,3}$ RESECTION

The pleural cavity is opened by a lateral approach in the fourth intercostal space.

The superior lobe is freed from the adhesions. The mediastinal pleura is cut over the cranial part of the root of the lung, and the left pulmonary artery is exposed. A_1, A_3, and A_2 are ligated and transected one by one (Fig. 168). Consideration should be given to the anatomical variants when four and even five arterial branches extend to $S_{1,2}$ and S_3. To avoid error, it is necessary to identify $A_{4,5}$ precisely. $B_{1,2,3}$ is prepared on the ventral surface of the root of the superior lobe, care being taken not to injure $V_{4,5}$ (Fig. 169).

With the veins transected, access is given to the segmental bronchi. In typical instances, $B_{1,2}$ and B_3 are exposed separately. The bronchi are transected, and their stumps sutured by hand (Fig. 170).

With the peripheral stumps of the bronchi being pulled on, the segments are removed in a single block. The wound surface of the lingular segments is sutured only if air stasis is insufficient.

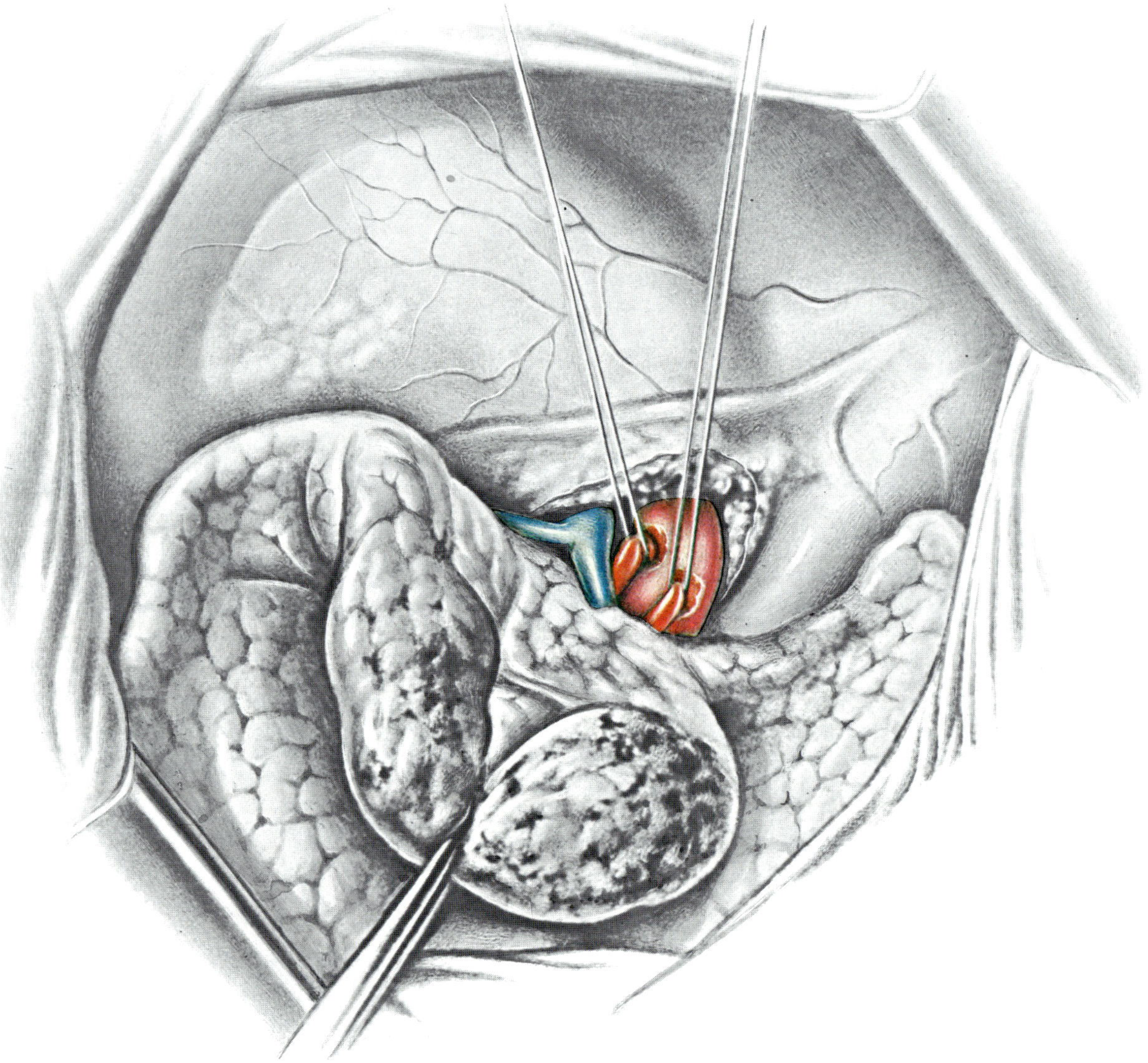

Fig. 168. Ligatures are brought under A_1 and A_2.

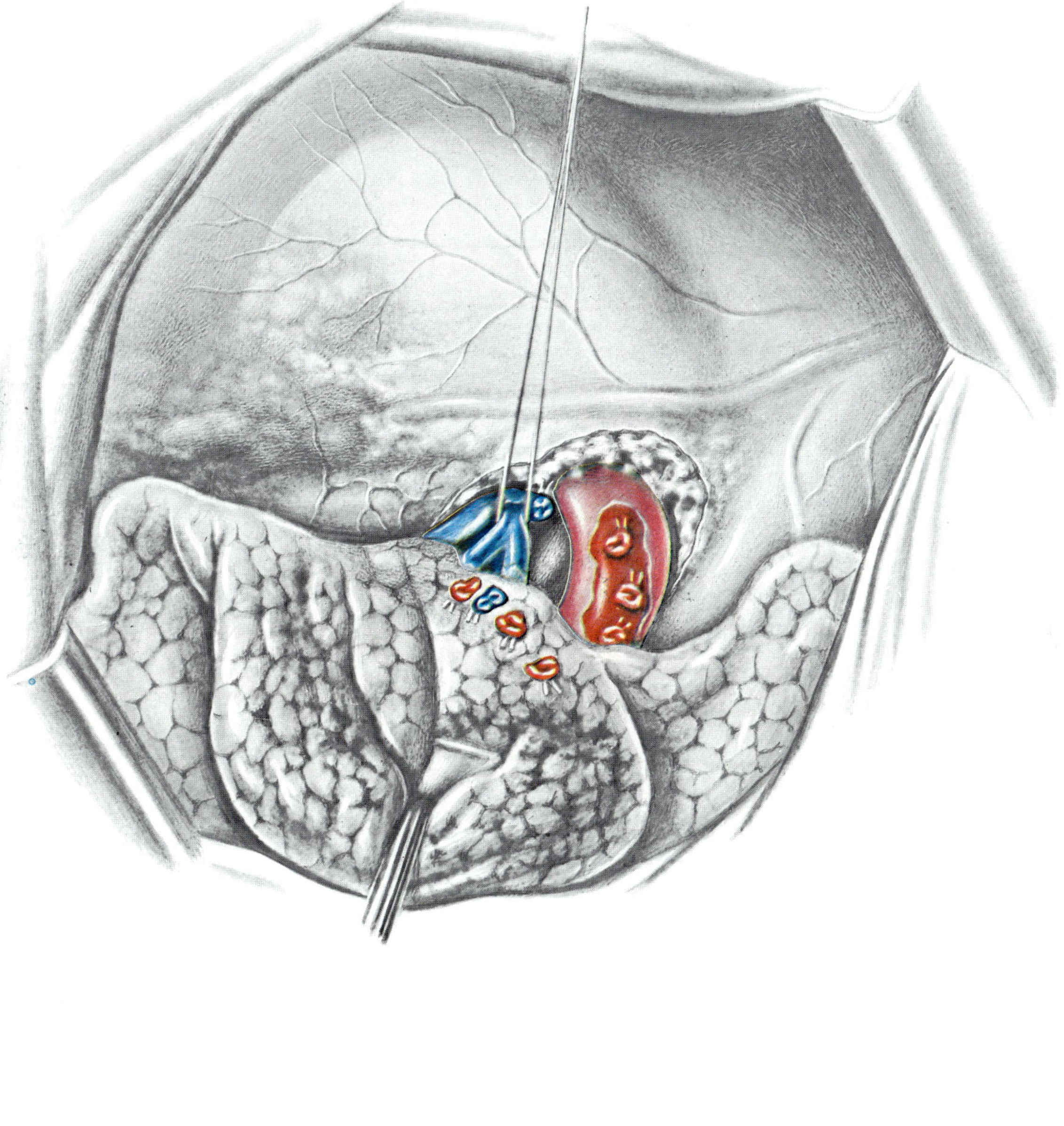

Fig. 169. Treatment of $B_{1,2}$. $A_{1,2,3}$ have been transected.

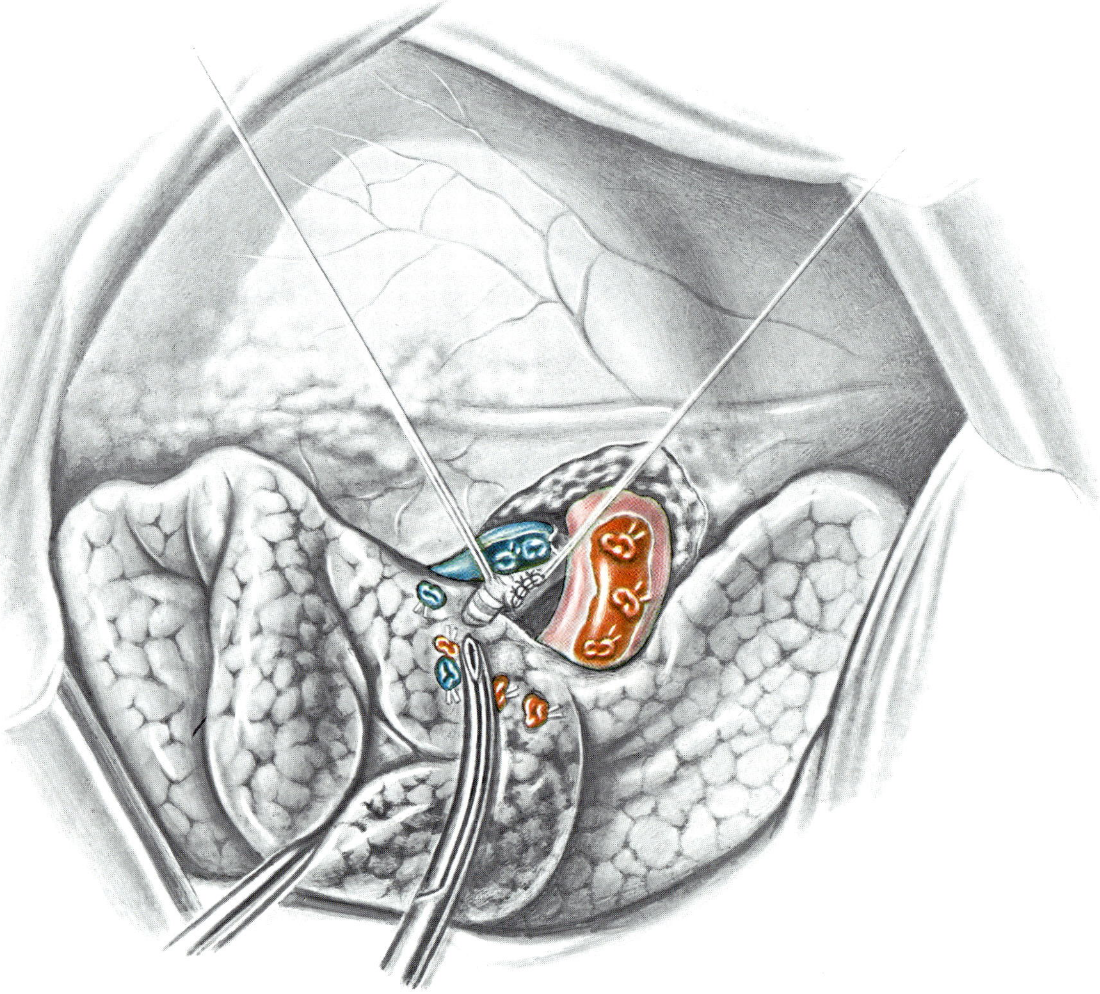

Fig. 170. B_3 is separated and held with loops. $B_{1,2}$ has been transected and its stump sutured.

$S_{4,5}$ RESECTION

The pleural cavity is opened by anterolateral or lateral approach in the fourth intercostal space.

The lingular segments are pulled away laterally. $V_{4,5}$, the most caudal branch of the superior pulmonary vein, is prepared (Fig. 171).

$B_{4,5}$ is found immediately under the vein and prepared. The bronchus of the lingular segments is exposed by the blunt techniques down to the orifice of B_3. To avoid constriction of the latter, the stump of $B_{4,5}$ is made no shorter than 0.5 cm (Fig. 172). During preparation of the dorsal bronchial wall the adjacent $A_{4,5}$ should be protected from damage. $B_{4,5}$ is transected, and its stump closed with interrupted sutures or tied with a circular ligature.

When the bronchus has been treated, access is gained to $A_{4,5}$ stretching along its dorsal wall. The artery is treated by the ligature method (Fig. 173).

With the peripheral bronchial stump being pulled on, the lingular segments are removed. The intersegmental venous communications are ligated. The wound surface of S_3 is not sutured, as a rule.

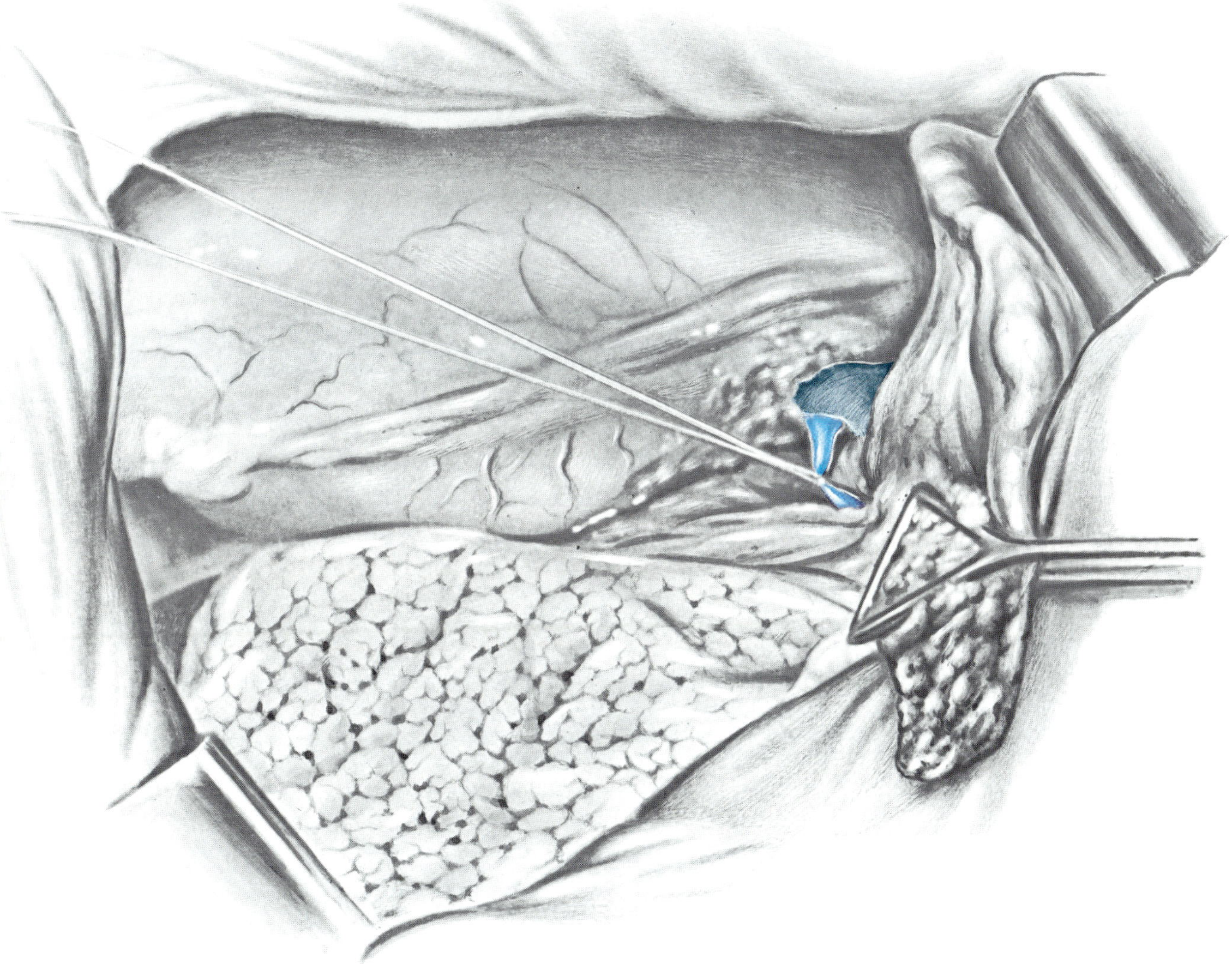

Fig. 171. Separation of vein of lingular segments.

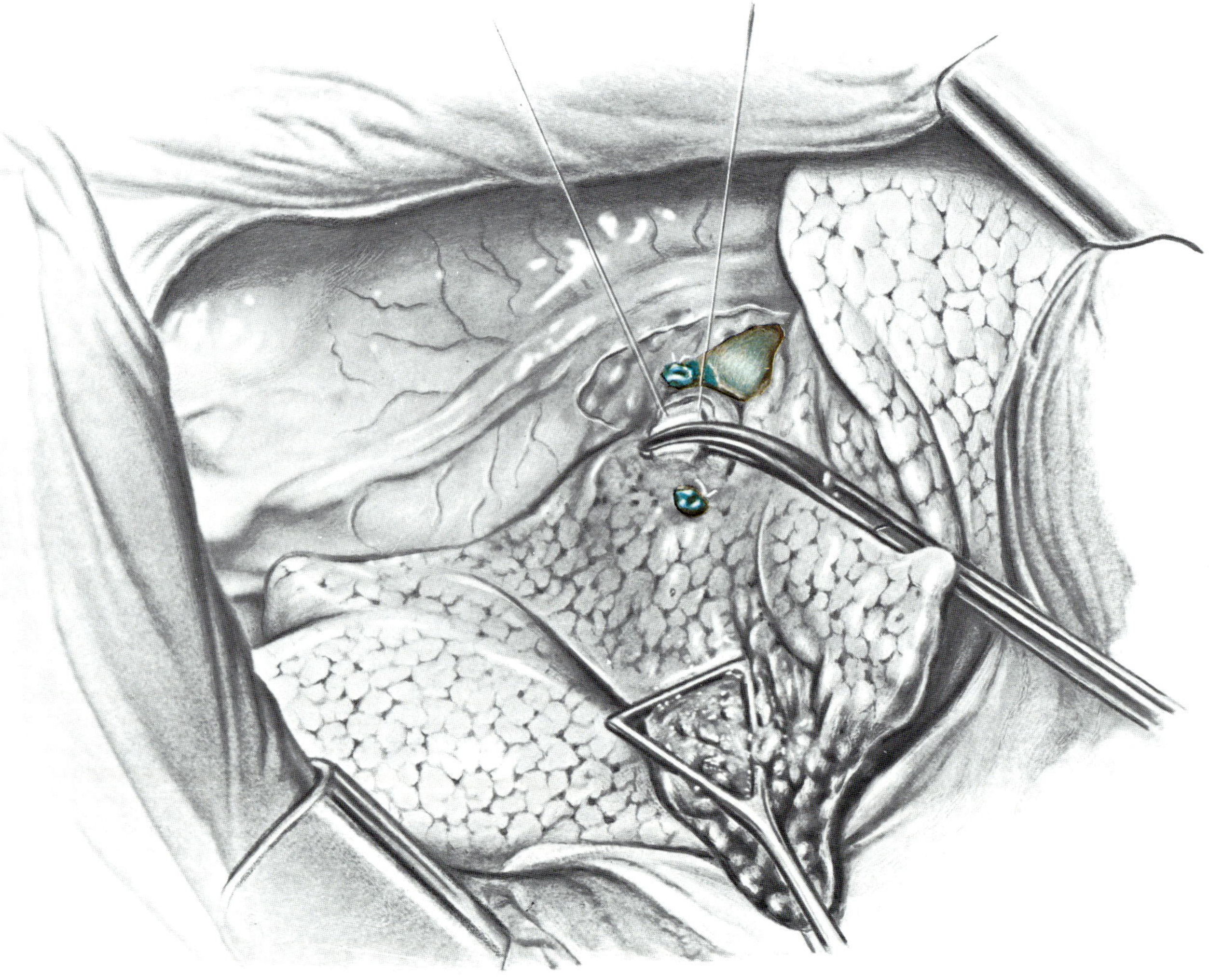

Fig. 172. Traction sutures have been applied to bronchus of lingular segments. $V_{4,5}$ has been transected.

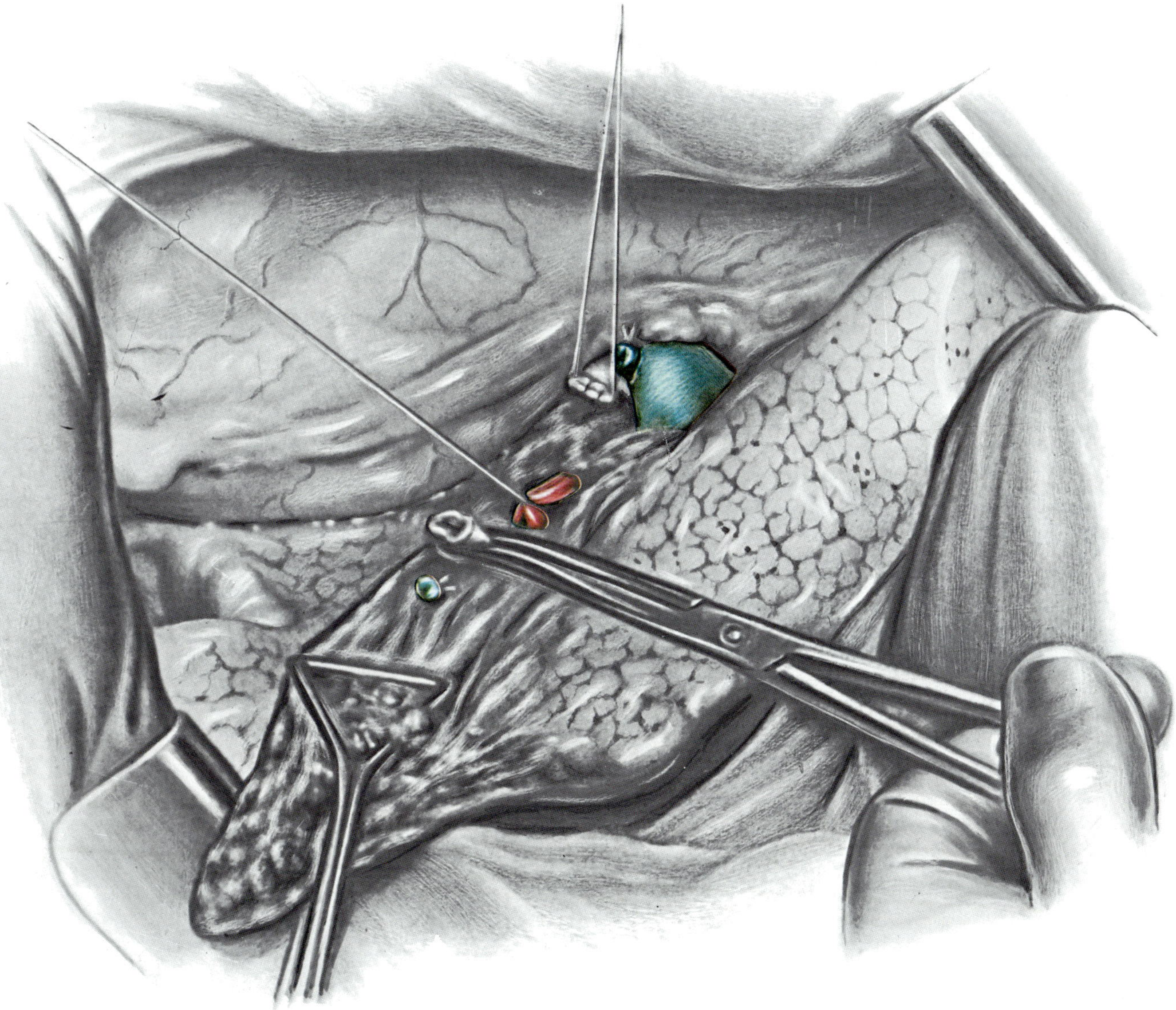

Fig. 173. Preparation of $A_{4,5}$. Bronchus of lingular segments has been transected and its stump sutured.

S_6 RESECTION

The pleural cavity is opened by a lateral, posterolateral, or anterolateral approach in the fifth intercostal space.

The components of the segmental root may be treated from the side of the main interlobar fissure as it is described in the case of S_6 on the right, or from the side of the dorsal surface of the lung as described below.

The inferior lobe is freed from the adhesions and pulled away ventrally and medially. The mediastinal pleura is cut over the artery of the inferior lobe. A_6 is found at the upper edge of the interlobar fissure between S_2 and S_6 and treated (Fig. 174). In rare cases the artery of the basal segment gives off an accessory branch to S_6, which is also ligated and transected.

B_6 is found immediately under the artery and is prepared, transected, and its stump treated by hand (Fig. 175).

The inferior pulmonary vein is exposed, and its cranial branch, V_6, is treated by the ligature method (Fig. 176).

With the peripheral stumps of the bronchi and vessels being pulled on, S_6 is removed while the small intersegmental veins are ligated. The wound surface of the basal segment is not sutured.

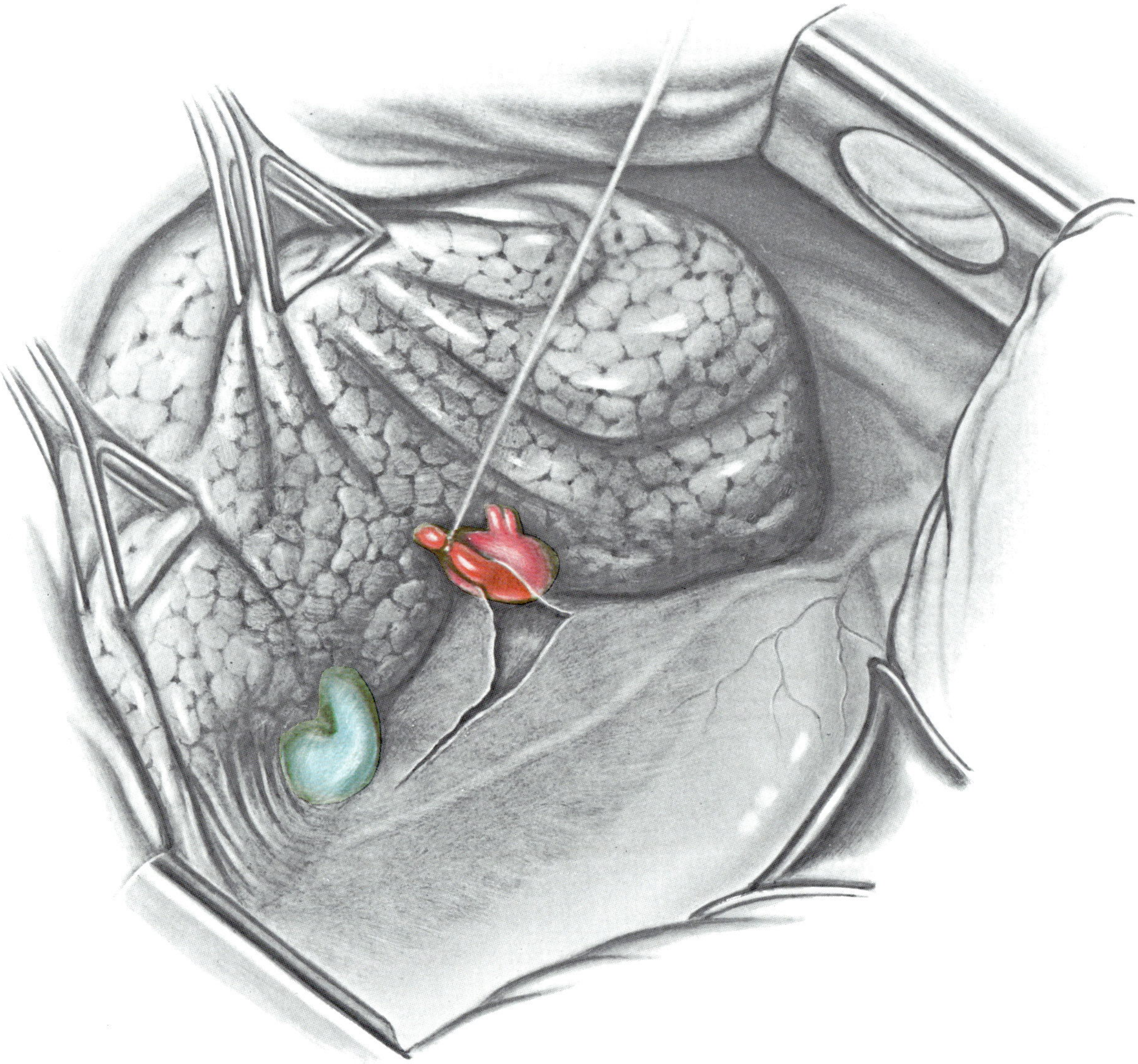

Fig. 174. Separation and ligation of A_6 from dorsal surface of lung, which has been drawn away ventrally.

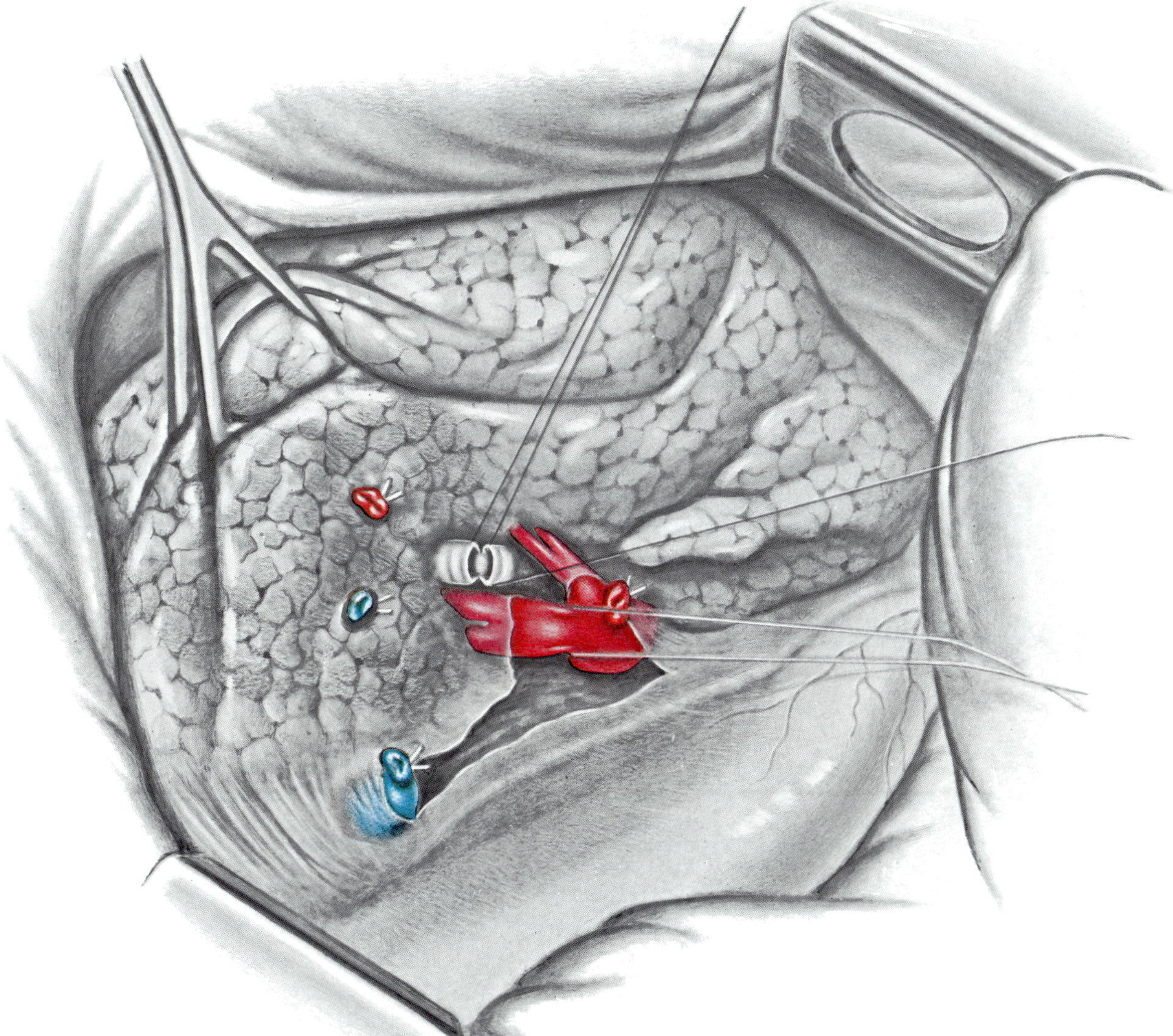

Fig. 175. B_6 is held with loops and transected. Relaxation ligature is applied to artery of basal segments. Veins and artery of sixth segment have been transected.

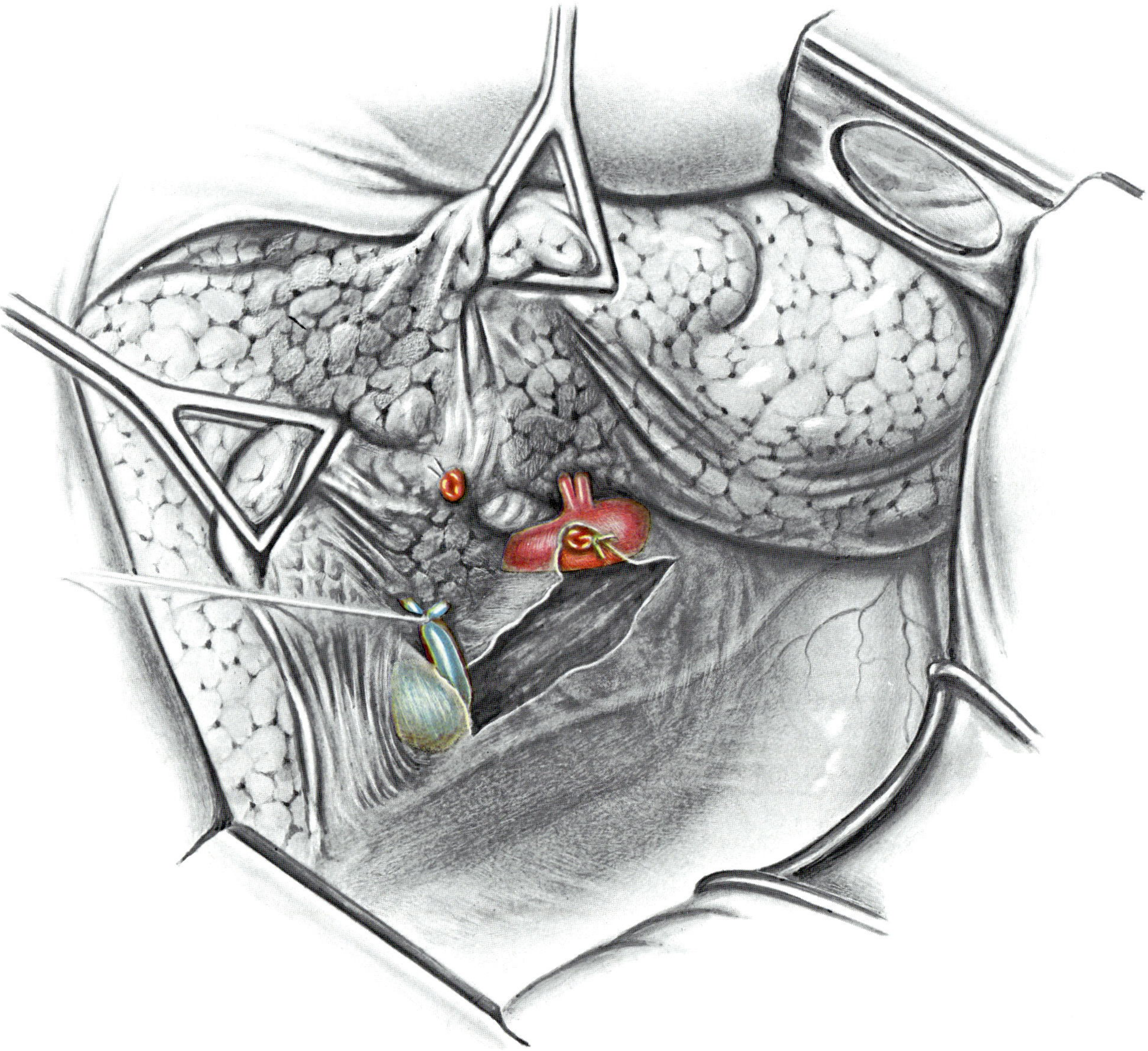

Fig. 176. Separation and ligation of V_6.

$S_{9,10}$ RESECTION

The pleural cavity is opened by a lateral or posterior approach in the sixth intercostal space.

The inferior lobe is freed from the adhesions, and the pulmonary ligament is cut. The artery of the basal segment is exposed from the side of the main interlobar fissure in its middle third. Its segmental branches are carefully identified. $A_{9,10}$, located between A_6 and A_8, are prepared (Fig. 177).

$B_{9,10}$ are found immediately under the arteries and are exposed. The common trunk of these bronchi is short. That is why it is preferable to expose $B_{9,10}$ as far to the periphery as possible. The bronchi are transected so as to form a single stump, which is closed with sutures applied by hand (Fig. 178).

Since $S_{9,10}$ are located between S_6 and S_8 they have to be exposed in two stages. First, depending on the

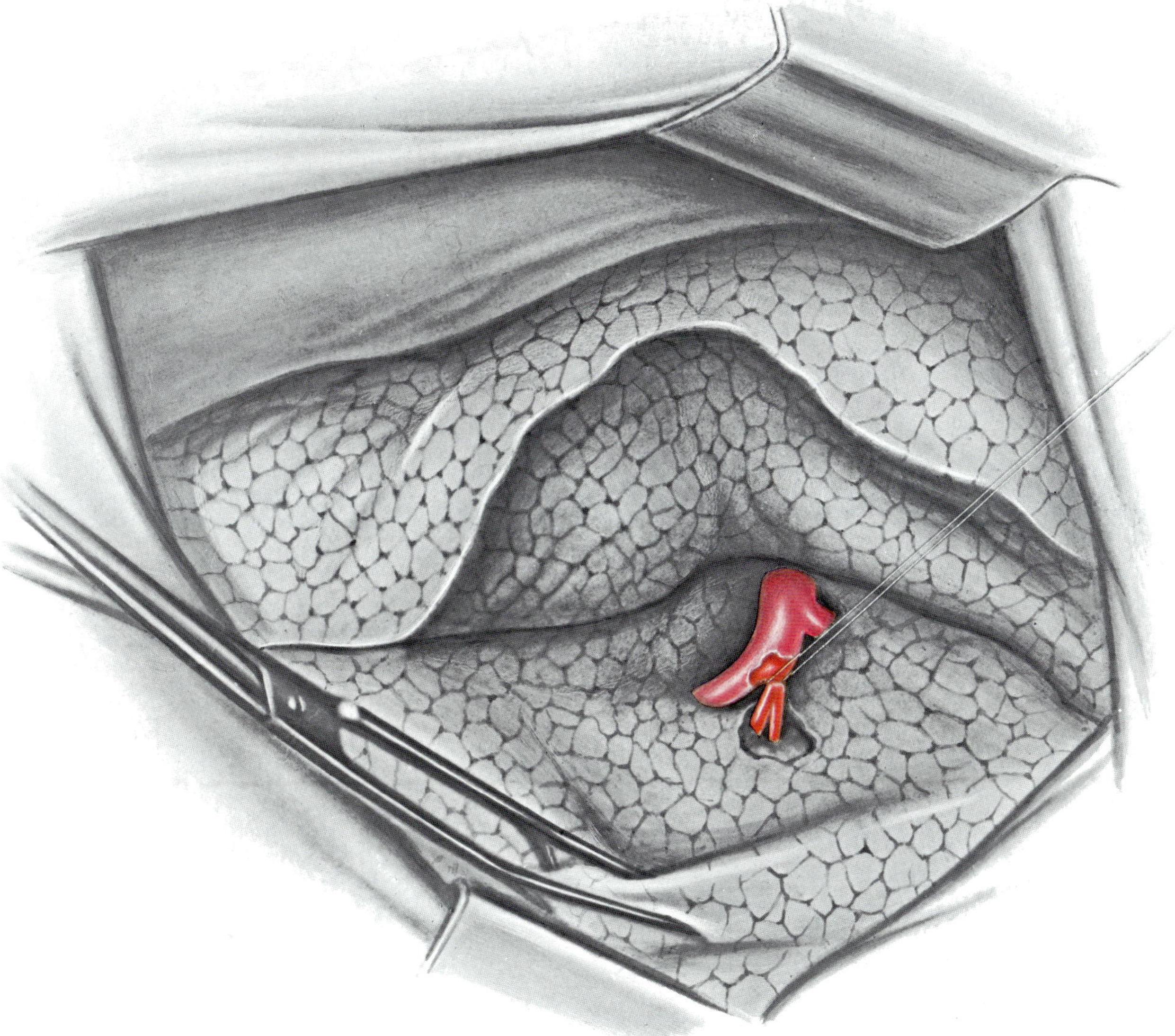

Fig. 177. Separation and ligation of $A_{9,10}$ from side of main interlobar fissure.

individual operative situation, $S_{9,10}$ are separated from one of these segments. For this purpose the pulmonary pleura is cut along the presumable boundary of the resection, the part of the lobe being removed is folded over on the hand, and with the peripheral stumps of the bronchi and arteries being pulled on. $S_{9,10}$ are detached. In the second stage the connections between the other part of the inferior lobe and $S_{9,10}$ are disconnected. The defect thus formed in the parenchyma of the inferior lobe is repaired by stitching S_6 and S_8 together (Fig. 179).

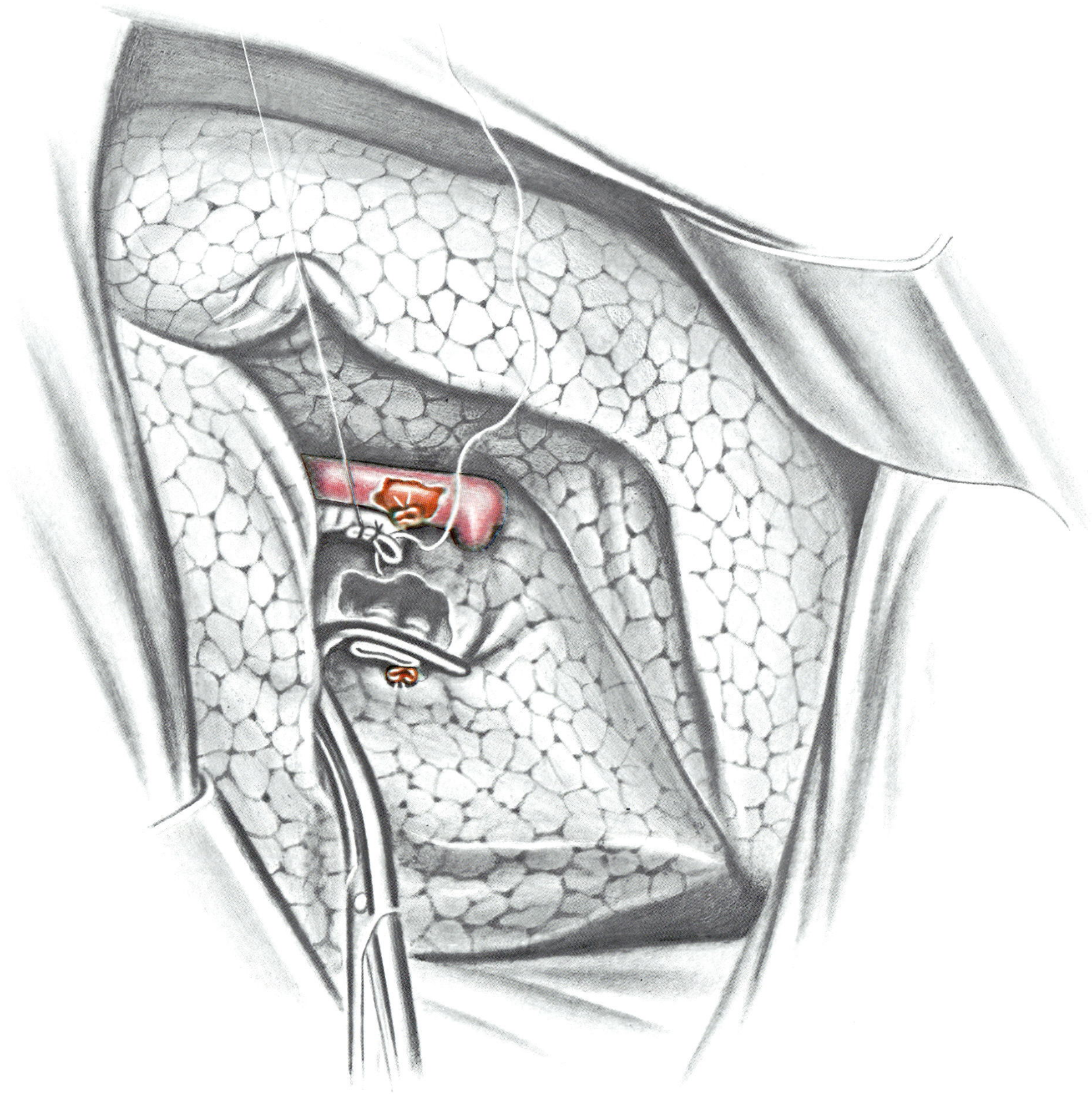

Fig. 178. Transection of $B_{9,10}$ and closure of stump with sutures.

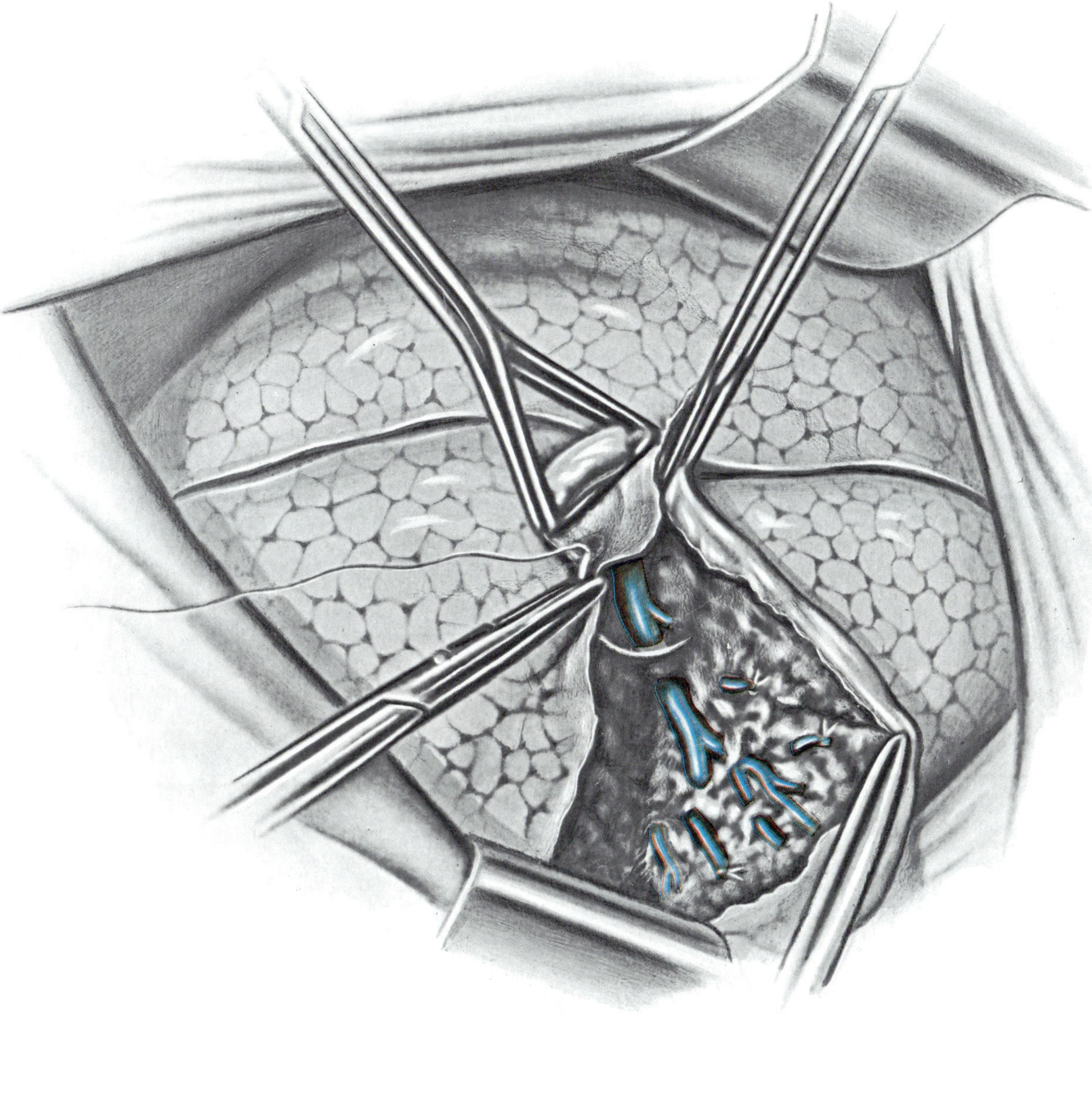

Fig. 179. Edges of S_6 and S_8 are stitched together after removal of $S_{9,10}$.

RESECTION OF $S_{8,9,10}$ (BASAL SEGMENTS)

The pleural cavity is opened by a lateral approach in the fifth intercostal space. The inferior lobe is freed from the adhesions, and the pulmonary ligament is transected. The interlobar fissure is opened. The artery of the basal segments is found on its floor at the junction of the dorsal and middle thirds and is prepared (Fig. 180).

Quite often, $A_{4,5}$ arises from the artery of the basal segments caudal to A_6. This is why each segmental branch should be clearly identified before the arteries are ligated.

With the inferior lobe pulled aside laterally the mediastinal pleura is cut over the inferior pulmonary vein. The vein of the basal segments is prepared (Fig. 181).

The communications between the basal and lingular segments are divided, and the bronchus of the basal segments is then exposed from the side of the interlobar

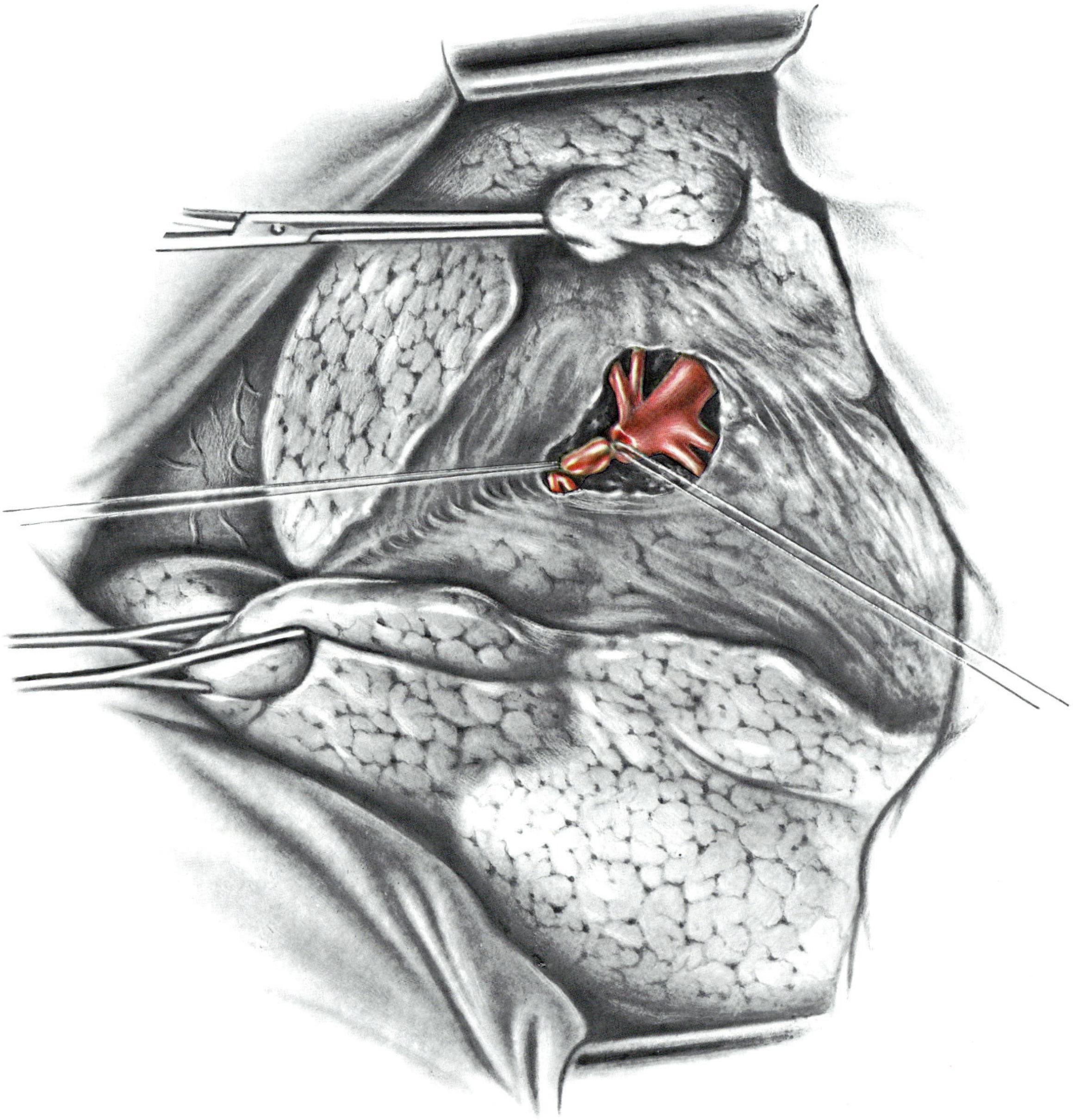

Fig. 180. Ligation of artery of basal segment on side of main interlobar fissure.

fissure (Fig. 182). When the dorsal wall of the bronchus of the basal segments is being separated, B_6 adjoining it is protected from injury. The bronchus is transected, and its stump treated by hand.

With the peripheral stumps of the bronchus and vessels being pulled on, the basal segments are removed with an effort to strip a flap of visceral pleura from them (Fig. 183). The flap is placed on the wound surface of S_6 and fastened to its edges with interrupted sutures (Fig. 184). S_6 is stitched to S_2.

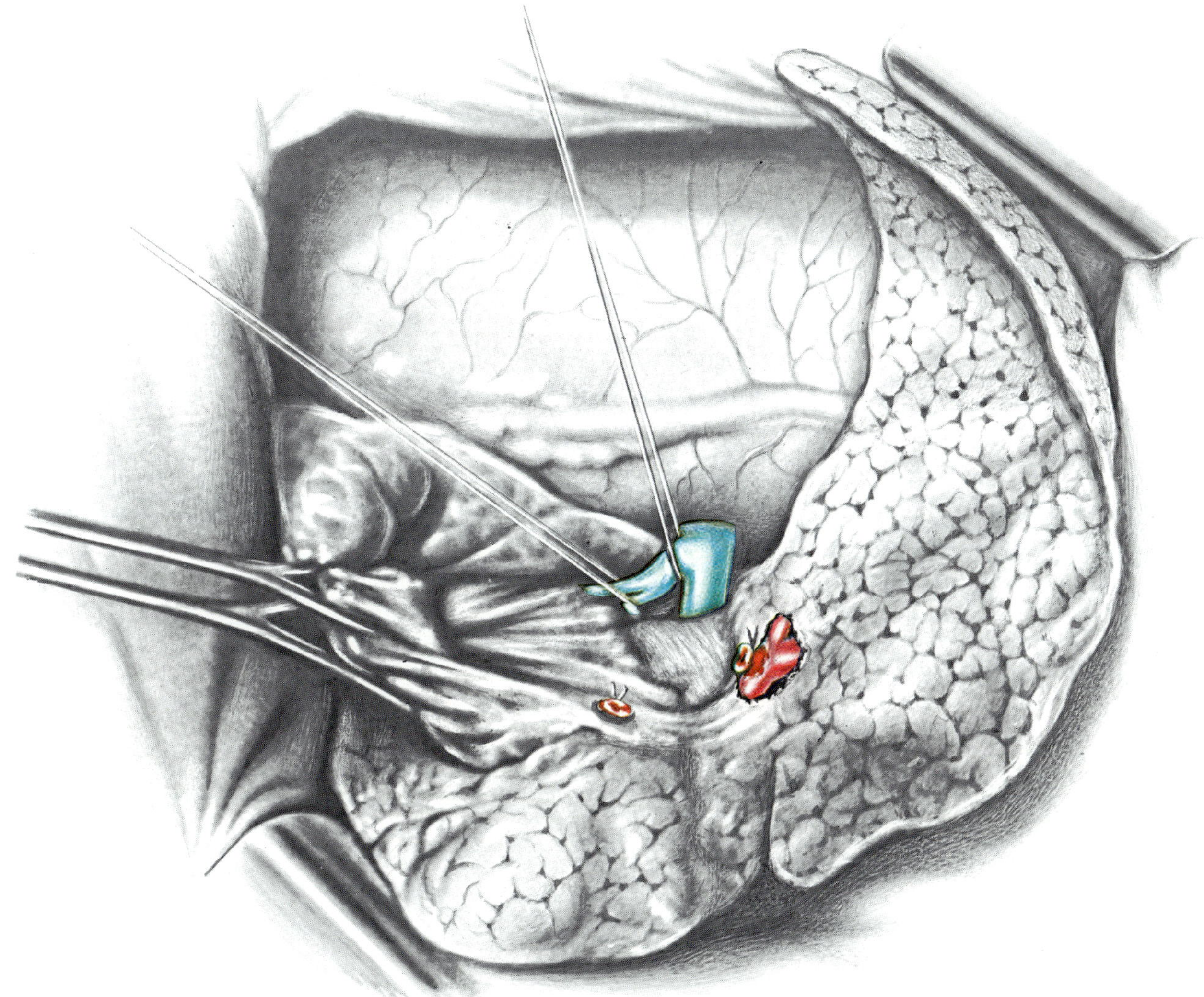

Fig. 181. Preparation and ligation of vein of basal segments.

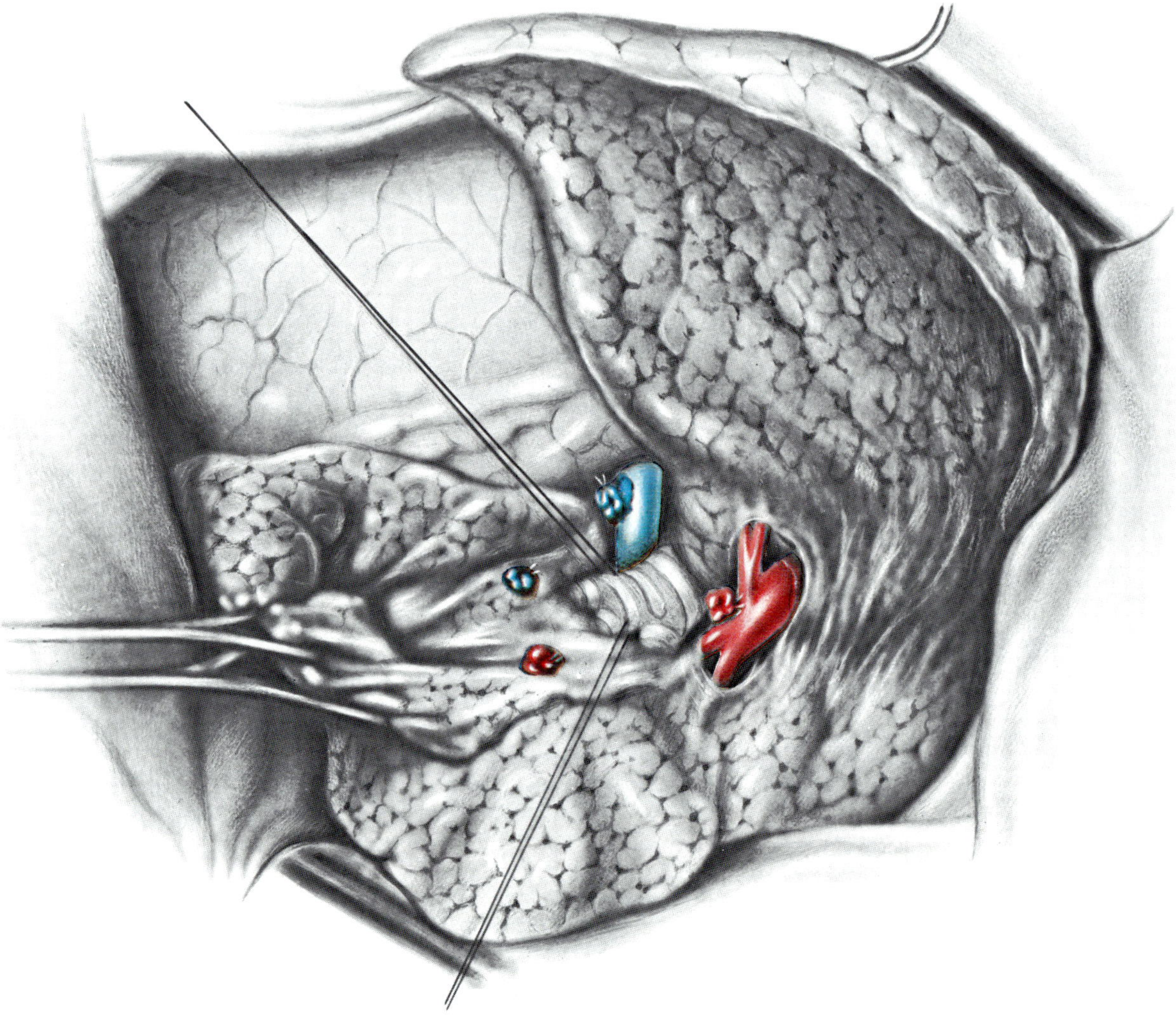

Fig. 182. Bronchus of basal segments is prepared and held with traction sutures. Artery and vein of segments have been transected.

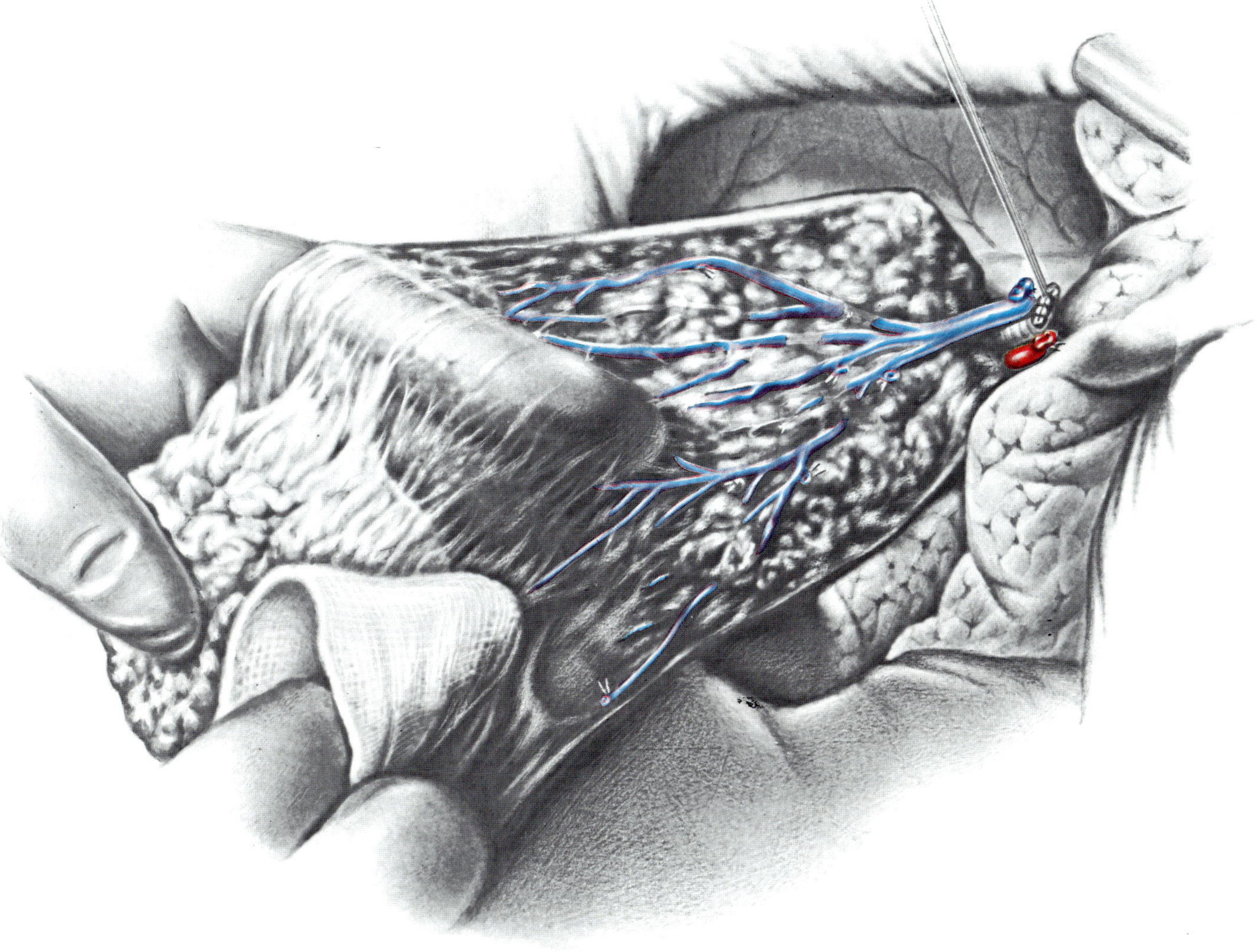

Fig. 183. Basal segments are separated from S_6 and flap of pulmonary pleura is stripped off.

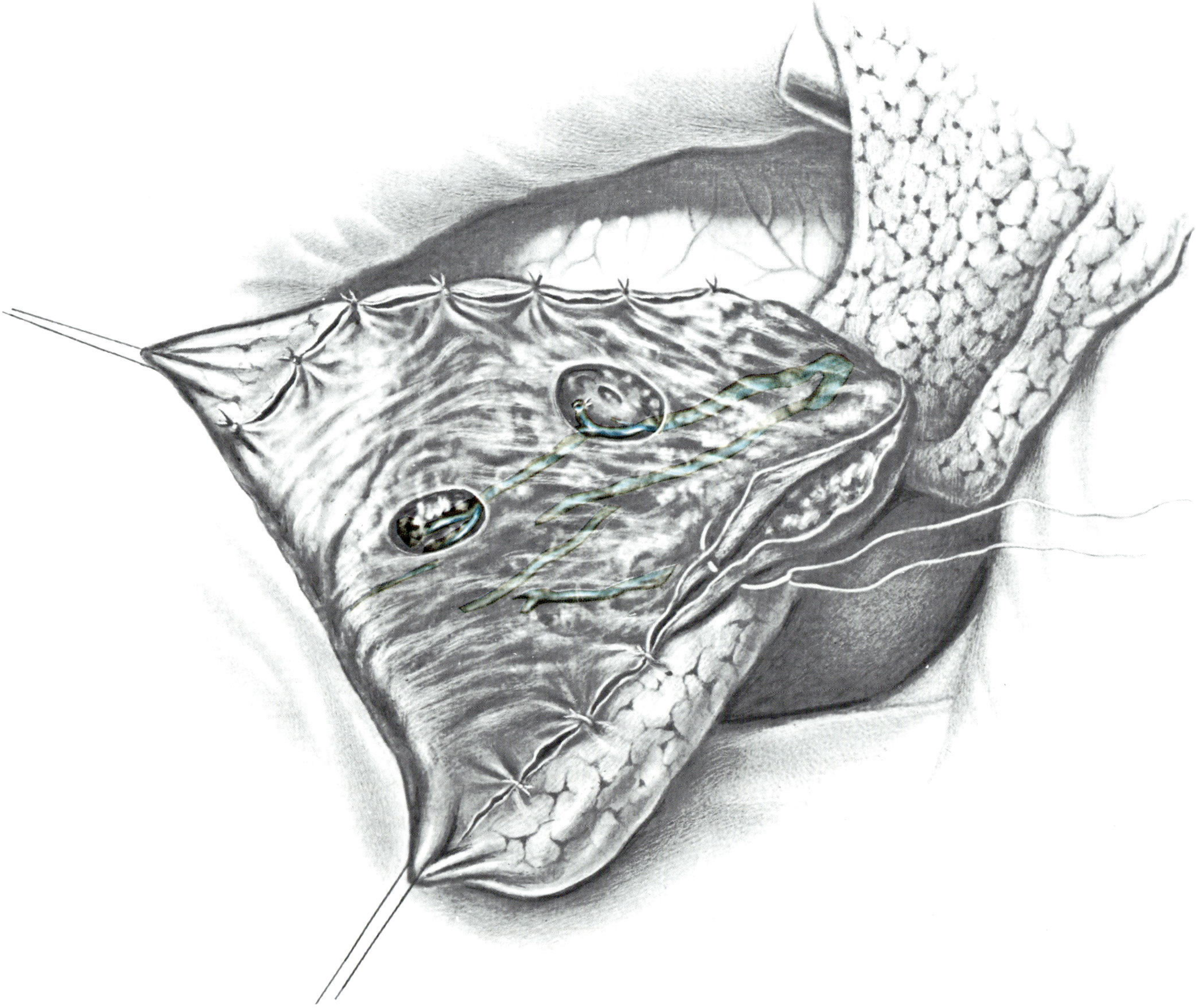

Fig. 184. Flap of pulmonary pleura is stitched to margins of S_6.

Operations on the trachea and main bronchi

*SLEEVE RESECTION OF THE THORACIC TRACHEA

The operation is performed through a lateral approach in the fourth intercostal space or a posterior approach in the fifth intercostal space on the right.

The lung is moved laterally and ventrally. The arch of the azygos vein is transected between ligatures. The mediastinal pleura is cut longitudinally over the trachea. The vagus nerve is held with loops and drawn aside laterally. The thoracic trachea and the right and left main bronchi are separated by the blunt and sharp techniques successively (with due caution for the recurrent laryngeal nerves) and are held with loops.

Two traction sutures are applied to the membranous

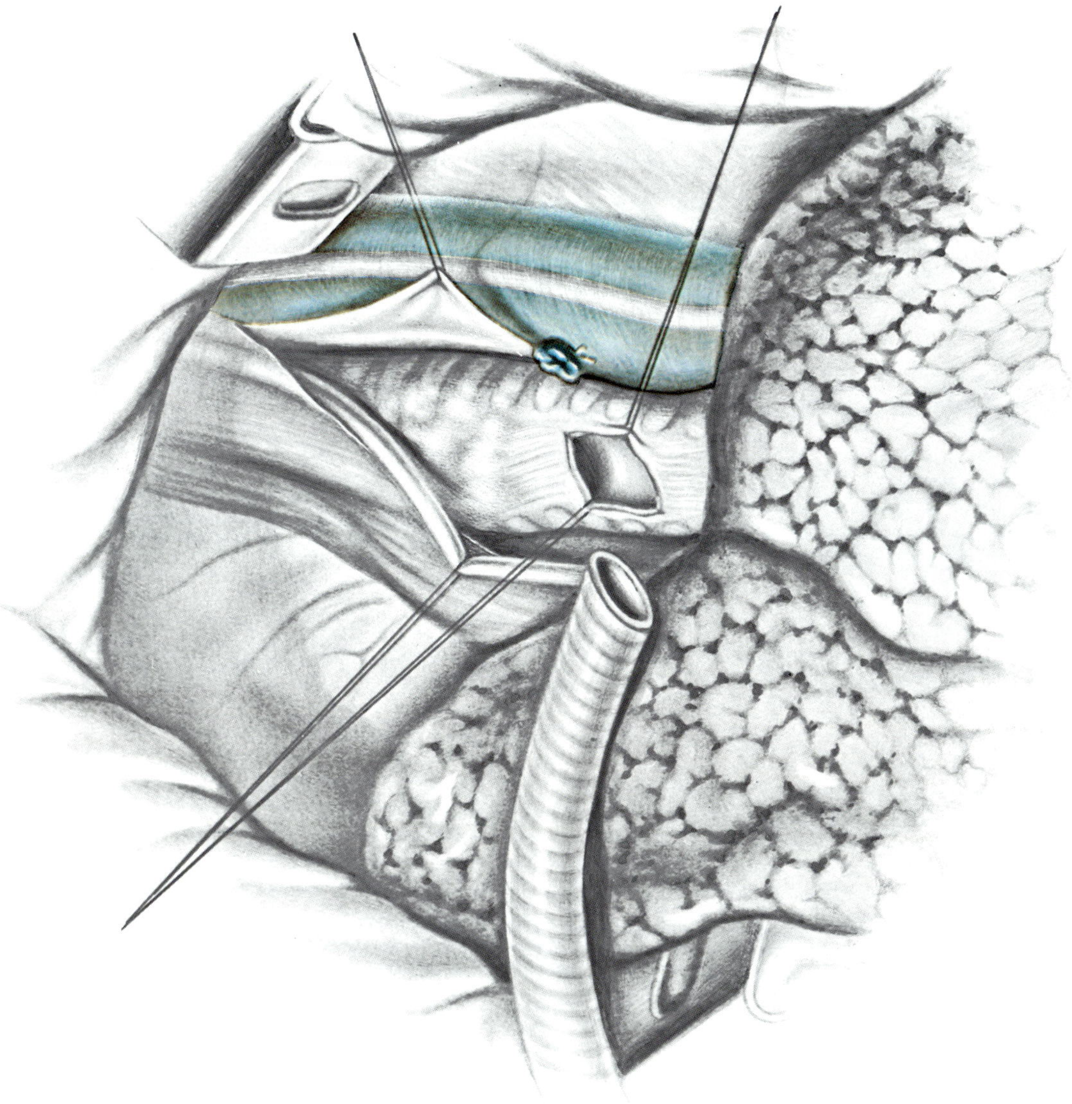

Fig. 185. Right main bronchus is opened with oblique incision in membranous part for introduction of intubation tube. Carina and orifice of left main bronchus are visible.

part of the right main bronchus 1 cm from the bifurcation. The bronchus is cut obliquely between them for 1 cm. The contents of the bronchus are removed with an aspirator. A sterile armored intubation tube fitted with an inflatable cuff is introduced into the opening formed and advanced beyond the carina into the left main bronchus and connected to the system of shunt-respiration (Fig. 185). Ventilation through the orotracheal tube is stopped. All further stages of the operation are carried out with only the left lung ventilated.

Two traction sutures are applied at the junction of the cartilaginous and membranous parts of the trachea, caudal to the lesion. The trachea is opened with a transverse incision through the membranous part, caudal to the tumor (Fig. 186). The tracheal lumen is inspected and, if necessary, palpated with the finger to determine the level of the cranial pole of the tumor exactly.

A sleeve resection of the affected portion of the trachea is carried out (Fig. 187). If the tracheal ends have to be stretched to bring them together, the thoracic tra-

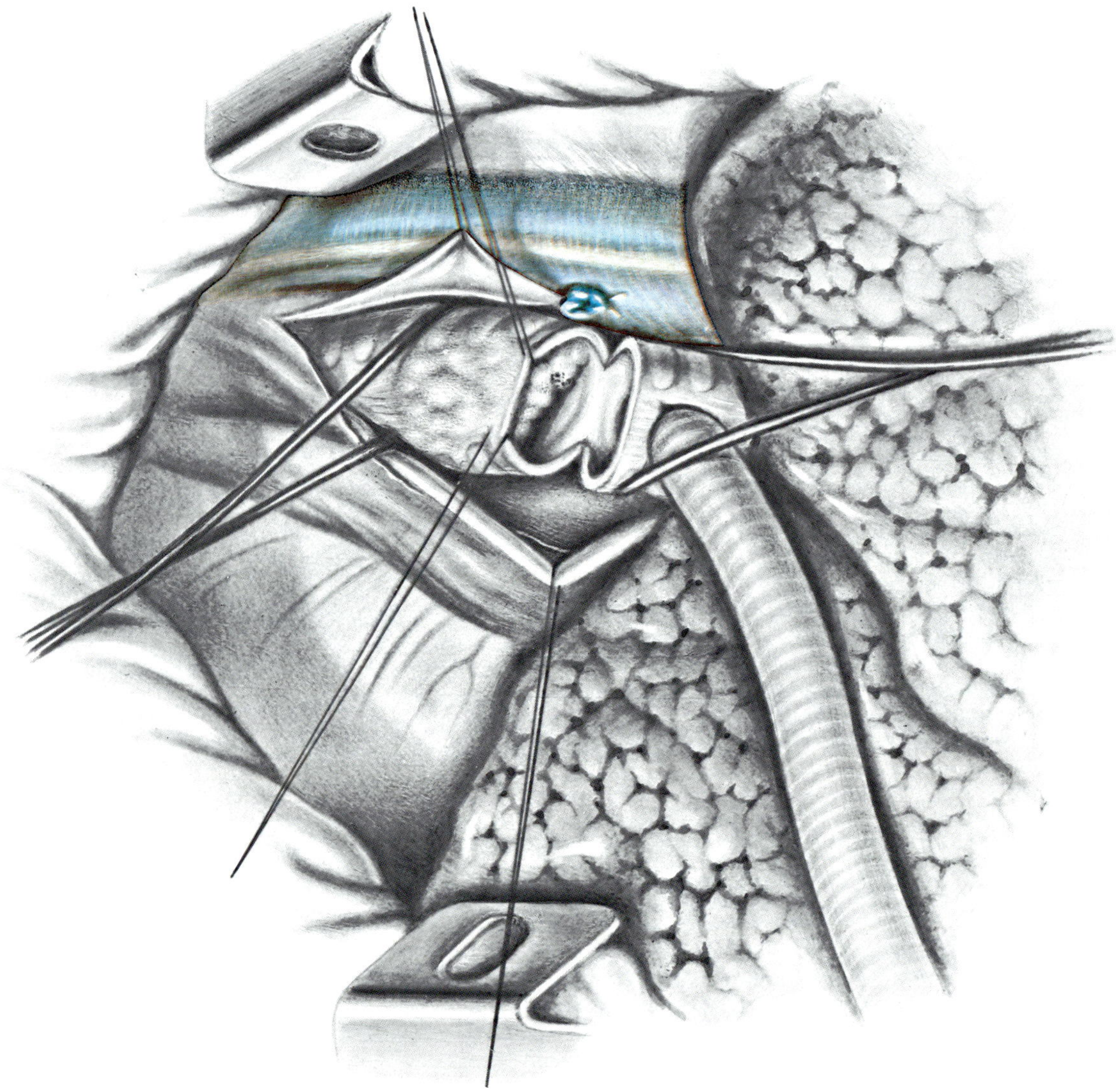

Fig. 186. Trachea is held by traction sutures and opened by a transverse incision. Border of tumor is visible in lumen.

chea and the region of the bifurcation are mobilized additionally. To reduce the strain, the patient's chin is made to rest on the chest. End-to-end anastomosis is created between the tracheal segments with interrupted sutures, tying the knots on the outside. The tracheal wall is stitched through all its coats. The posterior wall of the anastomosis is first sutured (Fig. 188). Before suturing the anterior wall of the anastomosis, relaxation interrupted sutures are applied, which are then tied on the outside one by one (Fig. 189). With the anastomosis created, ventilation of the lungs through the orotracheal tube is resumed, pressure of the gaseous-anesthetic mixture in the tracheobronchial tree is raised, and the anastomosis is tested for airtightness.

The intubation tube is removed from the left main bronchus. The opening in the right bronchus is closed with interrupted or Halsted sutures. Airtightness of the bronchial suture is tested under fluid. The region of the intertracheal anastomosis is covered by stitching together the medial and lateral pleural sheets (Fig. 190). Two drains, upper and lower, are left in the pleural cavity. The wound in the thoracic wall is sutured layer by layer.

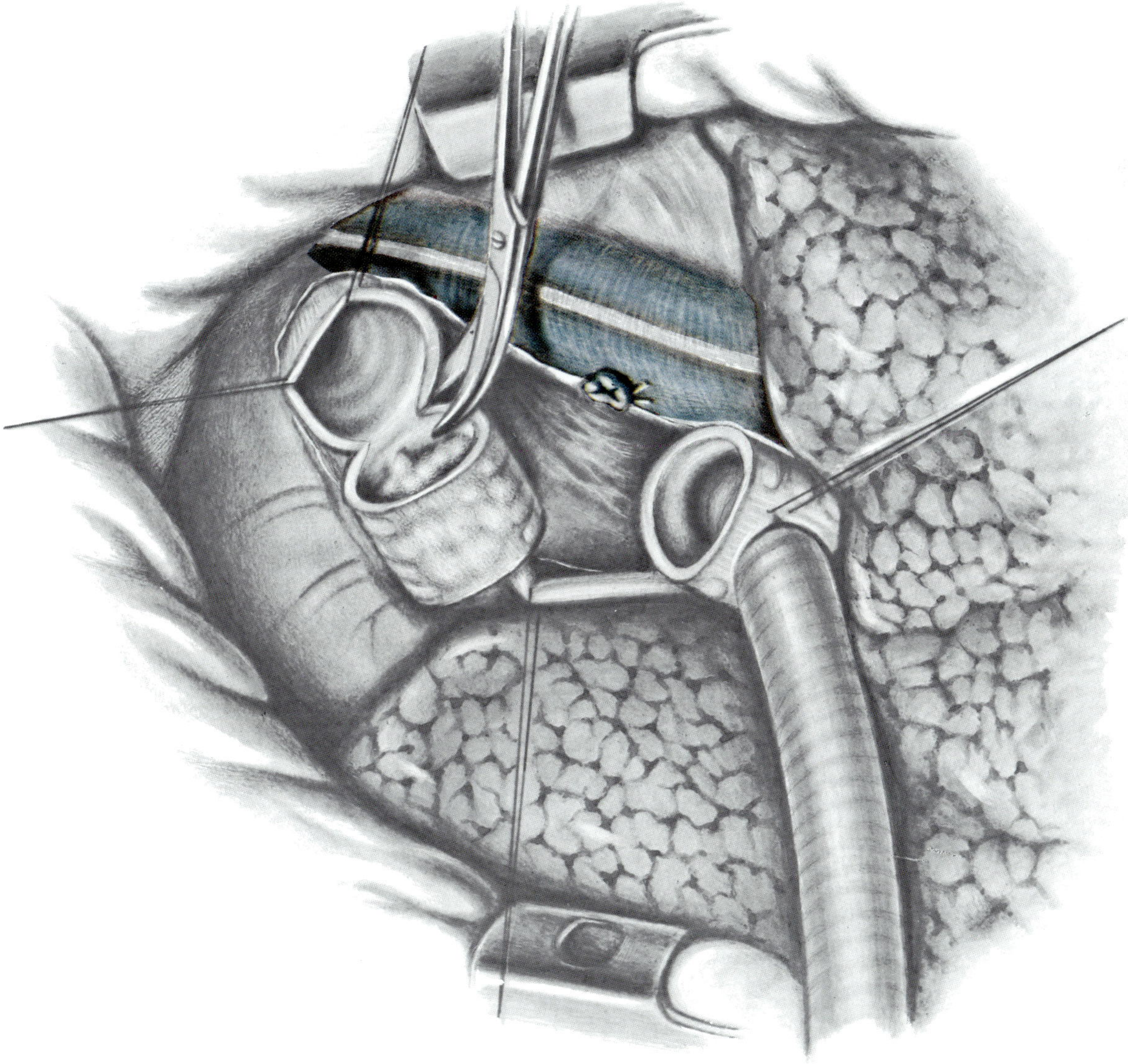

Fig. 187. Sleeve resection of trachea with tumor.

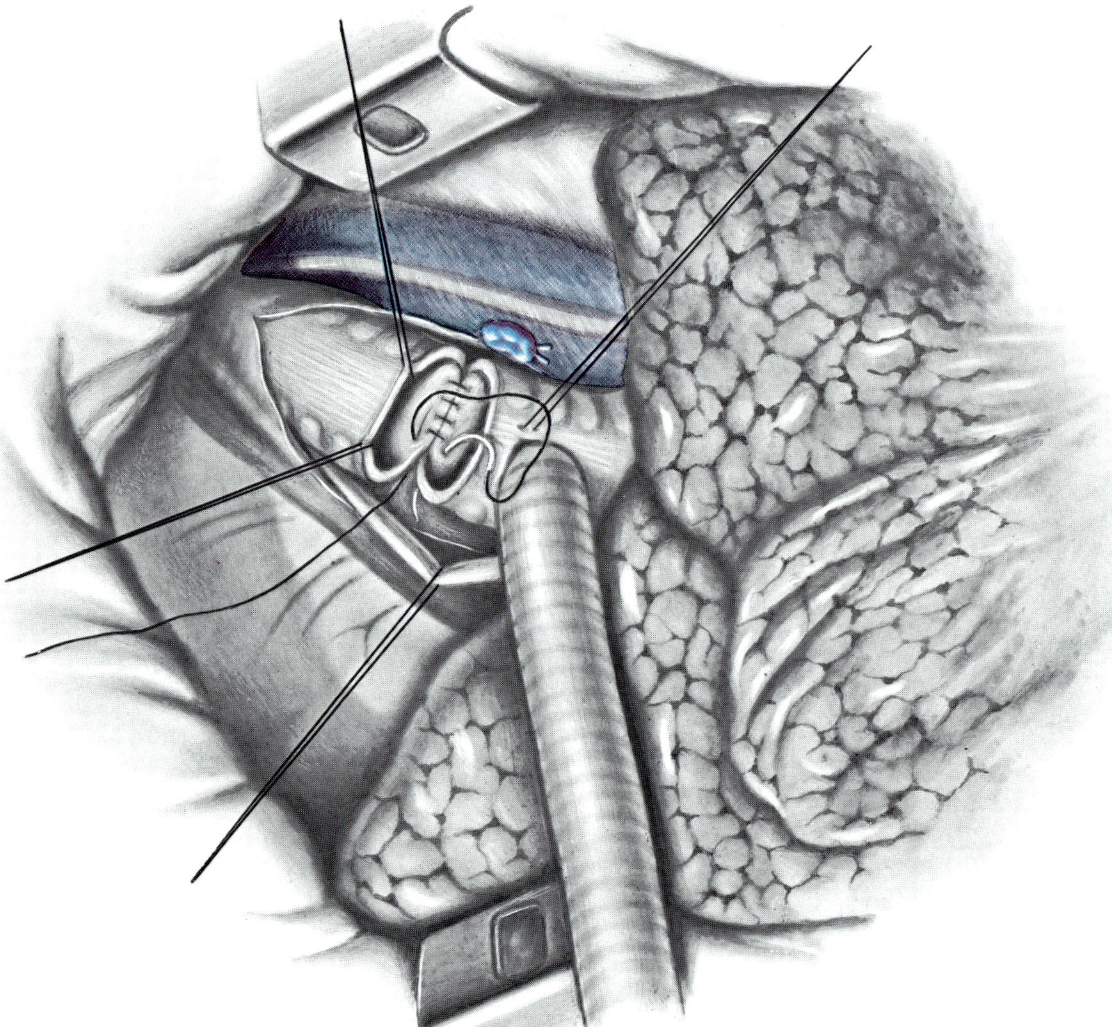

Fig. 188. Sutures are applied to posterior wall of intertracheal anastomosis.

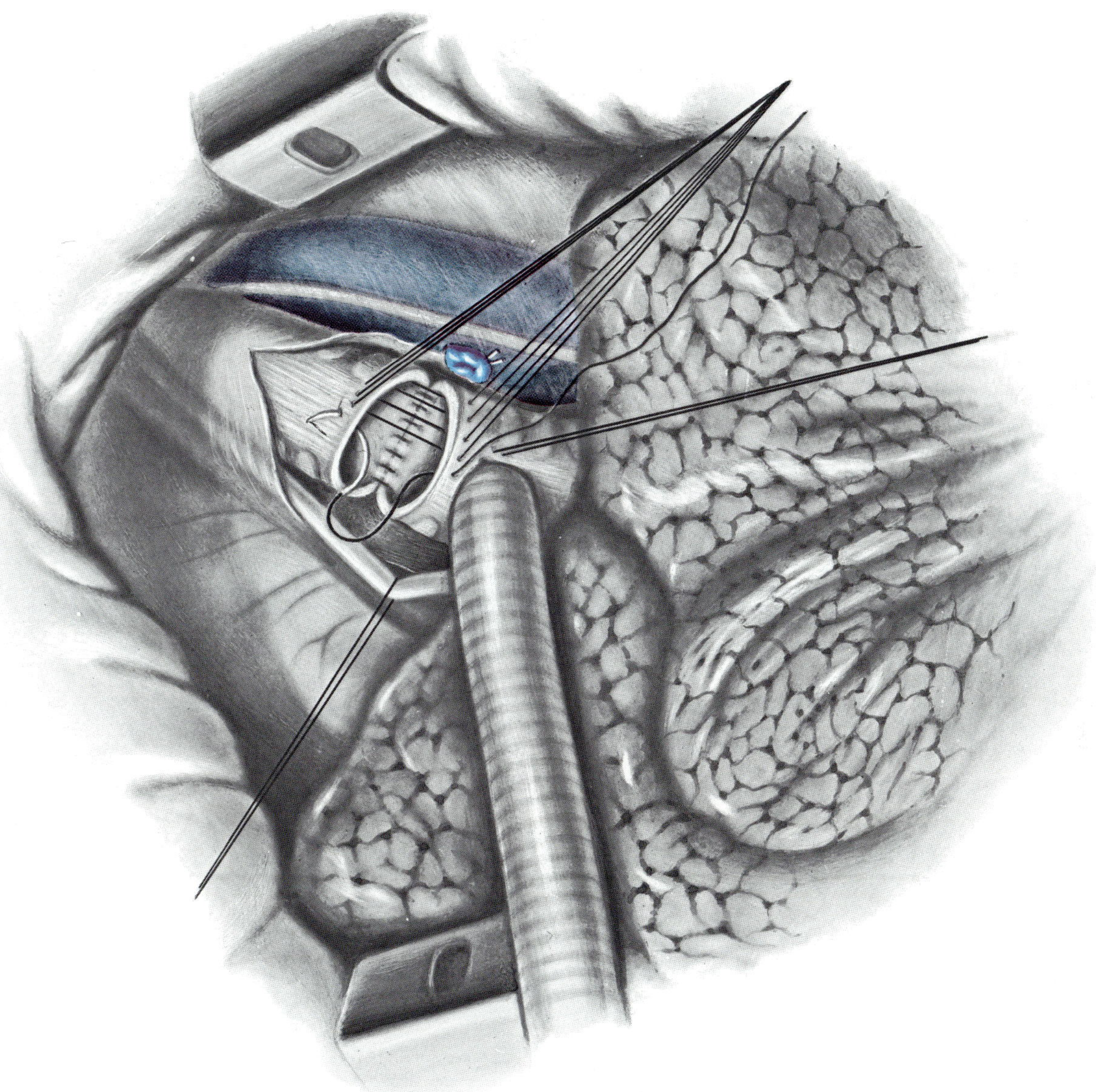

Fig. 189. Sutures are applied to anterior wall of intertracheal anastomosis.

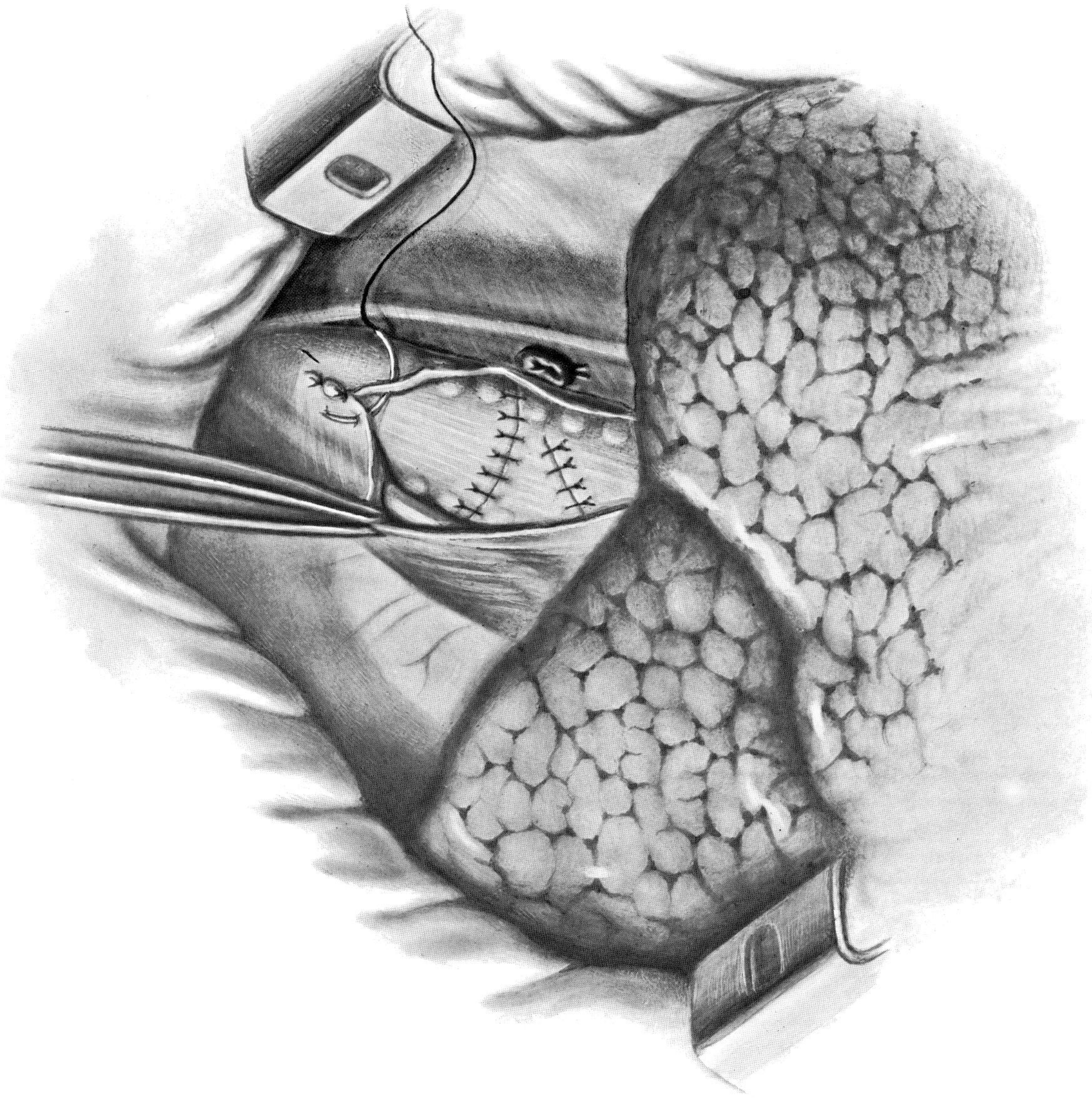

Fig. 190. Intertracheal anastomosis has been created. Opening in right main bronchus has been sutured. Region of anastomosis is covered with pleura.

*RESECTION OF THE BIFURCATION OF THE TRACHEA

The operation is carried out through a posterior approach on the right in the fourth intercostal space with resection of the necks of the fourth and fifth ribs; the patient is placed in a prone position.

The lung is drawn aside laterally and ventrally. The arch of the azygos vein is ligated and transected between the ligatures. The mediastinal pleura is cut longitudinally for 12 to 14 cm between the vagus nerve and the esophagus. The vagus nerve is drawn aside laterally with a loop. With extreme care being taken not to injure the recurrent laryngeal nerves, the thoracic trachea and the right and left main bronchi are successively separated by the blunt and sharp techniques and held with rubber loops. The bifurcation of the trachea is freed from the adhesions, and the pericardiacotracheal ligament is cut. Two traction sutures are applied to the left main bronchus, which is then cut off from the trachea. A sterile intubation tube is introduced into the bronchus and is connected to the shunt-respiration system (Fig. 191).

All further stages of the operation are performed with only the left lung ventilated. Two traction sutures are applied at the junction between the cartilaginous and membranous parts of the trachea, cranial to the lesion, and another two traction sutures are placed on the right

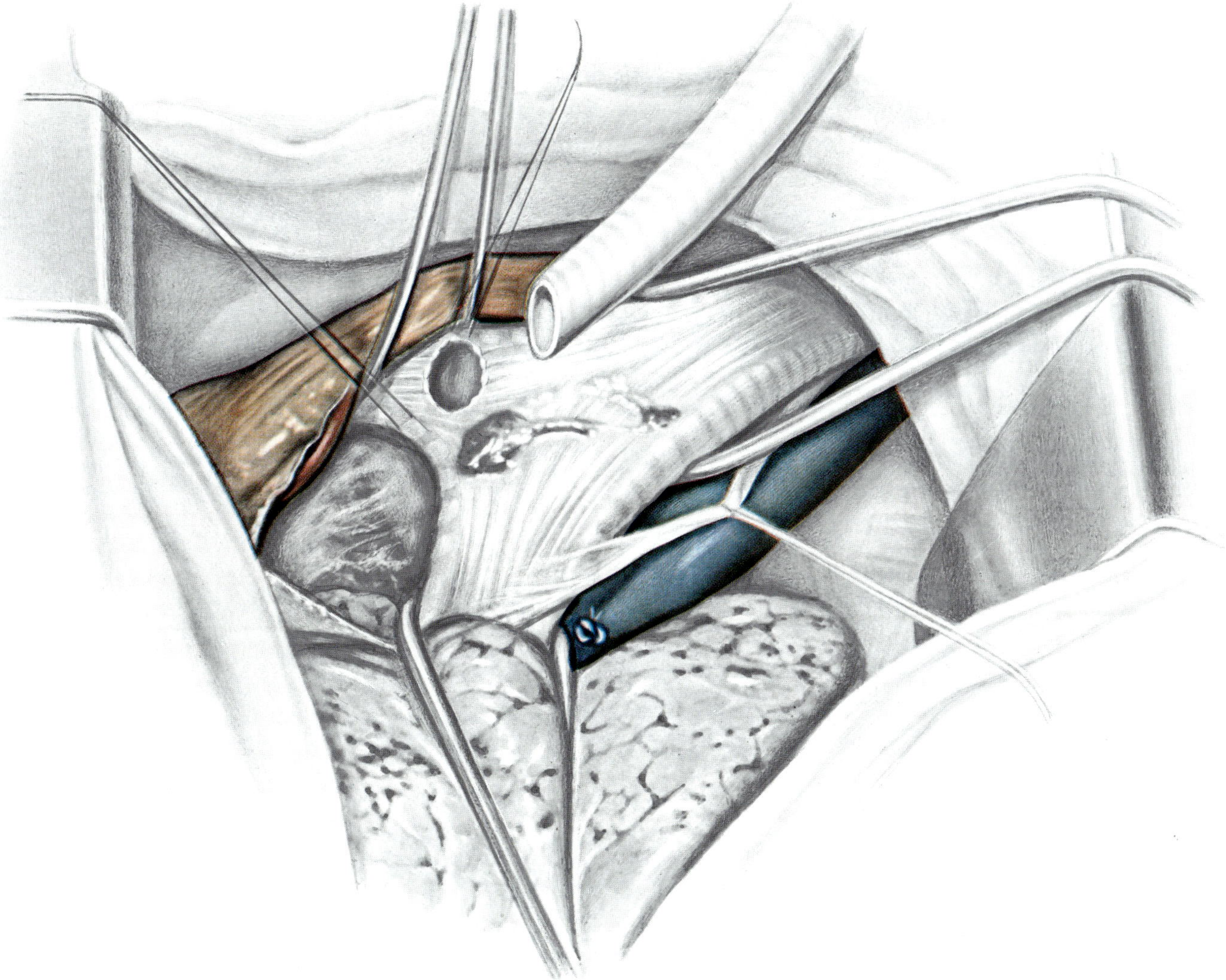

Fig. 191. Introduction of intubation tube into opening in left main bronchus. Region of bifurcation has been prepared. Trachea, both main bronchi, and right vagus nerve are held with loops. Esophagus and superior vena cava are visible.

main bronchus. The thoracic trachea and then the right main bronchus are transected (Fig. 192). The bifurcation of the trachea is removed. The tracheobronchial tree is reconstructed by one of three variants.

1. Anastomosis is created between the right main bronchus and the trachea with chromicized catgut sutures, tying the knots on the outside (Fig. 193). The anastomosis is first sutured on the ventral surfaces of the trachea and bronchus. With the anastomosis created, the orotracheal intubation tube is introduced into the right main bronchus. The sterile tube is removed from the left main bronchus. The right lung is ventilated. An oval window is formed with a scalpel and scissors on the medial wall of the intermediate bronchus in its cartilaginous and membranous parts. The opening corresponds to the lumen of the left main bronchus. The left main bronchus is pulled by the traction sutures into the right pleural cavity. The left main bronchus is joined end to side with the opening in the intermediate bronchus. The sutures are first applied to the ventral and then to the dorsal walls of the anastomosis (Fig. 194). The region of both anastomoses is covered, whenever possible, with the adjoining tissues and mediastinal pleura.

2. The intubation tube is removed from the left main bronchus and introduced into the right main bronchus from the side of the pleural cavity. The right lung is ven-

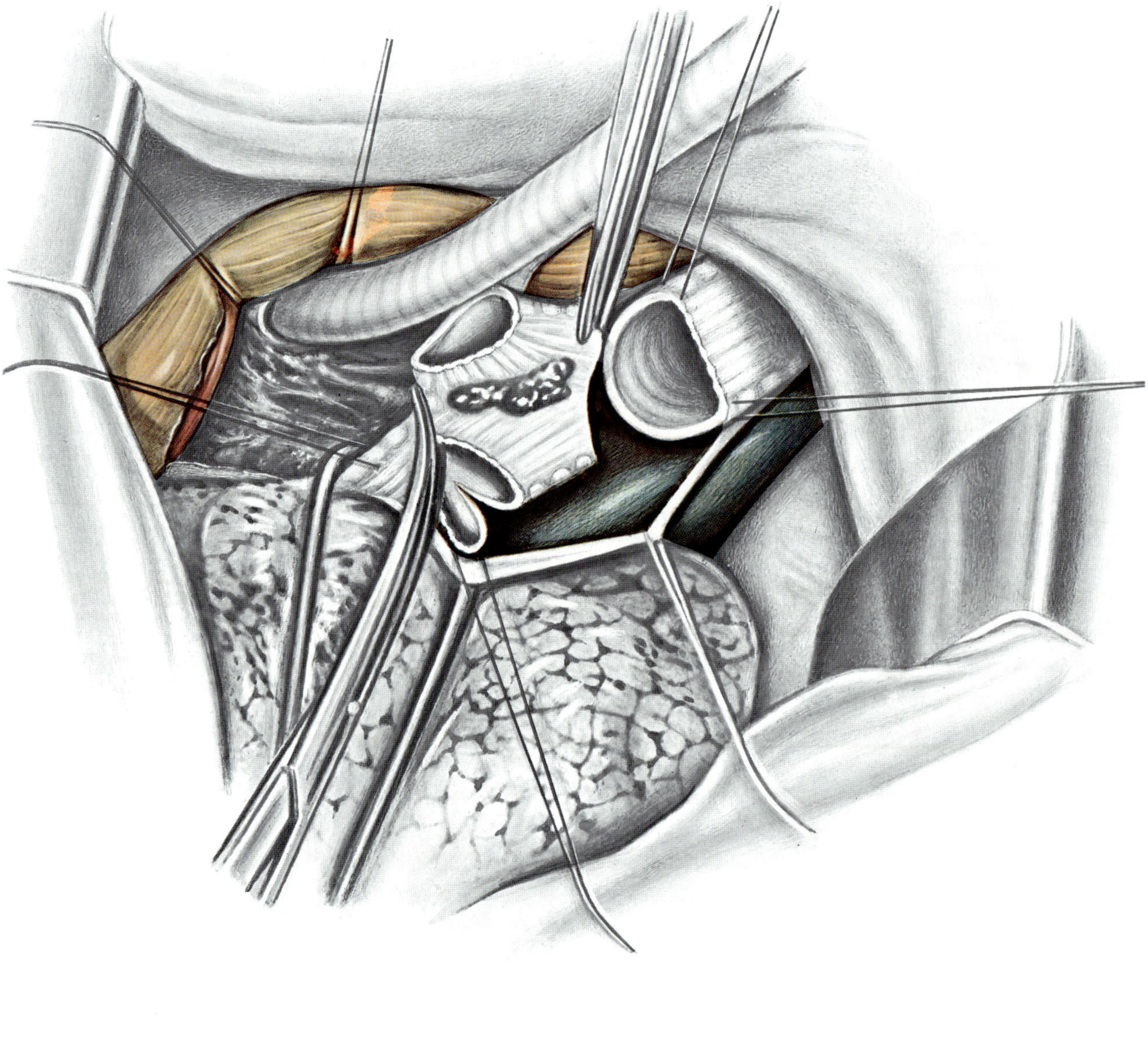

Fig. 192. Resection of bifurcation of trachea. Intubation tube for shunt-respiration system is in left main bronchus. Traction sutures have been applied to walls of trachea and right main bronchus.

tilated. The left main bronchus is pulled by the traction sutures into the right pleural cavity. Its stump is sutured tightly with interrupted chromicized catgut sutures. The left lung remains in a state of atelectasis. An anastomosis is created between the right main bronchus and the trachea, first stitching together the ventral surfaces of the trachea and bronchus. The intubation tube is removed from the right main bronchus, and an orotracheal tube is advanced into it. Sutures are then applied to the dorsal wall of the anastomosis. These sutures are tied over the orotracheal tube that had been introduced into the right main bronchus. The region of the anastomosis is covered with mediastinal pleura.

3. Semioval windows are formed with scissors in the edges of the medial walls of both main bronchi. The right and left main bronchi are stitched to each other by approximating the margins of these windows and shaping a new carina. End-to-end anastomosis is formed between the trachea and both the stitched-together bronchi. Sutures are applied to the ventral wall of the anastomosis, ventilating the left lung from time to time. The intubation tube is removed from the left main bronchus, into which the orotracheal tube is then advanced. Sutures are applied to the dorsal wall on the orotracheal intubation tube. The region of the anastomosis is covered by the surrounding tissues and mediastinal pleura.

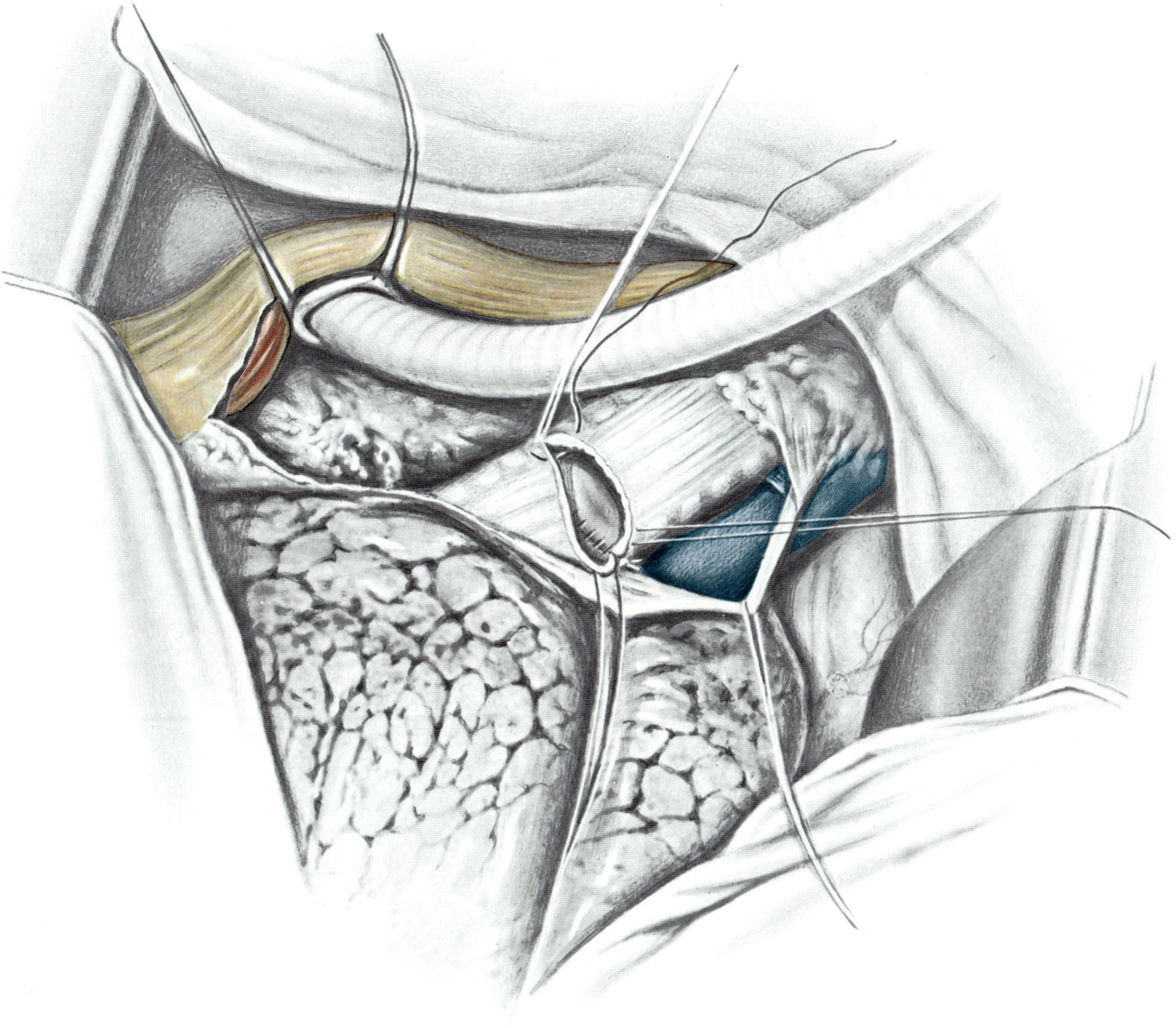

Fig. 193. Sutures are applied to dorsal wall of anastomosis between trachea and right main bronchus.

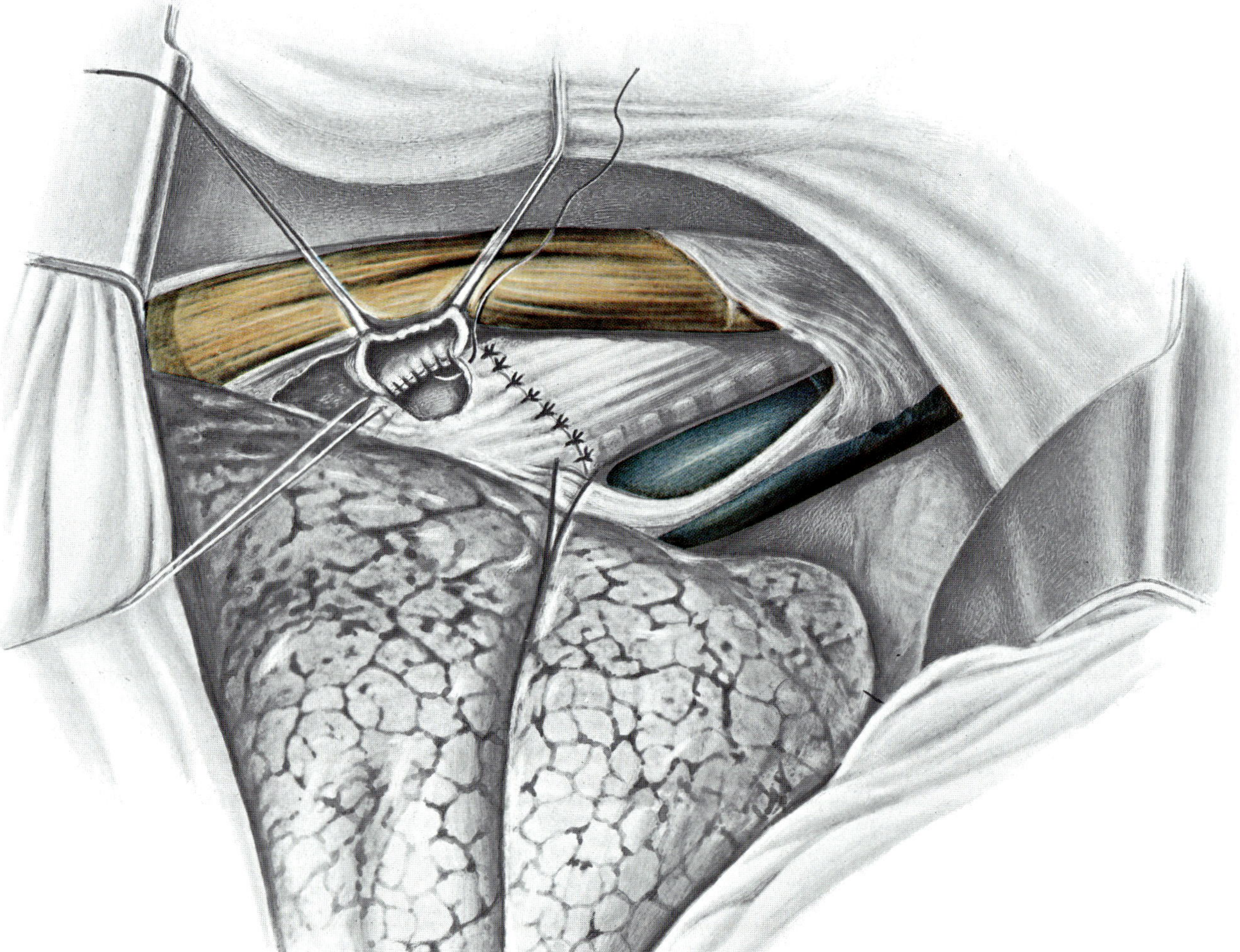

Fig. 194. Creation of end-to-side anastomosis between left main and intermediate bronchi. Intubation tube has been removed from left main bronchus.

SUPERIOR LOBECTOMY WITH SLEEVE RESECTION OF THE BRONCHUS

The pleural cavity is opened by a lateral approach in the sixth intercostal space.

The lung is freed from the adhesions, and the pulmonary ligament is transected between ligatures. The vessels of the superior lobe are treated as in routine lobectomy. The main and inferior lobar (on the right the intermediate) bronchi are exposed and held with rubber loops. The vagus nerve and bronchial vessels are separated from the membranous part of the main bronchus and drawn aside on a thick thread. In resection for cancer the bronchial vessels located cranially and caudally to the site of the intended transection of the bronchus are separated with a dissector, ligated, and cut. Two traction sutures are applied to the edges of each of the future cranial and caudal stumps. Careful hemostasis is accomplished, and isolating gauze napkins are inserted under the bronchus.

The left lung is disconnected from ventilation, and excision of the diseased bronchial segment is begun. The main bronchus is transected in the intercartilaginous

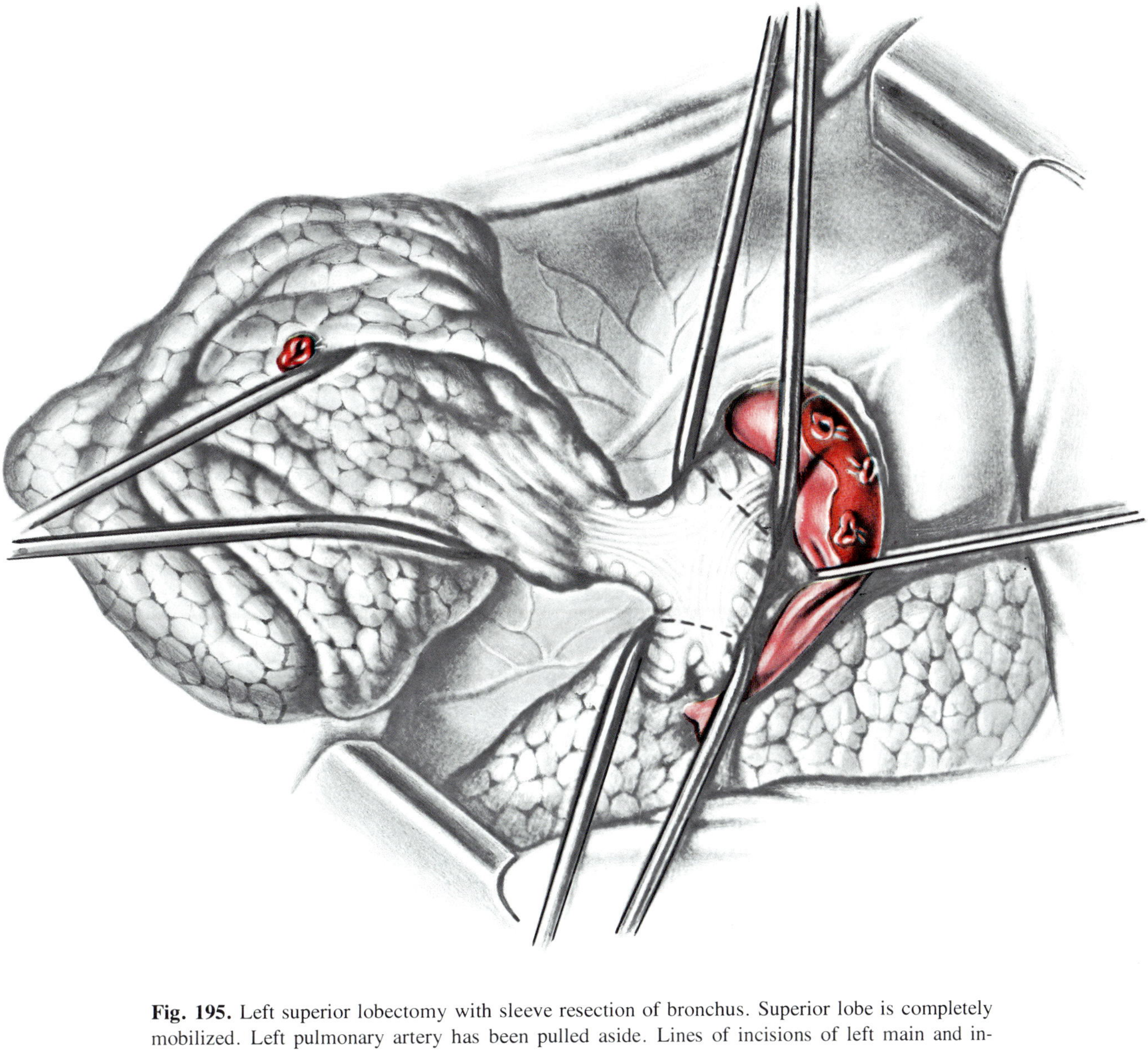

Fig. 195. Left superior lobectomy with sleeve resection of bronchus. Superior lobe is completely mobilized. Left pulmonary artery has been pulled aside. Lines of incisions of left main and inferior lobar bronchi are marked.

space. After that the inferior lobar bronchus (on the right the intermediate bronchus) is transected 2 to 3 mm cranial to the orifice of the sixth segmental bronchus. To reduce the discrepancy in the bronchial openings the bronchus of lesser diameter may be transected obliquely. It is advisable to cut the cartilaginous part of the bronchus with a scalpel with the traction sutures drawn apart and the lung drawn aside laterally. The membranous part is cut with scissors. The superior lobe with the segments of the resected bronchi is removed.

The creation of the anastomosis is begun from the medial angle between the cartilaginous and membranous parts of the bronchial wall. The first suture is applied to the cartilaginous part, after which sutures are successively placed and immediately tied on the posterior and lateral walls. It is advisable to apply the anterior sutures as relaxation sutures and then to tie them consecutively. The number of interrupted sutures for interbronchial anastomosis varies from 15 to 18. In applying a bronchial suture the thread is stitched through all the coats of the wall, but as little as possible of the mucous membrane is included. The sutures are placed at intervals of

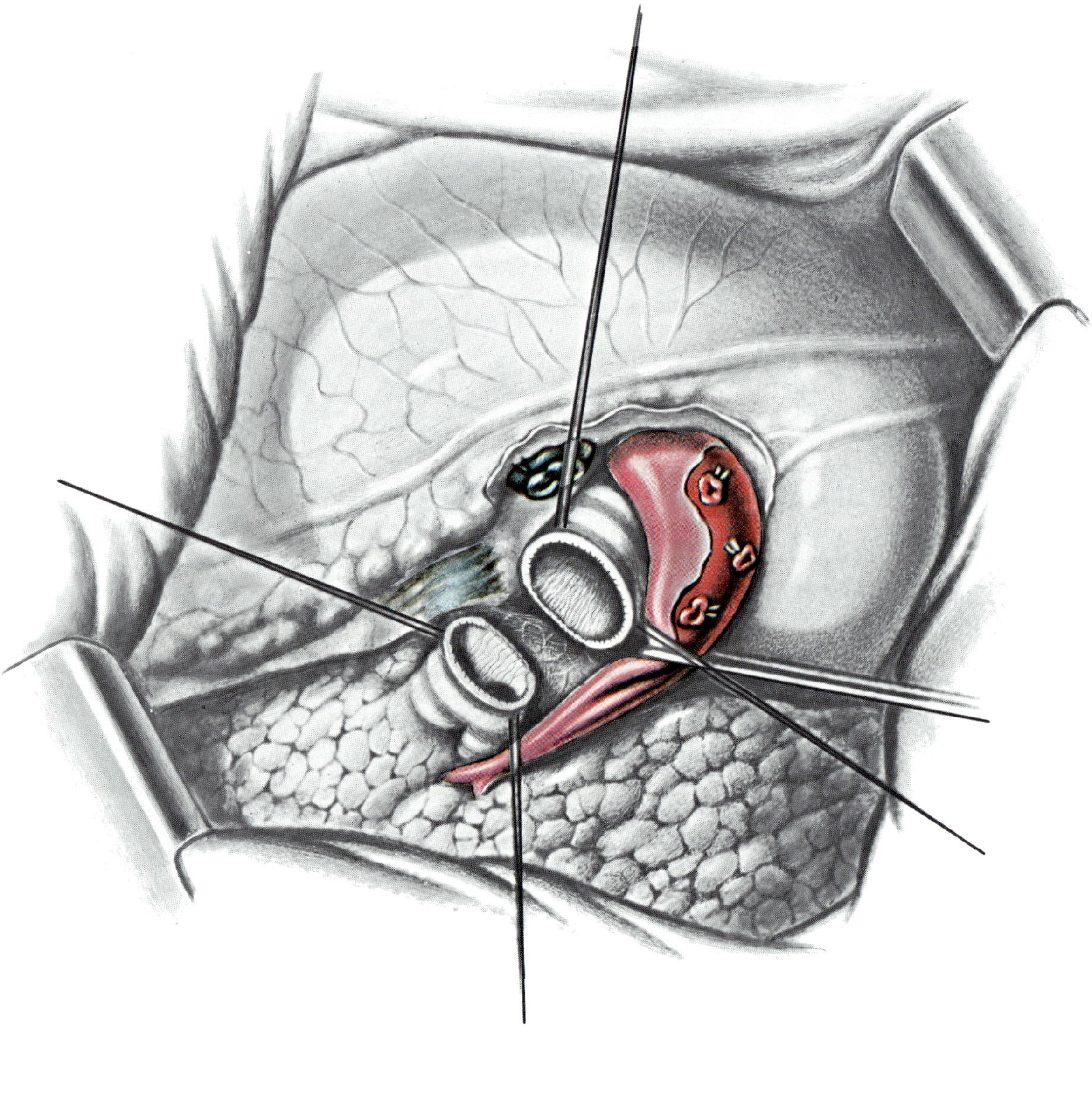

Fig. 196. Superior lobe of left lung with segments of main and inferior lobar bronchi removed.

3 to 4 mm. All the sutures are tied only on the outside. After creation of the interbronchial anastomosis the lung on the side of the operation is ventilated and fully inflated. The pleural cavity is filled with warm physiological saline solution. The airtightness of the anastomosis and pulmonary tissue is tested by raising the pressure in the system of the anesthetic machine to 40 to 50 mm Hg.

If possible, the region of the interbronchial anastomosis is covered with the pleura, applying three or four interrupted or Halsted sutures.

The stages of right and left superior lobectomy with sleeve resection of the bronchus are shown in Figs. 195 to 201.

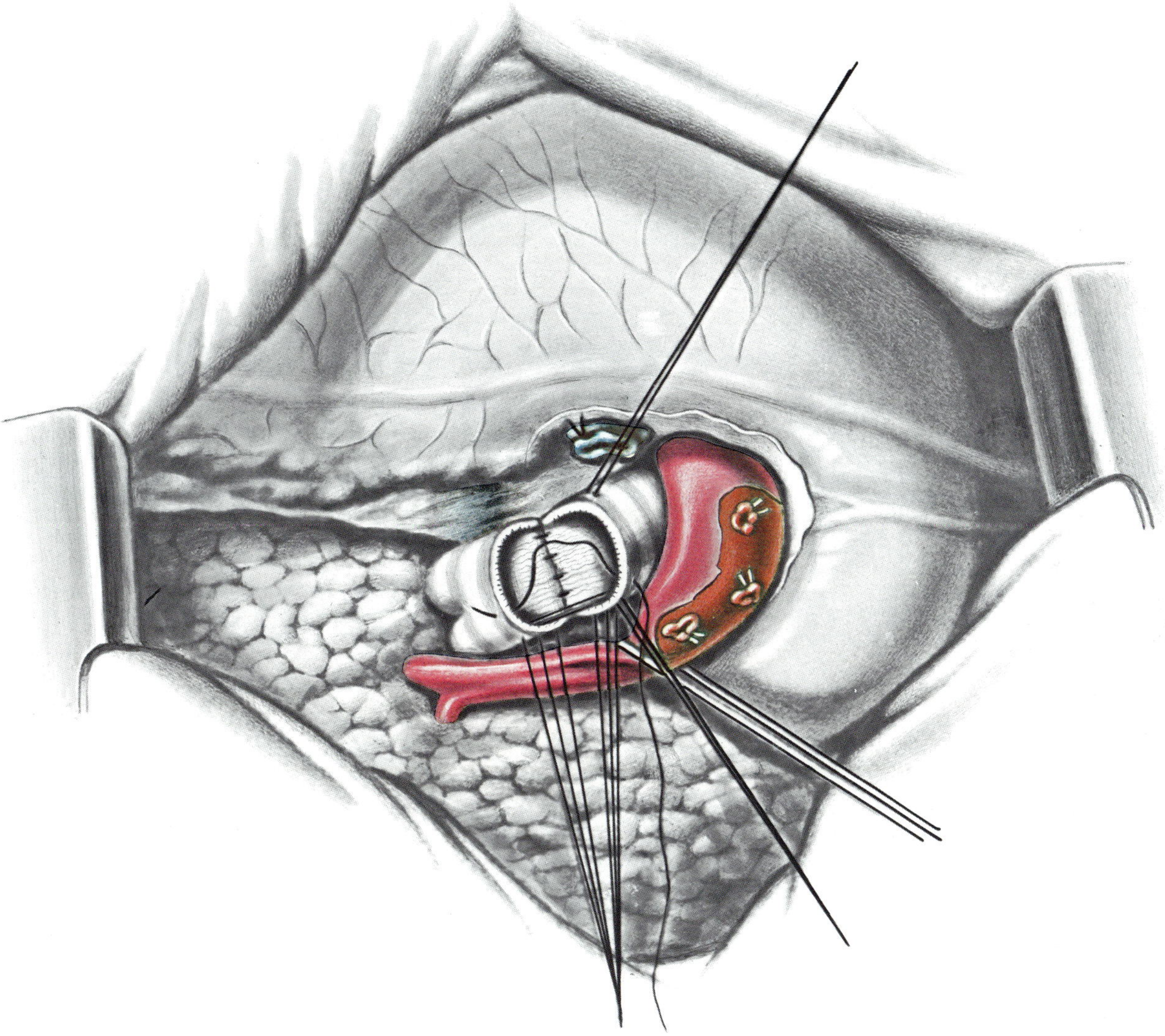

Fig. 197. Sutures are applied to ventral wall of interbronchial anastomosis. Stitches on dorsal wall are visible.

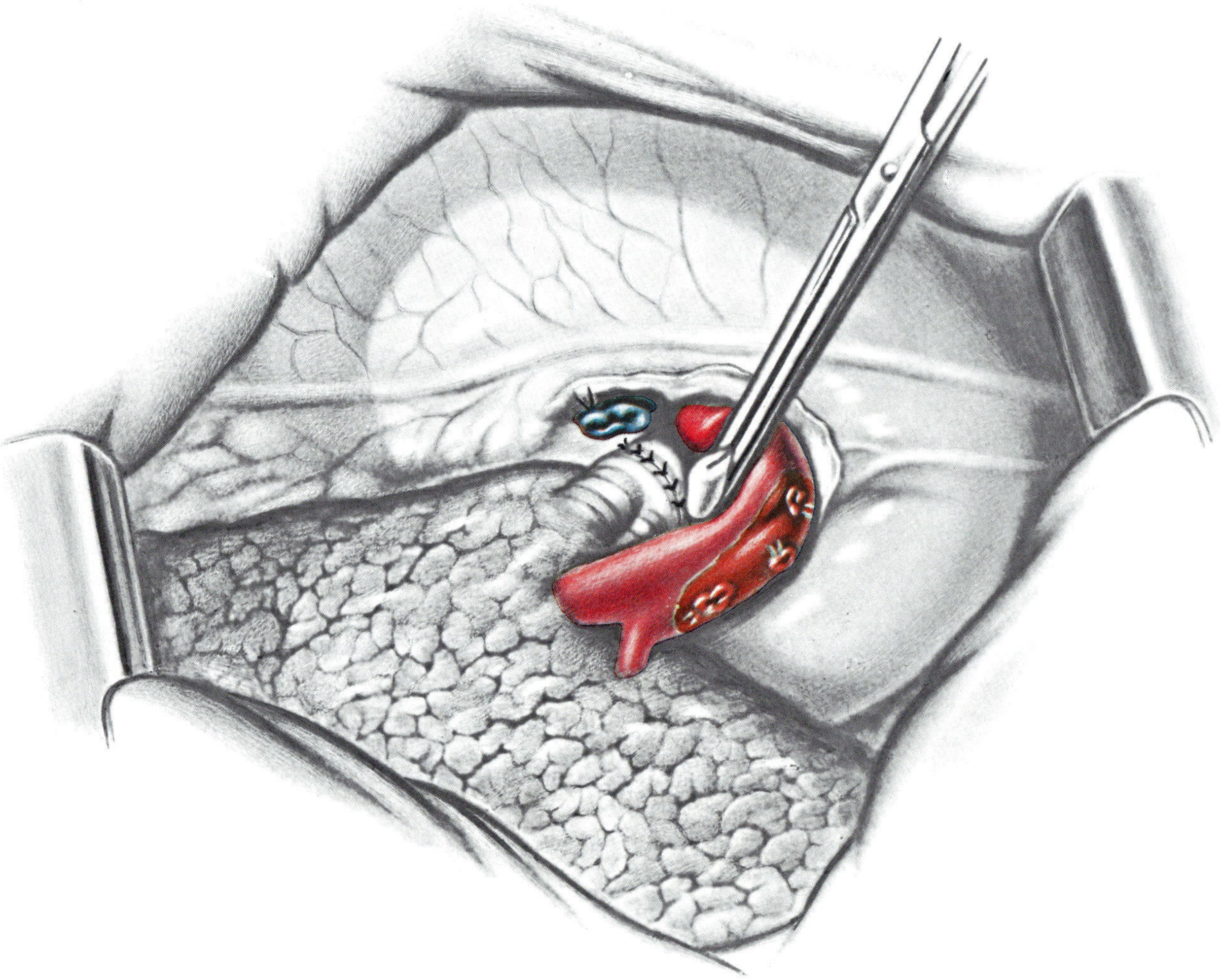

Fig. 198. Anastomosis between left main and inferior lobar bronchi has been formed.

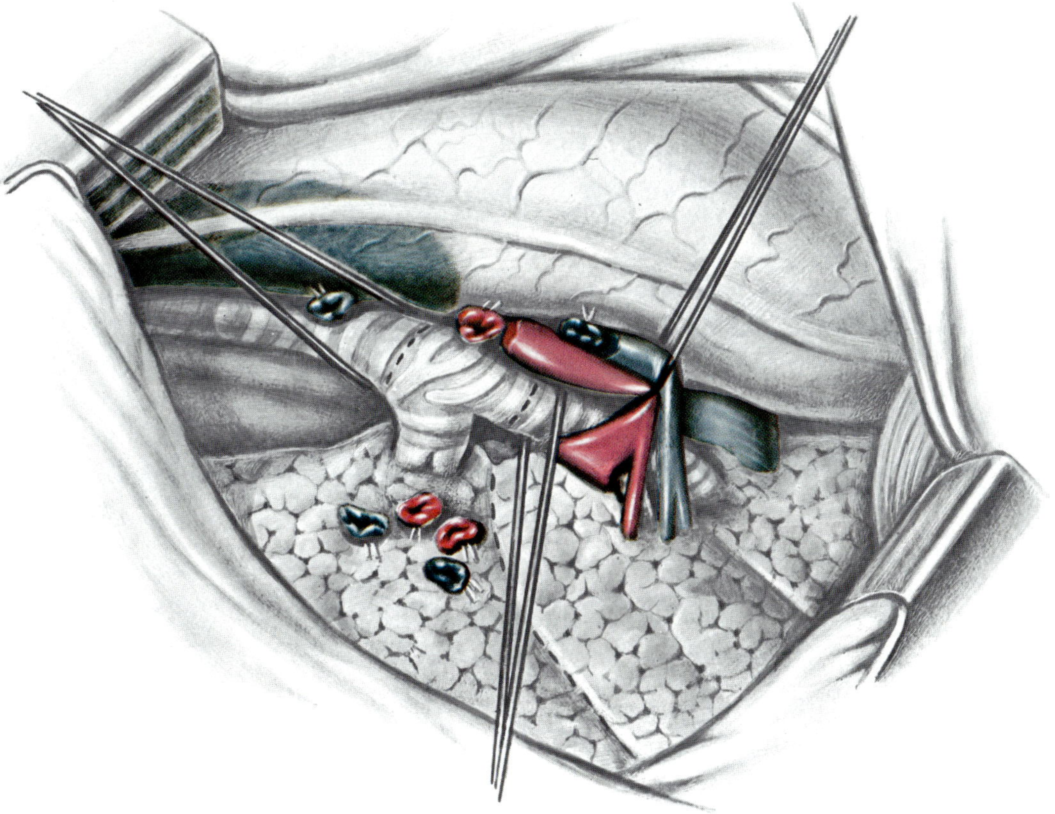

Fig. 199. Right superior lobectomy with sleeve resection of bronchus. Descending part of right pulmonary artery and vein of middle lobe are drawn aside medially. Lines of incisions of right main and intermediate bronchi are marked. Stumps of arch of azygos vein, anterior trunk of pulmonary artery, and $V_{1,2,3}$ are visible.

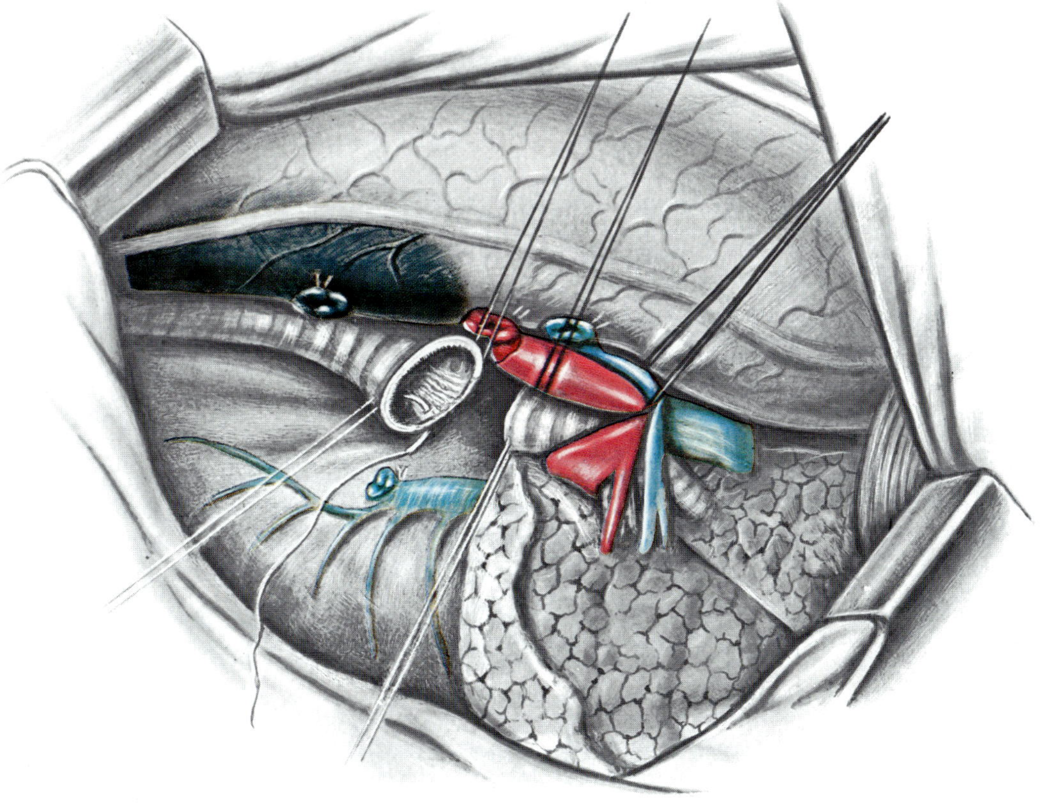

Fig. 200. Stumps of main and intermediate bronchi as viewed before they are anastomosed.

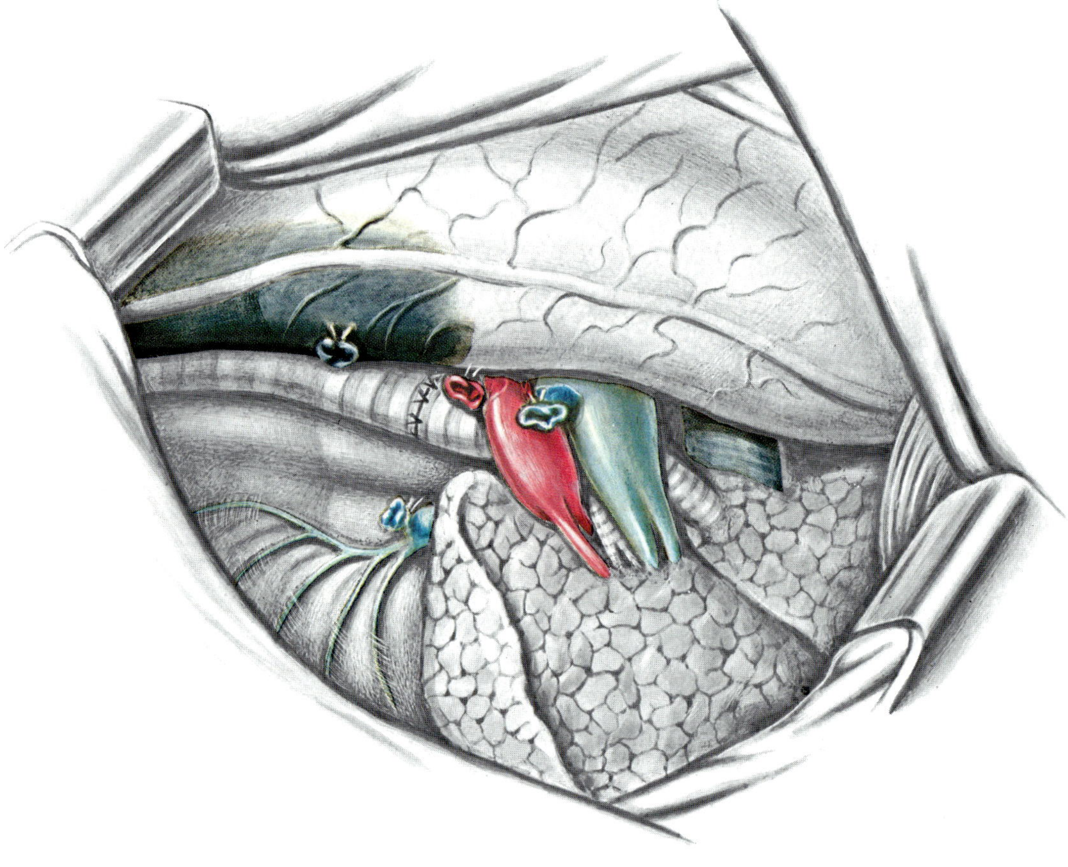

Fig. 201. Anastomosis between right main and intermediate bronchi has been created.

OPERATION FOR FISTULA OF THE STUMP OF THE MAIN BRONCHUS BY TRANSSTERNAL APPROACH

A skin incision is made from the jugular fossa to the tip of the xiphoid process. Typical longitudinal sternotomy is carried out with Gigli's saw or a sternotome. In cases with a large xiphoid process, access is gained into the retrosternal space from below, not along the midline, but through the sheath of the rectus abdominis muscle. The pleural reflection on the side of the lung is separated laterally. The sternal edges are drawn apart with a retractor. The *right* main bronchus is approached on the right of the ascending aorta within the limits of a rectangle, the sides of which are the right border of the ascending aorta and the initial part of the brachiocephalic artery on the left, the superior vena cava on the right, the left brachiocephalic vein above, and the pericardial reflection corresponding to the superior border of the right pulmonary artery below. The superior vena cava, ascending aorta, and brachiocephalic artery are drawn apart to the sides. The bifurcation of the trachea and the base of the stump of the right main bronchus are palpated on the floor of the rectangle thus formed.

The base of the stump of the right main bronchus is separated by the sharp and blunt techniques. A rubber loop is drawn under the tracheobronchial angle from the side of the right pulmonary artery, by means of which

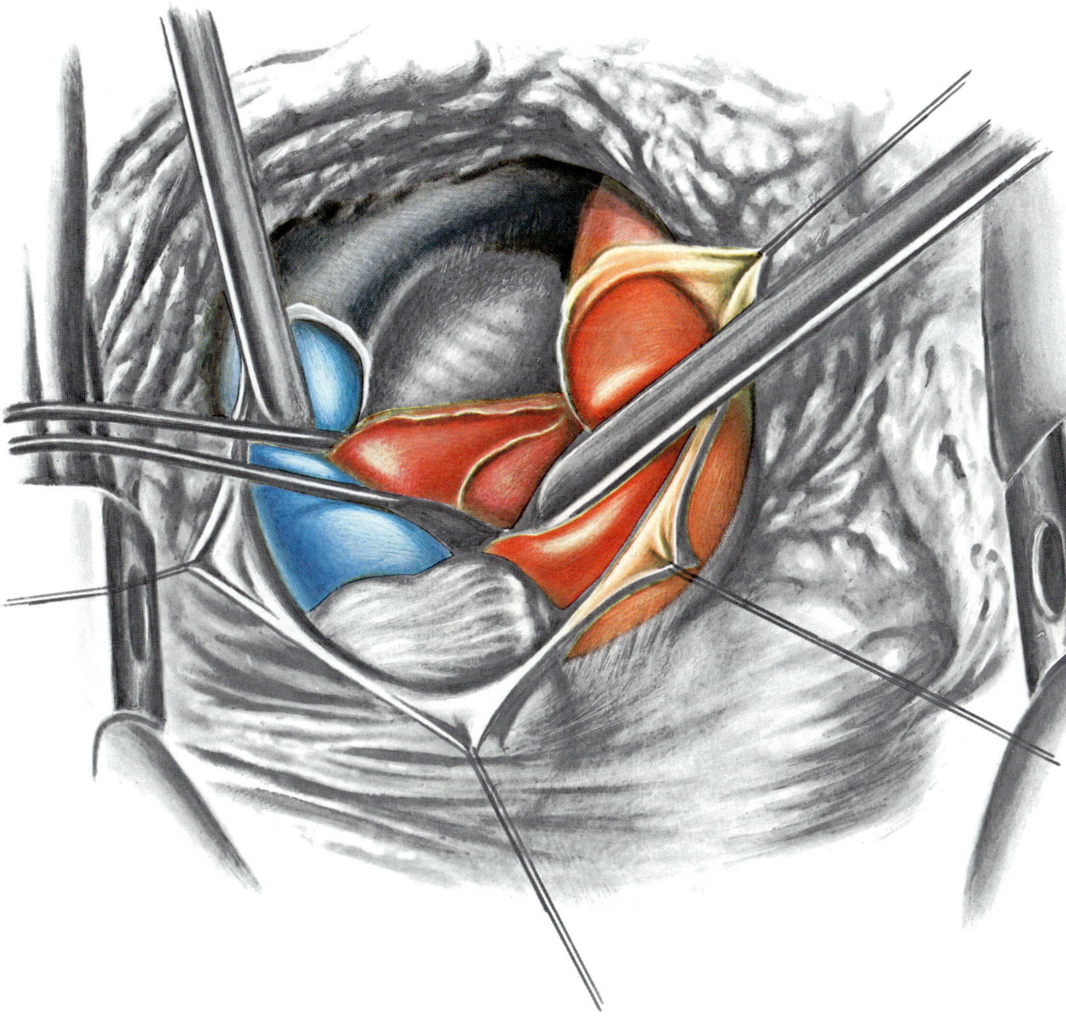

Fig. 202. Superior vena cava and ascending aorta with brachiocephalic artery are drawn apart to sides. Base of stump of right main bronchus is visible. Pericardium has been opened. Stump of right pulmonary artery is held with loop.

the bronchus is pulled into the wound. Holder sutures are applied to the lateral wall and the bifurcation of the trachea. The *YO* instrument is brought under the separated base of the bronchial stump, and a mechanical suture is applied as laterally as possible. The sutured bronchial stump is cut away from the trachea.

To achieve greater mobility of the region of the tracheobronchial angle, the intubation tube is removed from the main bronchus and advanced into the trachea. The bifurcation of the trachea is pulled ventrally by means of previously applied traction sutures, turned medially, and brought up as closely as possible to the operating surgeon. The opening in the trachea is closed with interrupted sutures passed through all the layers. To provide ventilation during application of the sutures, the opening in the trachea is closed from time to time with a moistened tampon.

A wider approach may be gained to the stump of the right main bronchus by opening the pericardium (Fig. 202) and reamputating the stump of the right pulmonary artery (Fig. 203). It is easier to suture the opening in the trachea after this manipulation (Fig. 204).

To expose the base of the stump of the *left* main bronchus, an approach through the pericardial cavity to the left of the ascending aorta is more convenient.

Following longitudinal sternotomy, the pericardium is opened at the level of the left auricle with an incision 10 to 12 cm long extended ventrally and parallel to the left phrenic nerve. The edges of the incision are drawn apart by means of traction sutures. The operating table

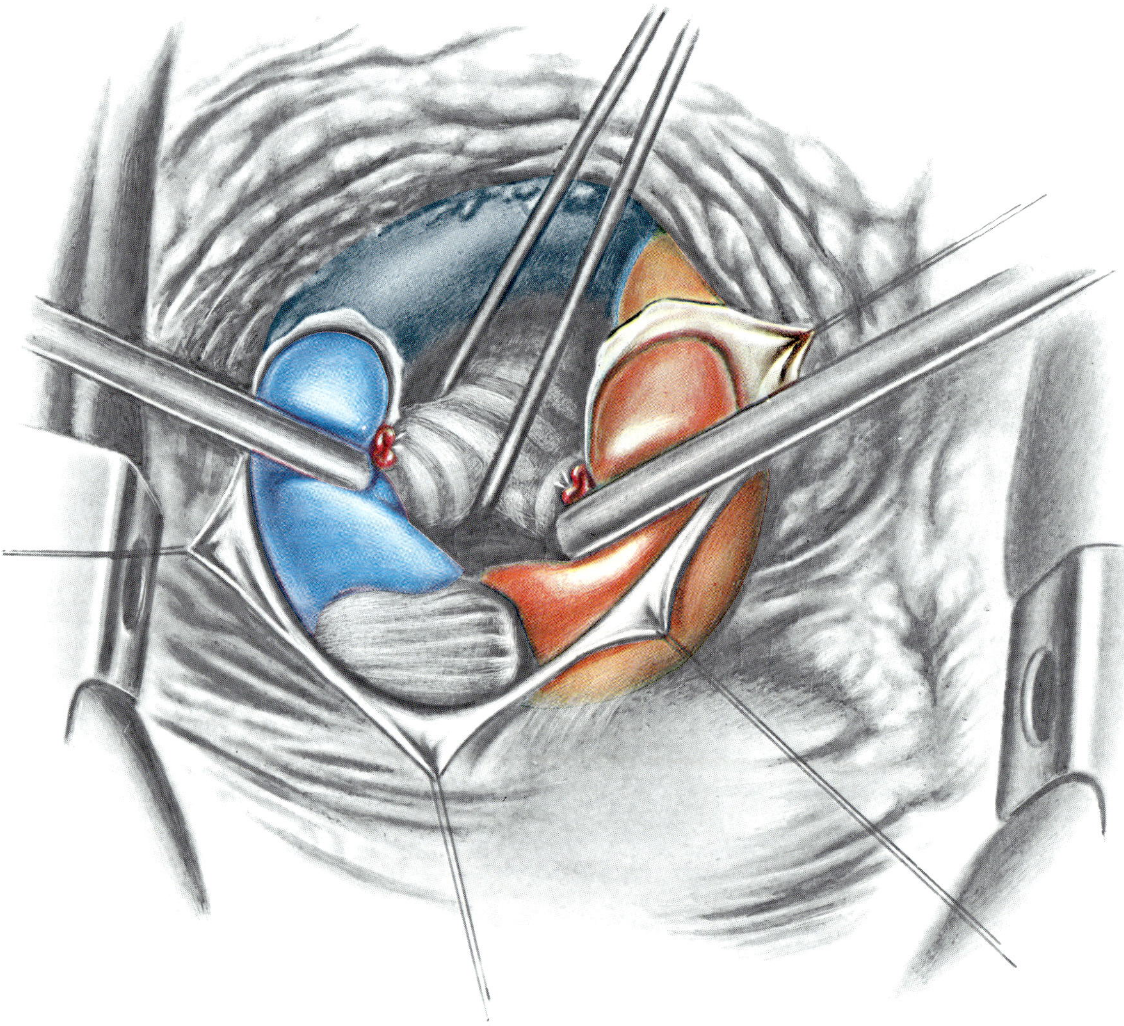

Fig. 203. Stump of right pulmonary artery has been reamputated. Base of stump of right main bronchus is held with a rubber loop.

is inclined to the right side; the heart is moved to the right, and the posterior pericardial wall is opened (Fig. 205). The stump of the left pulmonary artery is ligated intrapericardially as far in the central direction as possible. The opening in the posterior pericardial wall is widened, and the stump of the left main bronchus exposed. It is treated by the same method as on the right (Fig. 206).

The operation is completed by inserting a rubber drain into the region of the bifurcation of the trachea. The other end of the drain is brought out through the floor of the pericardial cavity. A second drain is placed in the anterior mediastinum and also brought out through a special incision made near the xiphoid process. The sternum is sutured with tantalum wire or plastic threads, and the periosteum with interrupted catgut sutures.

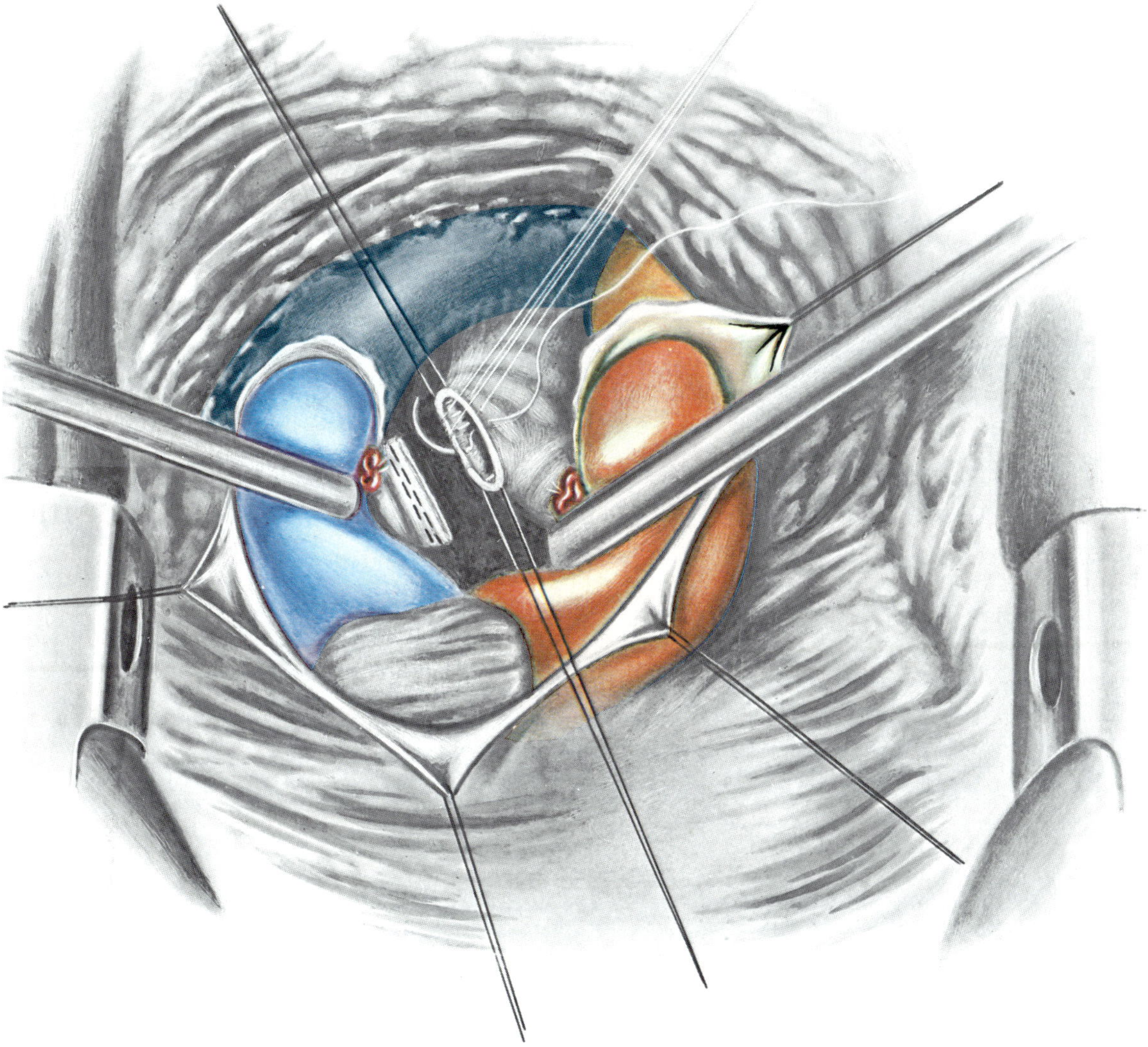

Fig. 204. Suturation of opening in trachea formed after removal of stump of right main bronchus, which had been stitched through with the *YO* instrument.

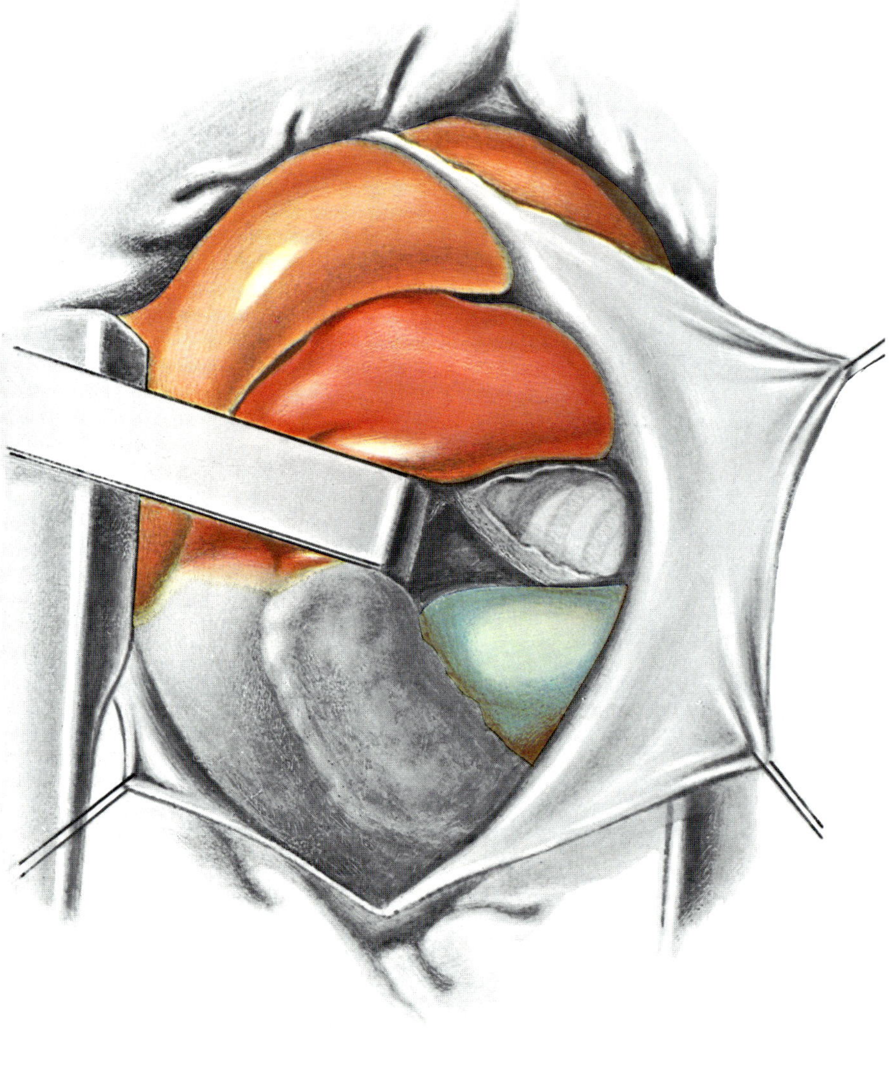

Fig. 205. Approach to stump of left main bronchus through pericardial cavity. Pulmonary artery has been displaced to right. Dorsal wall of pericardium has been cut over stump of left main bronchus.

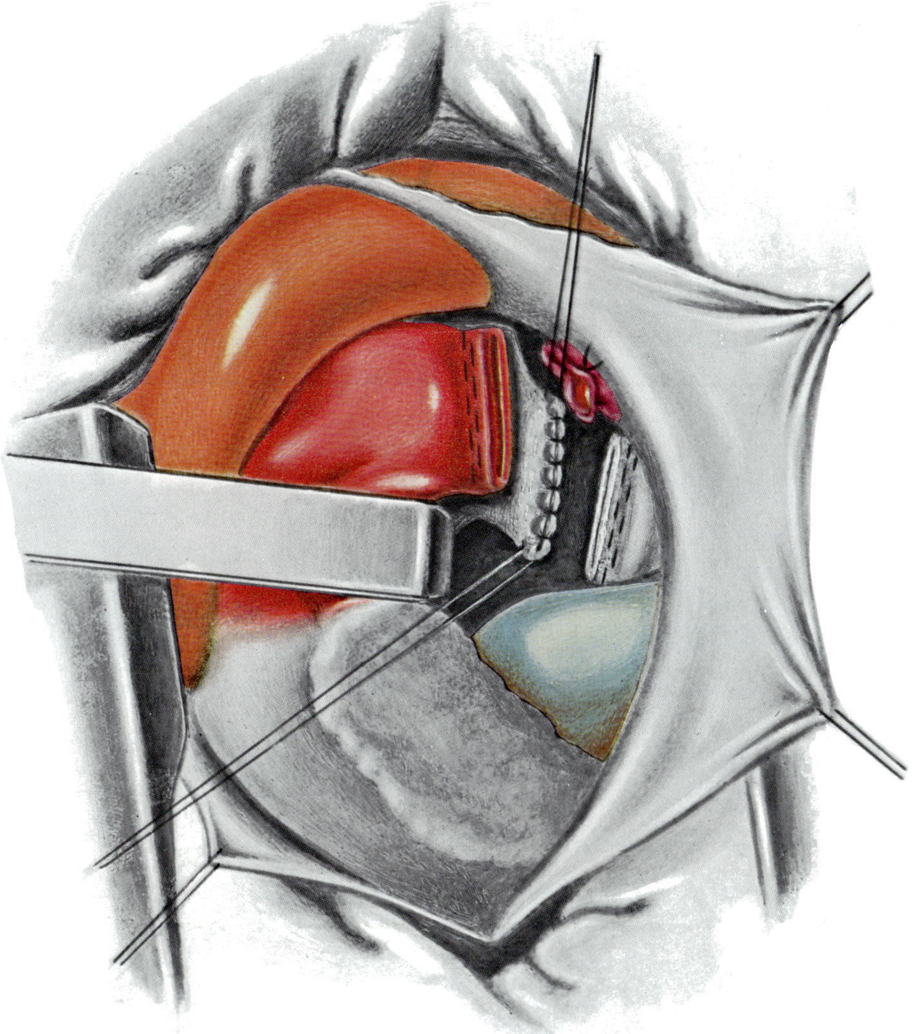

Fig. 206. Stump of left pulmonary artery has been reamputated. Stumps of left main bronchus have been closed with sutures.

SEVERANCE OF THE STUMP OF THE LEFT MAIN BRONCHUS BY RIGHT POSTERIOR APPROACH

With the patient lying prone, posterior thoracotomy in the right fifth intercostal space with resection of the necks of the fifth and sixth ribs is carried out. The lung is moved laterally and caudally. The mediastinal pleura is cut longitudinally over the inferior portion of the trachea. The arch of the azygos vein is ligated and transected between ligatures. The vagus nerve is drawn aside laterally with a loop. The lower portion of the trachea above the bifurcation and the right main bronchus are mobilized by the blunt techniques with the finger and Satinsky's clamp and held with rubber loops. Pulling by these loops, exposure of the bifurcation of the trachea is begun. Any adhesions between the esophagus and the trachea here are cut under visual control.

The next stage consists in the exposure of the base of the stump of the left main bronchus. If the stump is long enough, this can be done with the finger. If the stump is short and there are scars, it is best to bypass the left tra-

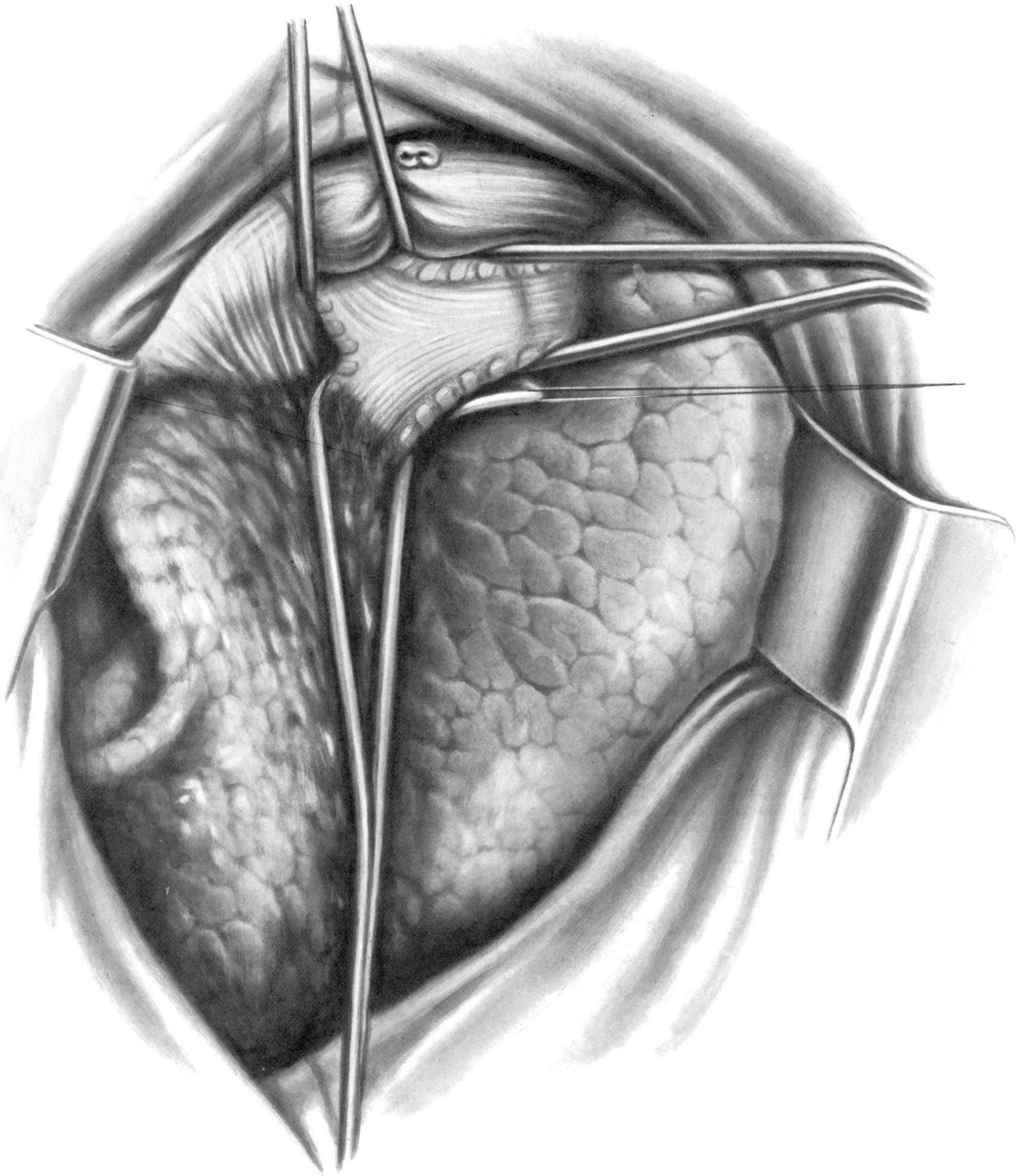

Fig. 207. Trachea, right main bronchus, and stump of left main bronchus are held with rubber loops.

cheobronchial angle with Fedorov's clamp. The exposed base of the stump of the left main bronchus is also held with a rubber loop (Fig. 207).

Traction sutures are applied to the cartilaginous parts of the left tracheobronchial angle: two sutures to the lateral tracheal walls and the carina and another two to the superior and inferior walls of the stump of the left main bronchus. The stump is severed from the trachea between the two pairs of sutures (Fig. 208). The opening in the trachea is closed with interrupted sutures (Fig. 209).

The stump of the left main bronchus is pulled by the traction sutures, and its mucous membrane is treated with a 33% solution of silver nitrate. The opening in the stump is closed with interrupted sutures passed through all its layers (Fig. 210).

If there is a narrow communication between the bronchial stump and the residual pleural cavity, it is expedient to expose the stump and remove it after the isthmus connecting the stump with the residual cavity of the empyema is stitched through and ligated.

The line of the suture on the trachea is covered with a pedicle graft of parietal pleura. One drain is left in the pleural cavity.

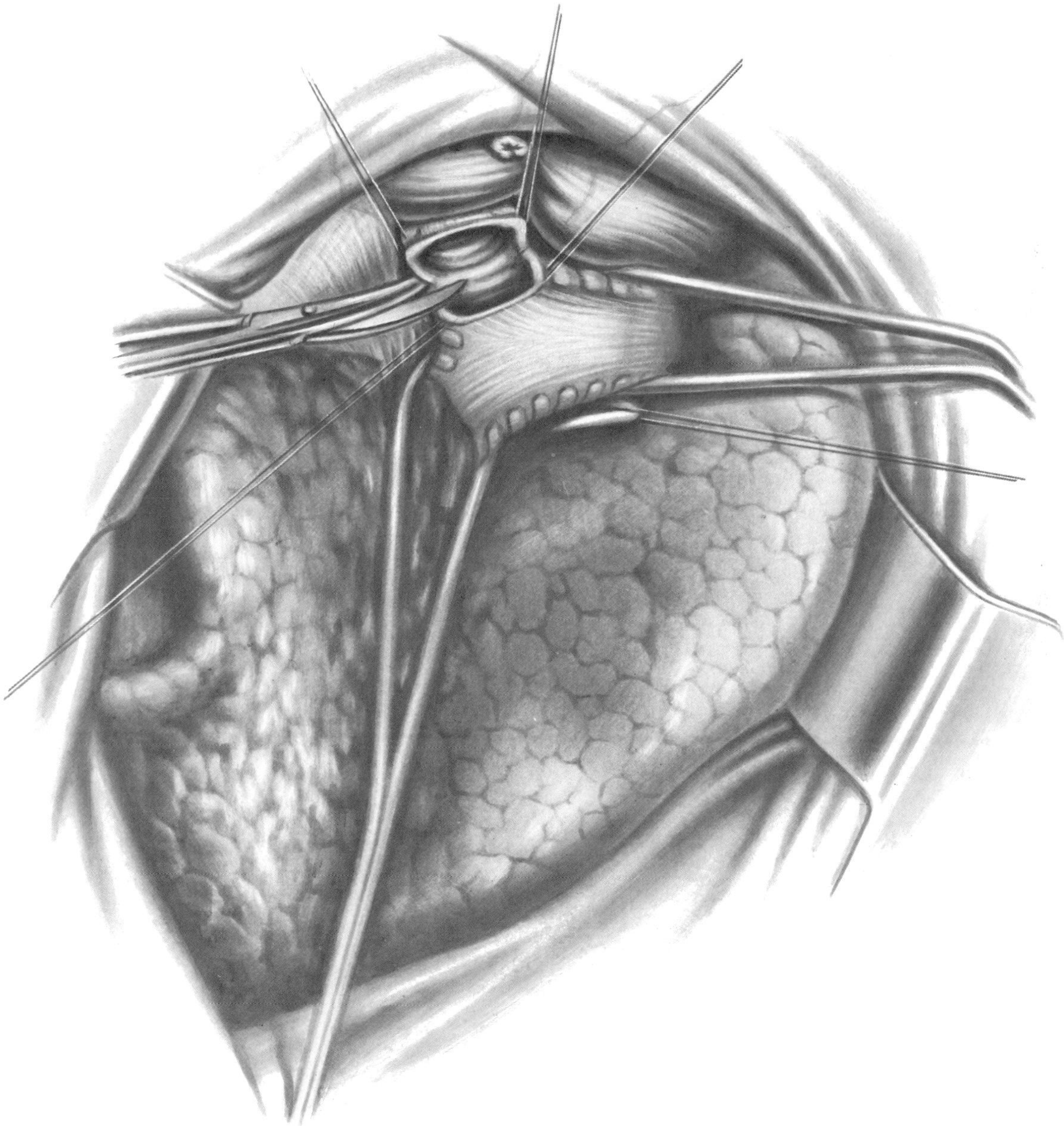

Fig. 208. Stump of left main bronchus is severed from trachea.

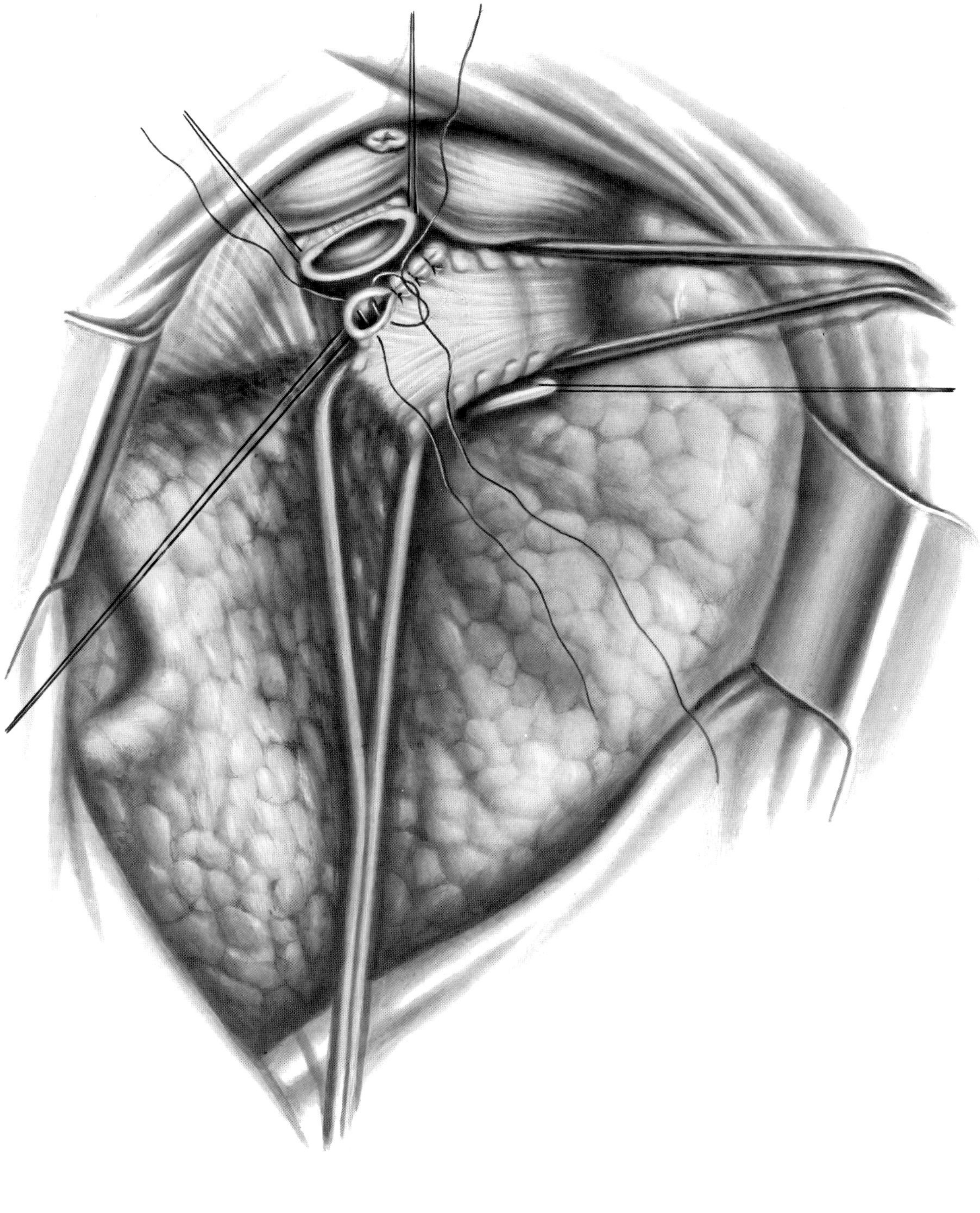

Fig. 209. Opening in trachea is sutured. Lumen of stump of left main bronchus is visible.

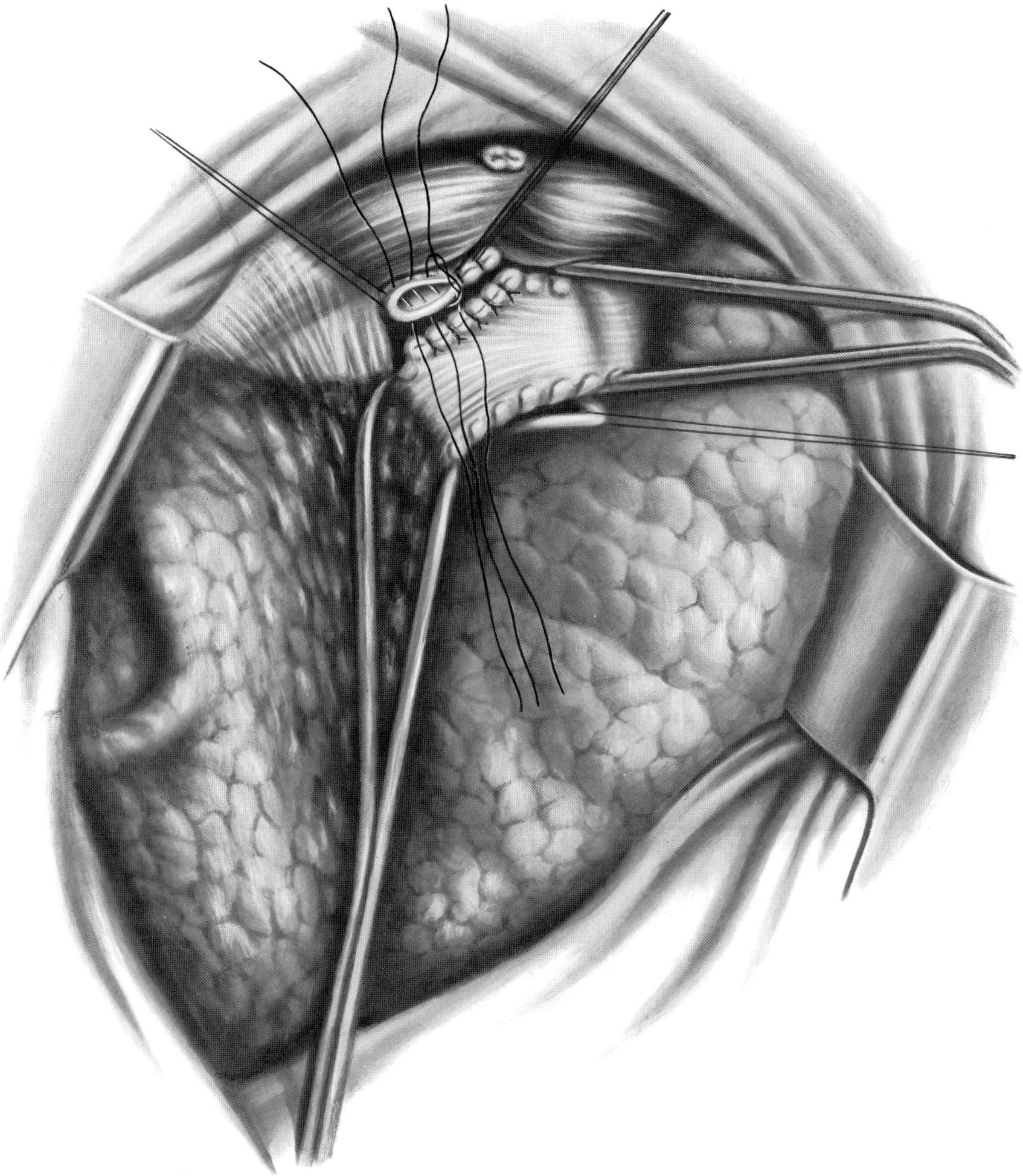

Fig. 210. Opening in stump of left main bronchus is sutured.

Pleurectomy with decortication of the lung

The operation is carried out by a lateral approach, usually with resection of the fifth or sixth rib.

The thick parietal pleura is separated from the thoracic wall by the blunt technique, with a finger or a tampon held by dressing forceps. A retractor is introduced into the wound. Separation of the parietal pleura is continued, and the ribs are drawn apart as far as possible. Those portions of the pleural sac which strip away most easily are separated first. After that the parietal wall of the pleural sac is detached: up to the thoracic dome cranially, down to the diaphragm caudally, to the root of the lung ventrally, and to the vertebral column dorsally. Bleeding is arrested by tamponade and electrocoagulation. Ventral palpation determines the place where the parietal wall of the pleural sac is continuous with the visceral. The reflection of the parietal pleura is gradually cut with a scalpel or scissors, pressing away the lung with a tampon held by dressing forceps (Fig. 211). Forceps for grasping the pleura are applied to the edge of the pleural sac. The dorsally located reflection is found by palpation and cut. The thoracic aorta may serve as an orientation point. The visceral wall of the pleural sac is then detached from the lung in all directions with a tampon held by dressing forceps (Fig. 212). Thicker adhesions are cut with scissors (Fig. 213). The greatest difficulties are encountered in separating the pleural sac

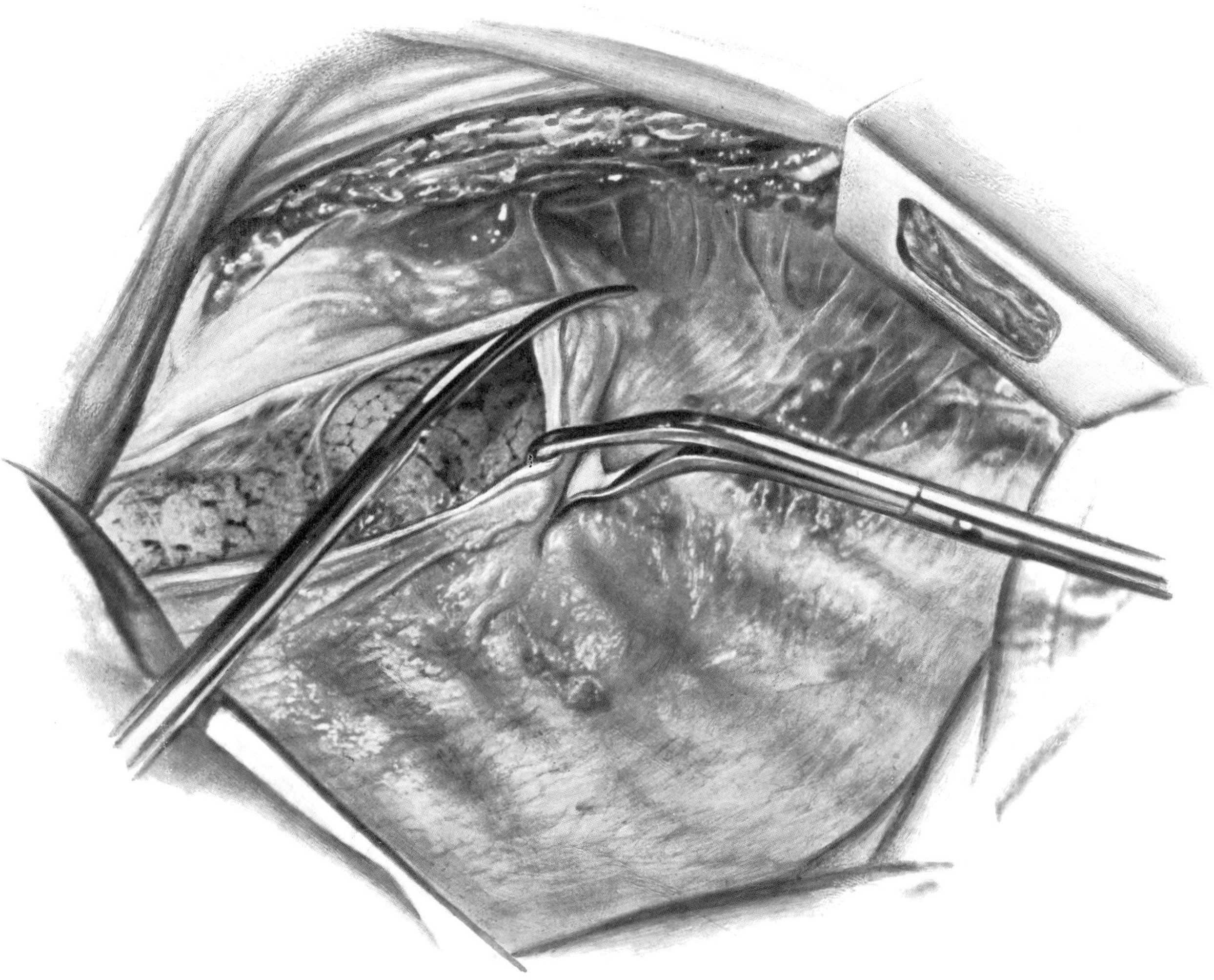

Fig. 211. Reflection of parietal pleura is cut at ventral margin of purulent sac.

in the region of the thoracic dome and the diaphragm. Great care is taken when the pleural sac is detached from the dome, taking into account the immediate proximity of the subclavian vessels. Just as much caution should be exercised when manipulating on the right in the dorsal part of the thoracic cavity and above the root of the lung where the azygos vein passes, and also in the region of the superior and inferior venae cavae. On the left, attention should be focussed on the thoracic aorta and hemiazygos vein.

In detaching the pleural sac from the pericardium, the phrenic nerve must be left intact.

Detachment of the pleural sac from the diaphragm is mostly accomplished by the sharp technique, with strong scissors.

The entire pleural sac separated from the lung and diaphragm is removed.

The lung is inflated, and to obtain better expansion, final decortication, removal of fibrous deposits from the lung surface, is conducted (Fig. 214).

The places where air escapes from the lung are sutured with fine thread on atraumatic needles.

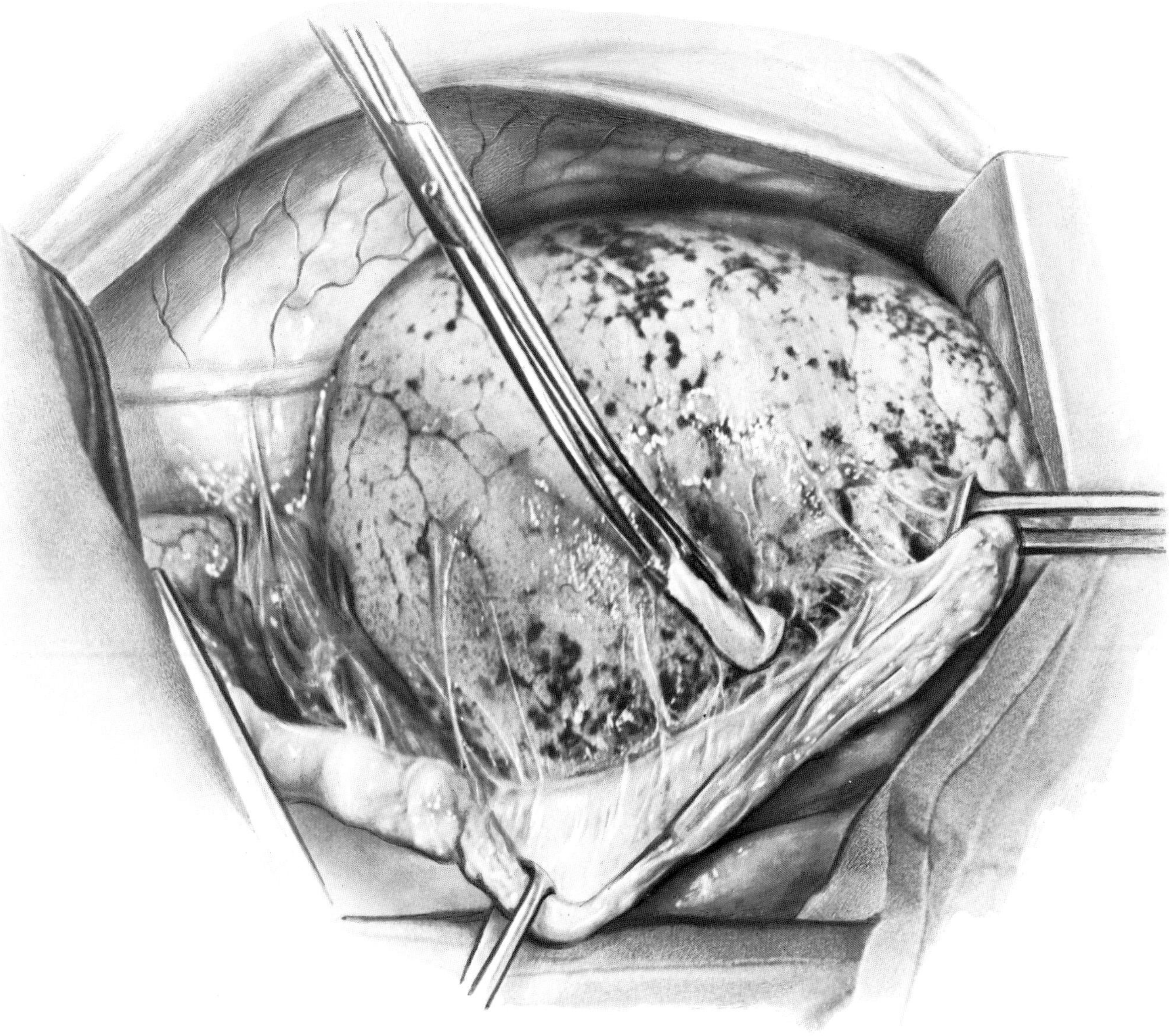

Fig. 212. Sac of empyema is detached from lung with tampon held with dressing forceps.

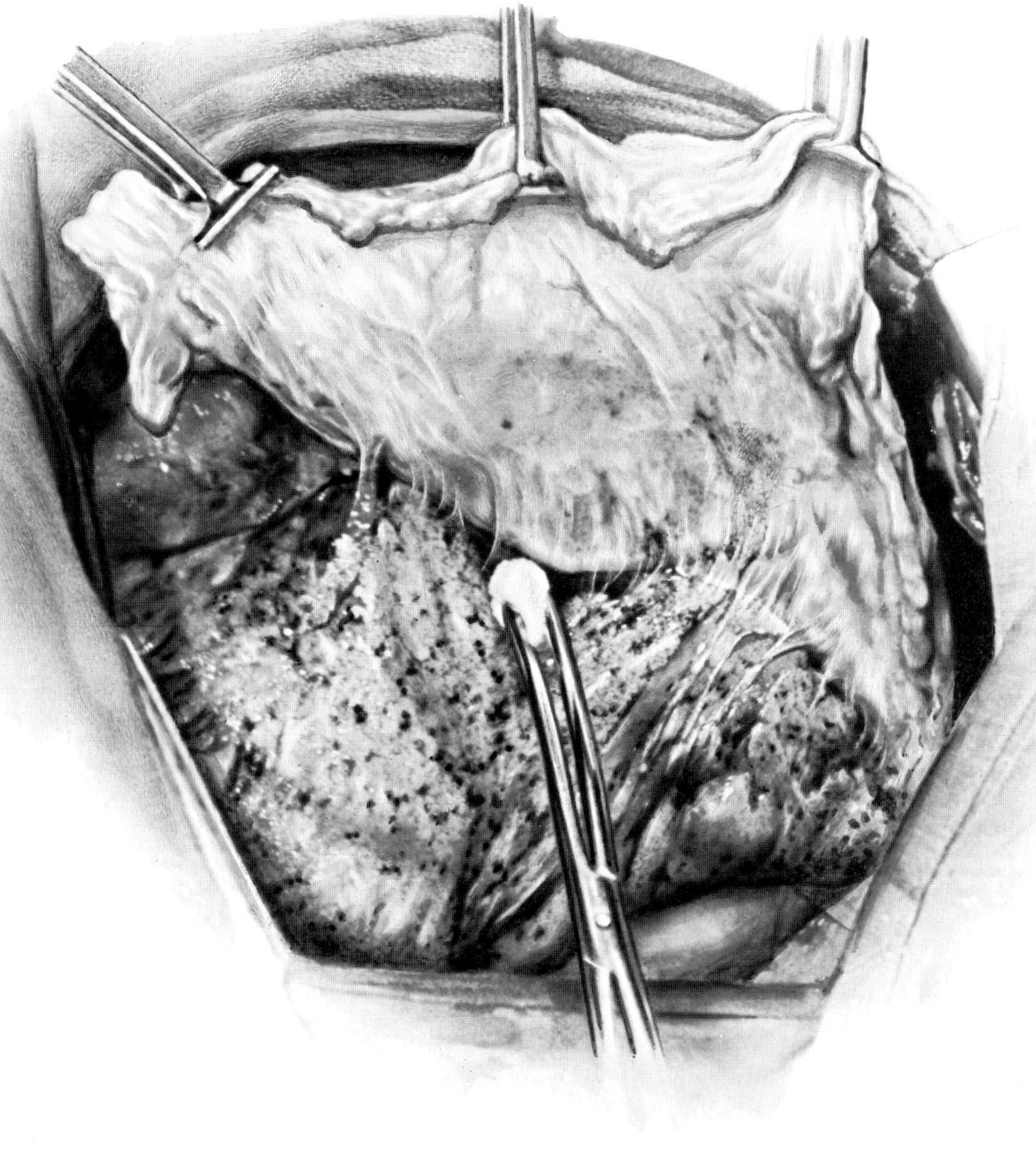

Fig. 213. Pleural sac is cut away from dorsal surface of lung.

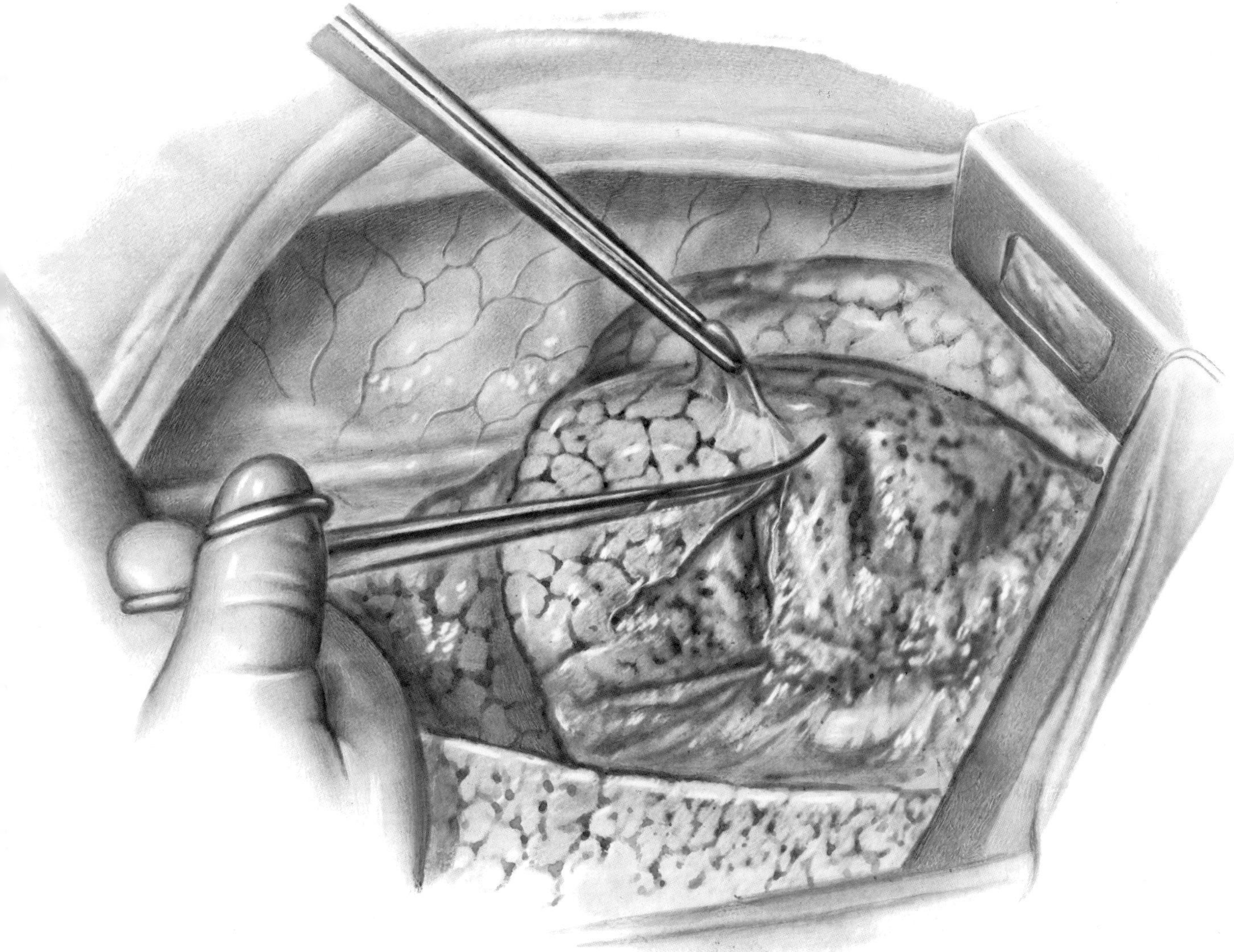

Fig. 214. Removal of fibrous deposits from surface of lung, the final stage of decortication. Empyema sac has been removed.

Opening a residual pleural cavity

An incision is made through the skin, subcutaneous fat, and muscles down to the ribs on a level with the floor of the residual cavity from the scapular to the midaxillary line. The removal of the eighth and ninth ribs is most typical. After detachment of the periosteum, the rib is resected subperiosteally for a distance of 10 to 12 cm (Fig. 215). The intercostal nerves are excised, and the intercostal vessels ligated and transected. The posterior sheet of the periosteum and the parietal pleura are then cut.

The pleural cavity is opened wide, and its contents are removed with an aspirator. The edges of the pleural cavity are stitched to the skin (Fig. 216).

A "window" is thus formed in the pleural cavity that permits inspection and treatment when the dressing is changed (Fig. 217). Tampons with Vishnevskii's ointment are placed into the cavity.

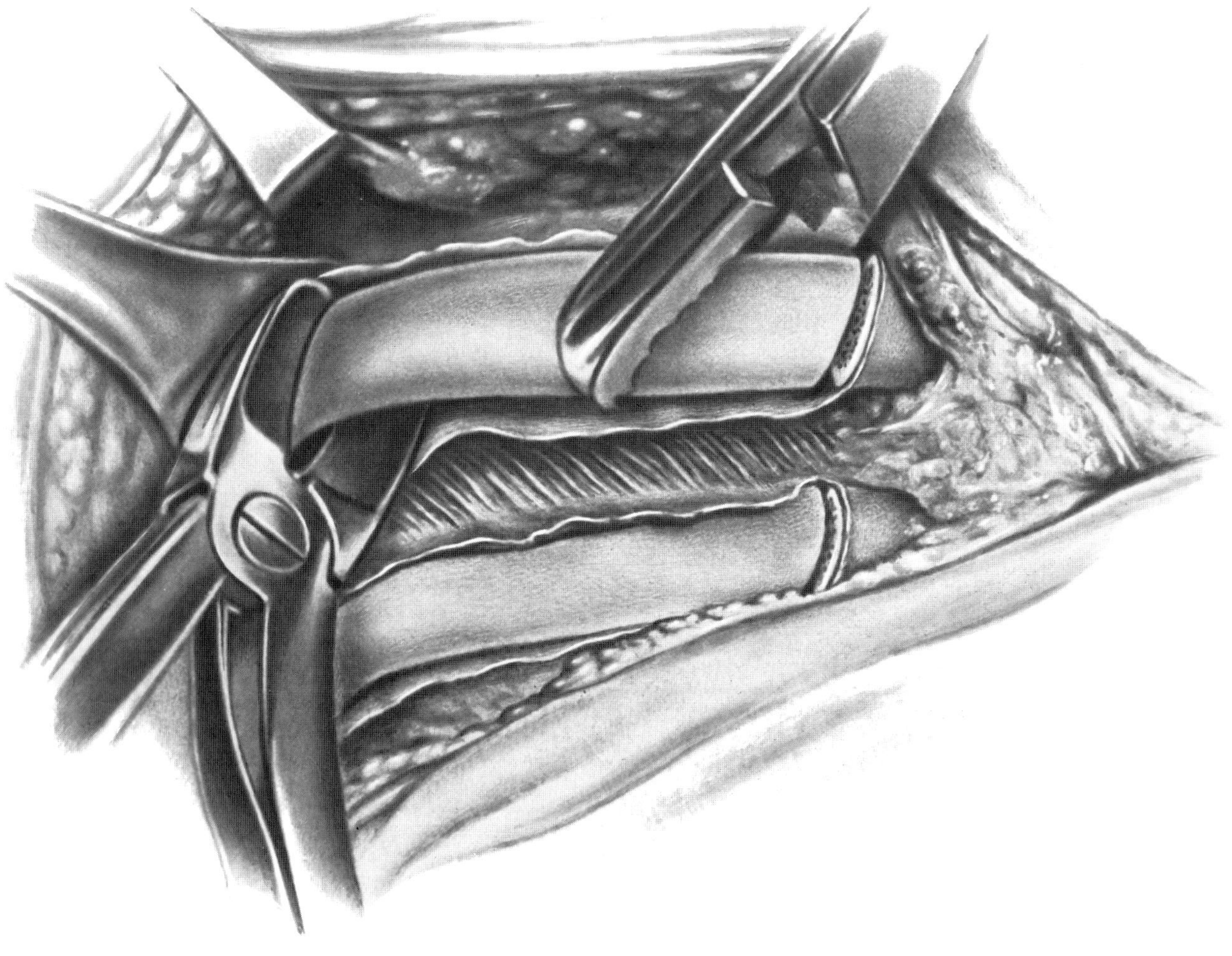

Fig. 215. Periosteum of eighth and ninth ribs has been separated. Eighth rib is being cut.

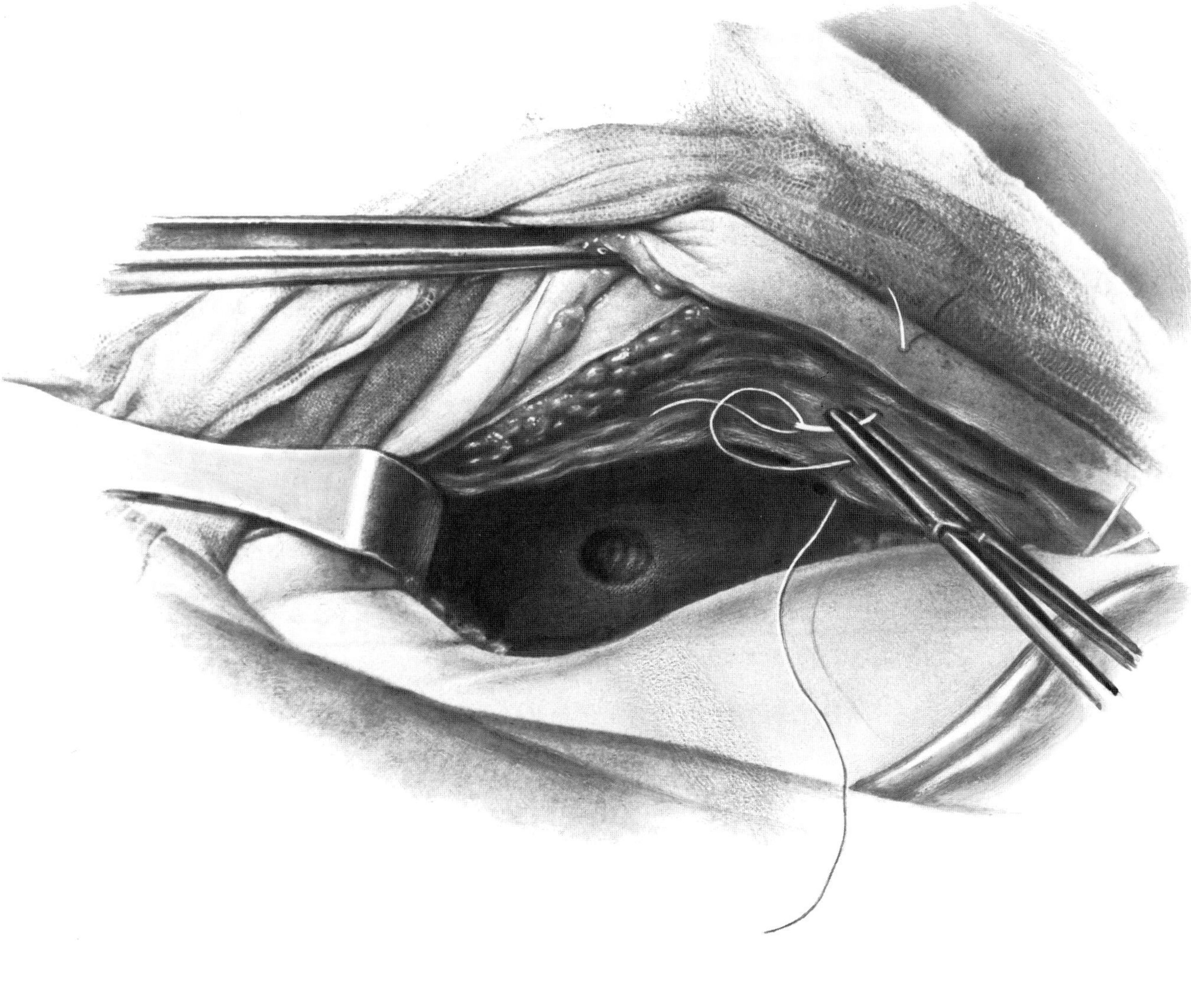

Fig. 216. Pleural cavity has been opened. Its edges are stitched to skin.

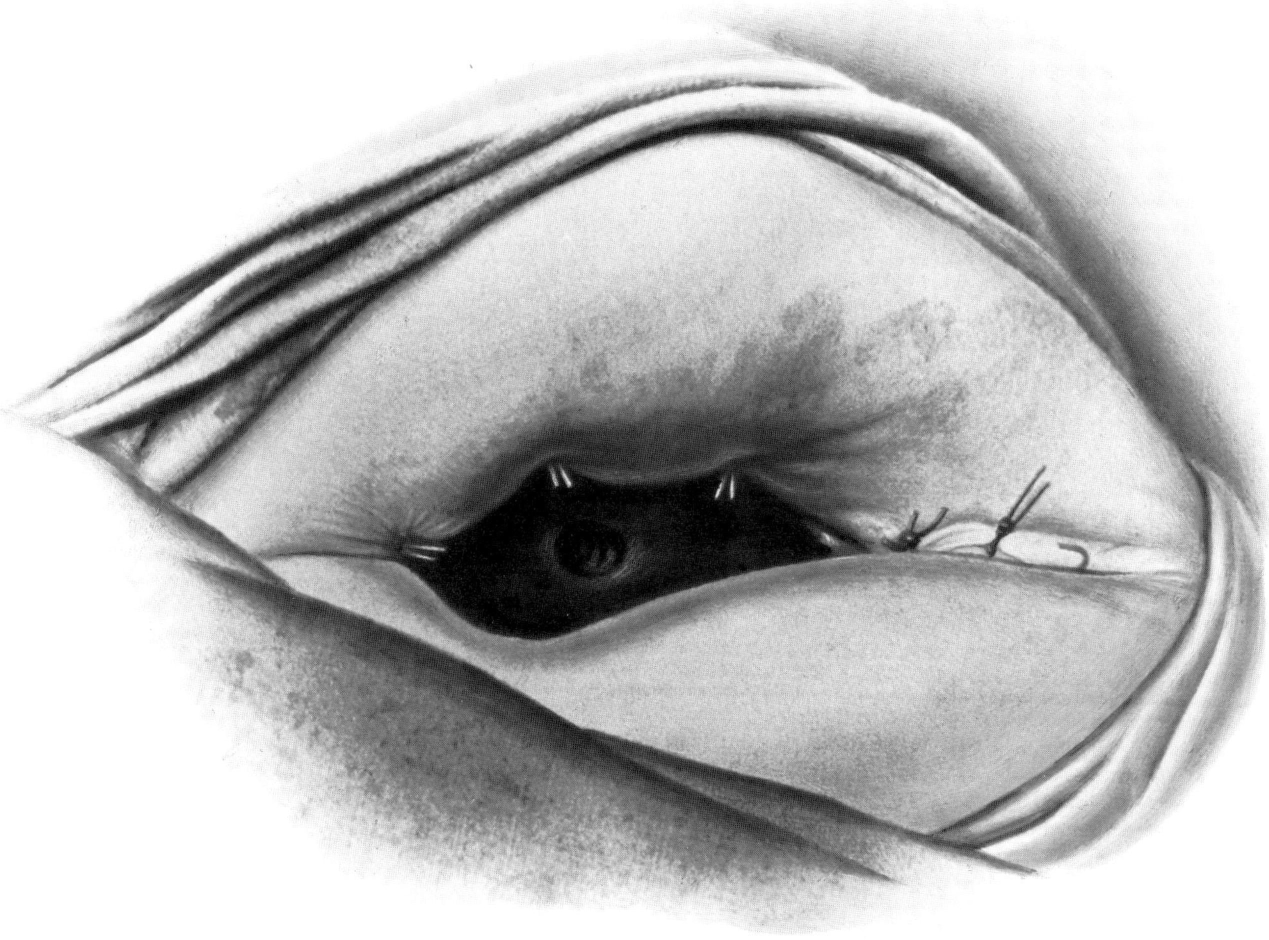

Fig. 217. Edges of skin have been stitched to wall of residual pleural cavity. Bronchial fistula is visible on floor of pleural cavity.

Pneumonotomy

Segments 10 to 12 cm long are resected periosteally from two or three ribs over the abscess (cavern) in the axillary or subscapular region. The soft tissues of the intercostal spaces are excised between ligatures. The cavity in the lung is punctured through the posterior sheet of the rib periosteum. A thick needle and syringe, which is often filled with a fluid, are used for the puncture.

After aspiration of pus or air, the cavity of the abscess (cavern) is opened with an electrotome (Fig. 218). As much as possible of the external wall is resected. The cavity is wiped with tampons and treated with antiseptics. The edges of the cavity, which are usually marked by fibrous changes, are stitched to the margins of the skin incision (Fig. 219). Antibiotics and gauze tampons are put into the cavity.

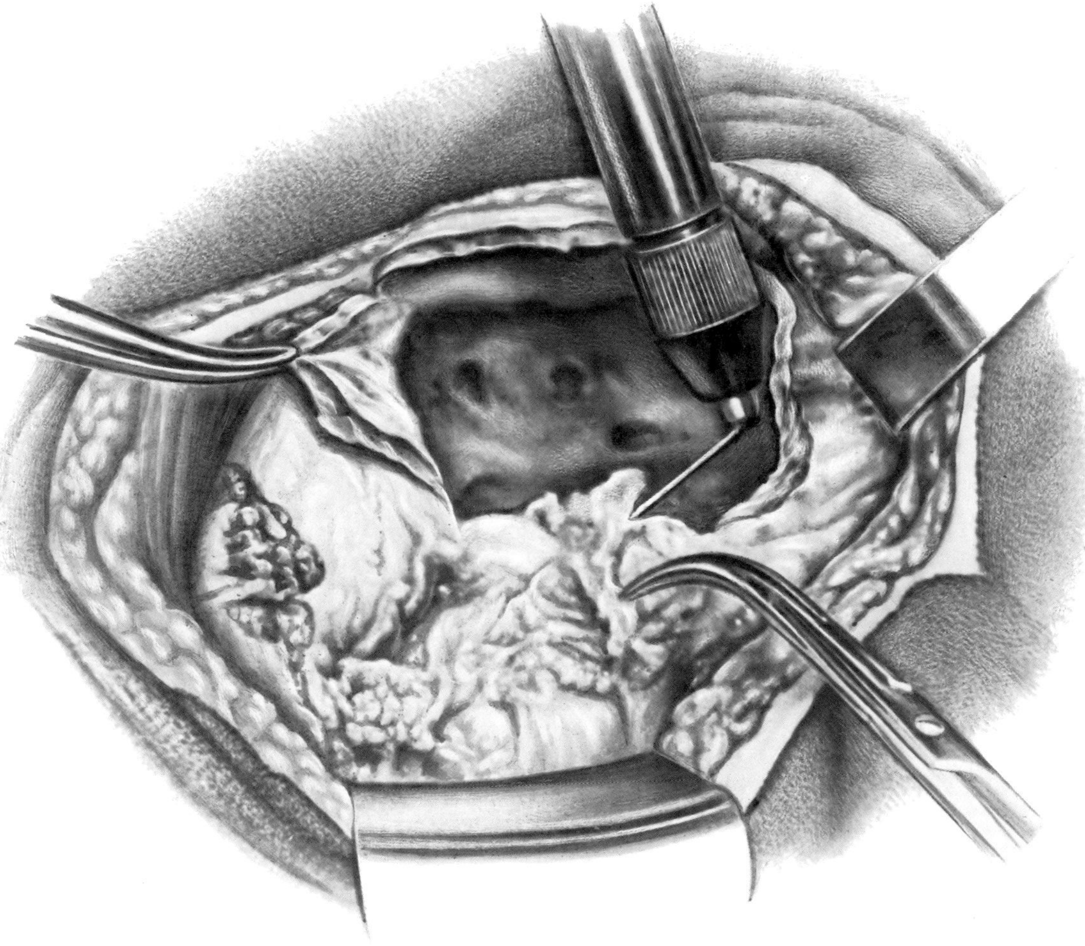

Fig. 218. Wall of residual pleural cavity is cut with electrotome.

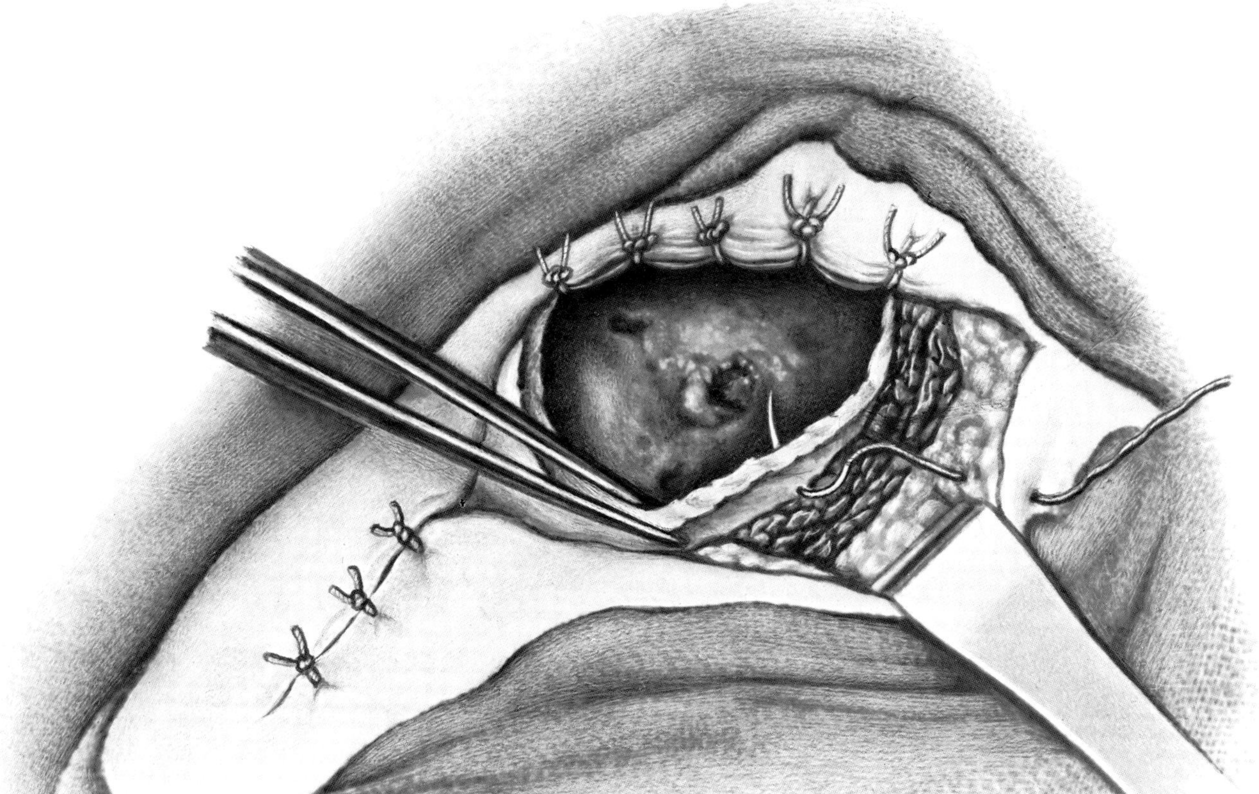

Fig. 219. Edges of residual pleural cavity are stitched to margins of skin incision.

Removal of caseous lymph nodes

The lymph nodes of the right paratracheal and bifurcation groups are usually removed.

The pleural cavity is opened by a lateral approach in the fourth intercostal space. The mediastinal pleura is cut over the caseous lymph nodes. If necessary, the arch of the azygos vein is ligated and transected. The vagus nerve, which is often involved in the inflammatory infiltration, is separated and held with a loop (Fig. 220). The lymph nodes are separated from the surrounding tissues by blunt and sharp techniques. Separation of adhesions

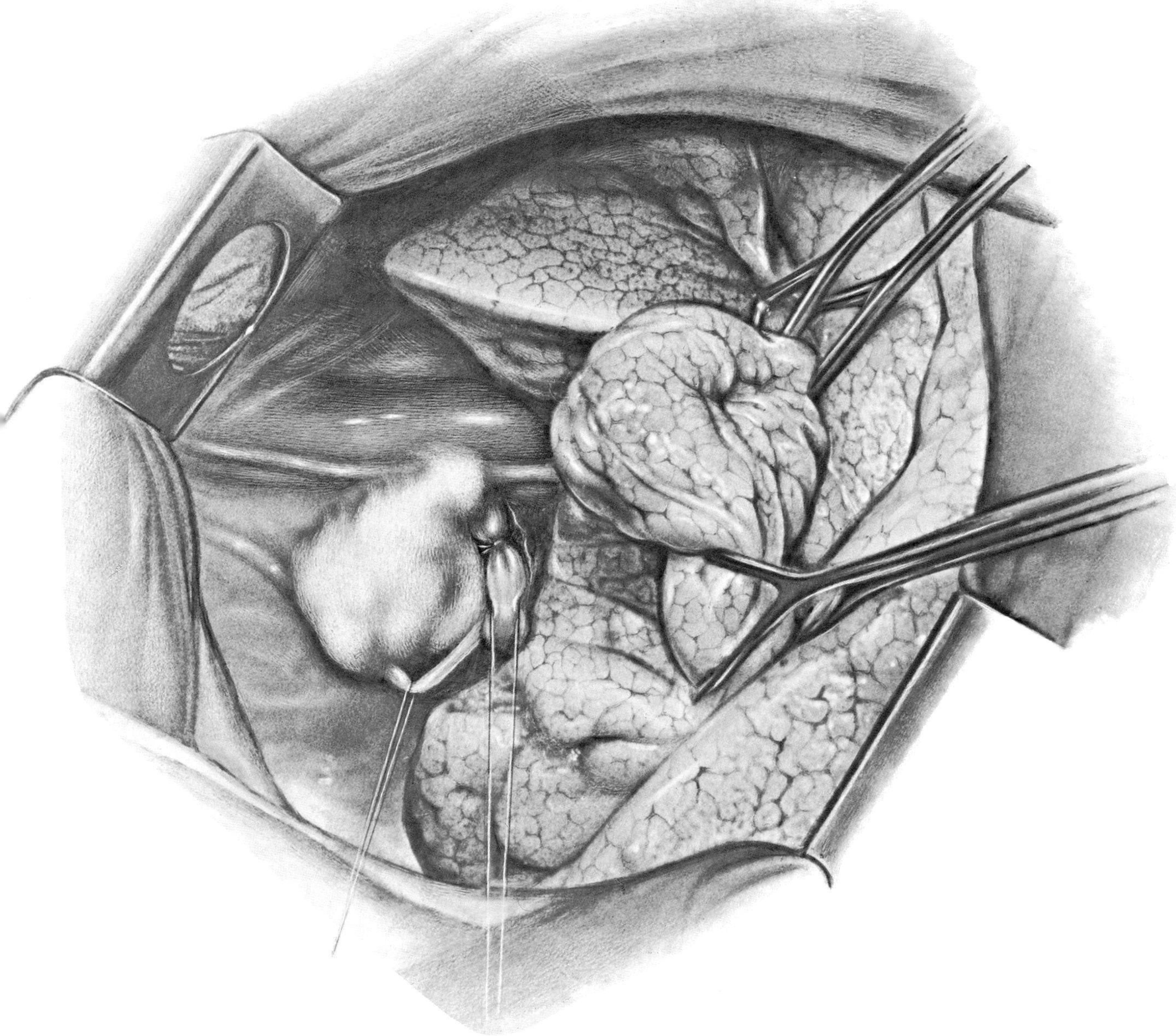

Fig. 220. Ligation of arch of azygos vein. Right vagus nerve is held with loop and drawn away from caseous paratracheal lymph node.

connecting the nodes with the superior vena cava presents certain technical difficulties and is fraught with the hazard of injury to its wall. To avoid this complication, the capsule of the lymph node may be opened, the caseous material removed, and the seat of the node scraped clean with a sharp spoon (Fig. 221). The remnants of the capsule fused with the superior vena cava are removed as much as possible (Fig. 222). The seat of the lymph nodes is powdered with streptomycin.

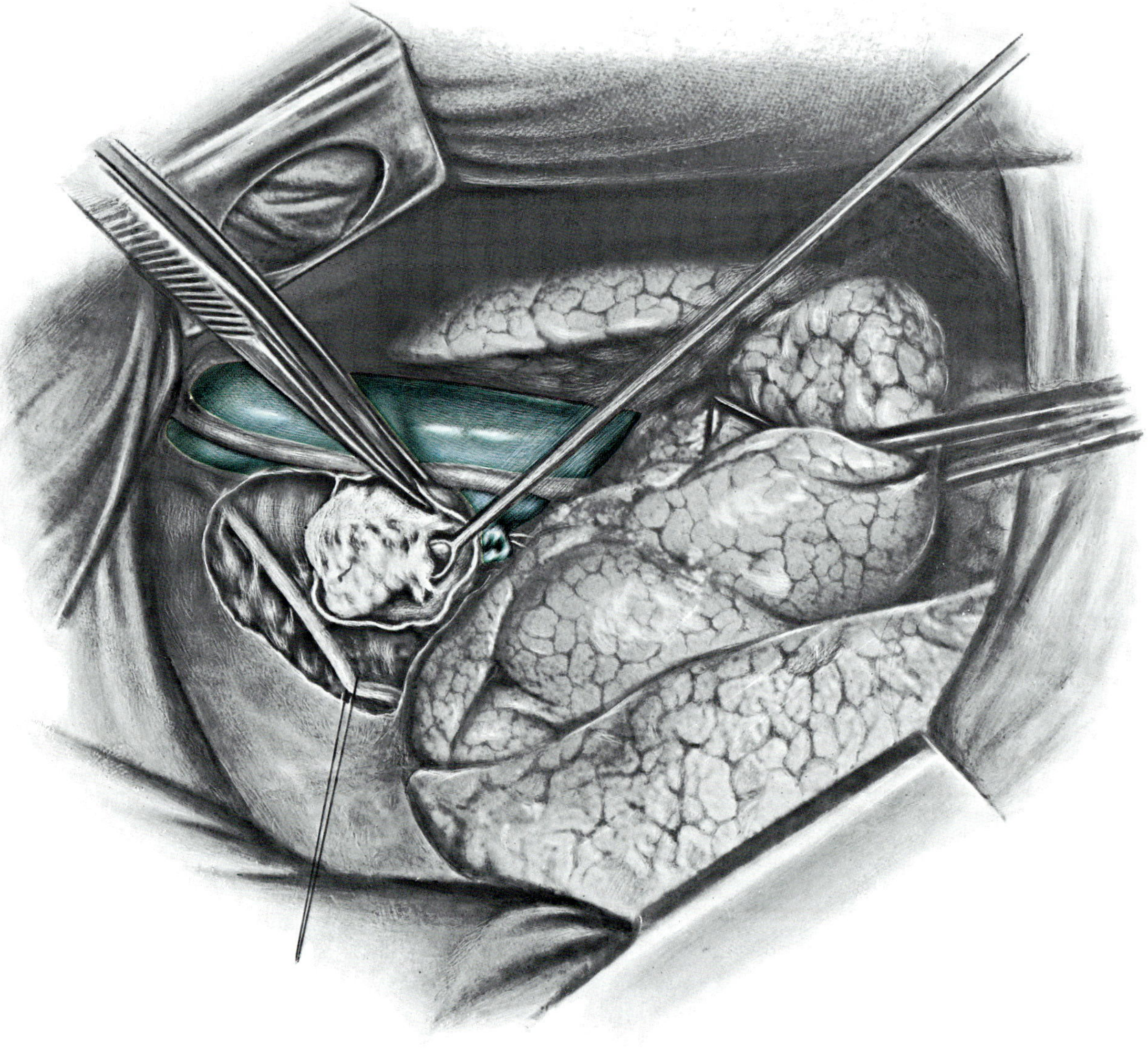

Fig. 221. Removal of caseous necrotic material of lymph node with spoon. Capsule of node has been partly excised.

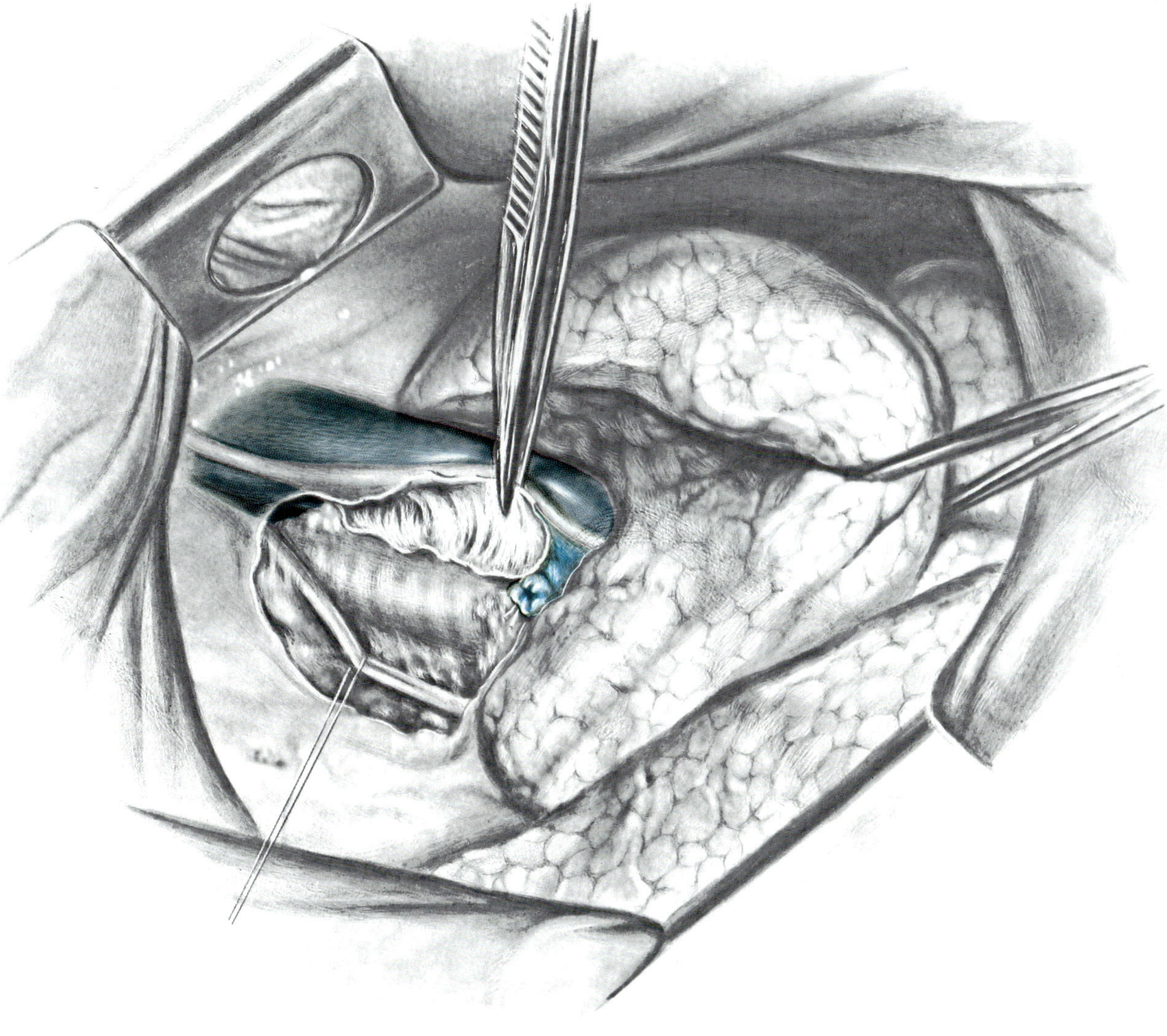

Fig. 222. Caseous necrotic material and most of lymph node have been removed. Remnants of node capsule fused with superior vena cava have been scraped away.

OPERATIONS ON THE HEART

General principles of operations on the heart

Operations on the heart are performed by various approaches. Left thoractomy in the fourth, fifth, or sixth intercostal space is usually undertaken. The sixth intercostal space is opened only when it is necessary to gain access to the apex of a hypertrophied left ventricle and to the diaphragm. The approach in the fourth intercostal space is most convenient for mitral commissurotomy on an individual with a hypersthenic type of thoracic cage. Such an approach provides for instrumental commissurotomy through the apex of the left ventricle with the heart dislocated from the pericardium. The same approach makes possible prosthetic replacement of the mitra! valve under conditions of extracorporeal circulation or the creation of intravascular anastomosis in Fallot's tetralogy.

In left thoracotomy on a narrow, asthenic thoracic cage and when it is presumed that there are adhesions in the left pleural cavity, it is most convenient to use the fifth intercostal space.

A right approach is almost always made in the fourth intercostal space. It provides a full view of the entire right half of the heart and the vessels on the right side stretching from the inferior vena cava and up to the cervical pleura.

Approaches to the heart that are more universal in character are preferable in cases when the diagnosis is questionable. The first among these approaches is longitudinal sternotomy, which is usually carried out extrapleurally. It provides for all operations on the heart, aorta, and pulmonary arteries.

The bipleural approach with transection of the sternum in the fourth intercostal space may cause more damage but, nonetheless, is still more universal. It combines the advantages of lateral thoracotomies and those of the transsternal approach.

The choice of the approach is guided by the type of the operation and also by the following considerations. In the event of possible complications the approach should guarantee the application of measures for their correction. It is difficult, for instance, to perform open-chest massage of the heart through a right thoracotomy approach when the right ventricle and right atrium are large. If atrioventricular block develops, it is difficult to suture the electrode to the right ventricular wall by this approach.

In cases with a large pulmonary artery and right ventricle it is sometimes difficult to reach the right cardiac auricle by access through the left side.

Though it is very traumatic, longitudinal or transverse sternotomy is most reliable in the event of unforeseen complications.

To approach the heart, the incisions in the pericardium are made corresponding to the heart chambers on which the intervention will be performed. The edges of the pericardial incision may be used for displacing the heart into the right and left pleural cavities and for pulling it up to the surface of the wound in a transsternal approach. Traction sutures applied to the inner surface of the pericardium help to draw out the apex of the right auricle into the left half of the thoracic cage in a left approach.

The pericardium is relatively rich in blood vessels, which are often the source of postoperative hemorrhage. Hemostasis is accomplished by electrocoagulation. It is not desirable to apply closely spaced sutures to the pericardium after an operation, because this hinders the drainage of blood and exudate into the pleural cavity. When longitudinal sternotomy is carried out in operations under extracorporeal circulation, a separate drain is inserted into the pericardial cavity and advanced to the apex of the left ventricle.

To prevent cardiac tamponade in longitudinal extrapleural transsternal approach, the right or left pleural cavity is opened at the end of the operation. As a result, the pericardial cavity drains into the pleural cavity. A drain tube is introduced into the pleural cavity according to common practice.

In surgical manipulations on the heart the surgeon constantly watches over the rhythm of cardiac contractions, their rate, and force. A sharp fall in the rate of the contractions, just as the development of polytopic extrasystoles and ventricular tachycardia, may herald ventricular fibrillation. These circumstances call for the cessation of traumatic manipulations on the heart and for the application of measures by the anesthetist: alteration of the depth of anesthesia, reduction of myocardial excitability, and correction of its hypoxia.

Ventricular fibrillation is usually consequent upon myocardial hypoxia and traumatic interventions on this background, cooling of the myocardium, and errors permitted in applying anesthesia. In such cases it is essential to begin direct massage of the cardiac ventricles without delay. The type of heart massage usually depends on the approach that had been used. The massage may be performed with one or both hands. Care should be taken that the surgeon's fingers compress the ventricles of the heart perpendicular to the septum and not along it.

In massage conducted from the left pleural cavity the heart may be compressed between the hand, brought under its dorsal surface, and the sternum. In poor tone of the myocardium and weak, small-wave fibrillation, 0.1 to 0.3 ml of 0.1% epinephrine solution is injected into the cavity of the left ventricle. Fibrillation is relieved by a defibrillator discharge of 2 to 3 kV. If defibrillation fails, it is repeated and measures are simultaneously taken to eliminate the cause of fibrillation.

During defibrillation care should be taken to provide close contact between the defibrillator electrodes and the myocardium; otherwise burns of the epicardium are possible.

Both in closed and open heart surgery the heart is punctured and cut in avascular areas. Bleeding from the site of ventricular puncture usually stops of itself. In increased venous pressure the sites of puncture of the right atrium may require the application of a Z-shaped suture with a fine atraumatic needle.

If a branch of the coronary artery is caught in the incision during operation on an open heart under conditions of extracorporeal circulation, it should be ligated separately because bleeding from the coronary arteries, apart from blood loss, leads to disorders of coronary circulation due to "escape" of blood from the system of the coronary vessels.

The sharp stretching of the ventricles is a dangerous moment in operations on the heart. This may occur in compression of passages along which the right or left ventricle is emptied, usually in operations performed under conditions of extracorporeal circulation with regurgitation through the aortic valve on the background of myocardial weakness. Distension of the ventricles calls for the rapid removal of the obstacle hindering blood drainage, additional heart massage, or the introduction of a drain to relieve the load carried by the distended ventricle.

To prevent air embolism of the vessels of vitally important organs and the coronary vessels, the danger of which is omnipresent in operations on an opened heart, the cavity of the heart is filled with blood or isotonic solution when its wounds are being sutured. The air left in the cavity is removed by puncture of the left ventricle in the region of its apex or at the very top of the cavity where air may accumulate.

When making incisions, particularly in the ventricles, it is borne in mind that the ventricular myocardium is sufficiently stretchable. With the hooks positioned correctly in the heart wound it is possible to inspect distant areas of the cavity through a relatively small opening.

Specific requirements are made to the illumination of the operative field in heart surgery. A head lamp is often used.

The application of sutures to the atrial and ventricular myocardium may differ depending on the thickness and the condition of the wall. The wall of the ventricle is usually closed with a double-row blanket suture, carefully tied. The atrial walls are mostly closed with mattress and blanket sutures on an atraumatic needle, approximating the endocardium of the atria. In hypertrophy of the wall of the left ventricle, the threads are not passed through the endocardium.

When the myocardium is sclerosed, plastic bolsters are sometimes used in applying the sutures. These bolsters, however, hinder the healing process and are, therefore, rarely used.

The technique of operation on the heart greatly differs from the techniques of interventions in other regions. The peculiarities are due to the contraction of the heart (a moving operative field), difficult access to certain intracardiac areas, and also to the flooding of the operation field with blood. Besides, it should be taken into account that the time factor in operations on the heart under conditions of artificial hypothermia and extracorporeal circulation is of vital importance for the results of the surgical intervention. Small atraumatic needles are used in most intracardiac interventions; this calls for precision and good visual estimation in the application of sutures.

The techniques in operations on the heart depend upon the skill and efficiency of teamwork more than in any other field of surgery; the success of this or that manipulation is often determined by the position of the hooks on the edges of the heart wound, by the coronary drain, and by the skill in grasping the tip of an atraumatic needle difficult to reach in the depth of the wound.

It is only natural that the specific problems of surgical techniques stem from the type of the pathological process, the type of operation, and the personal experience of the surgeon.

CLOSURE OF HEART WOUNDS

The approach to the heart in injury, or when a foreign body is embedded in it, depends on the localization of the wound canal and the x-ray findings. Right or left thoracotomy or longitudinal sternotomy may be applied. In transsternal or left thoracotomy the dorsal surface of the heart is examined after dislocating it from the pericardial cavity.

The heart wound is pressed with the finger (Fig. 223). Traction sutures are applied, and the edges of the wound are sutured with Halsted or blanket sutures (Fig. 224). In sclerosis of the ventricular myocardium plastic bolsters are used (Figs. 225 and 226).

Small wounds in the atrium or auricle may be closed with a Z-shaped or purse-string suture. After a heart wound has been sutured, drainage of the pericardial cavity is necessary.

In a transsternal approach the drain is introduced into the caudal corner of the pericardial incision (Fig. 227). In a left approach the pericardium is drained through an additional opening made in the region of the heart apex dorsal to the phrenic nerve.

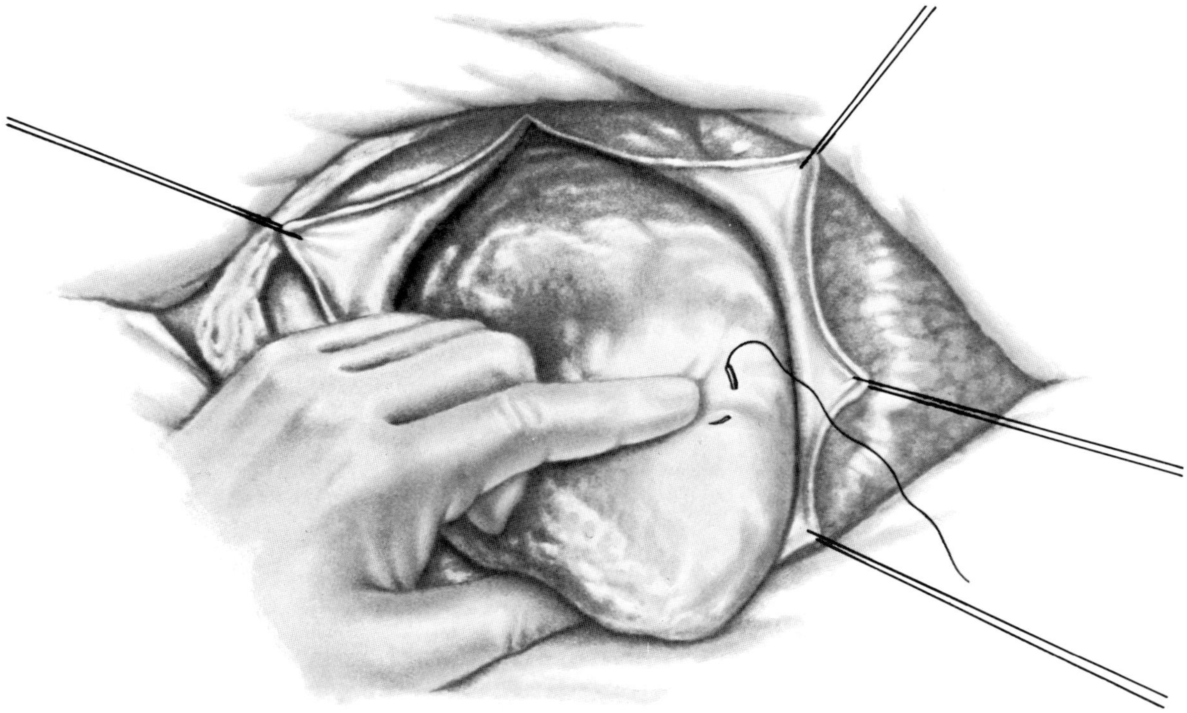

Fig. 223. Application of traction sutures to left ventricle in injury to heart. Wound is pressed with finger.

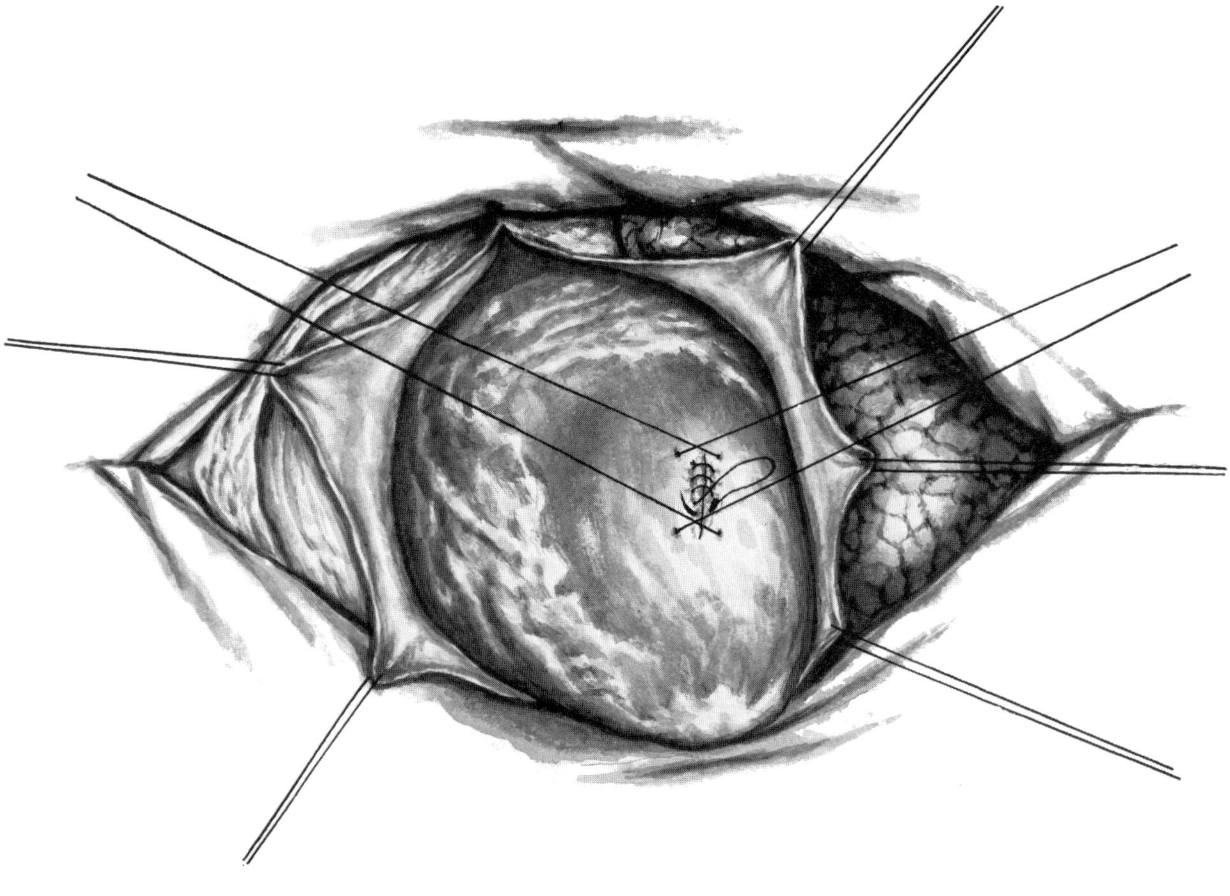

Fig. 224. Application of continuous blanket suture to heart wound. Edges of wound are approximated by means of Halsted-traction sutures.

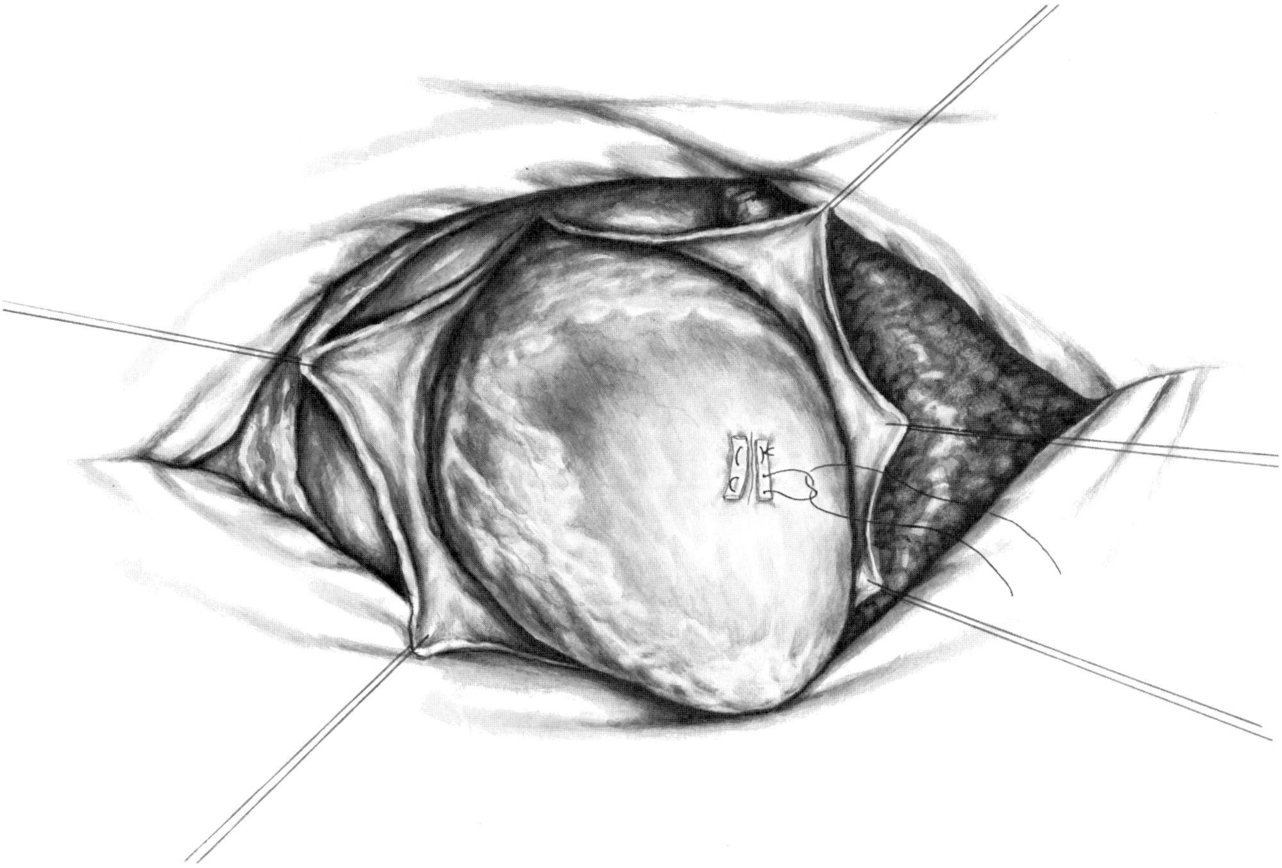

Fig. 225. Closure of wound in heart with mattress sutures and reinforcement of walls with Teflon bolsters.

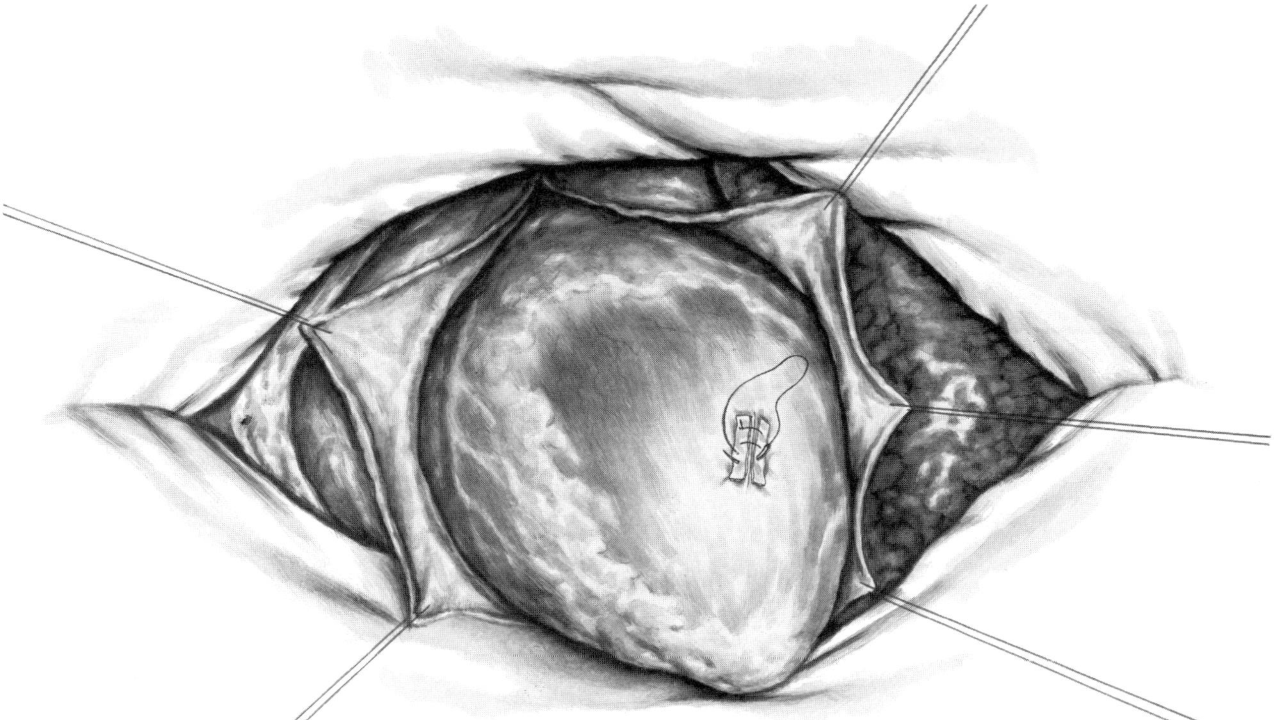

Fig. 226. Continuous blanket suture of left ventricle with use of Teflon bolsters.

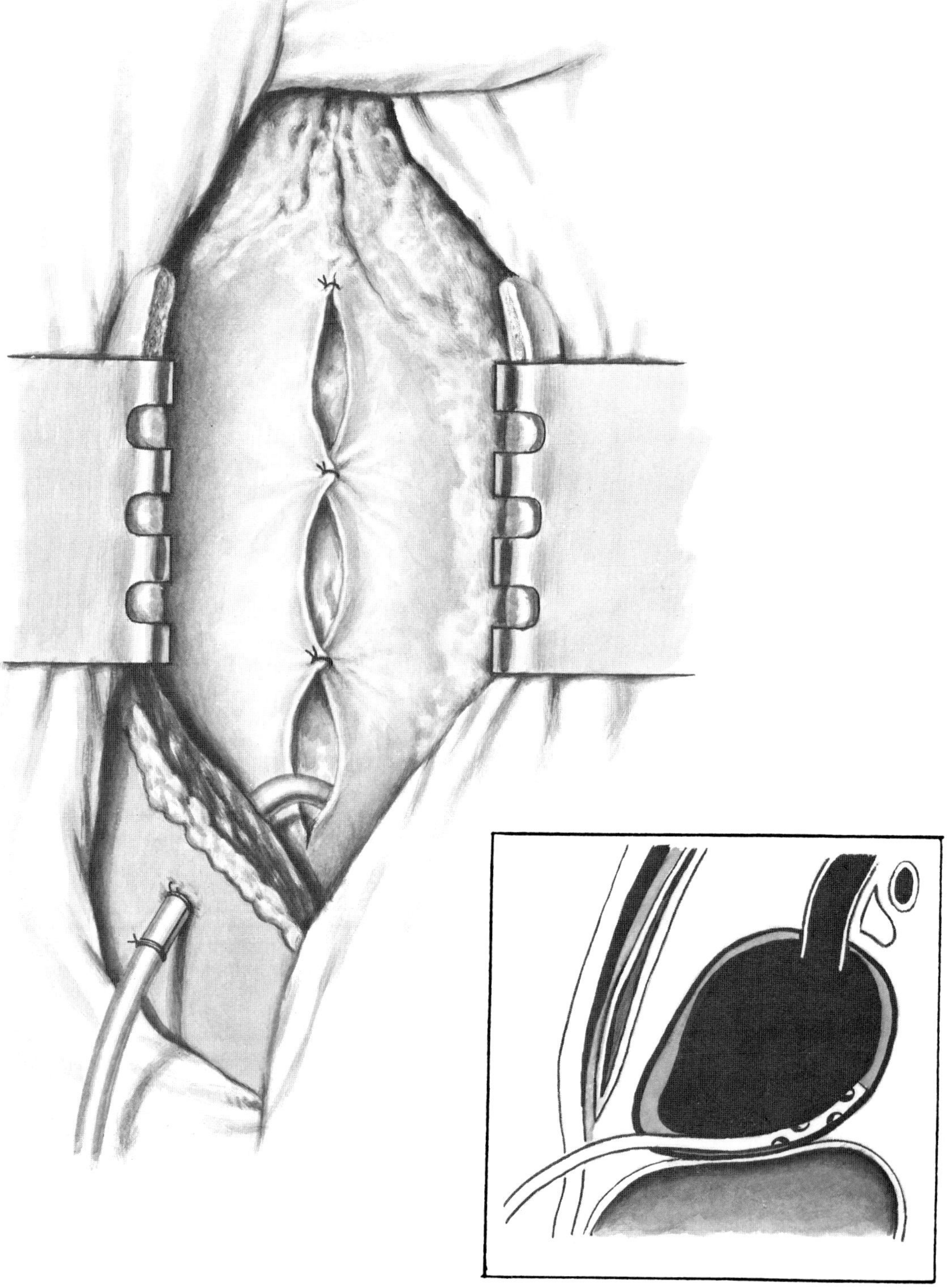

Fig. 227. Drainage of pericardial cavity in transsternal approach to heart. Pericardium has been closed with widely spaced sutures.

PERICARDICENTESIS

The pericardium is punctured in the space between the costal arch and the xiphoid process on the left with the patient's torso raised (Fig. 228). The needle is inserted at an angle of 45 degrees to the body surface. In abundant effusion the puncture may be performed in the fifth intercostal space on the left parasternal line (Fig. 229).

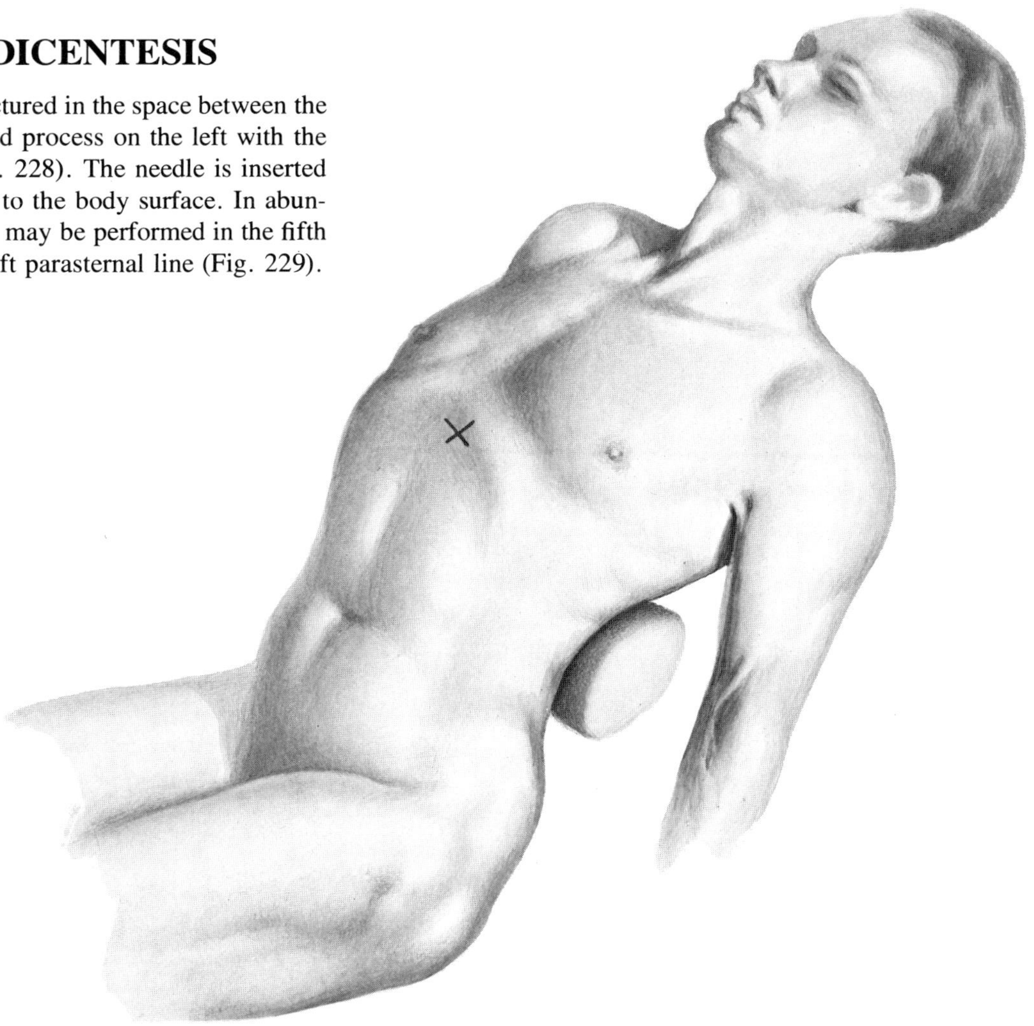

Fig. 228. Position of patient during pericardicentesis.

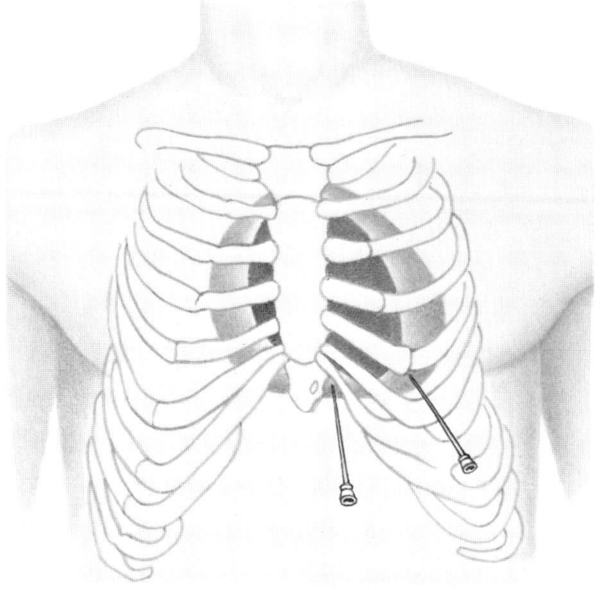

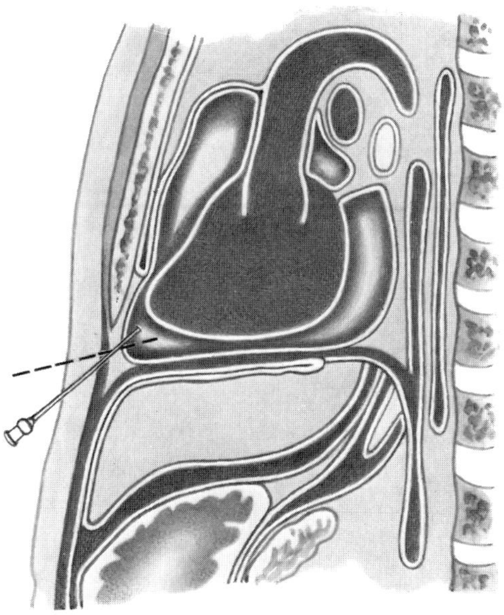

Fig. 229. Variants of pericardicentesis.

PERICARDIECTOMY

The operation is carried out by a left approach in the fifth intercostal space, longitudinal sternotomy, or transverse bipleural approach in the fourth intercostal space with transection of the sternum.

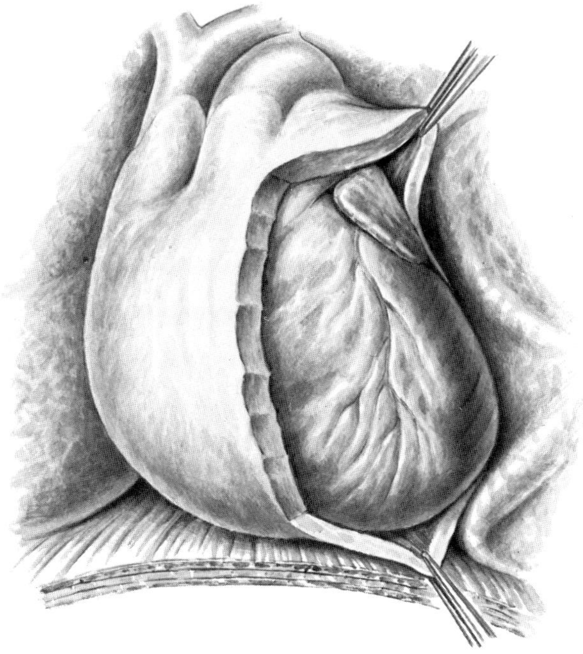

Fig. 230. Necessary extent of pericardiectomy through left approach.

In left thoracotomy the task consists in freeing the anterolateral surface of the left and part of the anterior surface of the right ventricle (Fig. 230). In longitudinal sternotomy the whole right ventricle and the anterior surface of the left ventricle, including the apex and the right atrium with the orifices of the venae cavae, are freed (Fig. 231). The bipleural approach makes it possible to perform subtotal resection of the pericardium (Figs. 232 and 233).

The pericardium is grasped with thumb forceps or toothed forceps and cut. The layer in which the pericardium will be separated from the epicardium is determined (Fig. 234). This manipulation is performed in portions, mostly by cutting (Fig. 235). Extra caution and thoroughness of sharp dissection are required in the region of the cellular tissue around the coronary arteries. The adhesions here are densest and calcified. Their blunt dissection is fraught with the danger of injury to the arteries. The thin wall of the right atrium may be damaged when separating the pericardium from it. The atrial wound is compressed with the finger; part of the wall surrounding it is carefully freed; and the opening is closed with one or two Halsted sutures. Bone forceps are used if the pericardium is drastically thickened or calcified.

The effectiveness of pericardiectomy is judged by the improvement of cardiac contractions and decrease in venous pressure.

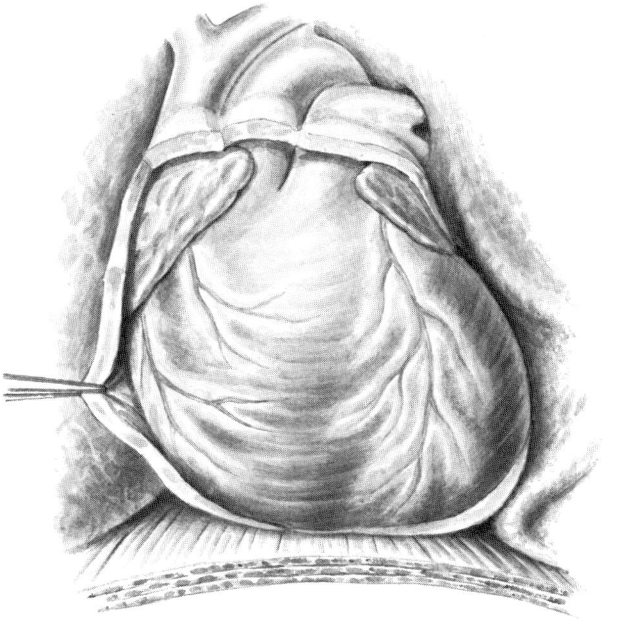

Fig. 231. Extent of pericardiectomy in longitudinal sternotomy.

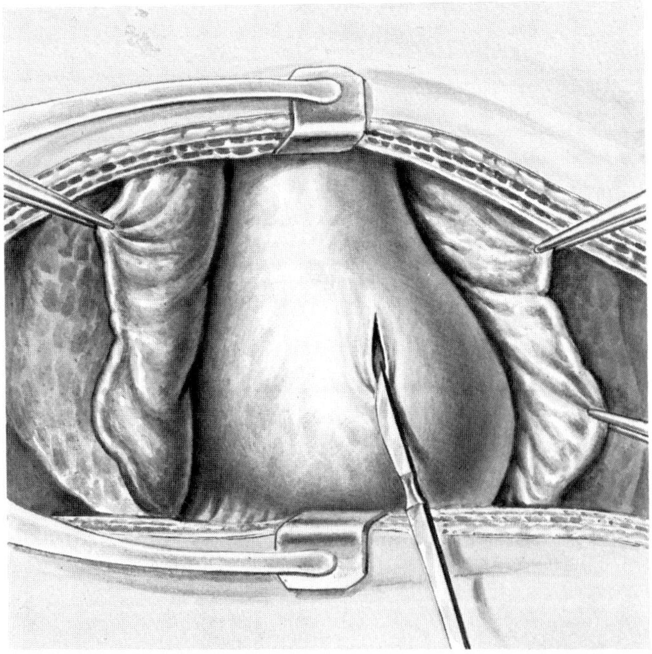

Fig. 232. Longitudinal division of pericardium and its separation through bipleural approach.

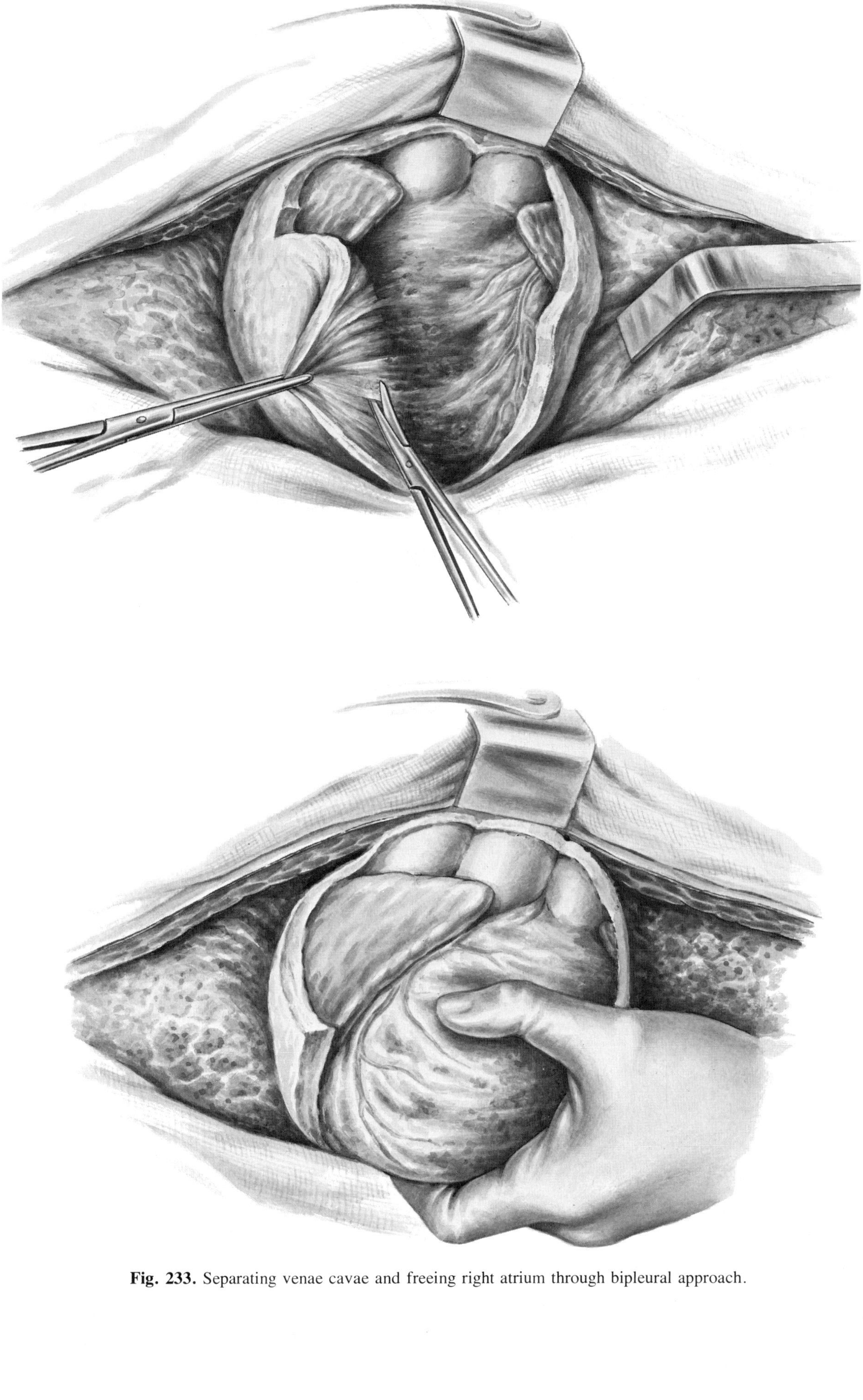

Fig. 233. Separating venae cavae and freeing right atrium through bipleural approach.

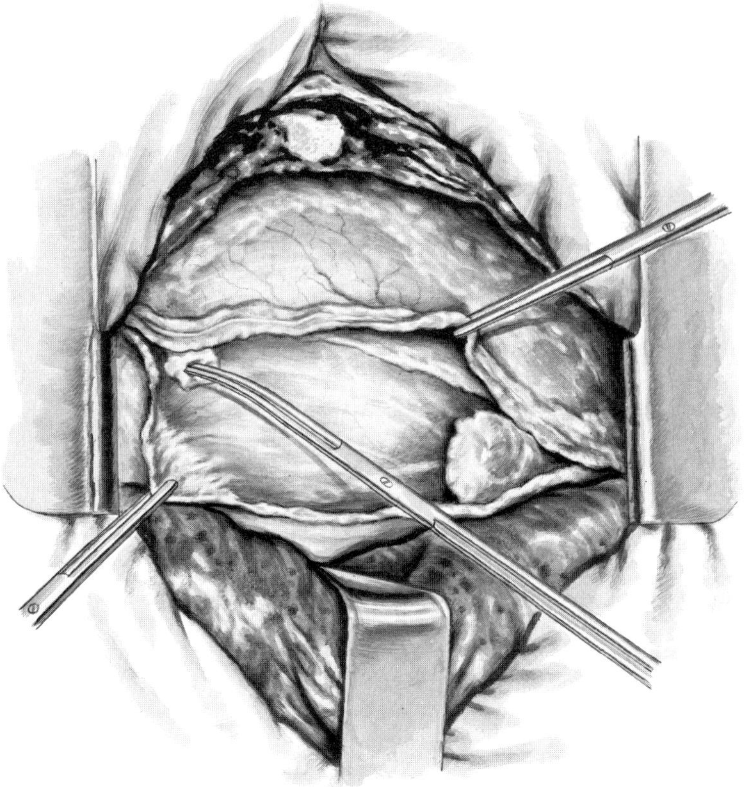

Fig. 234. Separation of thickened pericardium from epicardium in constrictive pericarditis by means of left approach.

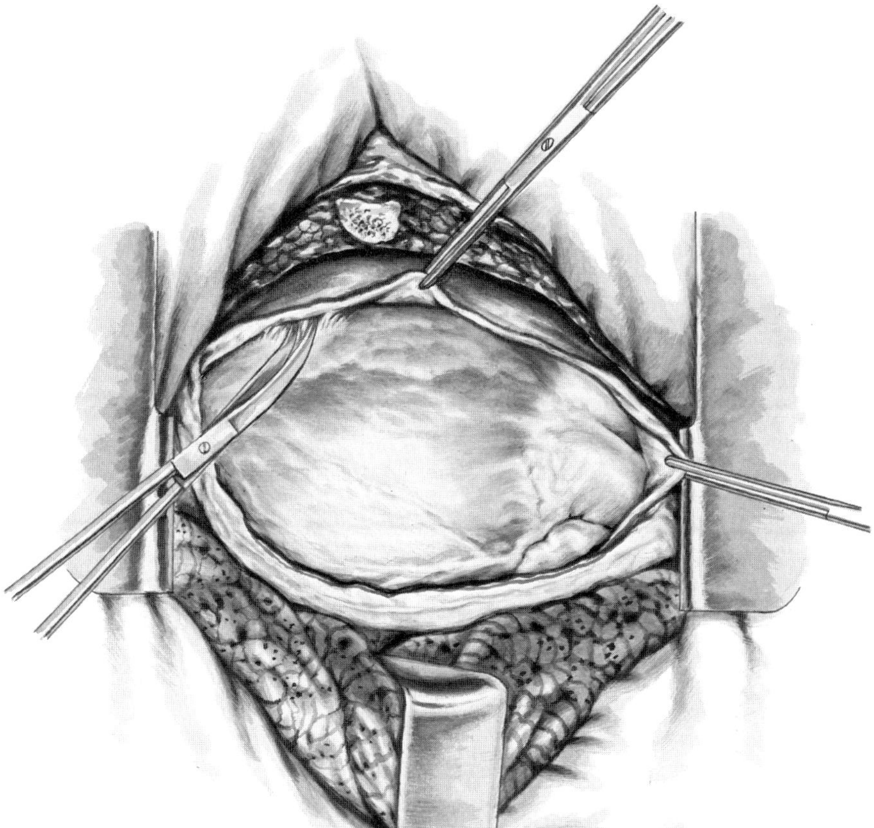

Fig. 235. Pericardium is cut away from epicardium.

Closed heart surgery

MITRAL COMMISSUROTOMY

DIGITAL COMMISSUROTOMY BY LEFT APPROACH

The operation is performed by a lateral or anterolateral approach in the fourth intercostal space. The lung is moved dorsally, and the pericardium is usually opened dorsal and parallel to the phrenic nerve (Fig. 236). If there are adhesions between the pericardium and the lung and also when the phrenic nerve is located directly on the root of the lung, the pericardium is incised ventrally to this nerve.

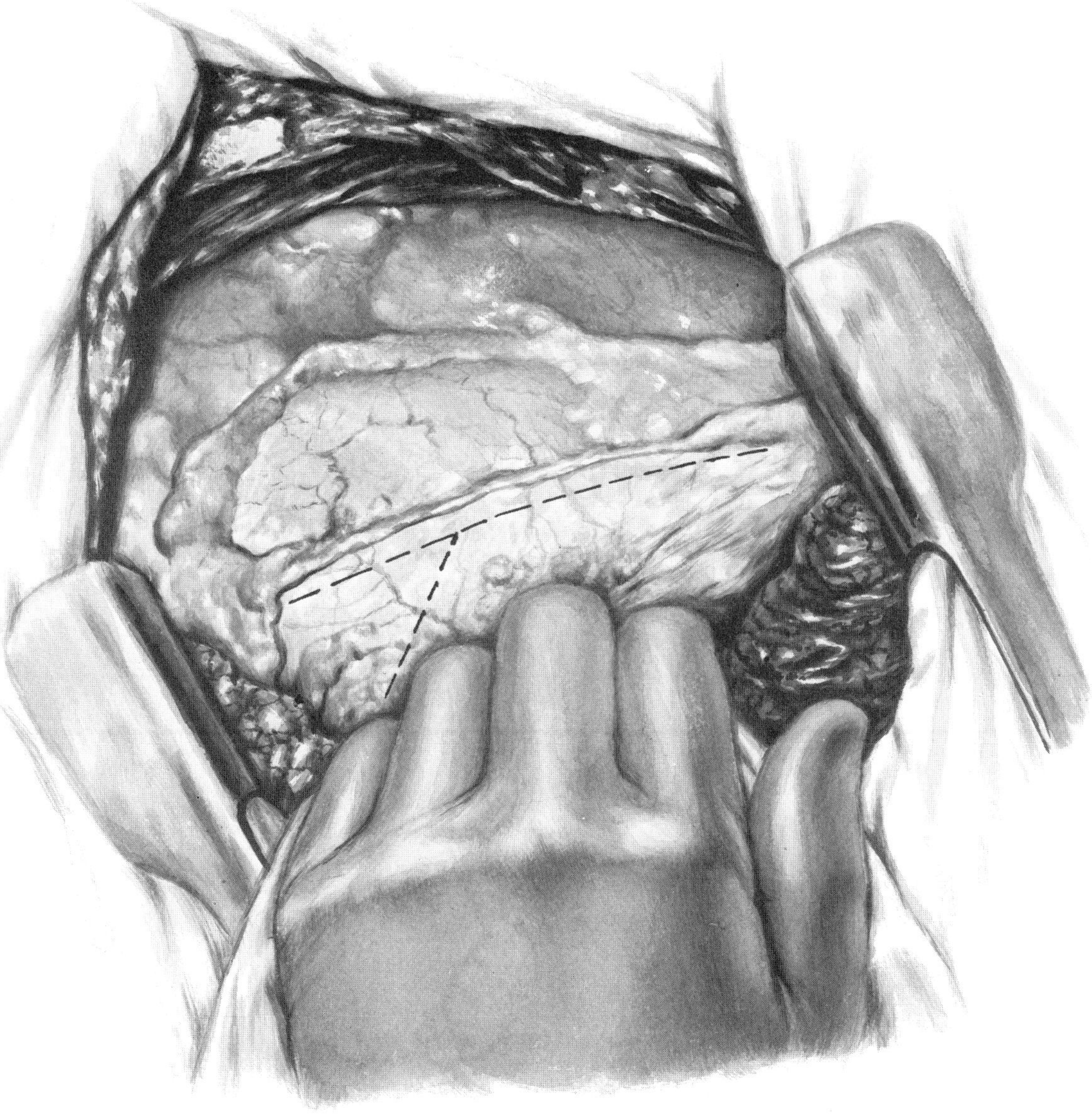

Fig. 236. Dashed line shows where incision in pericardium will be made. Lung has been shifted dorsally.

The first pericardial incision is supplemented by a second cut perpendicular to it and made in the dorsal flap parallel to and over the atrioventricular sulcus (Fig. 237). The pericardial cavity is drained adequately through this incision in the postoperative period.

Traction sutures are applied to the edges of the divided pericardium. Intraoperative inspection of the heart is conducted. In drastic mitral stenosis a dilated left atrium with an enlarged auricle and a difference in the color of the left atrium and ventricle are observed. The atrium is pink, while the ventricular myocardium is cyanotic (Kudas' sign) (Fig. 238). The pulmonary artery is dilated correspondingly to the degree of pulmonary hypertension. Diastolic thrill is palpated on the apex of the heart, which is a sign of mitral stenosis, and a systolic thrill on the wall of the left atrium, which is a sign of regurgitation in the mitral valve. Concomitant stenosis of the aortic orifice is determined by palpation of the root of the aorta in the transverse sinus of the pericardium.

The apex of the left auricle is grasped with triangular

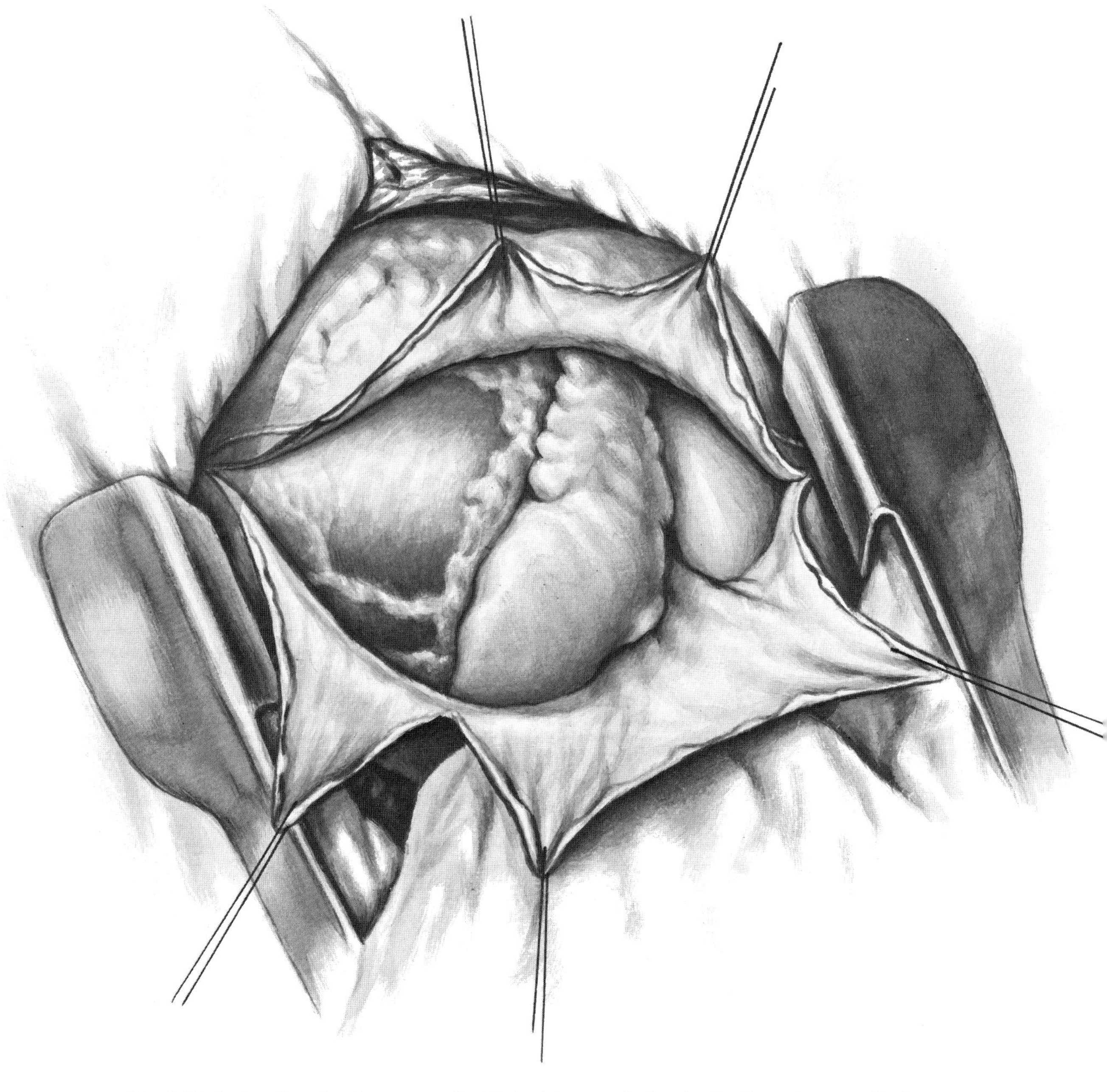

Fig. 237. Pericardium has been opened with incisions made longitudinally and perpendicular to phrenic nerve. Pericardium flaps have been drawn apart by means of traction sutures.

forceps. A purse-string suture is applied to the base of the auricle with a round needle, and the ends of the thread are passed through Rummel's tourniquet (Fig. 239). The purse-string suture with the tourniquet prevents bleeding from the left atrial auricle when the finger is advanced into it. This suture is not a ''must'' for a highly skilled surgeon.

The apex of the left auricle is clamped with Satinsky's clamp, and its cavity is opened with a crescent-shaped incision to accommodate the breadth of the surgeon's index finger. Traction blanket sutures are stitched to the edges of the incision through both walls (Fig. 240). Before inserting the finger into the incision in the left auricle, blood is carefully *aspirated* from its cavity and the auricle is washed out with physiological saline solution. The ungloved right index finger is inserted into the left atrial cavity, simultaneously removing Satinsky's clamp and holding the margins of the auricle fast by the applied threads. The dimensions of the left atrioventricular orifice, the development of the commissures, and the condition of the cusps of the mitral valve (calcified, thickened, mobile, retracted into the cavity of the left ventricle) are assessed by palpation (Fig. 241).

The anterior commissure is separated first, as a rule,

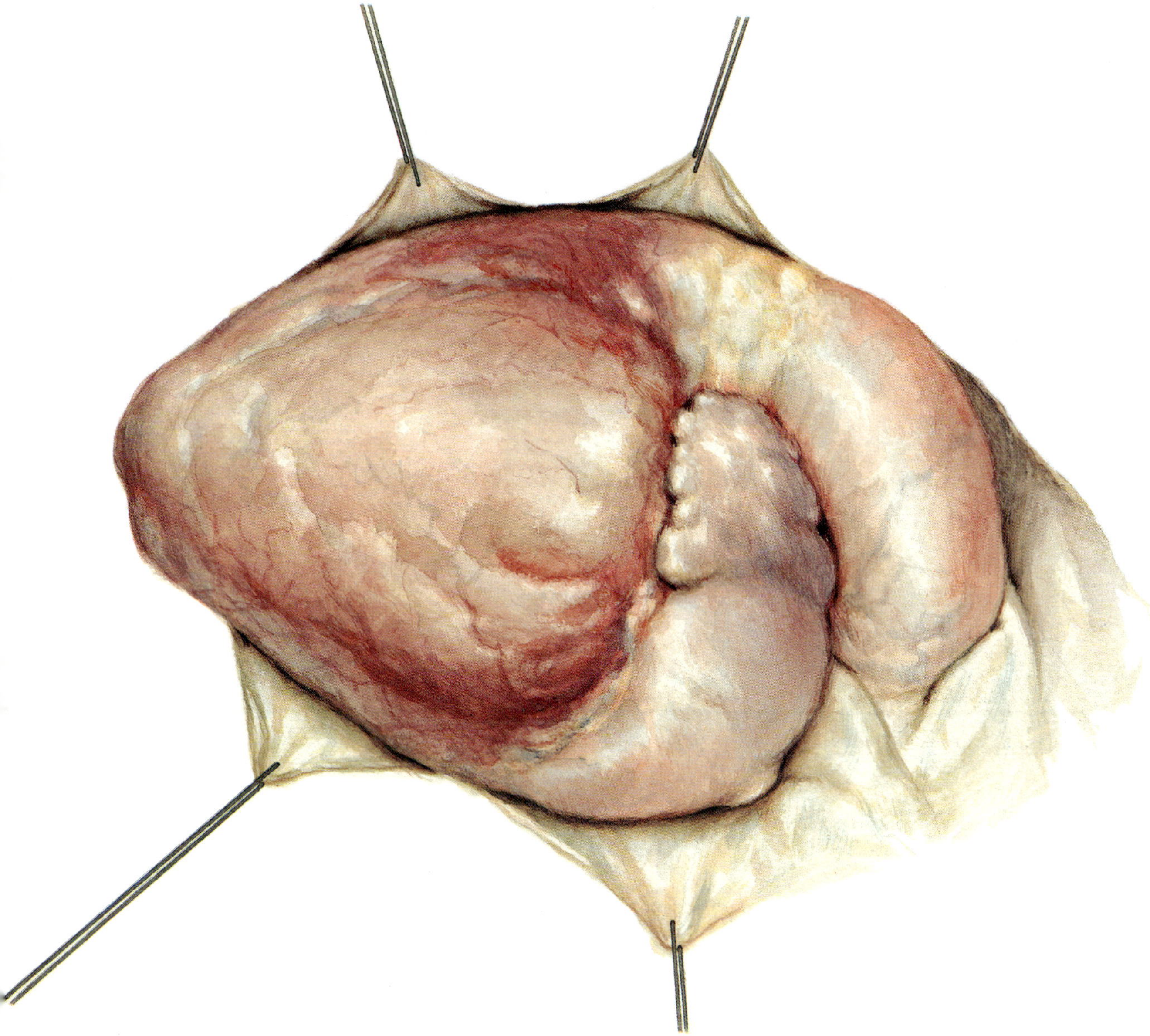

Fig. 238. Left atrium and auricle are enlarged in severe mitral stenosis. Atrium is pink, while myocardium of left ventricle is cyanotic (Kudas' sign).

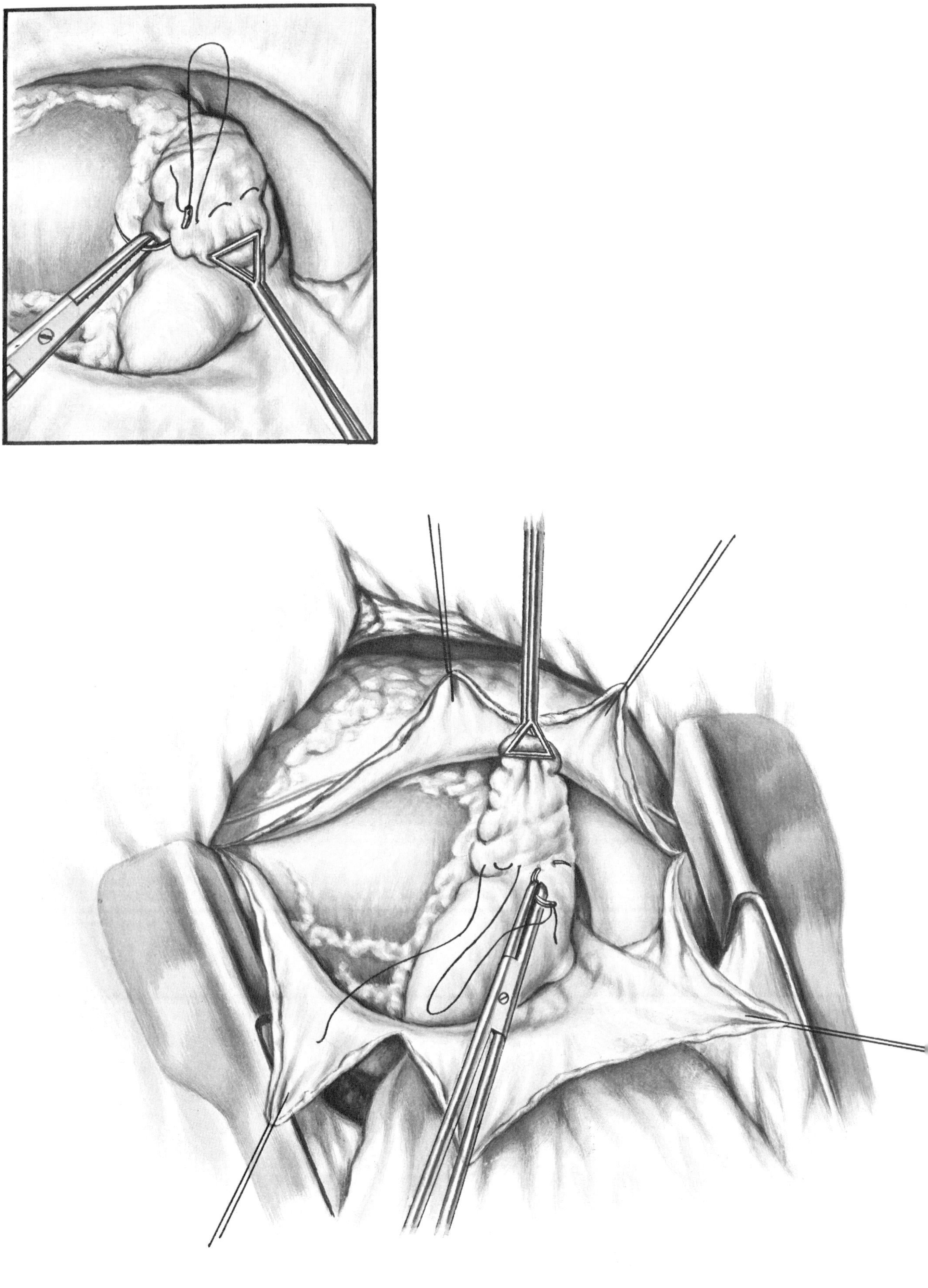

Fig. 239. Application of purse-string suture to base of left atrial auricle.

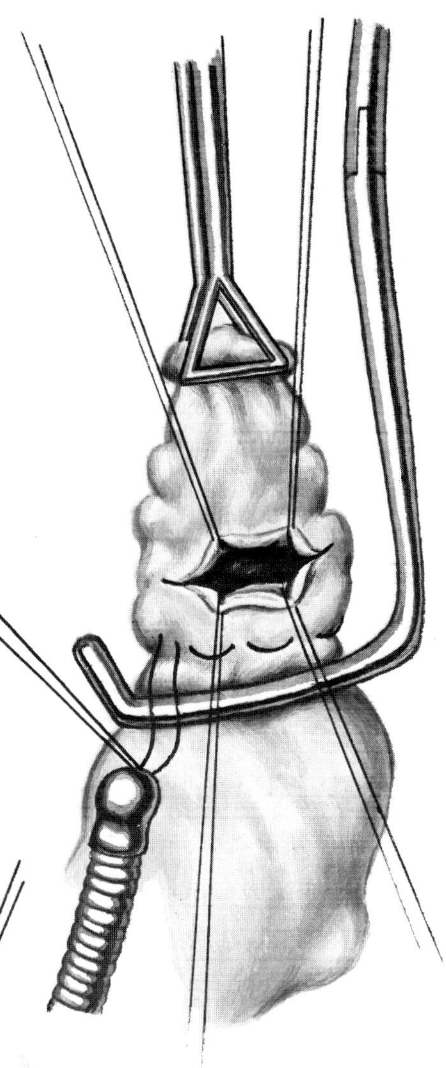

Fig. 240. Left atrial auricle is clamped with Satinsky's clamp; its cavity has been cut open and traction sutures applied to edges of incision.

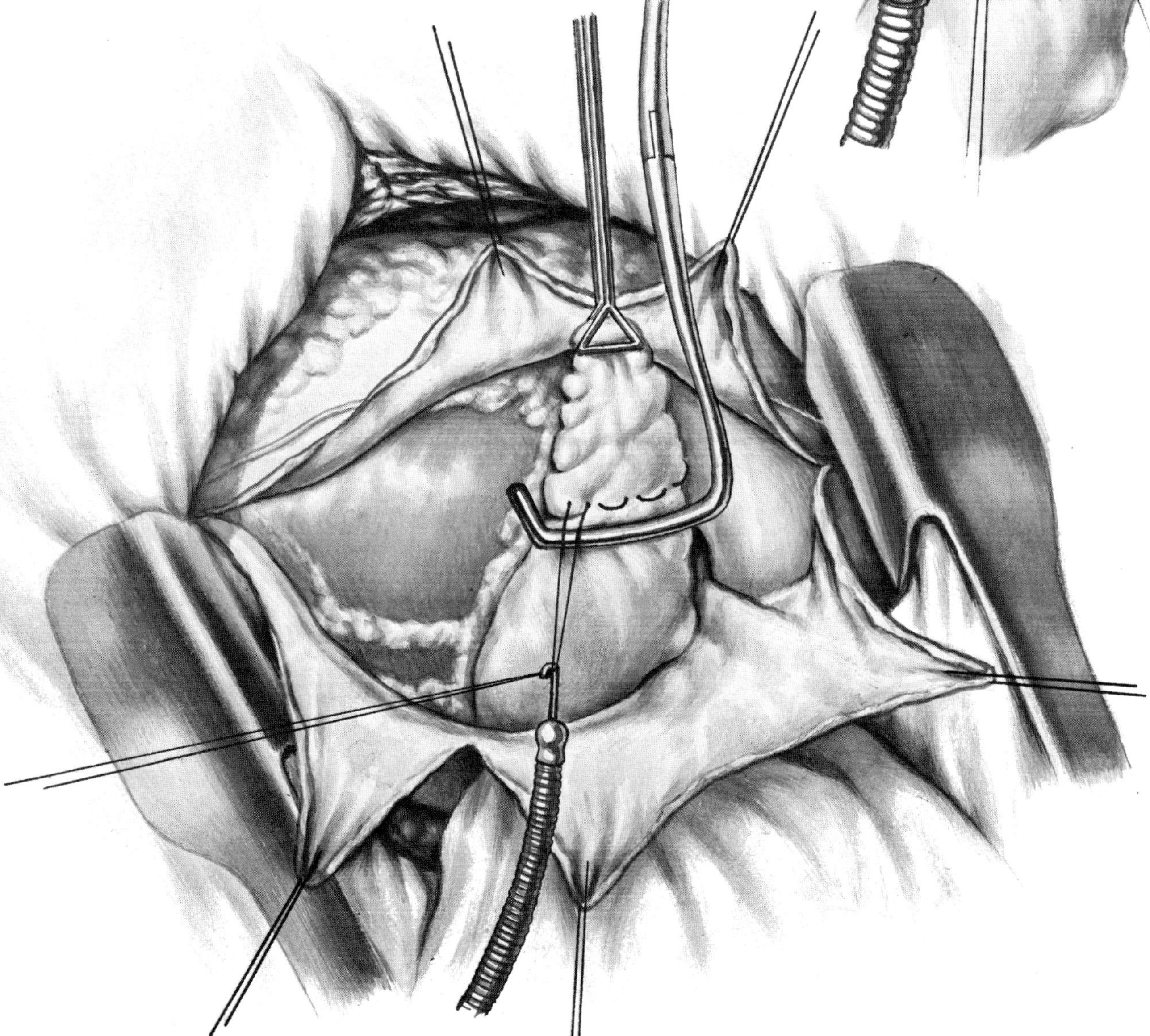

with the flexed distal phalanx (Fig. 242). Pressure is applied to the commissure along its length beginning with the margin of the stenosed orifice. When the rupture has been extended to the fibrous ring, the condition of the valvular apparatus is checked, and if need be, the fused chordae and papillary muscles are separated with extreme caution.

With the finger turned 180 degrees and straightened out, pressure is exerted along the length of the posterior commissure to separate it (Fig. 243). If this fails, an attempt is made to separate the commissure with the finger on supinating the hand. Harkin's manipulation may also be employed, in which event the surgeon goes to the other side of the table, stands facing the patient, and inserts his right index finger into the left atrium to separate the posterior commissure from this position.

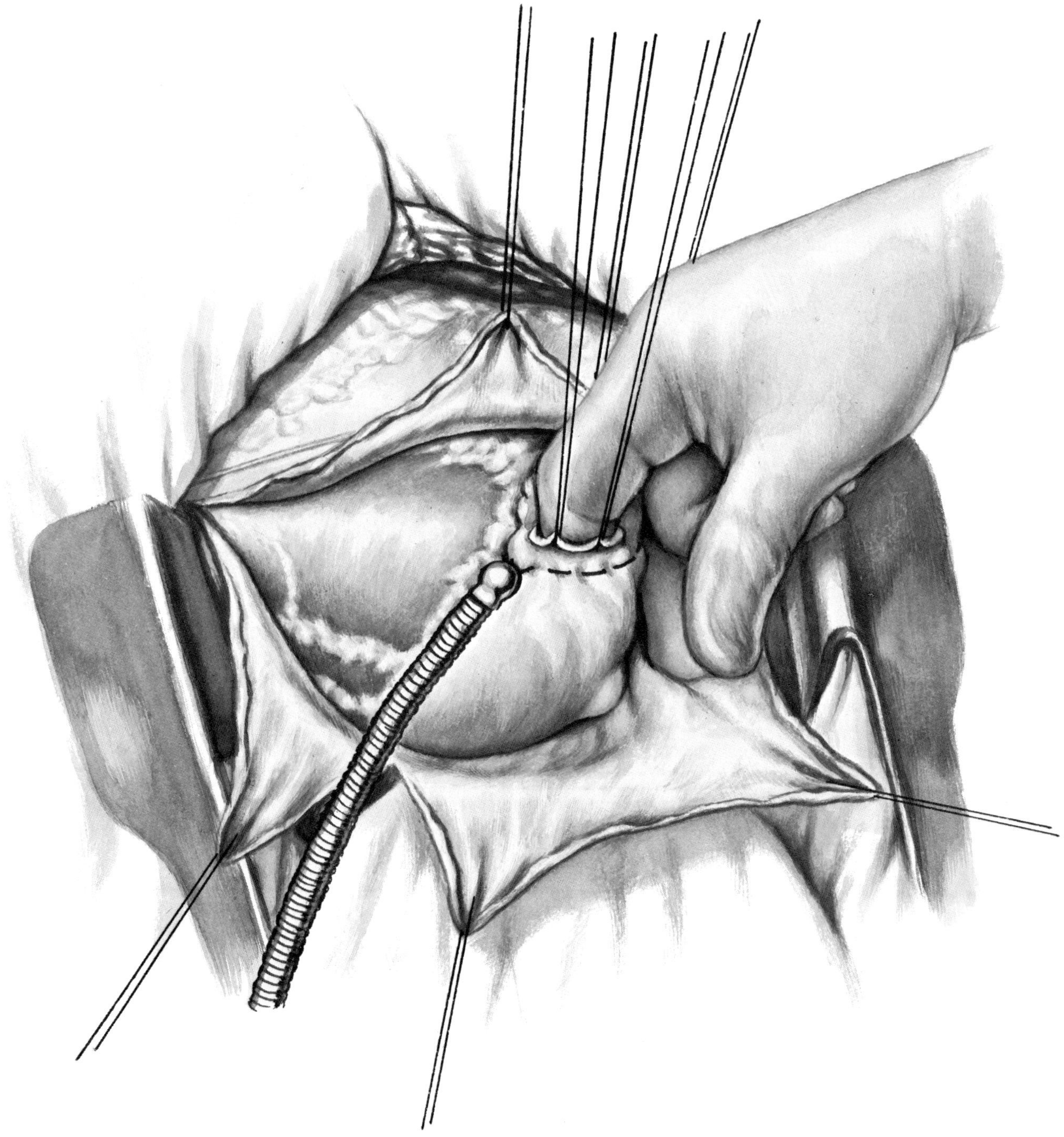

Fig. 241. Introduction of finger into left atrium and examination of mitral valve.

After commissurotomy is completed, a ligature is drawn around the base of the auricle, and the surgeon's finger within it. The surgeon's assistant ties this ligament as the surgeon's finger is withdrawn. The auricular tissue is cut away 1 cm above the applied ligature. Interrupted sutures are applied to the edges of the incision, and the purse-string suture is tied (Fig. 244). Spaced interrupted sutures are applied to the pericardium (Fig. 245). When the pericardium is opened ventrally to the phrenic nerve, a counter-aperture is formed in the region of the heart apex for draining the pericardial cavity.

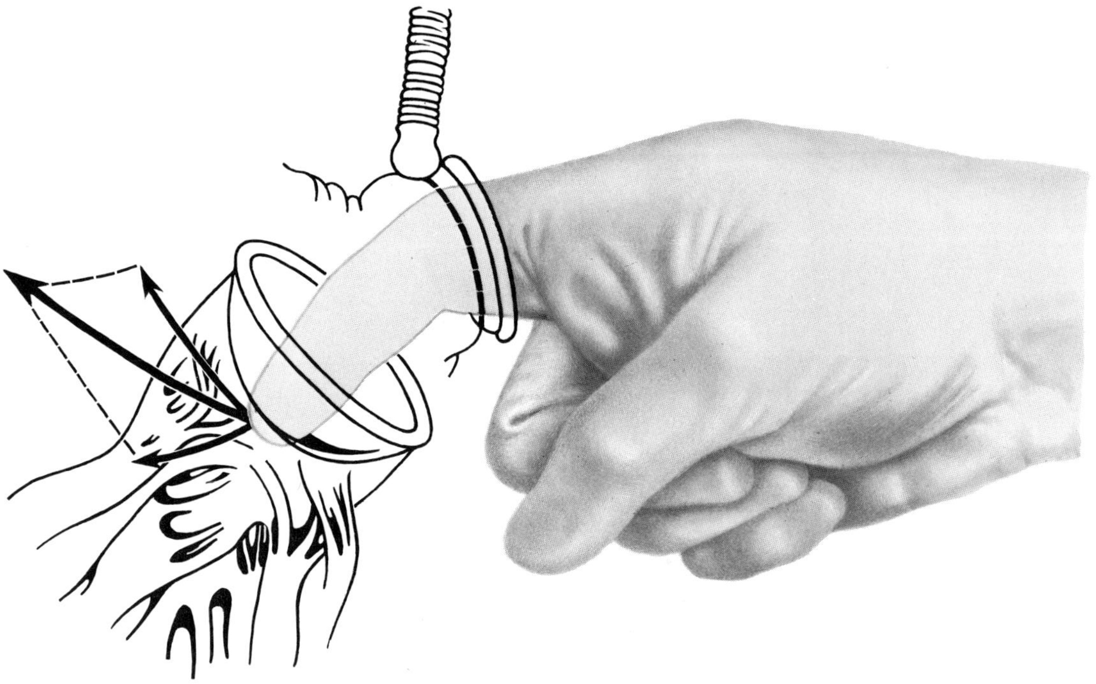

Fig. 242. Digital separation of anterior commissure. Arrows indicate direction of movements of distal phalanx.

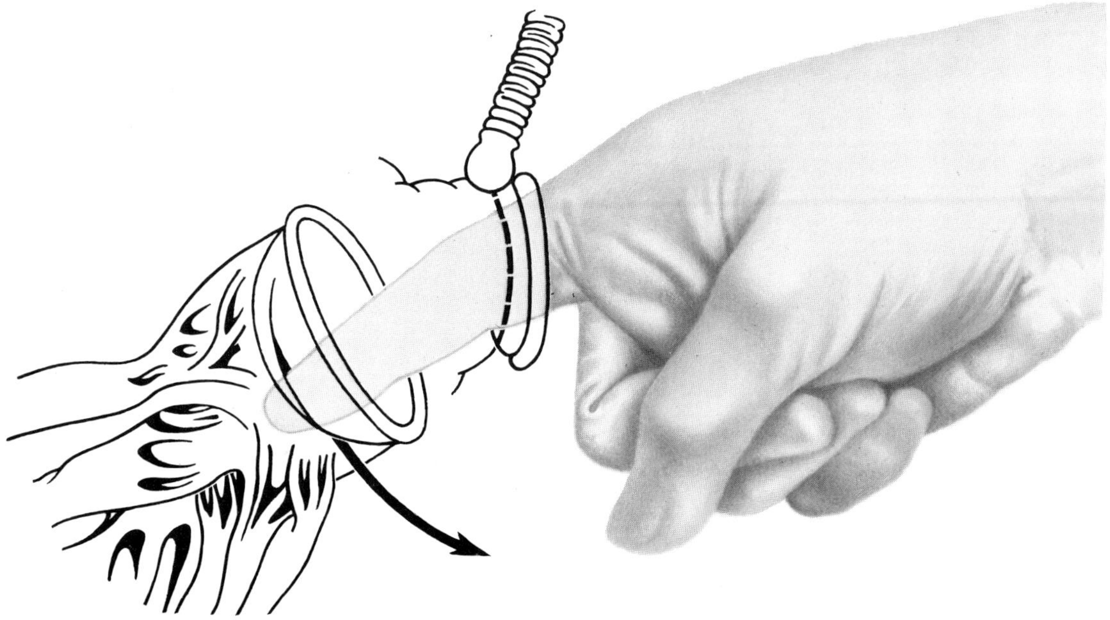

Fig. 243. Digital separation of posterior commissure.

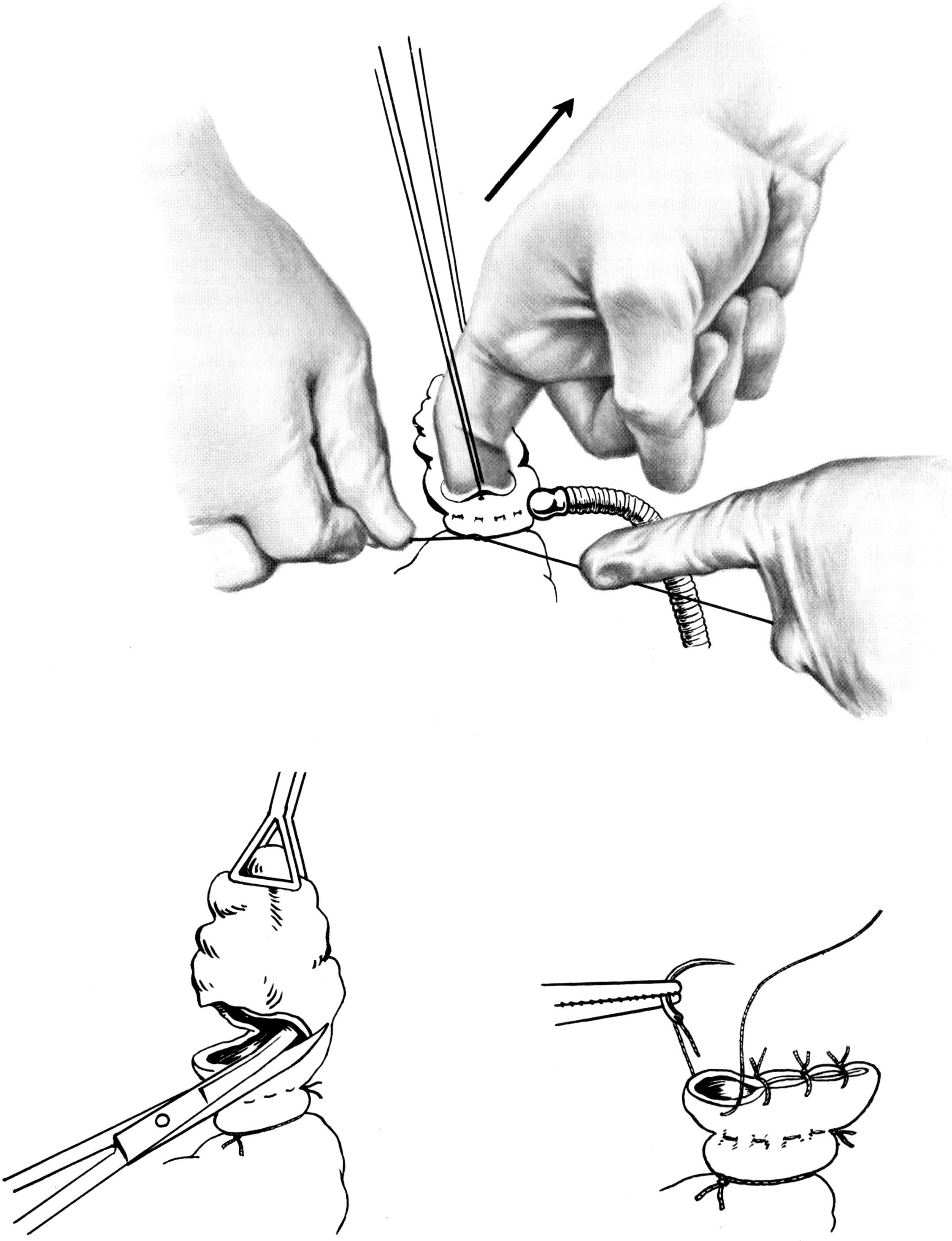

Fig. 244. Finger is withdrawn from left atrium and ligature is applied to base of auricle. Part of left auricle is cut away and its stump sutured.

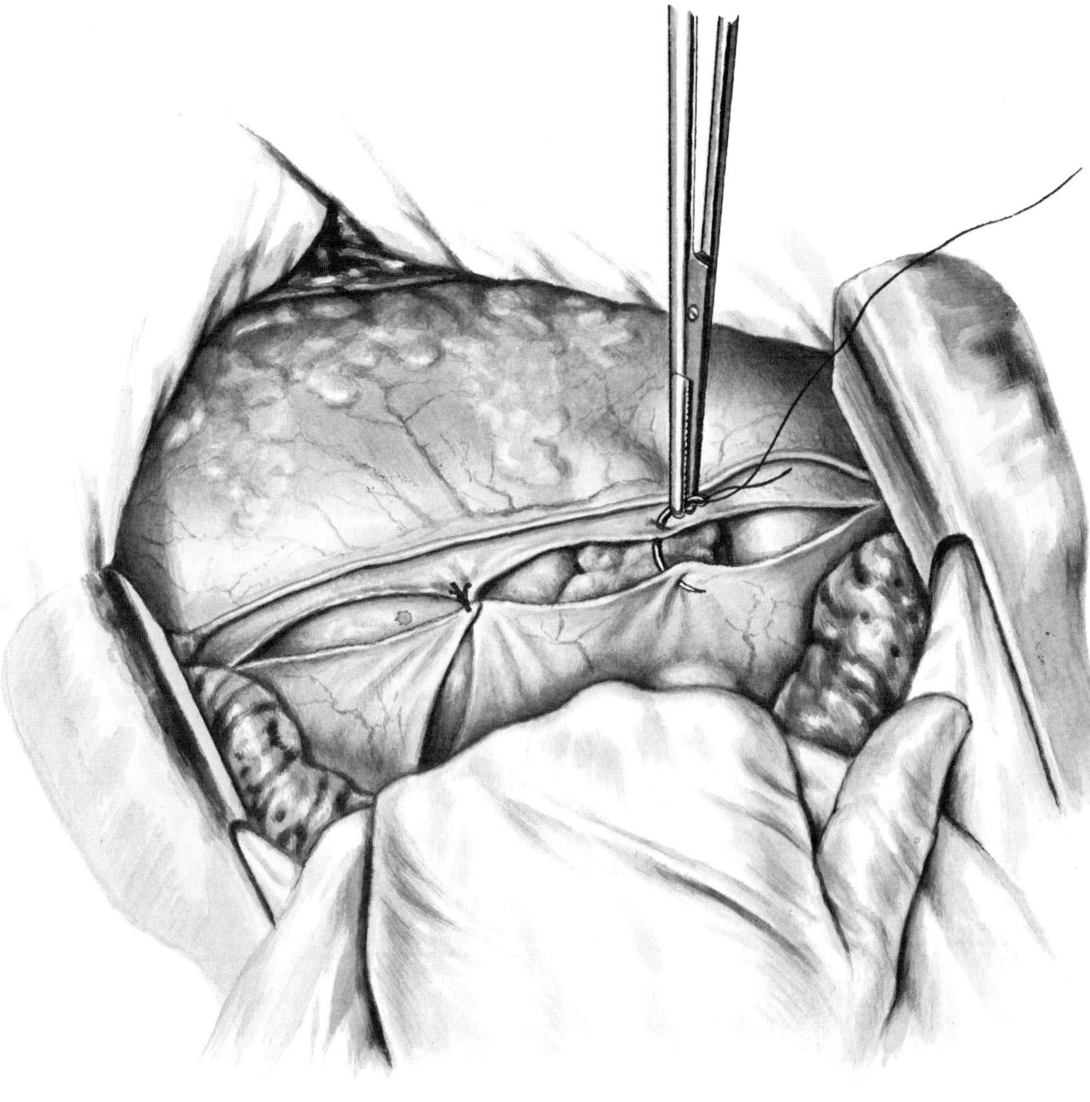

Fig. 245. Widely spaced interrupted sutures are applied to pericardium.

INSTRUMENTAL COMMISSUROTOMY BY LEFT APPROACH

If the attempt to separate the commissures by the digital method fails, the finger is withdrawn from the left atrium and Satinsky's clamp is again applied to the base of the auricle. The incision in the pericardium is extended to the apex of the heart. The apex is dislocated into the pericardial wound by putting one or two large gauze napkins under the posterior surface of the left ventricle. A Halsted suture is stitched through the wall of the left ventricle in an avascular zone close to the apex. A stab wound is made in the ventricular wall with a narrow scalpel (Fig. 246). The site of bleeding is compressed by the finger. The right index finger is inserted into the left atrium. Dubost's dilator is inserted by the left hand through the incision in the left ventricle. The limiter of the opening of the blades is set at 3.5 cm. The closed blades of the instrument, guided by the right index finger, are inserted into the cavity of the left atrium. The left atrioventricular orifice is dilated. In this manipulation the blades may be held either along the commissures or perpendicular to them (Fig. 247). If the blades are perpendicular, digital separation of the commissures is simultaneously performed. If no coarse

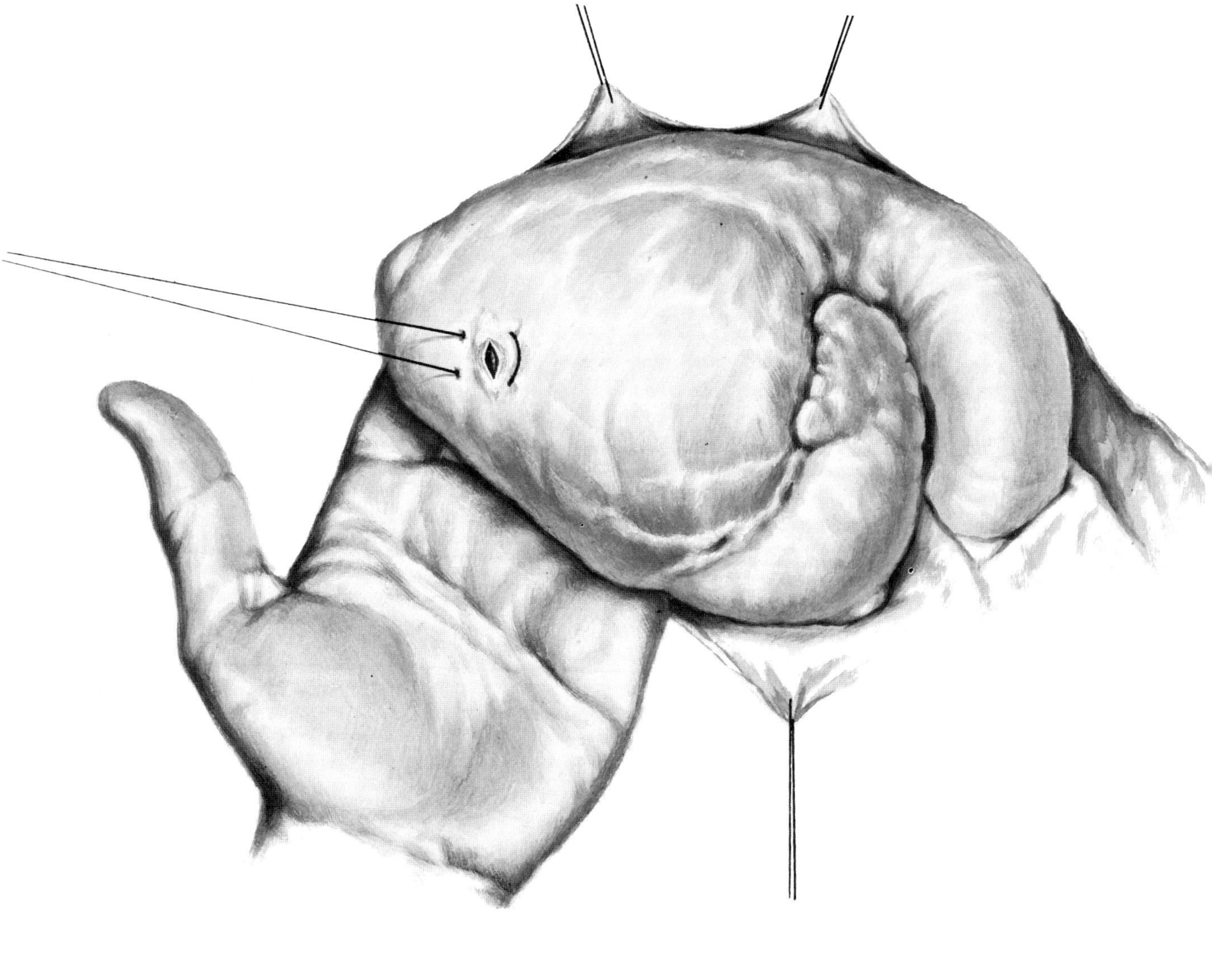

Fig. 246. Application of Halsted suture to anterior wall of left ventricle in lower third and formation of opening for introducing dilator.

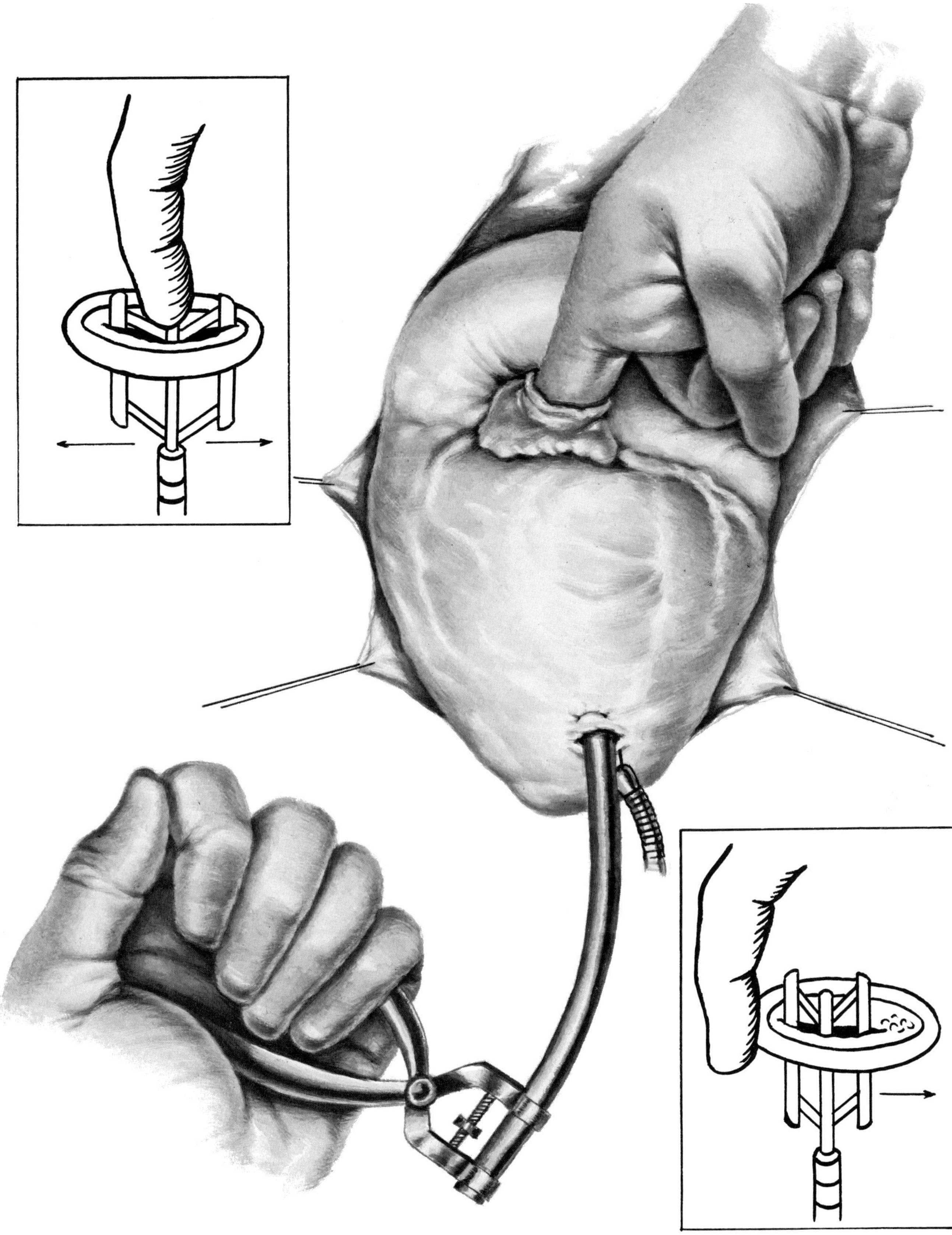

Fig. 247. Position of dilator and its blades during dilation of left atrioventricular orifice.

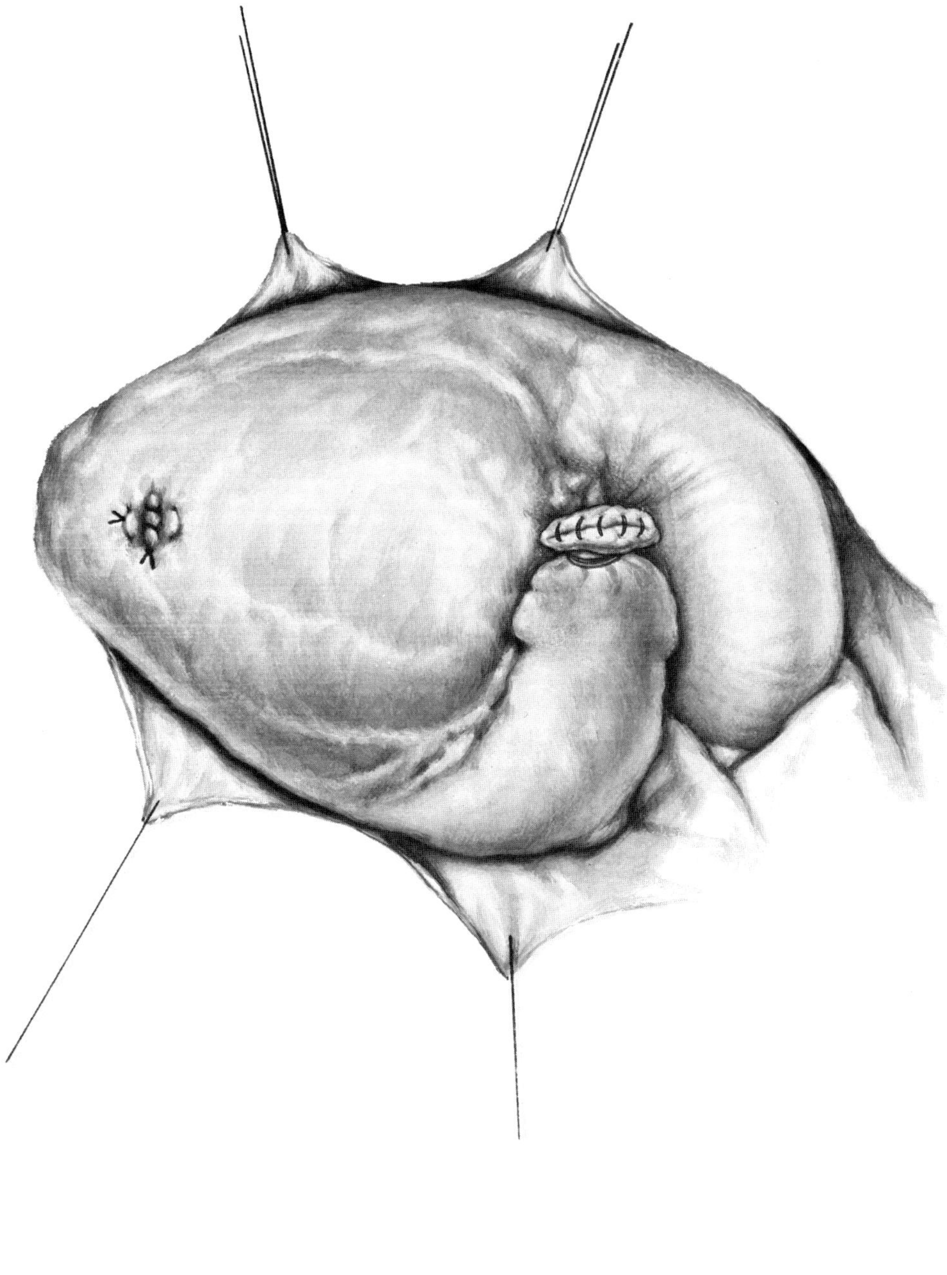

Fig. 248. Suture of left ventricle after instrumental commissurotomy.

regurgitation occurs after the commissures have been separated up to 3.5 cm, the blade limiter is set at 4 cm, and dilatation is repeated. With the blades closed, the dilator is withdrawn from the cavity of the left ventricle, while the traction sutures are crossed. The Halsted suture is tied. If necessary, additional interrupted sutures are applied with an atraumatic needle (Fig. 248).

Transventricular commissurotomy is not the only method. The stenosis may also be corrected with various commissurotomes inserted along the finger through the left atrial auricle. Of all these instruments, that of Petrovsky's design, which simultaneously dilates both commissures, is most efficient. Much bleeding is avoided when the instrument is inserted into the cavity of the left atrium, because it is flat (Fig. 249). The end of the dilator is passed into the cavity of the left ventricle. The separation of the commissure is accomplished under control of the finger in the left atrium.

In some cases, commissures may be separated by such instruments as a guillotine or ungual commissurotome (Figs. 250 and 251).

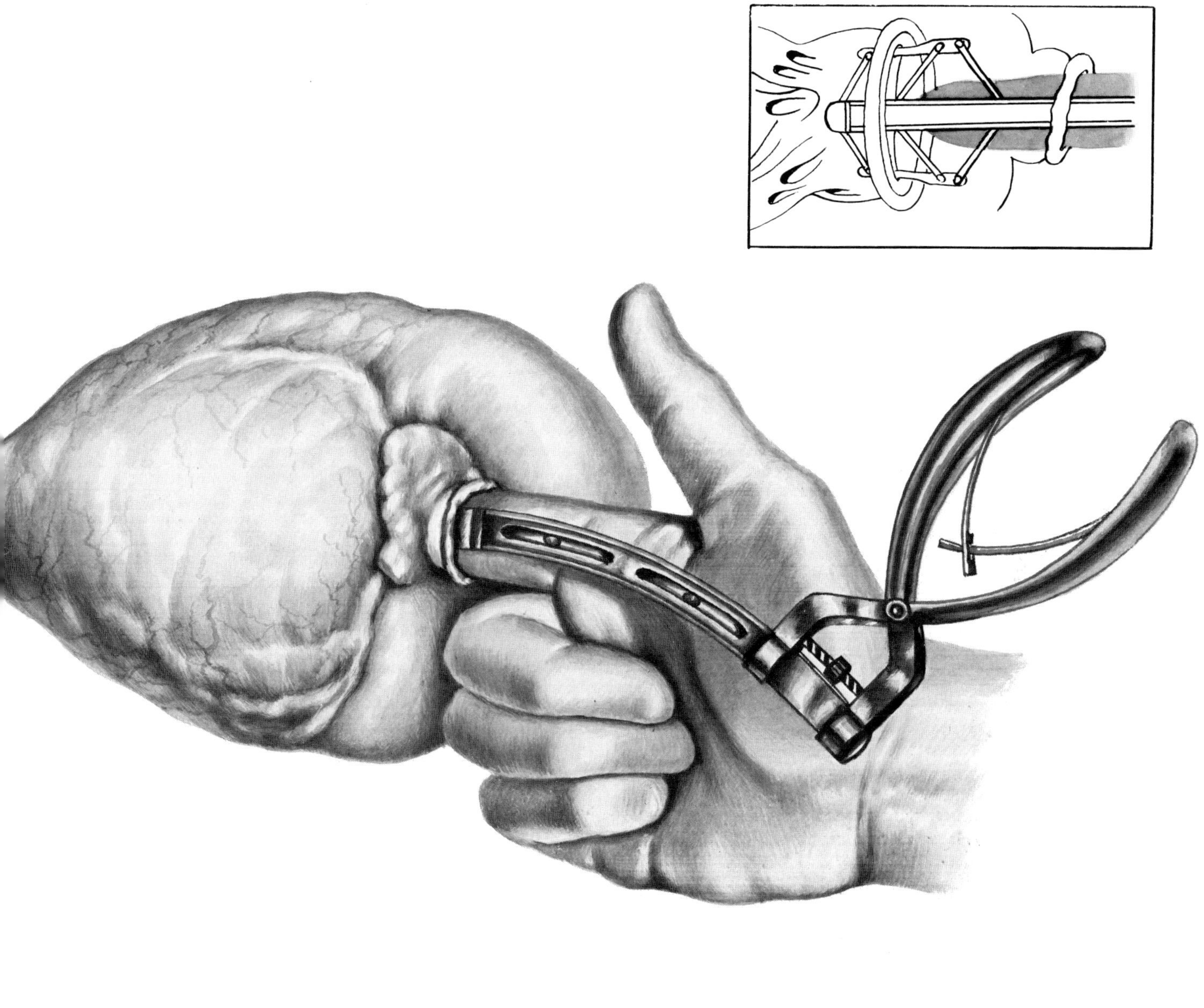

Fig. 249. Insertion of Petrovsky's dilator through left atrial auricle.

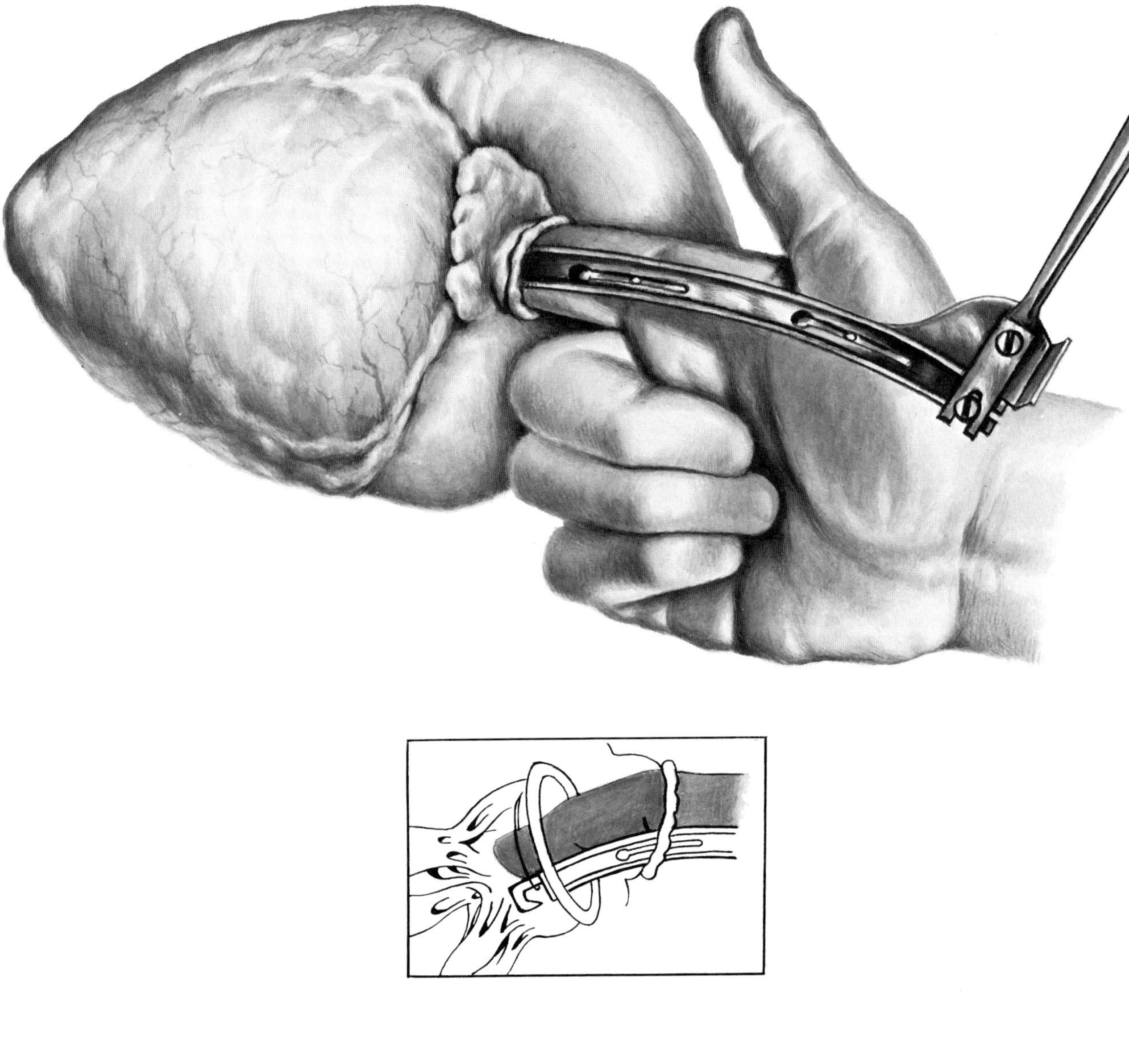

Fig. 250. Introduction of guillotine commissurotome through left atrial auricle.

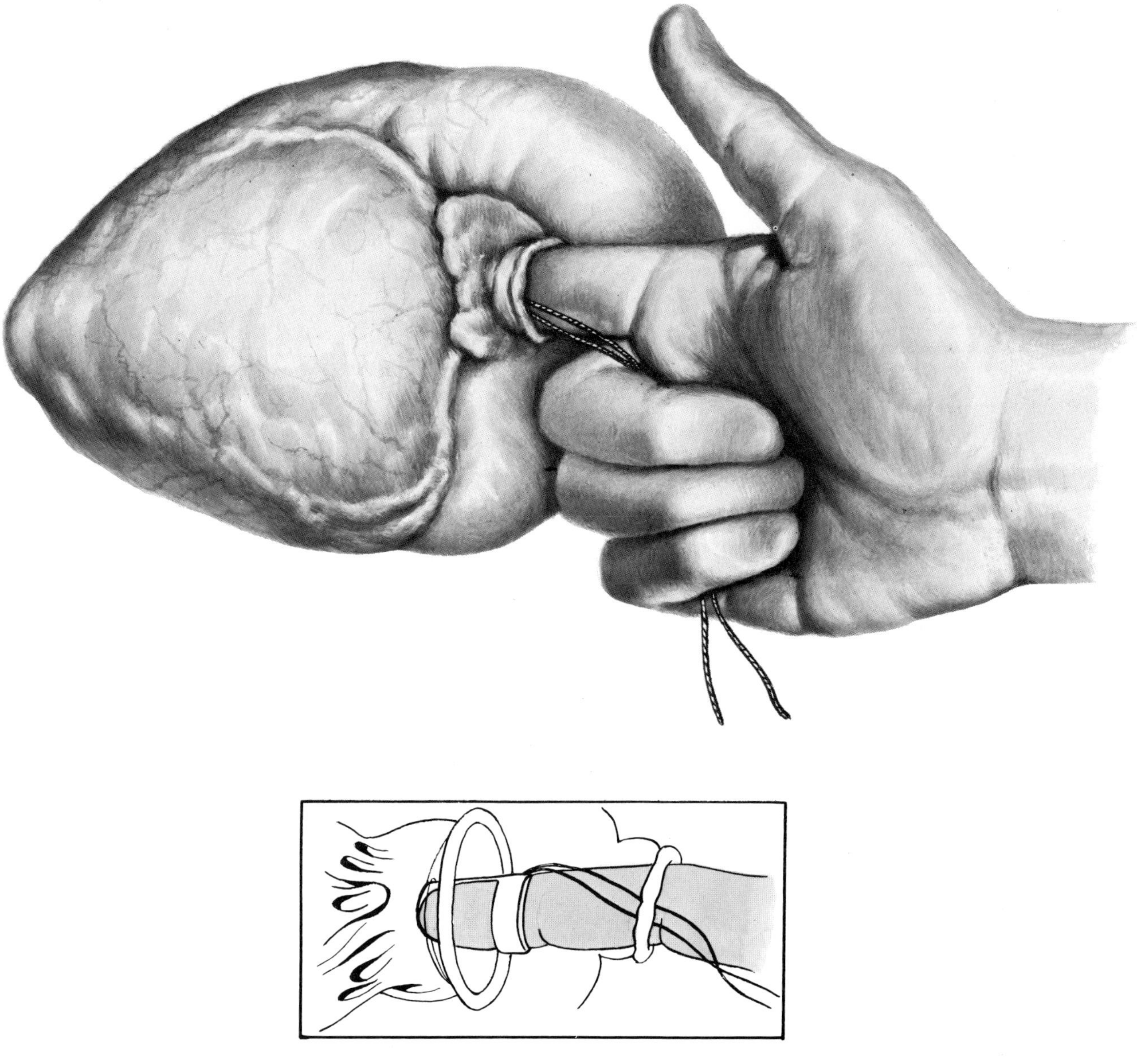

Fig. 251. Separation of mitral valve cusps by means of ungual commissurotome.

COMMISSUROTOMY BY RIGHT APPROACH

The operation is performed by an anterolateral approach in the fourth intercostal space.

The pericardium is opened ventral to the phrenic nerve with a Halsted incision forming a flap with the base at the phrenic nerve. Traction sutures are applied to the flap and the edges of the pericardium and are pulled to shift the heart slightly into the right pleural cavity (Fig. 252).

A 2 cm incision is made in the fatty cellular tissue of the atria ventral to the pulmonary vein, parallel and dorsal to the venae cavae; the interatrial septum is separated through this incision to a depth of 1 cm (Fig. 253). Silk traction sutures are applied to the edges of the incision. A purse-string and a wide Halsted suture are applied around the incision. The ends of the purse-string suture are drawn through Rummel's tourniquet (Fig. 254).

The left atrium is opened with a scalpel at the depth of the separated interatrial septum, and the left index finger is inserted into the incision (Fig. 255). The anterior commissure, which is easier for access, is usually separated first with the distal phalanx of the extended index finger (Fig. 256).

The separation of the posterior commissure is far more difficult. The commissurotomy is performed with a slightly flexed distal phalanx. If the atrium is large, the whole left index finger is sunk into its cavity. During this manipulation the surgeon places his right hand on the left side of the patient's chest making it easier to reach the posterior commissure of the stenosed left atrioventricular orifice and rupture it (see Fig. 256).

If the commissures cannot be separated by finger through the right approach, dilators and commissurot-

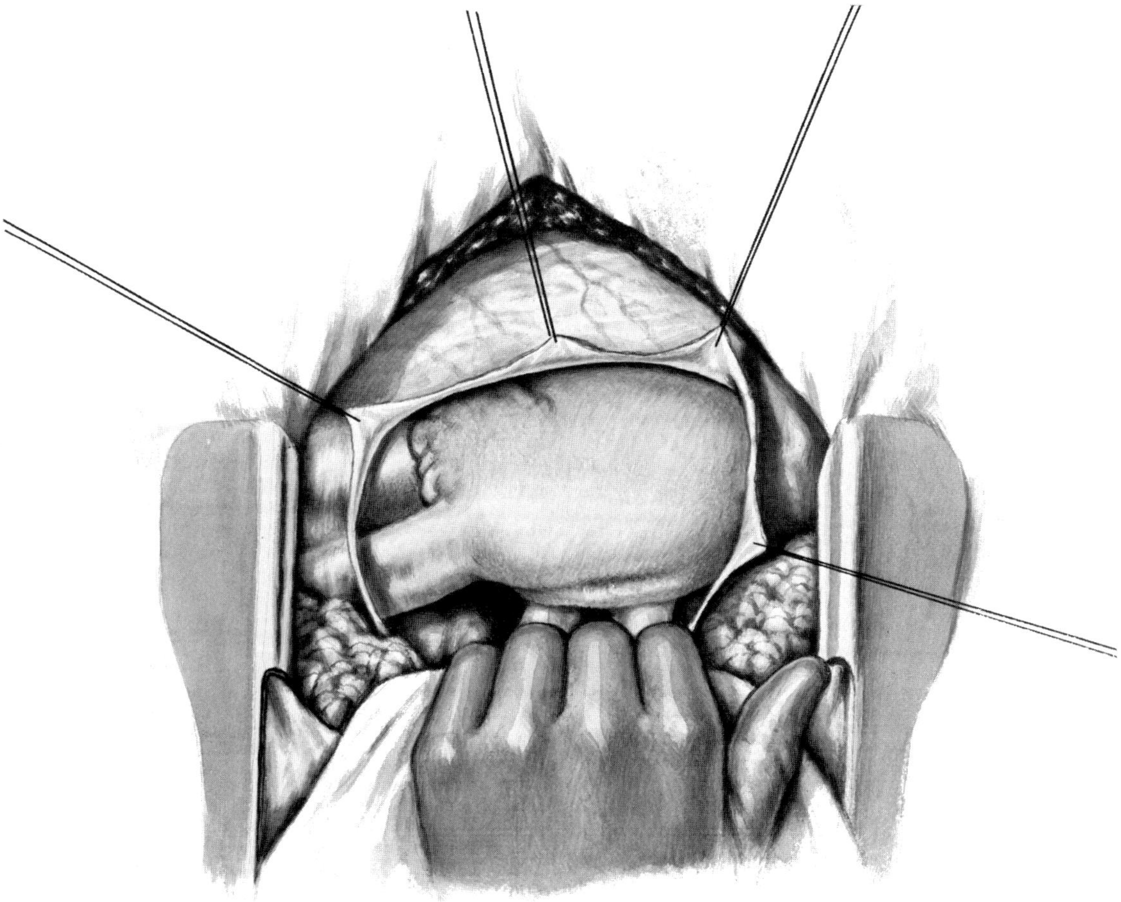

Fig. 252. Pericardium has been opened. Superior vena cava, part of ascending aorta, right auricle and atrium, part of right ventricle, and pulmonary veins are seen in its cavity.

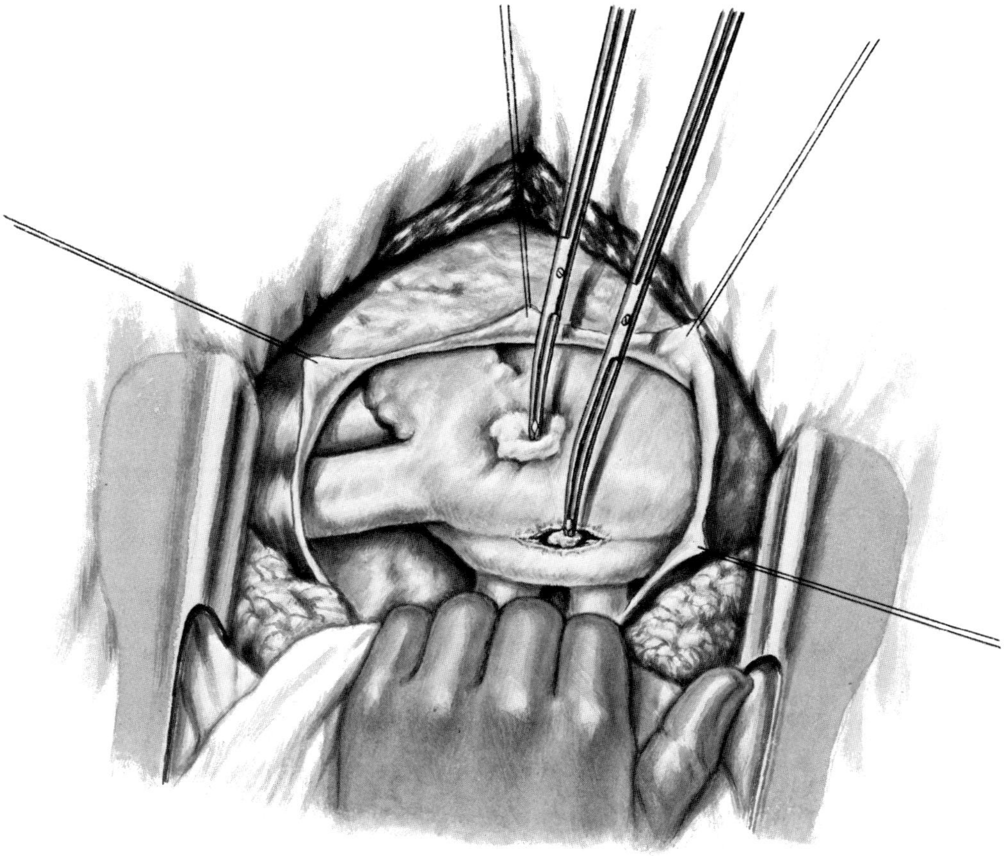

Fig. 253. Separation of interatrial septum ventral to pulmonary veins.

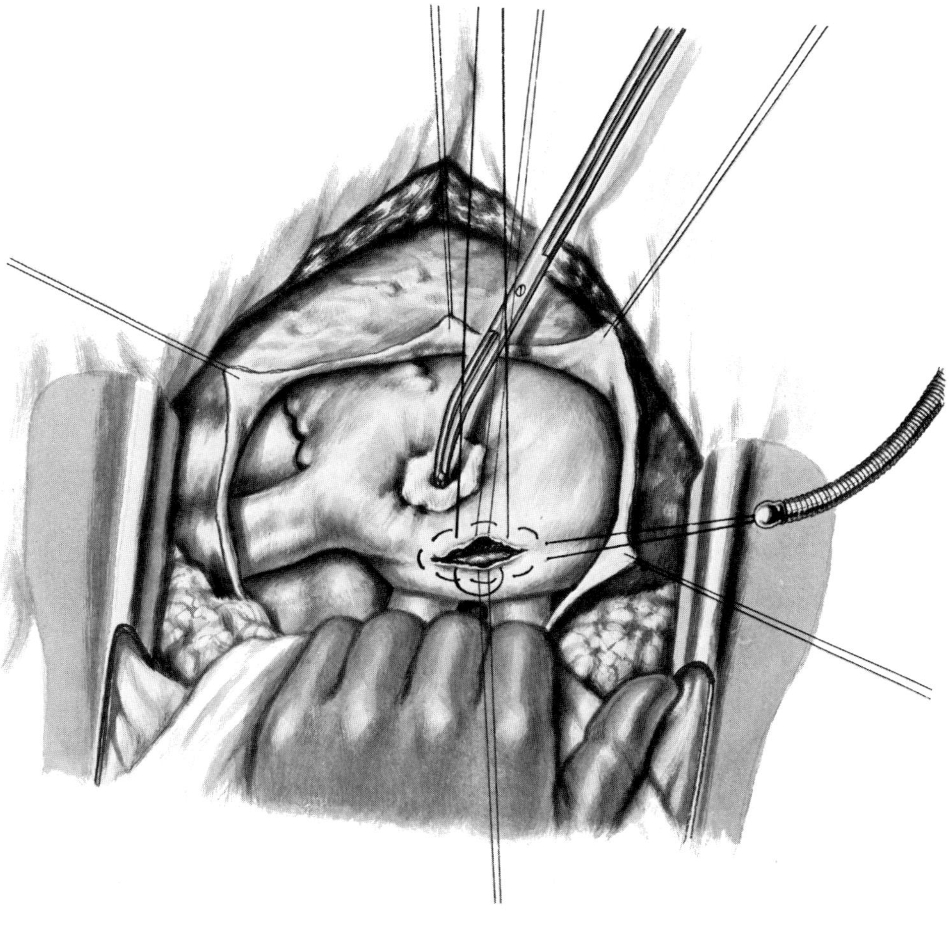

Fig. 254. Application of purse-string and Halsted sutures in region of opening formed in atrium.

omes are used. A dilator on a flexible line and Petrovsky's dilator are usually preferred. If these methods are also unsuccessful, the finger is withdrawn from the left atrium for some time, and the opening is clamped with a tourniquet. A small anterolateral thoracotomy is performed in the left fifth intercostal space, and the pericardium is opened in the region of the heart apex. After applying traction sutures and a Halsted suture, Dobost's dilator is introduced through the apex of the heart into the left ventricle and left atrium. The position of the instrument and the efficacy of dilatation are checked by the left index finger introduced into the left atrium through the separated interatrial septum.

The wound in the left atrium is closed by tying the Halsted and purse-string sutures as the finger is being withdrawn (Fig. 257). Additional interrupted sutures are usually unnecessary. The wound in the left ventricle is sutured as described above after the removal of the instrument.

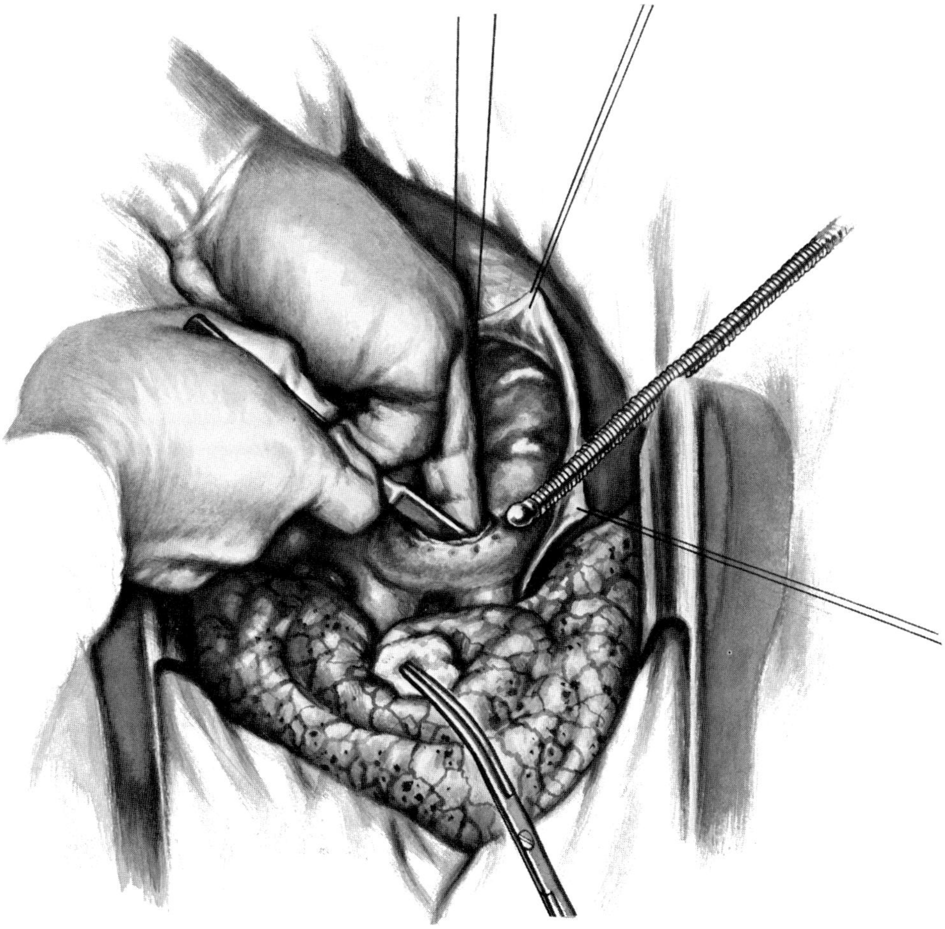

Fig. 255. Cavity of left atrium is opened with scalpel, and finger is inserted into incision.

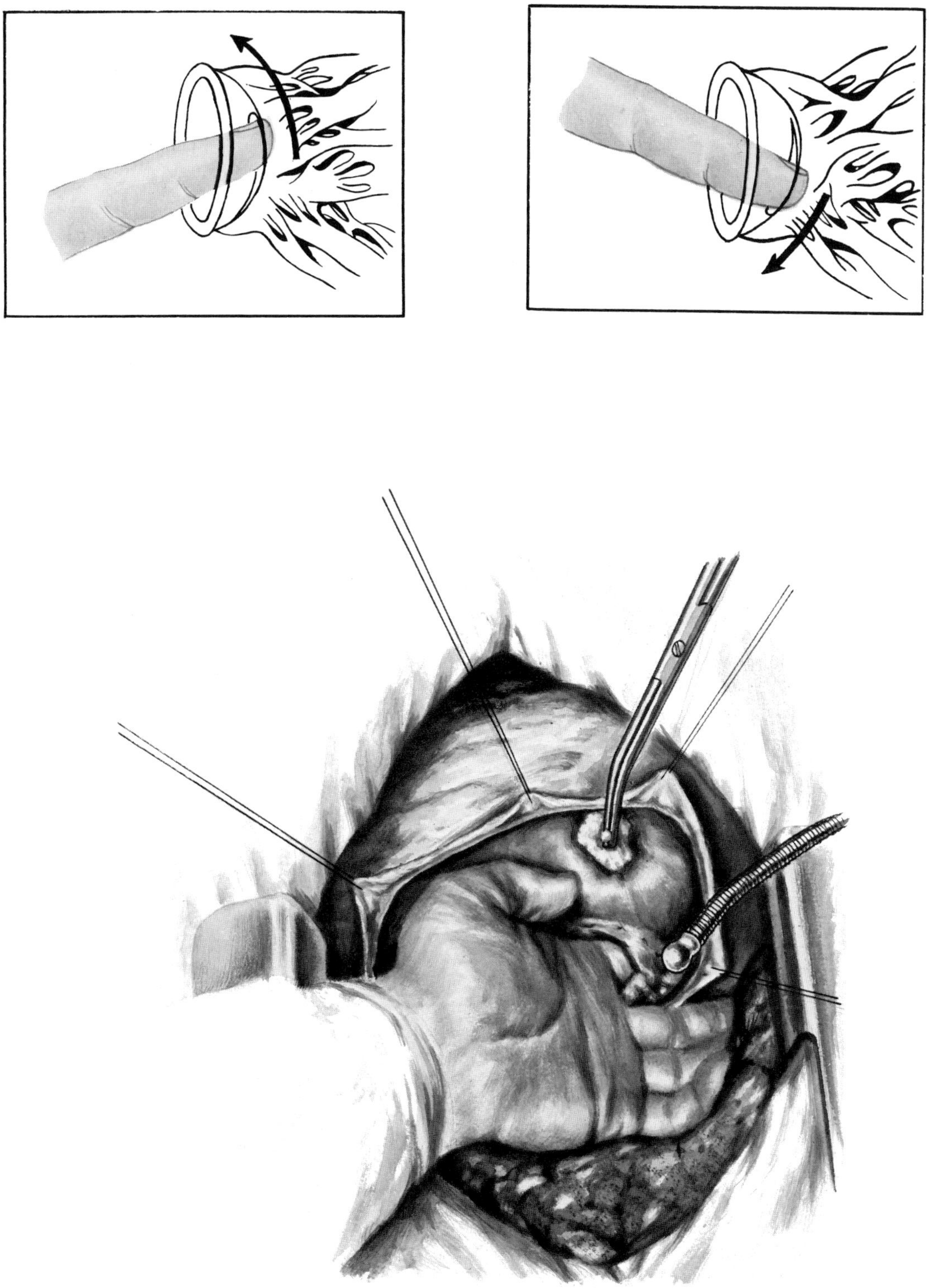

Fig. 256. Techniques of separation of mitral valve posterior and anterior commissures.

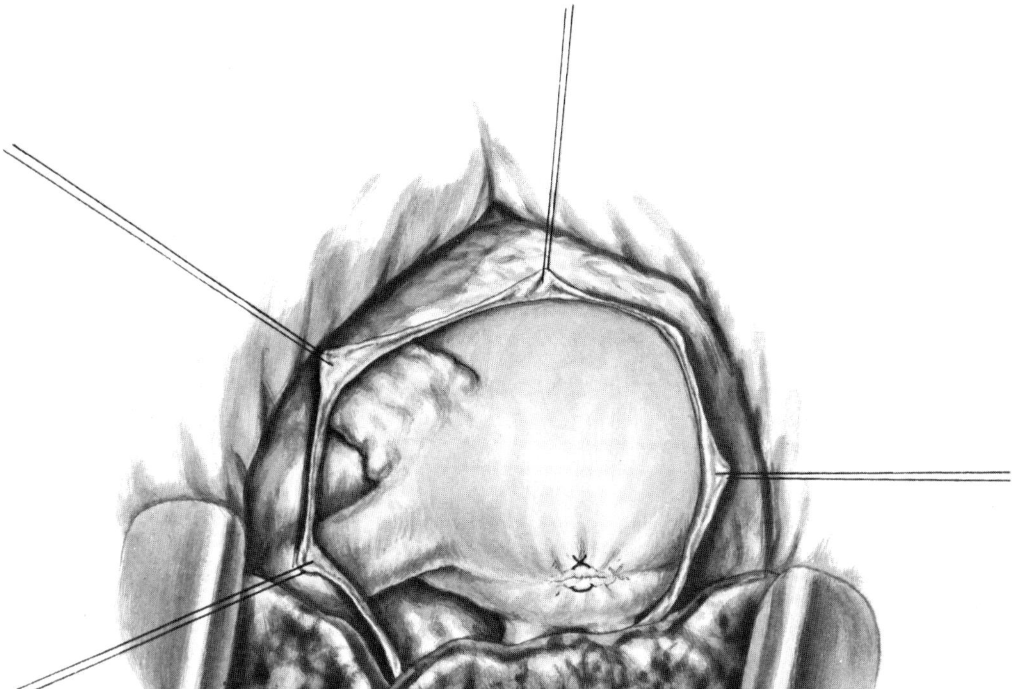

Fig. 257. Suture of left atrium after mitral commissurotomy.

CLOSURE OF RUPTURES IN AURICLE, ATRIUM, AND LEFT VENTRICLE IN MITRAL COMMISSUROTOMY

If the neck of the left auricle is narrow, it may be ruptured when the finger is inserted into the atrium, and commissurotomy is performed. The rupture often extends to the wall of the left atrium.

The line of the rupture is closed with the palmar surface of the index finger in the left atrium (Fig. 258). The ruptured walls of the atrium are closed with a continuous suture (Fig. 259). To accomplish this quicker, Satinsky's clamp may be applied to the base (Fig. 260). Coarse digital mitral commissurotomy may cause rupture of the anterior and, less frequently, of the posterior walls of the left ventricle in the region of the commissures directly below the circumflex branch of the left coronary artery. The rupture is also closed with the finger in the left ventricular cavity (Fig. 261). A suture is applied to the wall of the left ventricle with an atraumatic needle, using plastic bolsters, if possible. Care is taken to avoid injuring the coronary artery (Fig. 262).

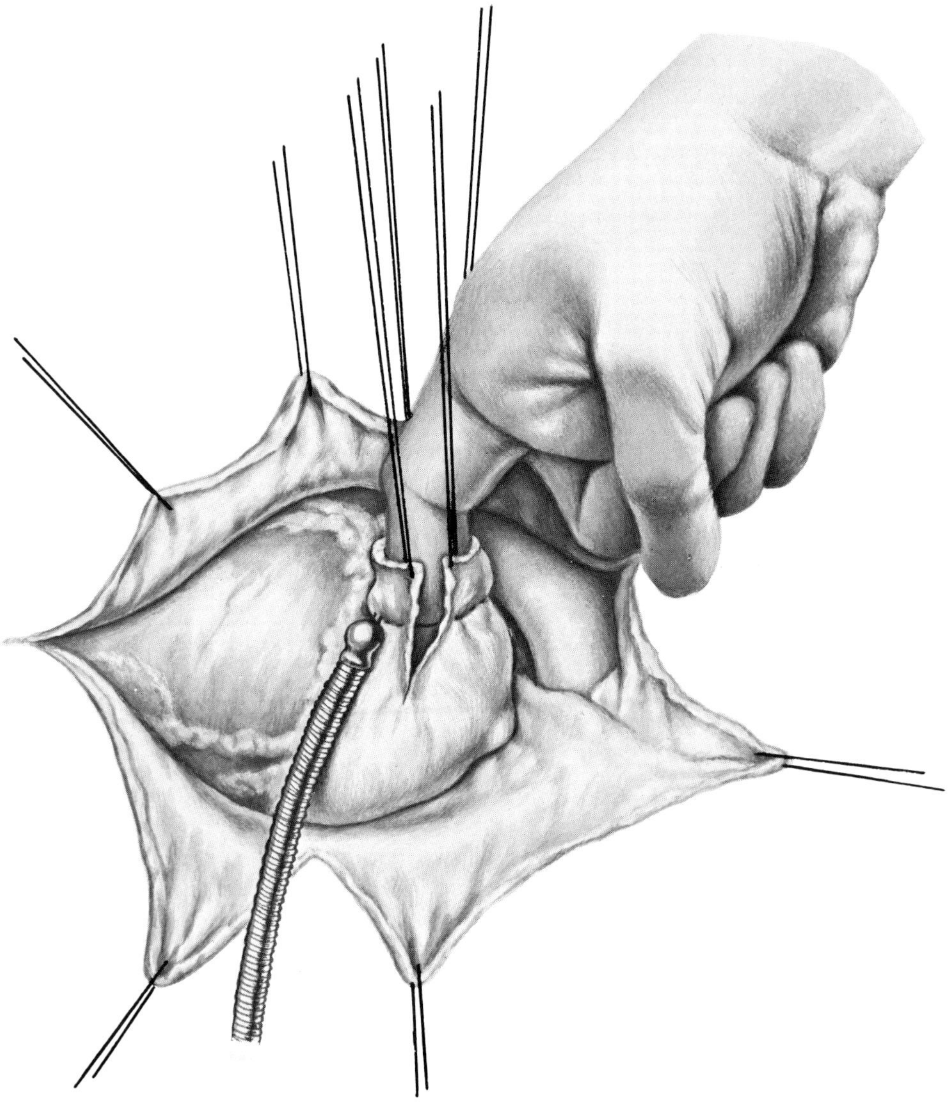

Fig. 258. Rupture in neck of auricle extending to wall of left atrium is compressed with finger.

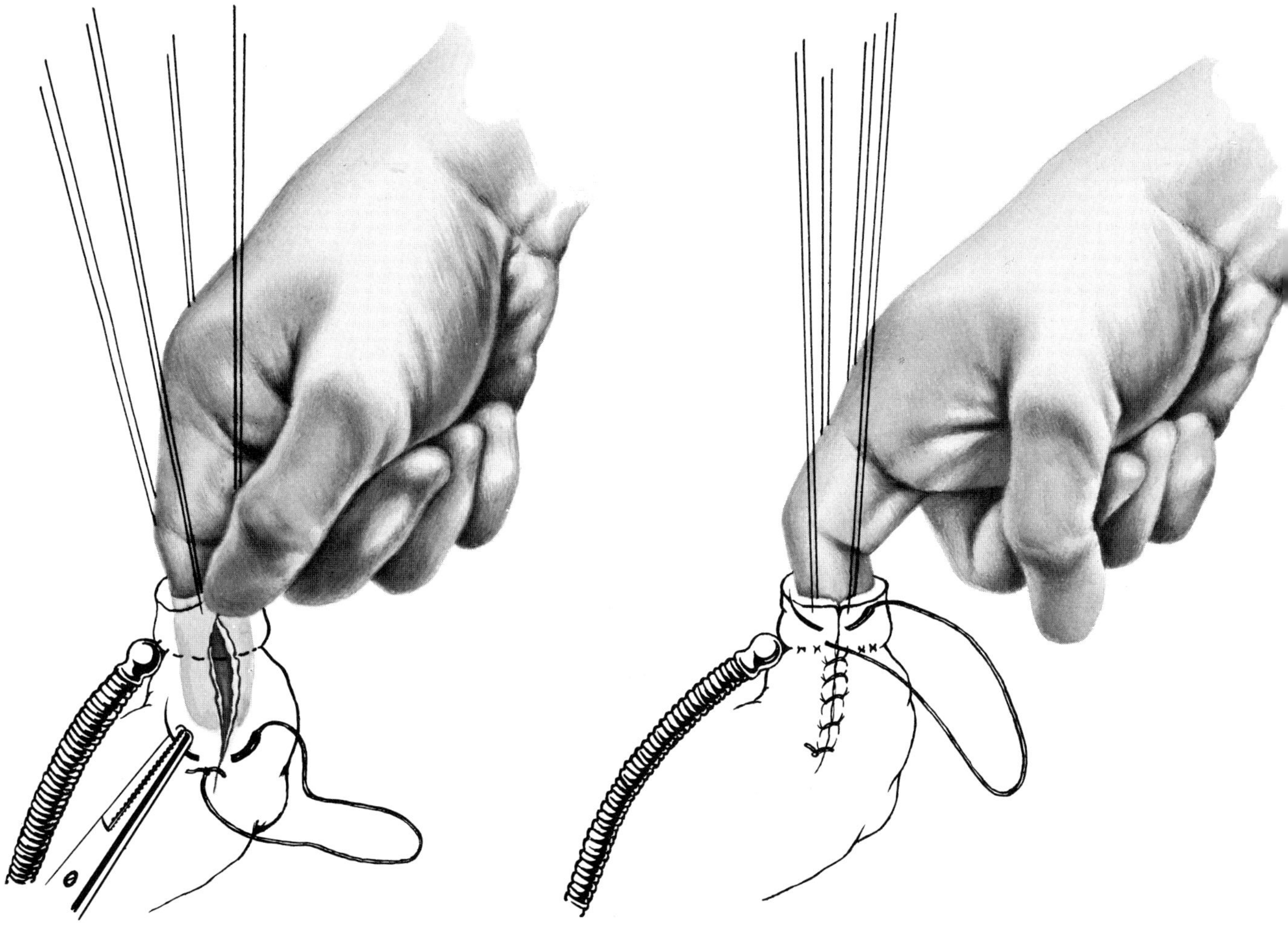

Fig. 259. Techniques of suturing rupture in left atrium and its auricle.

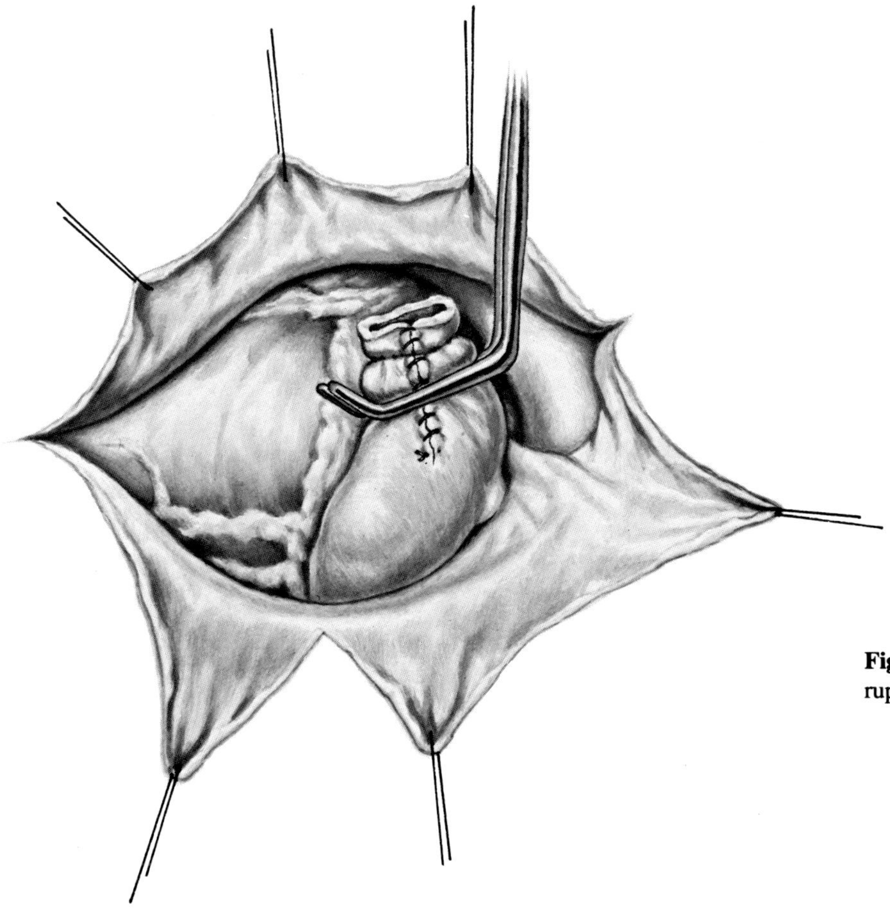

Fig. 260. Part of left atrium is clamped after rupture in its wall has been sutured.

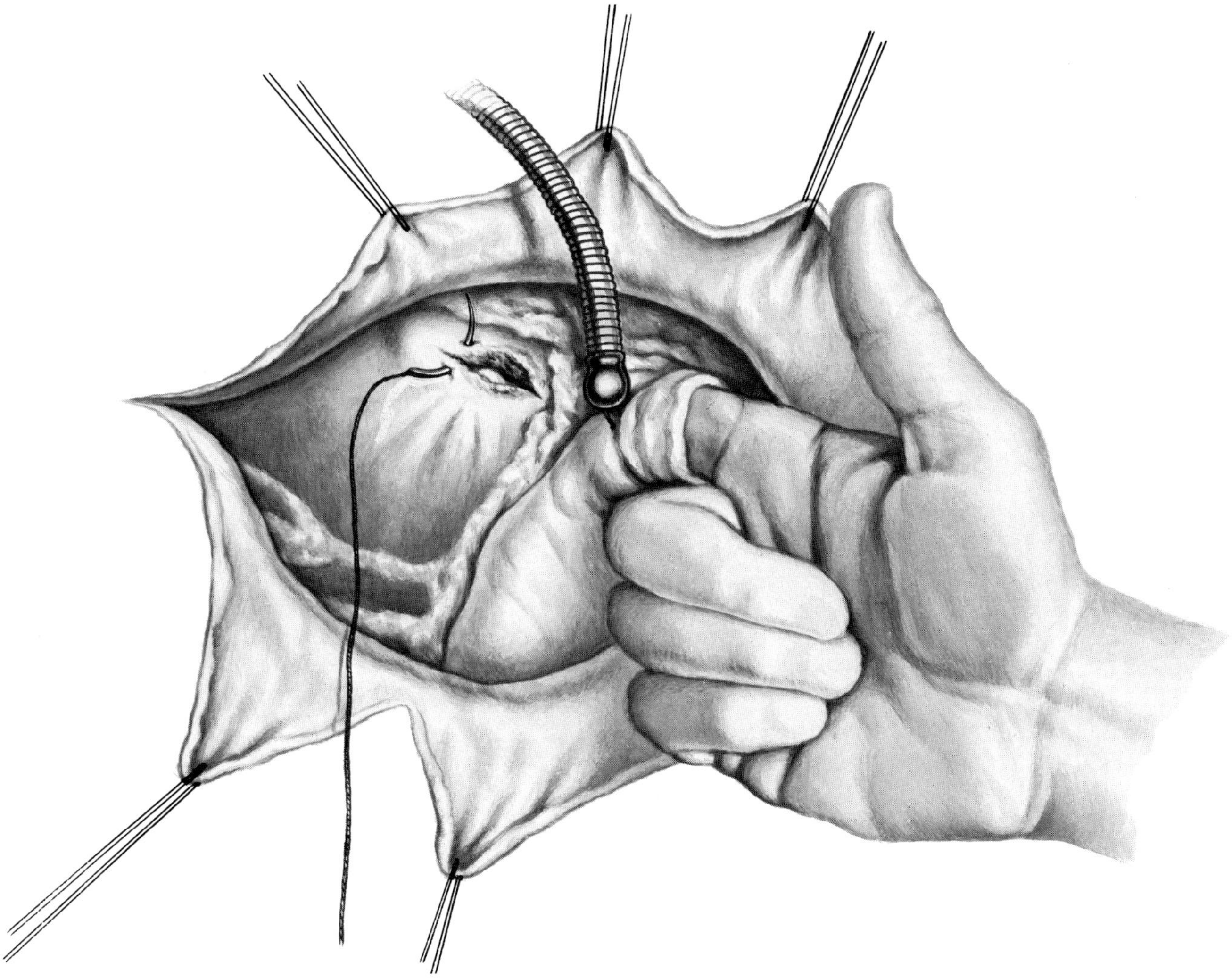

Fig. 261. Defect in ruptured left ventricle is closed with finger and repaired with sutures applied from its cavity.

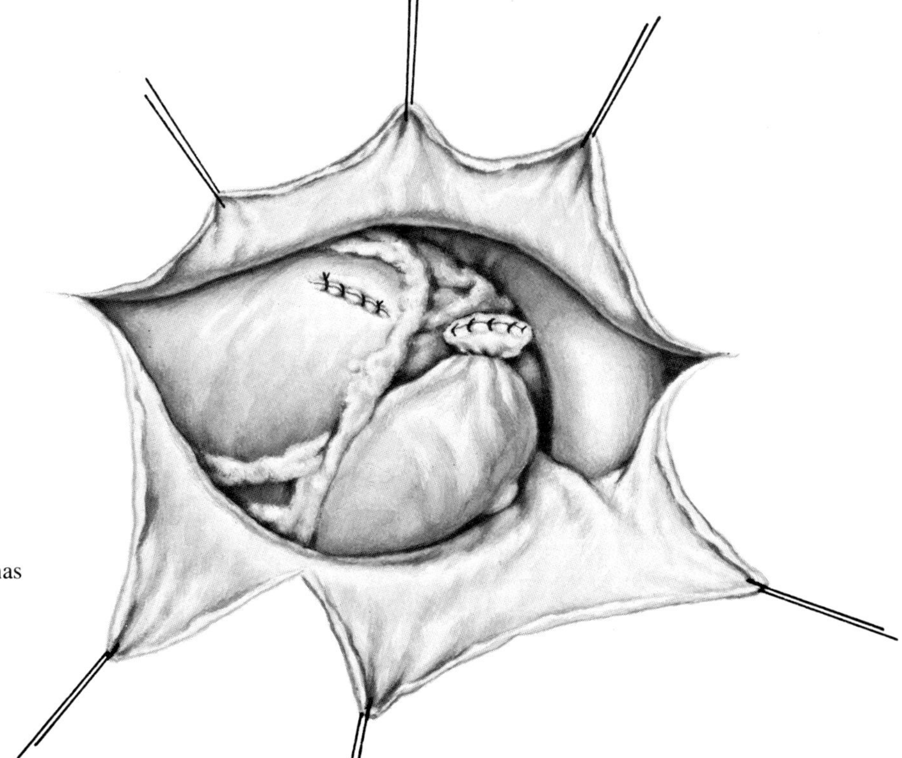

Fig. 262. Rupture in wall of left ventricle has been sutured.

COMMISSUROTOMY IN LEFT ATRIAL THROMBOSIS

The techniques of the operation consist in total or partial removal of the thrombus prior to mitral commissurotomy, or in the introduction of the finger bypassing the thrombus.

There are apical thrombi of the atrial auricle, mural thrombi of the atrium, total thrombi of the auricle, thrombi of the auricle extending to the left atrial wall, and pedicle thrombi and free spherical thrombi of the left atrium (Fig. 263). The diagnosis of thrombosis of the left atrial auricle is usually made on finding a wrinkled, whitish, and hard left auricle when the pericardium is opened (Fig. 264).

Fresh thrombi may not alter the appearance of the auricle and are only found by palpation. To avoid crushing fresh parts of the thrombus in the cardiac cavity, Satinsky's clamp is not used in treating the auricle, and the manipulation is begun with the application of a purse-string suture; care is taken to grasp the base of the

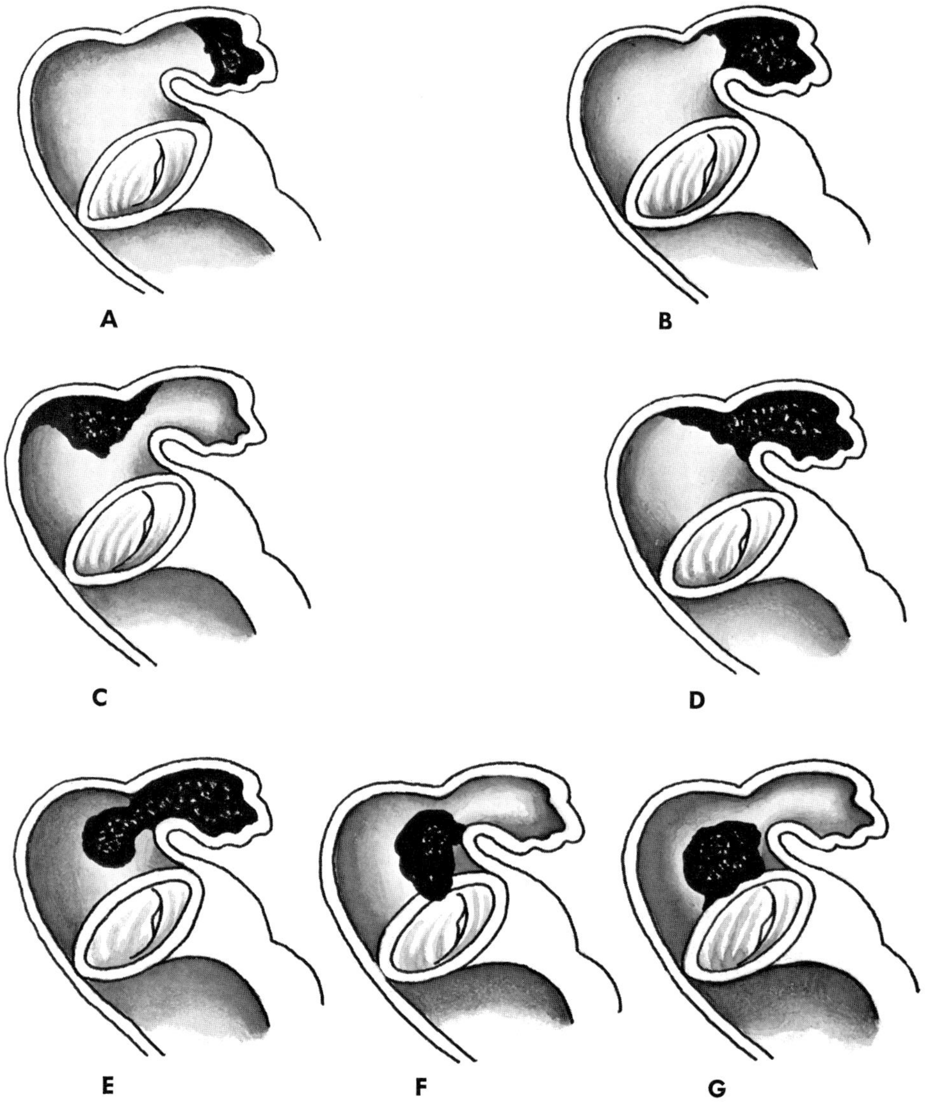

Fig. 263. Schema of various thrombi in left atrium. **A,** Apical. **B,** Total thrombus of left auricle. **C,** Fixed mural thrombus of left atrium. **D,** Fixed thrombus of auricle continued as mural thrombus of left atrium. **E,** Auricular thrombus connected by pedicle with mobile intracardiac thrombus. **F,** Spherical thrombus on pedicle. **G,** Free spherical thrombus.

wrinkled auricle as widely as possible (Fig. 265). Two traction threads are applied in the center of the purse-string suture, between which the auricular walls are cut as widely as possible (Fig. 266). The thrombus is separated from the wall with a spatula, and then entrance is gained into the atrial cavity between the border of the thrombus and the wall of the atrium. The loose parts of the thrombus are washed out with a jet of blood as the edges of the wound are drawn wide apart (Fig. 267). After this the finger is again introduced into the cavity of the left atrium, and the loose thrombotic masses suspended in the cavity, which are to be removed, are palpated. These are hooked with the distal phalanx, dislocated, and washed out of the atrial cavity with a jet of blood (Fig. 268). Massive blood loss occurring in thrombectomy is replaced by stream transfusion of blood.

Mitral stenosis is corrected only after removal of the

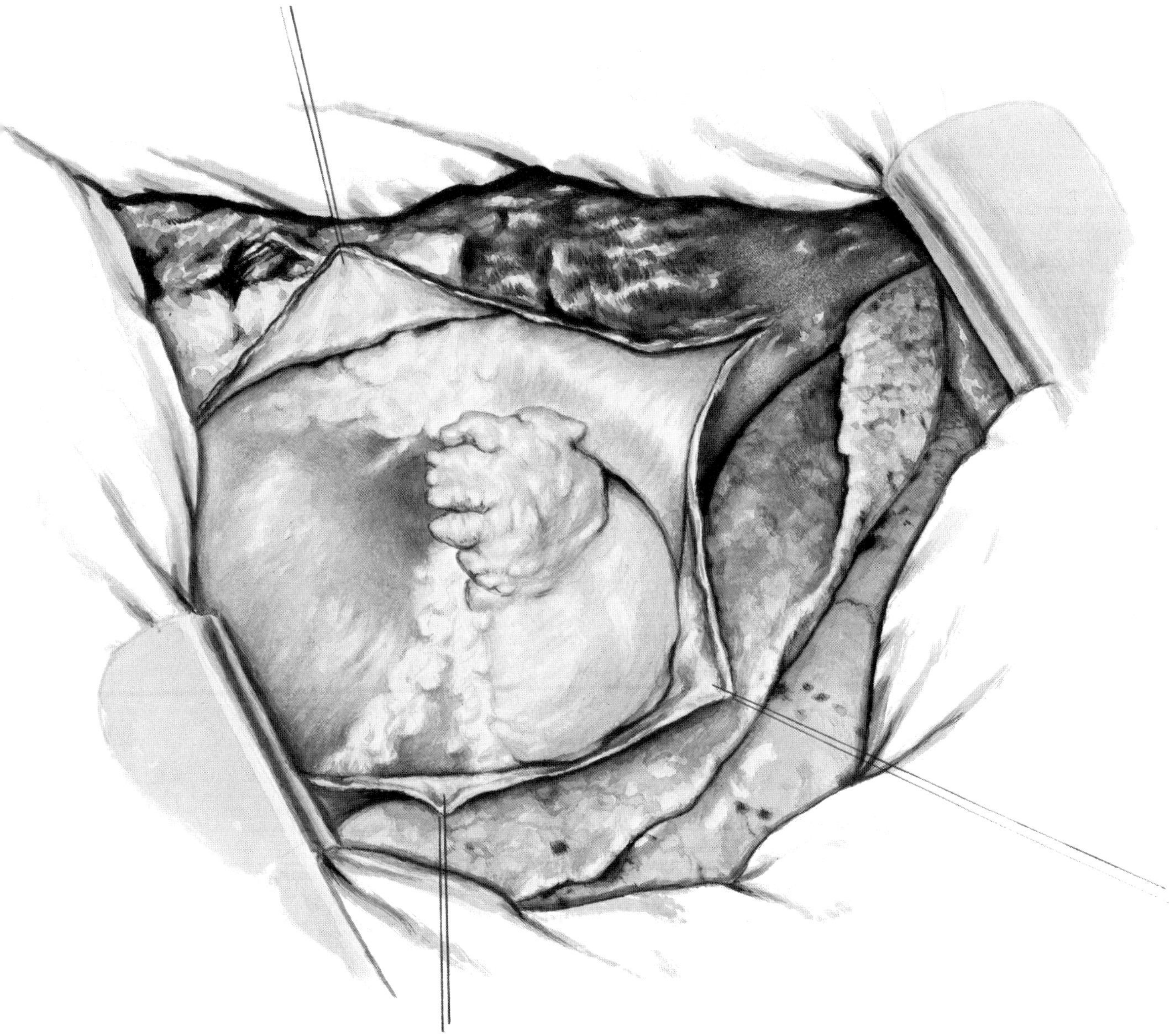

Fig. 264. Appearance of left atrium and its auricle in their thrombosis (auricle is sclerosed and wrinkled).

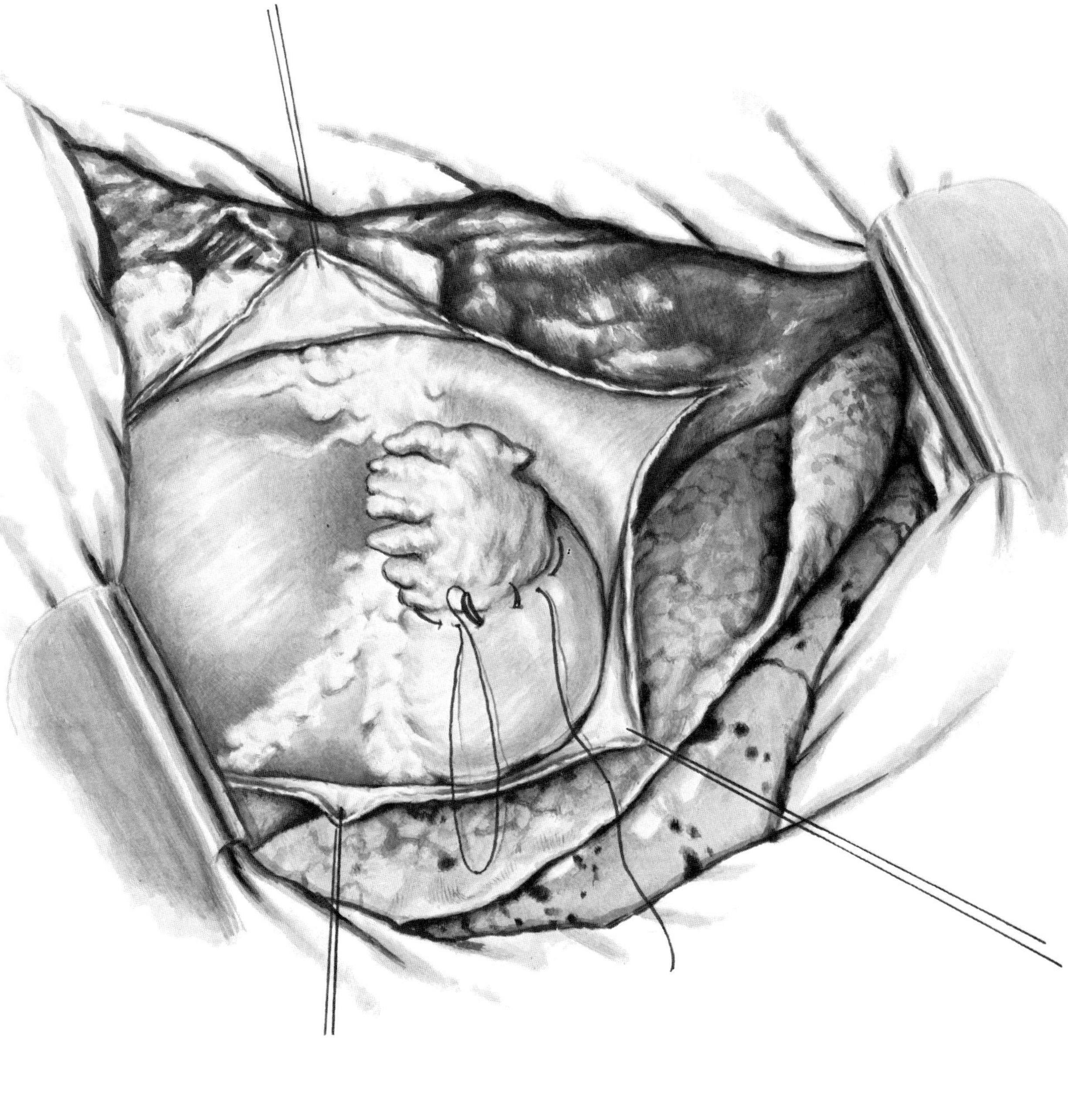

Fig. 265. Purse-string suture is applied around thrombosed auricle of left atrium.

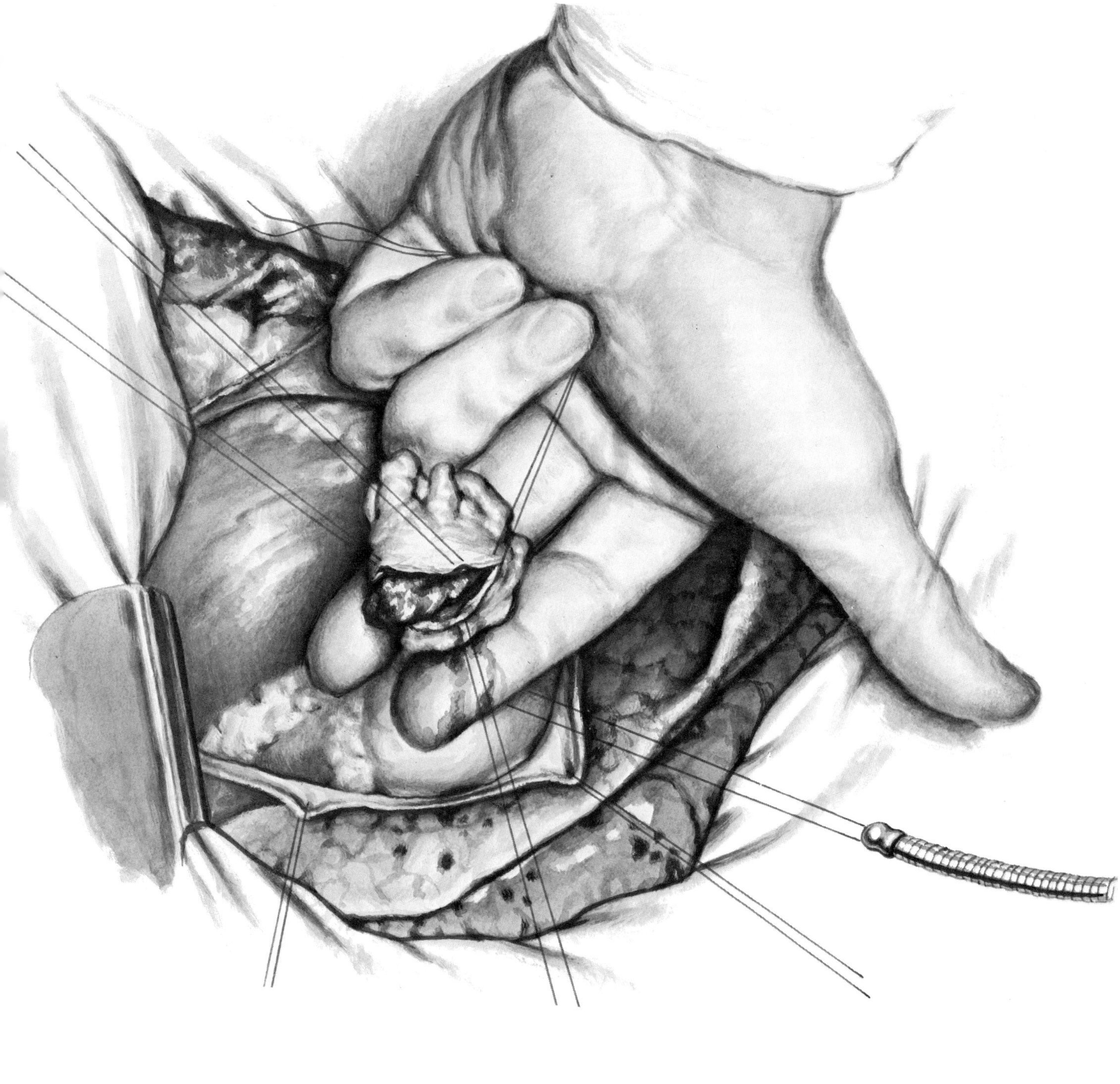

Fig. 266. Incision is made in auricle of thrombosed left atrium.

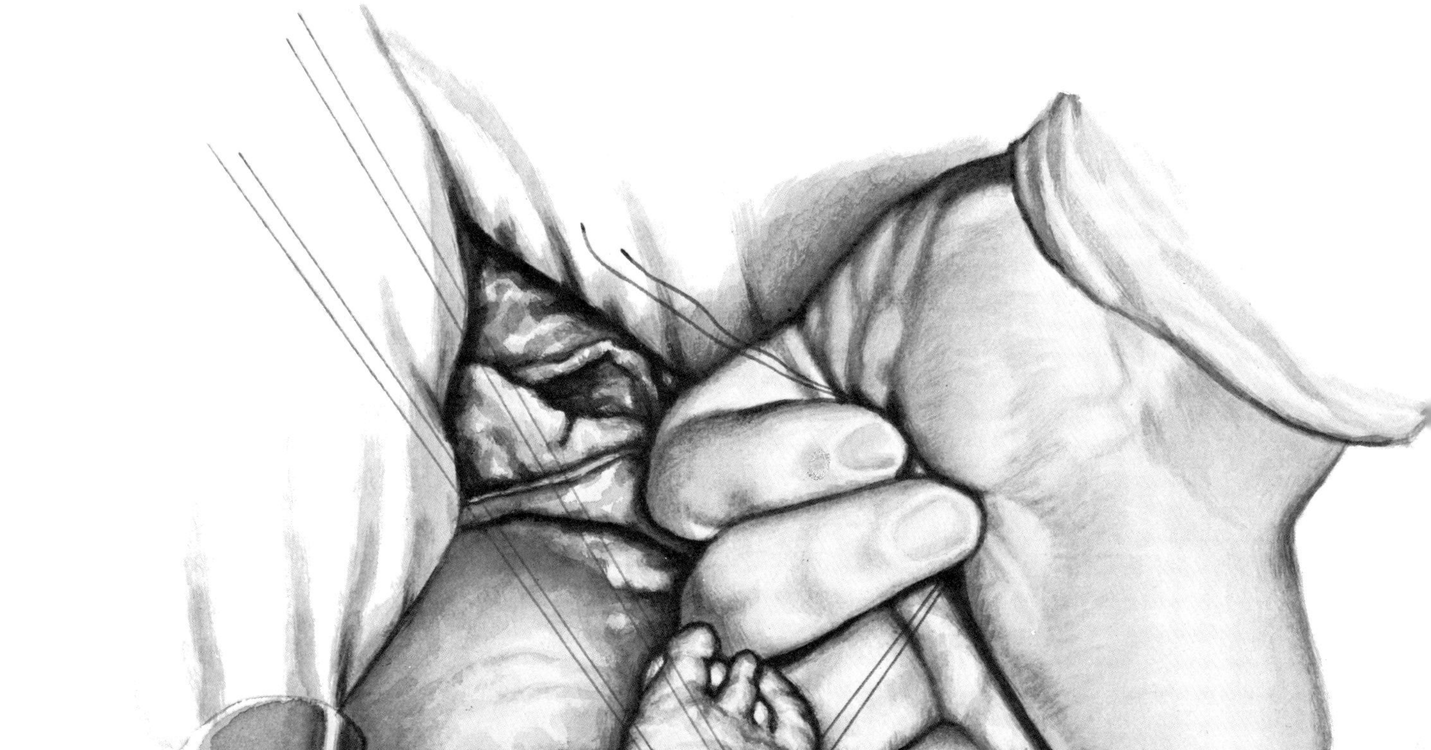

Fig. 267. Removal of thrombus from cavity of left atrium.

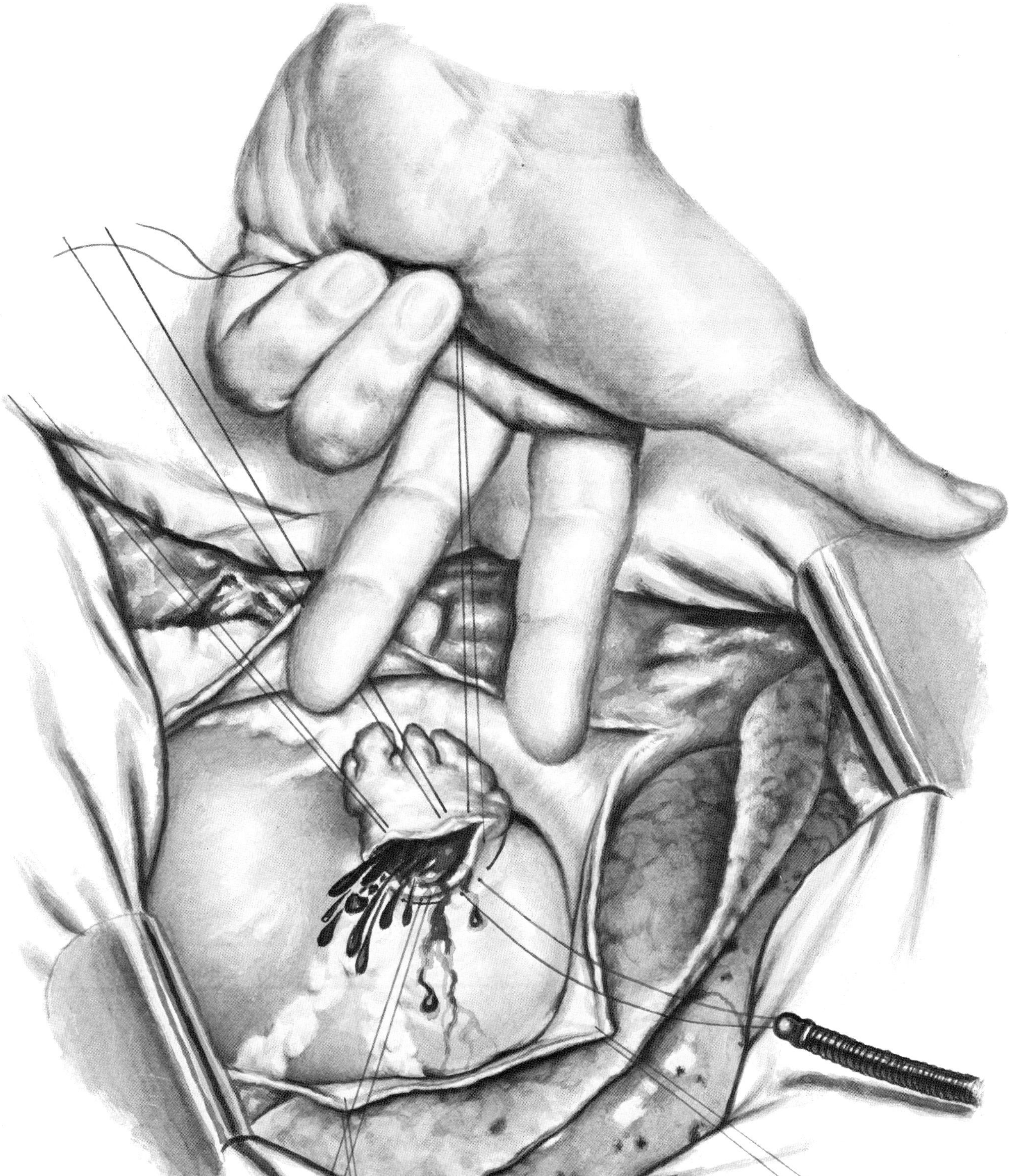

Fig. 268. Remnants of thrombus are expelled by jet of blood.

thrombi. The thrombi located on the posterior and superior walls of the left atrium are not removed in closed heart surgery.

In drastic wrinkling of the auricle the operation may be accomplished through the wall of the left atrium. In this case a purse-string and a wide Halsted suture are applied to the atrial wall between the auricle and the left pulmonary vein. Two traction threads are applied in the center of these sutures, and the ends of the purse-string suture are passed through Rummel's tourniquet (Figs. 269 and 270).

The wall of the left atrium is cut between the traction sutures, and when there is a free lumen in its cavity, the right index finger is inserted and the thrombus separated and removed (Fig. 271).

The left superior pulmonary vein may be used to by-

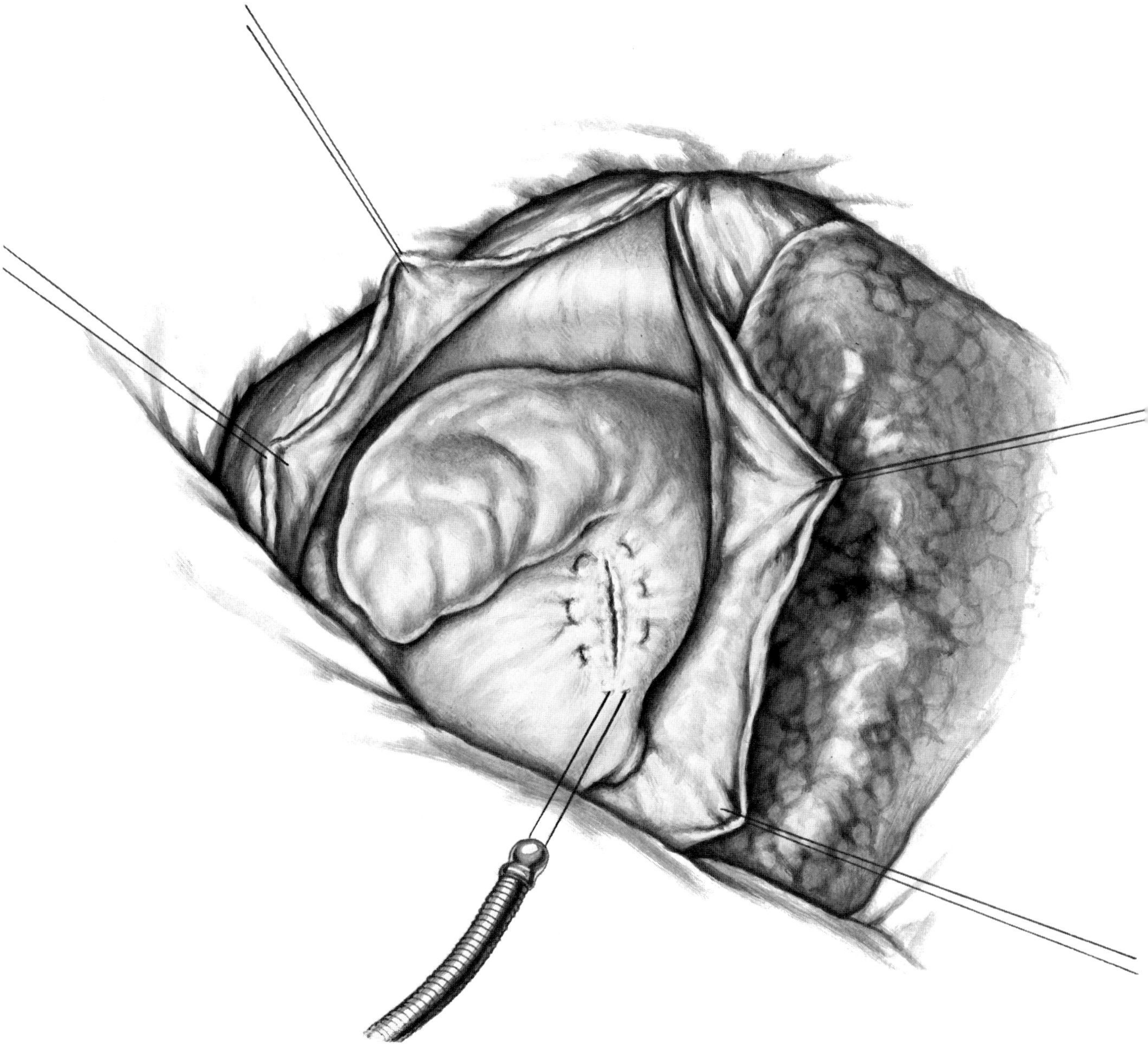

Fig. 269. Access into left atrium through its wall.

pass the thrombus with the finger, for which purpose a purse-string suture and traction sutures are applied to it (Fig. 272). After its wall is clamped lengthwise in the region of the traction sutures, the vein is opened. When the clamp is removed, the index finger is introduced into the vein and the left atrial cavity. Mitral commissurotomy is performed without touching the thrombi (Fig. 273). If necessary, the thrombi may be removed through an additional incision in the auricle with the finger introduced through the vein. In thrombosis many surgeons resort to commissurotomy from the right side.

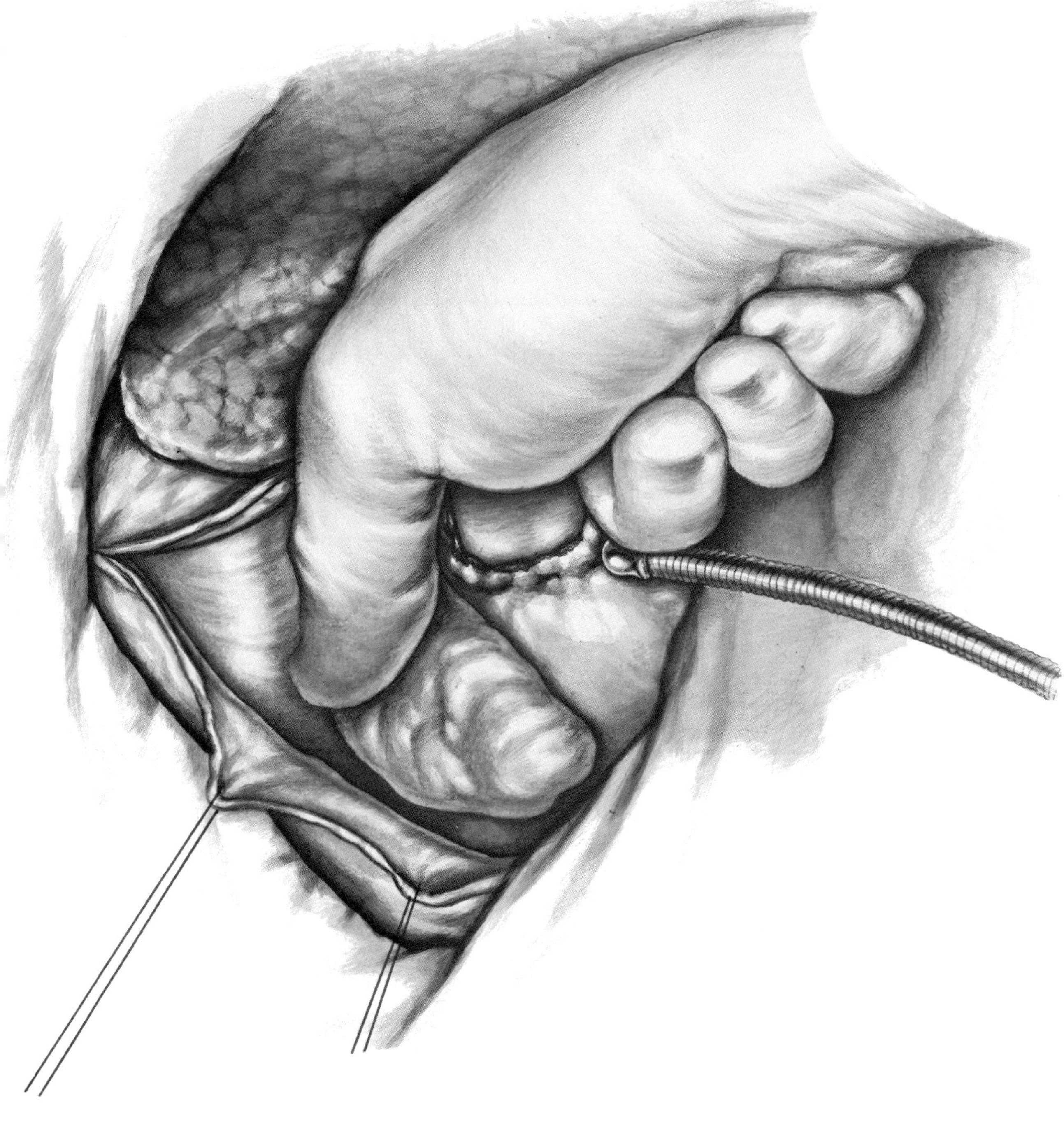

Fig. 270. Cavity of heart is explored through opening in wall of left atrium.

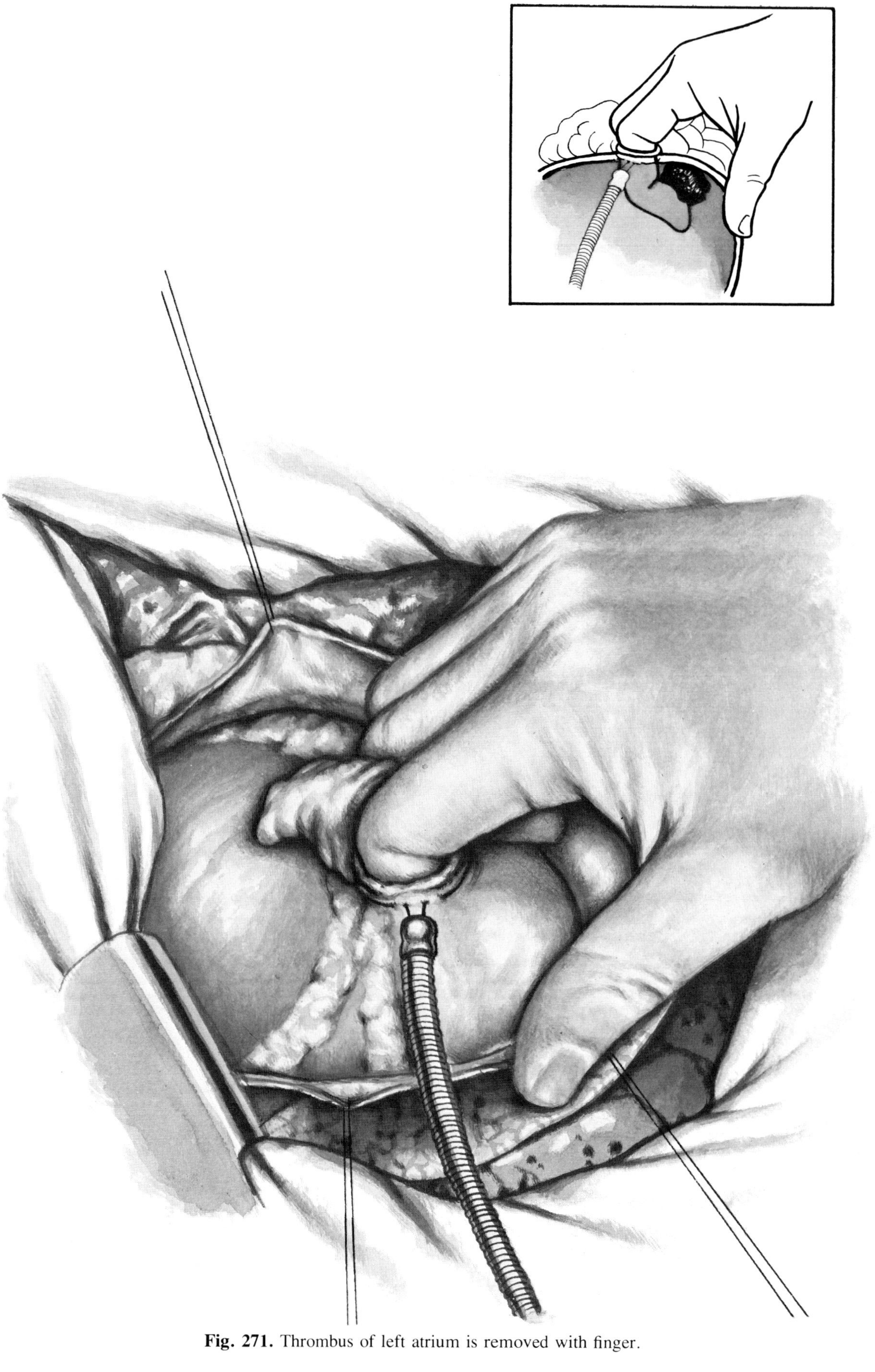

Fig. 271. Thrombus of left atrium is removed with finger.

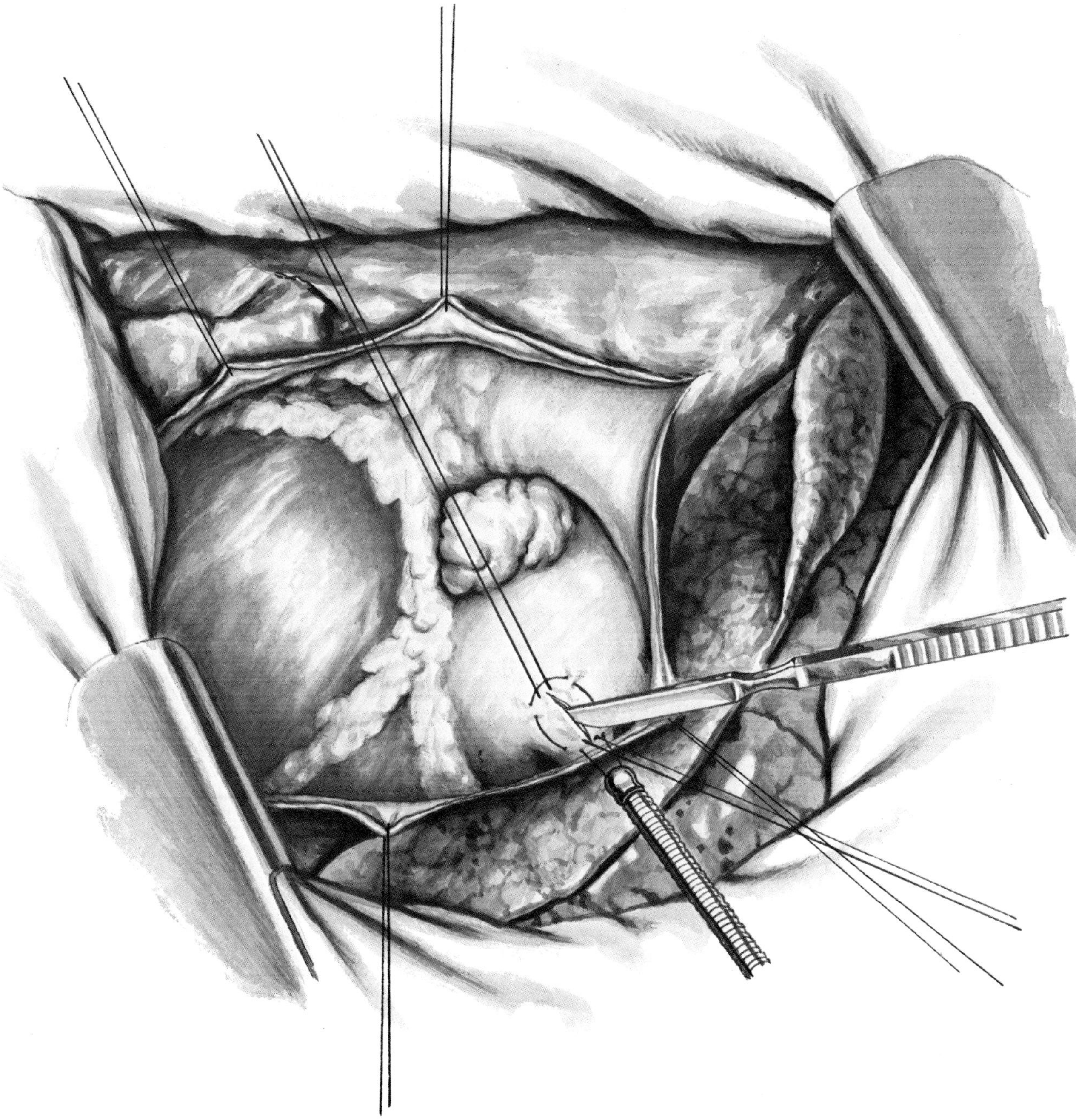

Fig. 272. Incision of left atrium for performing mitral commissurotomy through superior pulmonary vein.

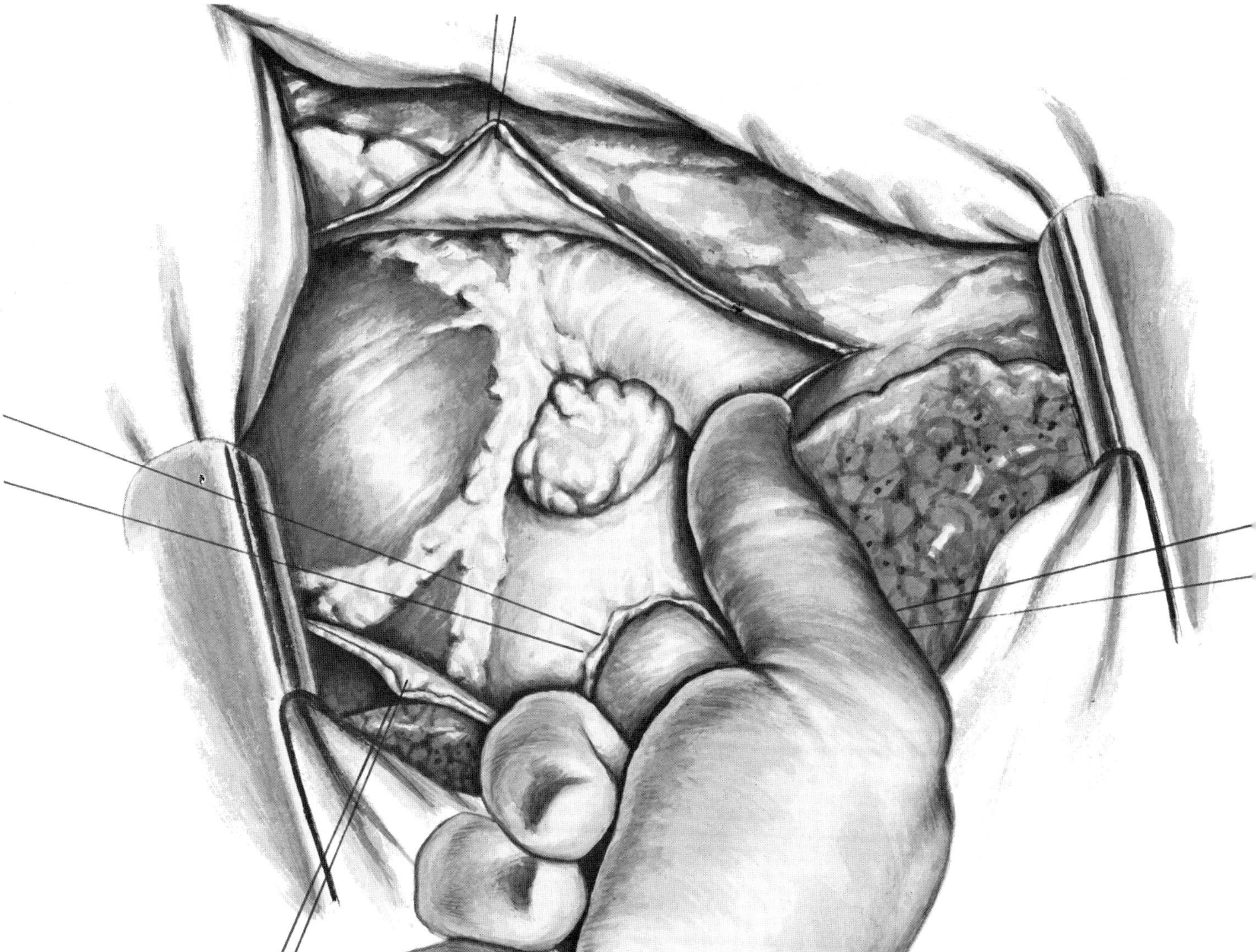

Fig. 273. Performance of mitral commissurotomy by approach through superior pulmonary vein in thrombosis of left atrium.

TRICUSPID COMMISSUROTOMY

Tricuspid commissurotomy may be carried out by a right, transsternal, or left approach. Isolated acquired stenosis of the tricuspid valve is never encountered, and the operation is usually part of an intervention conducted for the defects of other valves. In right thoracotomy in the fourth intercostal space the pericardium is opened with a Halsted incision. The finger may be introduced into the right atrium through the apex of its auricle, but in defects of the tricuspid valve the right atrium is enlarged and the apex of the auricle is displaced retrosternally. This is why manipulations with the finger introduced through the auricle are rather limited. An approach through the lateral wall of the right atrium is used more frequently. For this purpose a purse-string suture is applied with an atraumatic needle, and its ends are passed through a tourniquet (Fig. 274). Two traction sutures are applied in the center of the suture. Since the wall of the right atrium is thin, it is punctured with a needle in the region of pink bands, which correspond to the trabecular thickenings here. Satinsky's clamp is applied to the right atrial wall in the region of the purse-string suture, and a cut is made between the traction sutures (Fig. 275).

The left index finger is introduced into the atrium,

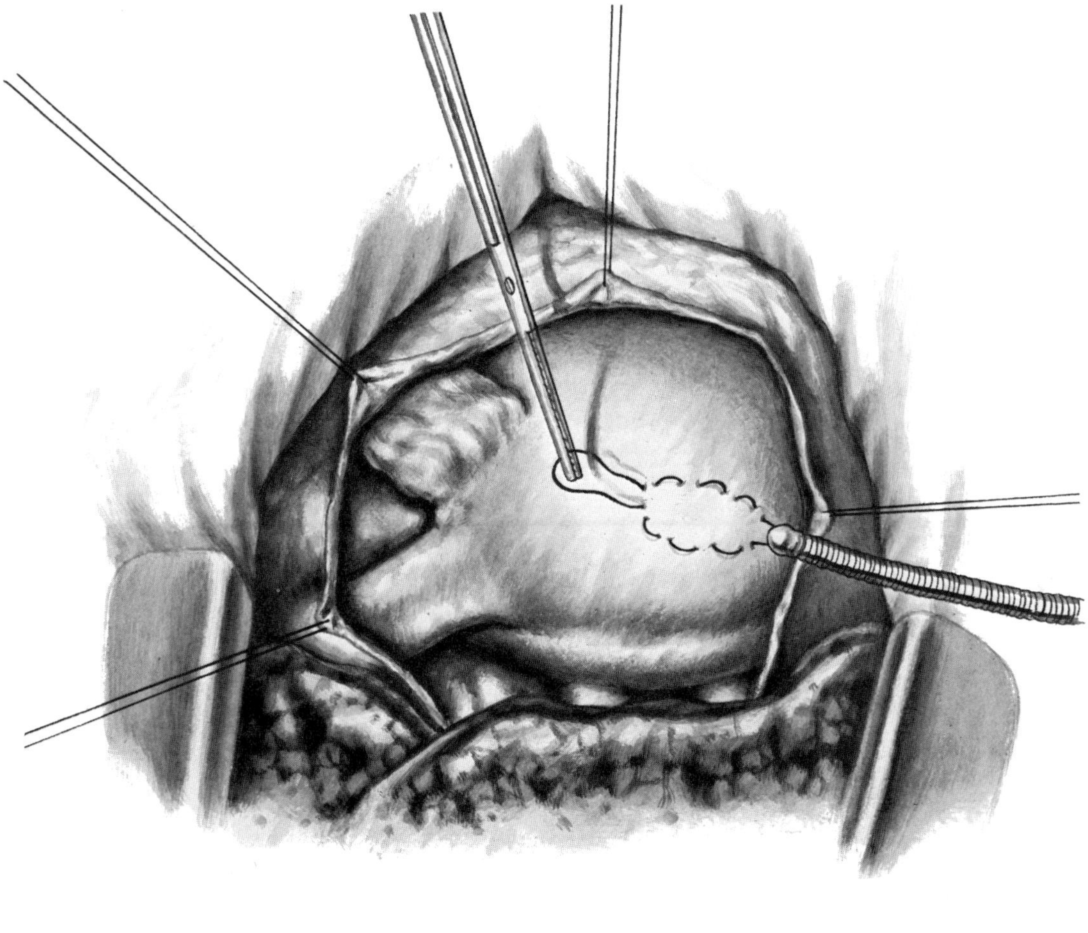

Fig. 274. Purse-string suture is applied to wall of right atrium.

and two commissures are usually separated with it (Fig. 276). Separation of all three commissures usually causes regurgitation. The atrial wound is sutured (Fig. 277).

In the transsternal approach, access to the tricuspid valve is most frequently gained through the auricle.

In mitral commissurotomy by a left approach, stenosis of the right atrioventricular orifice may be suspected when there is a diastolic thrill on the right ventricle. In such cases, stenosis of the tricuspid valve may be corrected from the left pleural cavity. The right auricle may be reached when the pericardium is opened widely. The incision in the pericardium is made ventrally to the phrenic nerve, and the apex of the right auricle is pulled out into the left pleural cavity by everting traction sutures (Figs. 278 and 279). The same may be accomplished through an additional incision of the pericardium behind the sternum.

The apex of the right auricle is held with a triangular clamp, and a purse-string suture is applied with an atraumatic needle (Fig. 280).

The auricle is opened by the routine method after applying Satinsky's clamp, its edges are held with the threads of blanket sutures, and the finger is introduced into the atrial cavity (Fig. 281). If the tricuspid valve is inaccessible by digital commissurotomy, instrumental separation of the commissures is carried out through the lower third of the anterior wall of the right ventricle.

The blades are opened up to 4.5 to 5 cm. The position of the end of the instrument and the result of the manipulation are checked by a finger inserted into the right auricle.

A ligature is placed on the right auricle below the purse-string suture. In transventricular commissurotomy the wound in the right ventricle is closed by tying the Halsted suture and with additional interrupted sutures applied with an atraumatic needle.

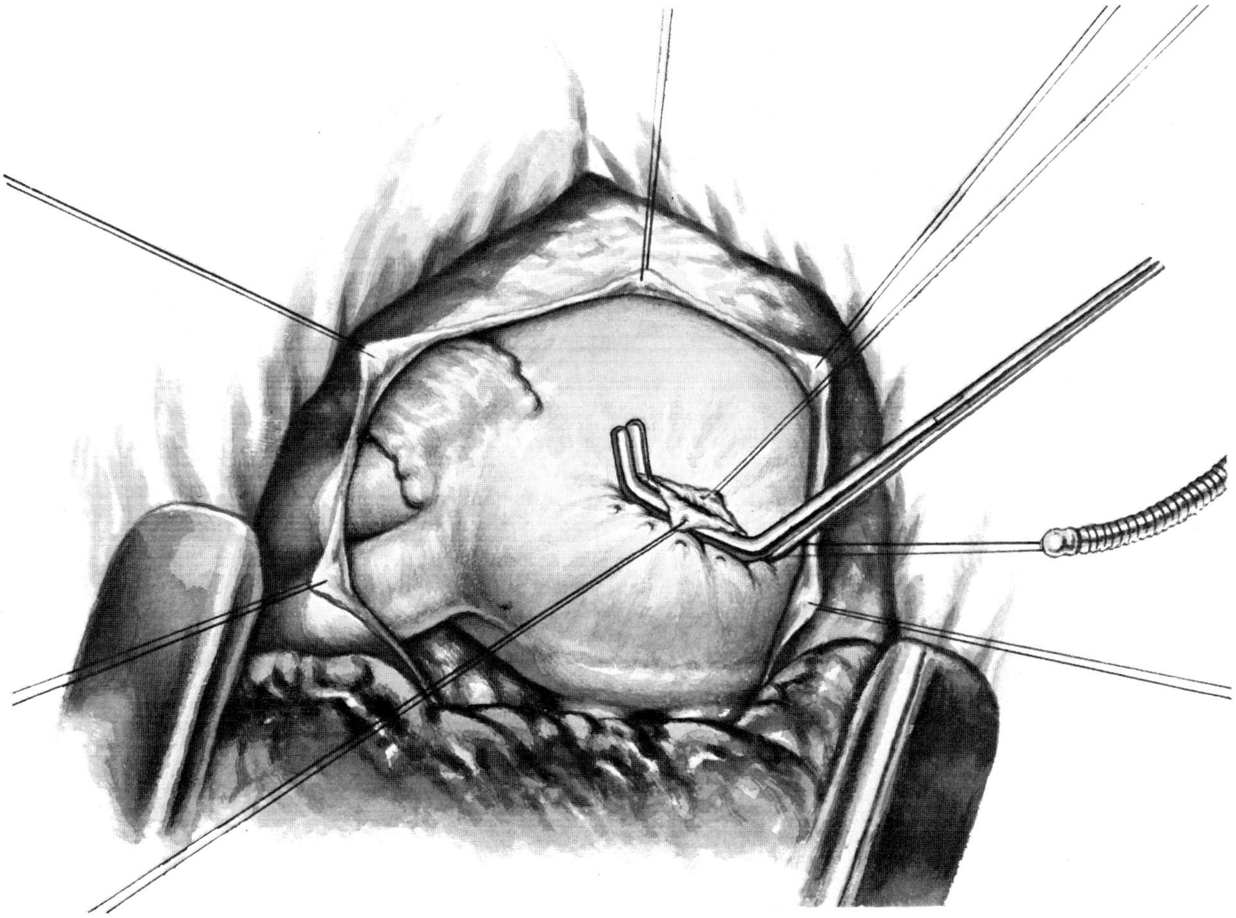

Fig. 275. Right atrial wall in region of purse-string suture is compressed with Satinsky's clamp and opened between traction sutures.

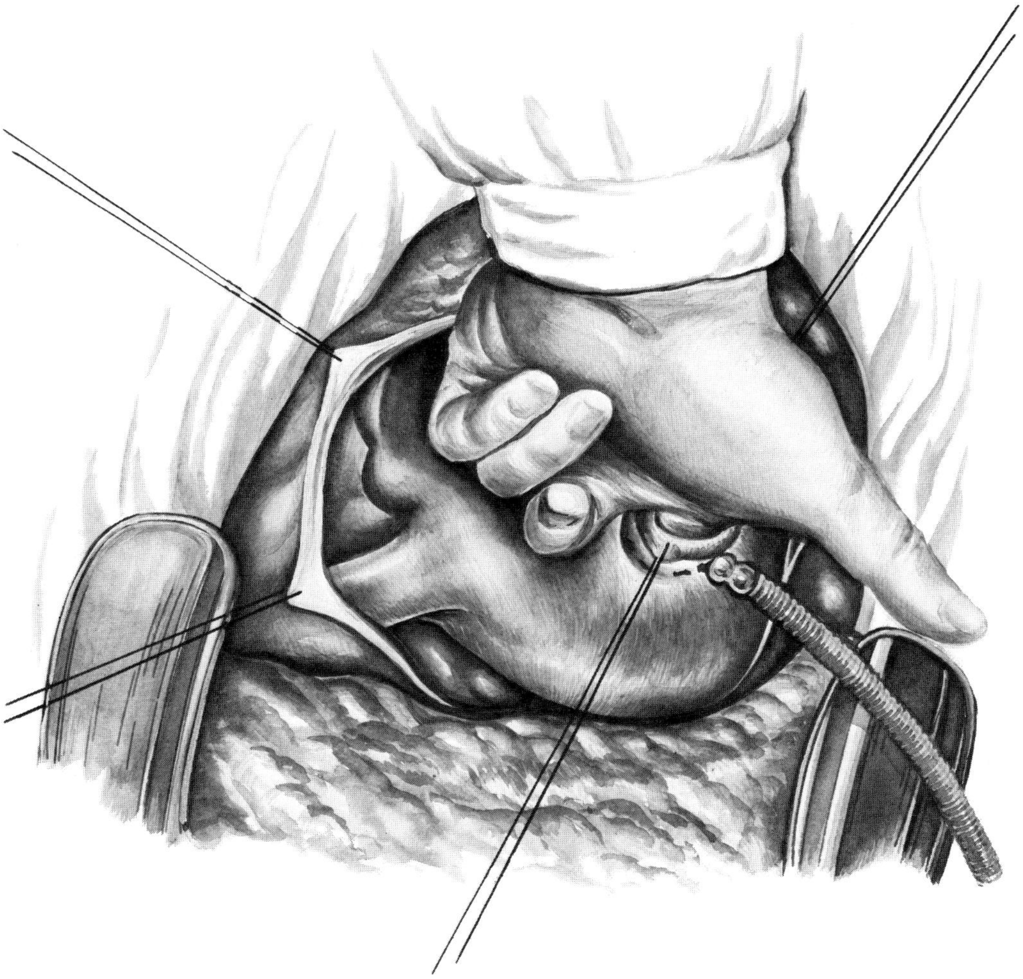

Fig. 276. Separation of commissures of tricuspid valve.

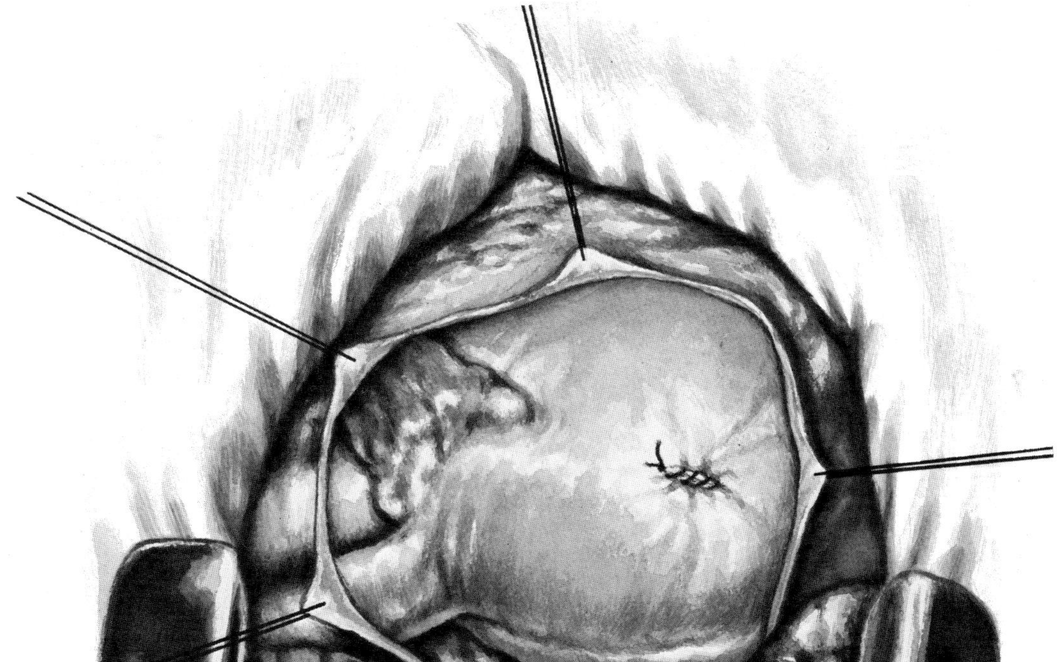

Fig. 277. Closure of wound in right atrium.

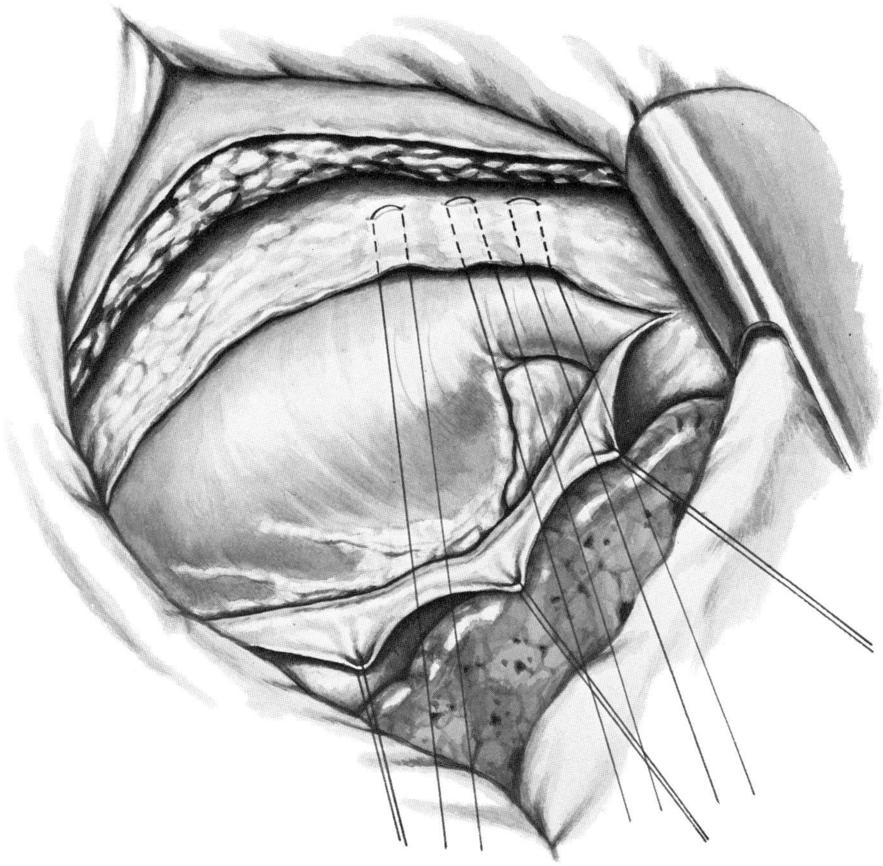

Fig. 278. Pericardium is opened, and everting traction sutures are applied in left approach.

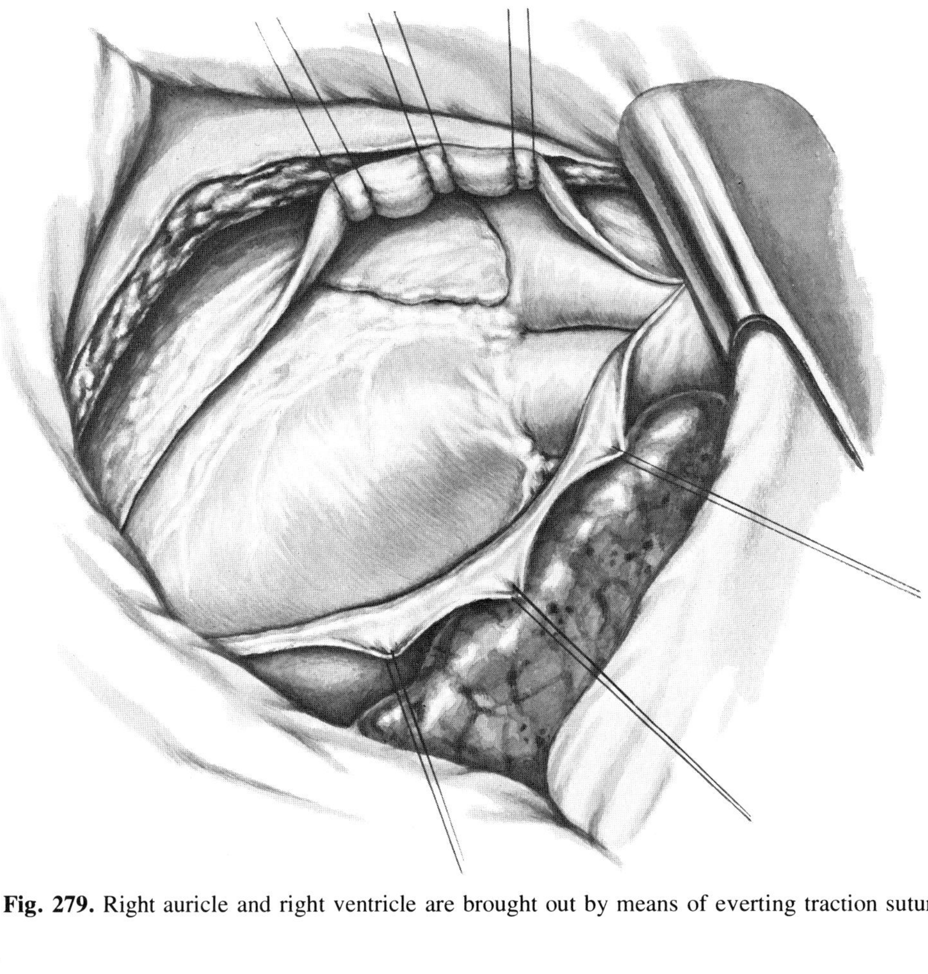

Fig. 279. Right auricle and right ventricle are brought out by means of everting traction sutures.

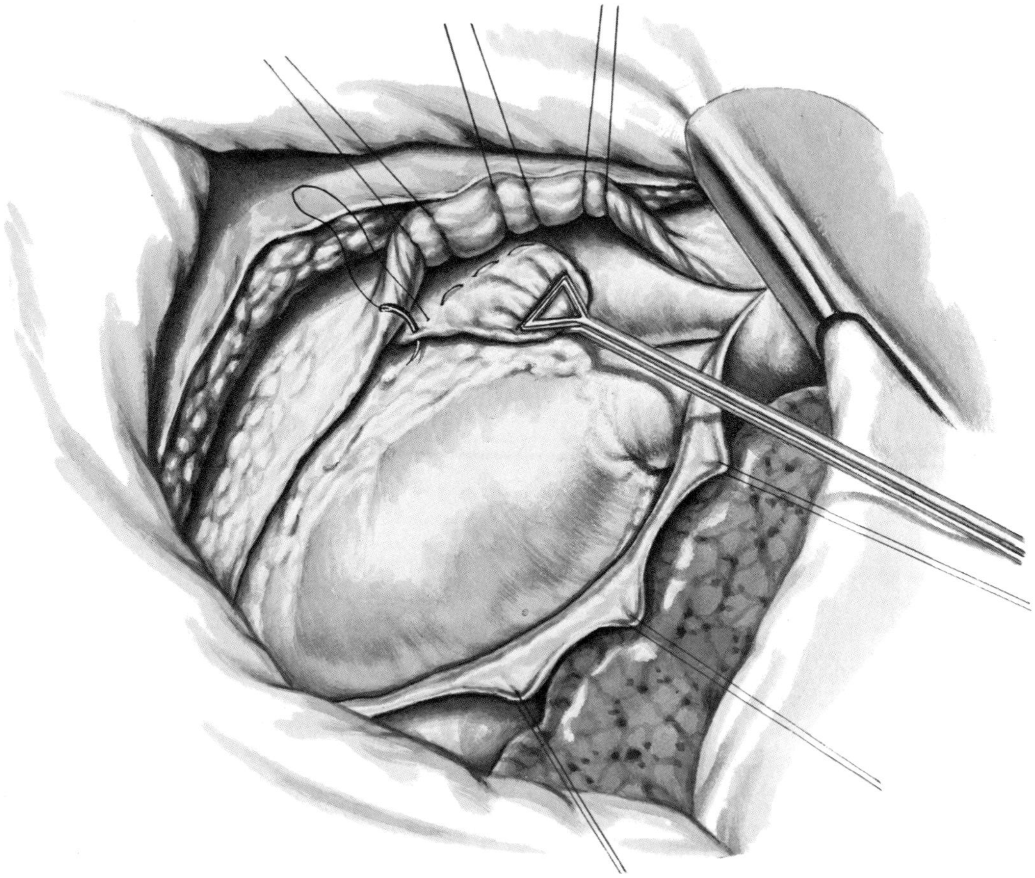

Fig. 280. Purse-string suture is applied to right auricle.

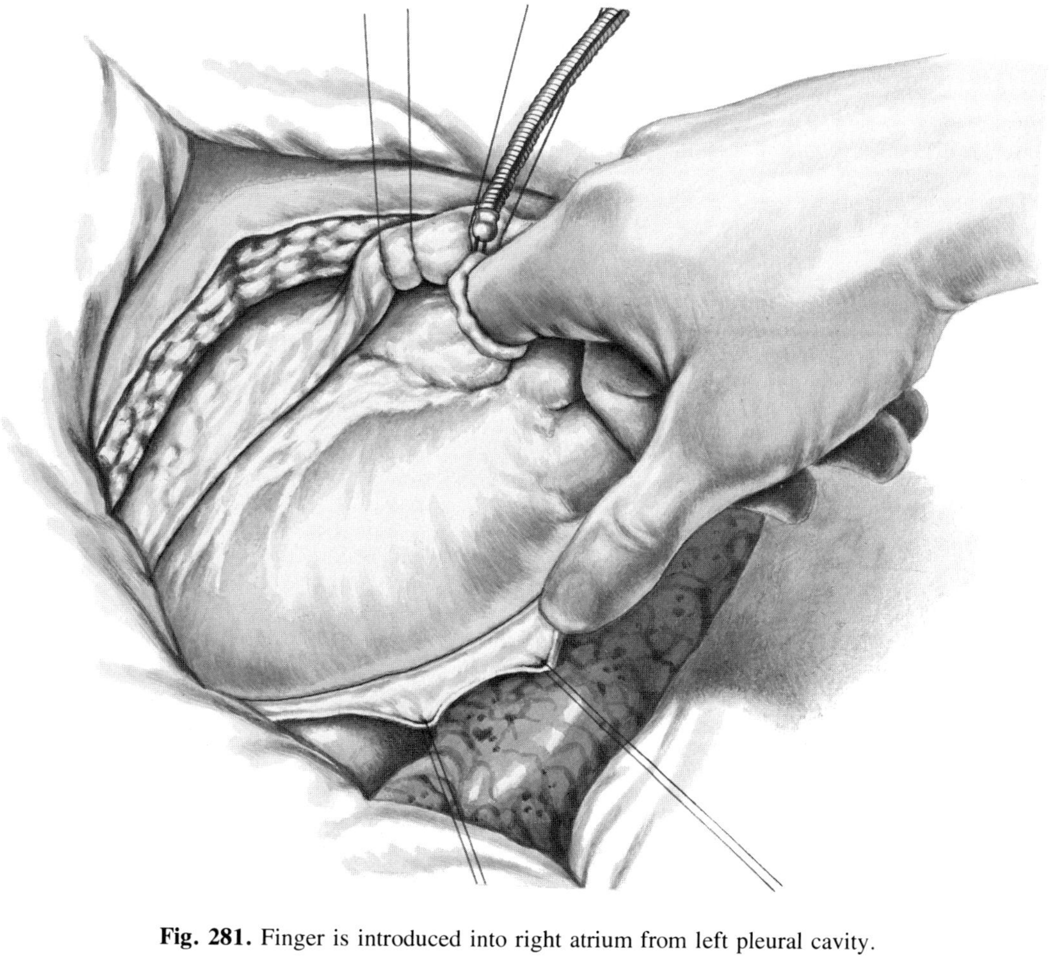

Fig. 281. Finger is introduced into right atrium from left pleural cavity.

INSTRUMENTAL AORTIC COMMISSUROTOMY

The operation is conducted through a left anterolateral or lateral approach in the fifth intercostal space.

The pericardium is opened wide ventral and parallel to the phrenic nerve, and the apex of the left ventricle is dislocated into the pericardial incision by putting two large gauze napkins under the posterior surface of the heart. A Halsted or purse-string suture is placed in the avascular zone of the left ventricular apex. If the myocardium is sclerosed, Teflon bolsters are used when applying the Halsted suture to prevent the thread from cutting through the tissues.

A stab wound is made in the left ventricular wall in the center of the purse-string suture between the traction sutures; care must be taken to prevent the scalpel from invading the cavity (Fig. 282). A triple-blade dilator is introduced through this wound into the left ventricle; the position of the blades should correspond to that of the aortic commissures (Fig. 283). The position of the end of the instrument is checked by palpating it in the aortic lumen through the transverse sinus of the pericardium. The aortic orifice is dilated, and the dilator removed.

The wound in the left ventricle is sutured by the method described.

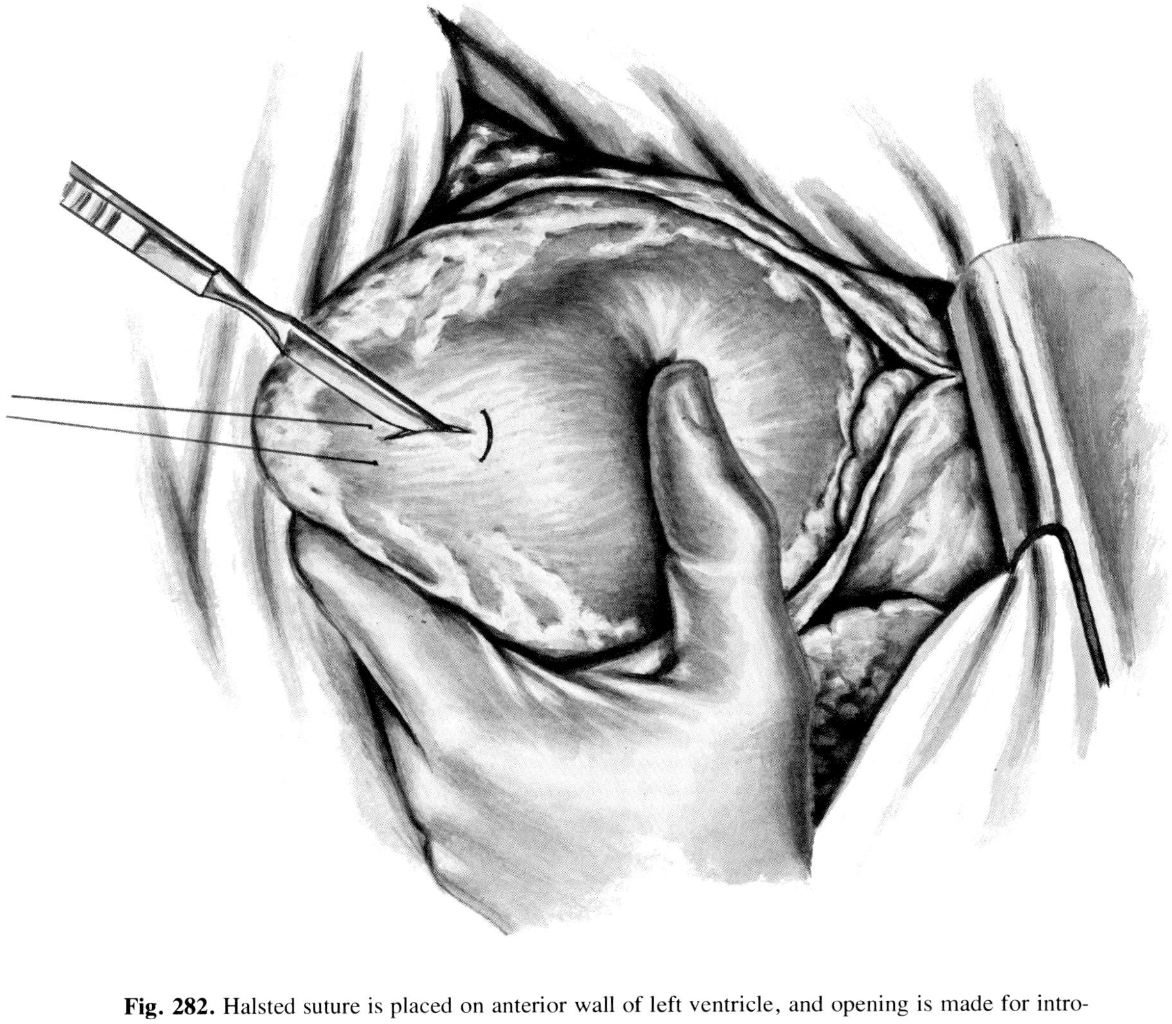

Fig. 282. Halsted suture is placed on anterior wall of left ventricle, and opening is made for introducing dilator.

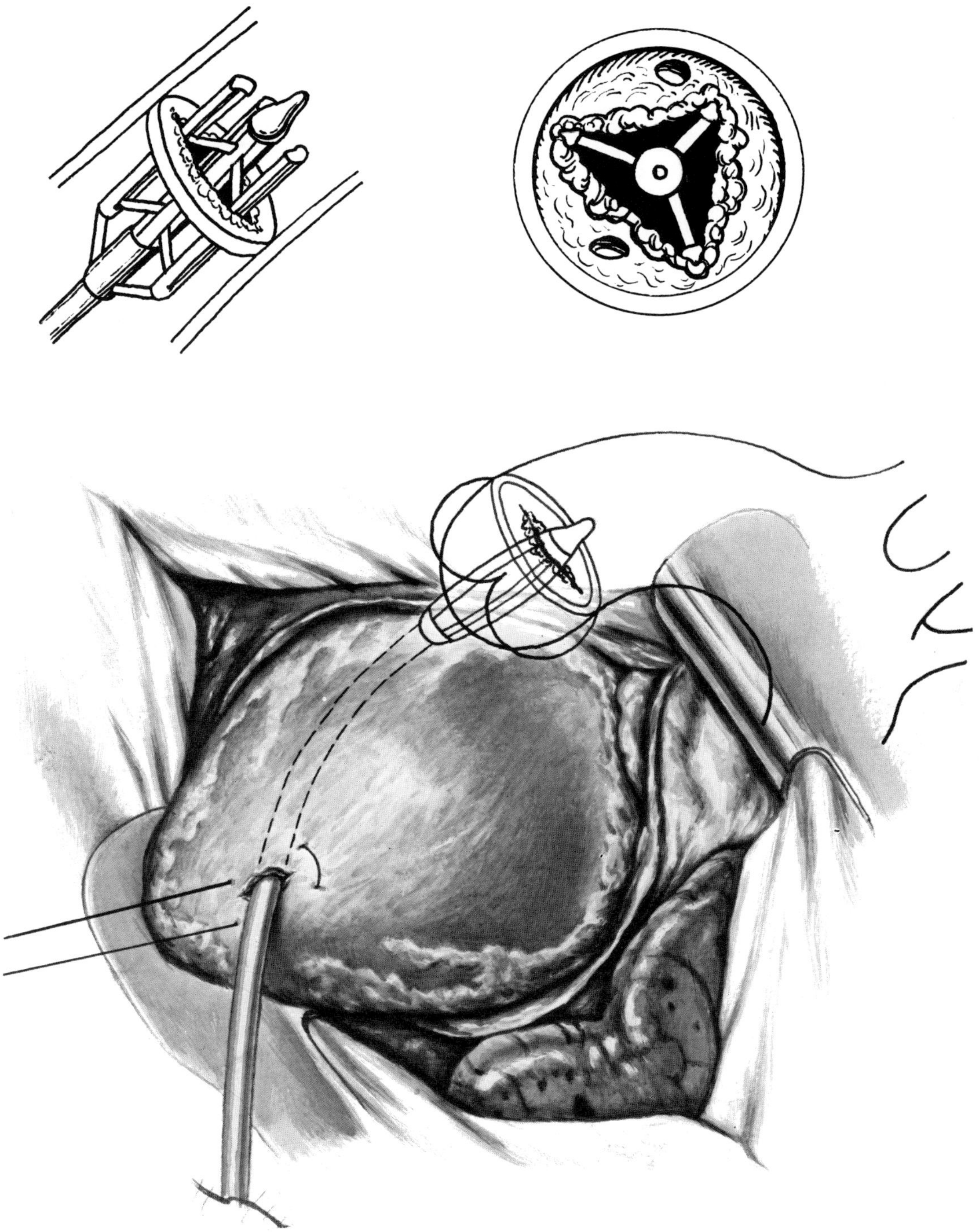

Fig. 283. Position of dilator and its blades at moment when aortic orifice is dilated.

CORRECTION OF PATENT DUCTUS ARTERIOSUS

The operation is carried out through left lateral or posterolateral thoracotomy. The lung is moved ventrally and caudally. The mediastinal pleura overlying the aorta in the region of the patent ductus arteriosus is opened by means of hydraulic procaine dissection or without it (Fig. 284). The aorta is slightly dilated in the region of the duct.

The presence of the duct is determined by the incessant systolic-diastolic thrill over the pulmonary trunk and the left pulmonary artery. The vagus nerve is separated from the cellular tissue of the posterior mediastinum over the aortic arch medial to the origin of the left subclavian artery with a dissector, and a loop is applied to draw it away.

The ductus arteriosus is freed by blunt and sharp dissection. A small dissector is brought around its dorsal wall, and two silk ligatures are drawn under the duct. Trial clamping of the duct is performed, which arrests the systolic-diastolic murmur. Simultaneously, the state of hemodynamics is examined, and the absence of cyanosis is confirmed. Clamping of the duct may cause cyanosis if it is attendant to tetralogy of Fallot.

The duct is tied with a thick silk ligature, first at the aortic and then at the pulmonary end. After that a thread is stitched through it between the ligatures and tied on both sides (Figs. 285 to 287).

When the ductus arteriosus is wide and its wall is

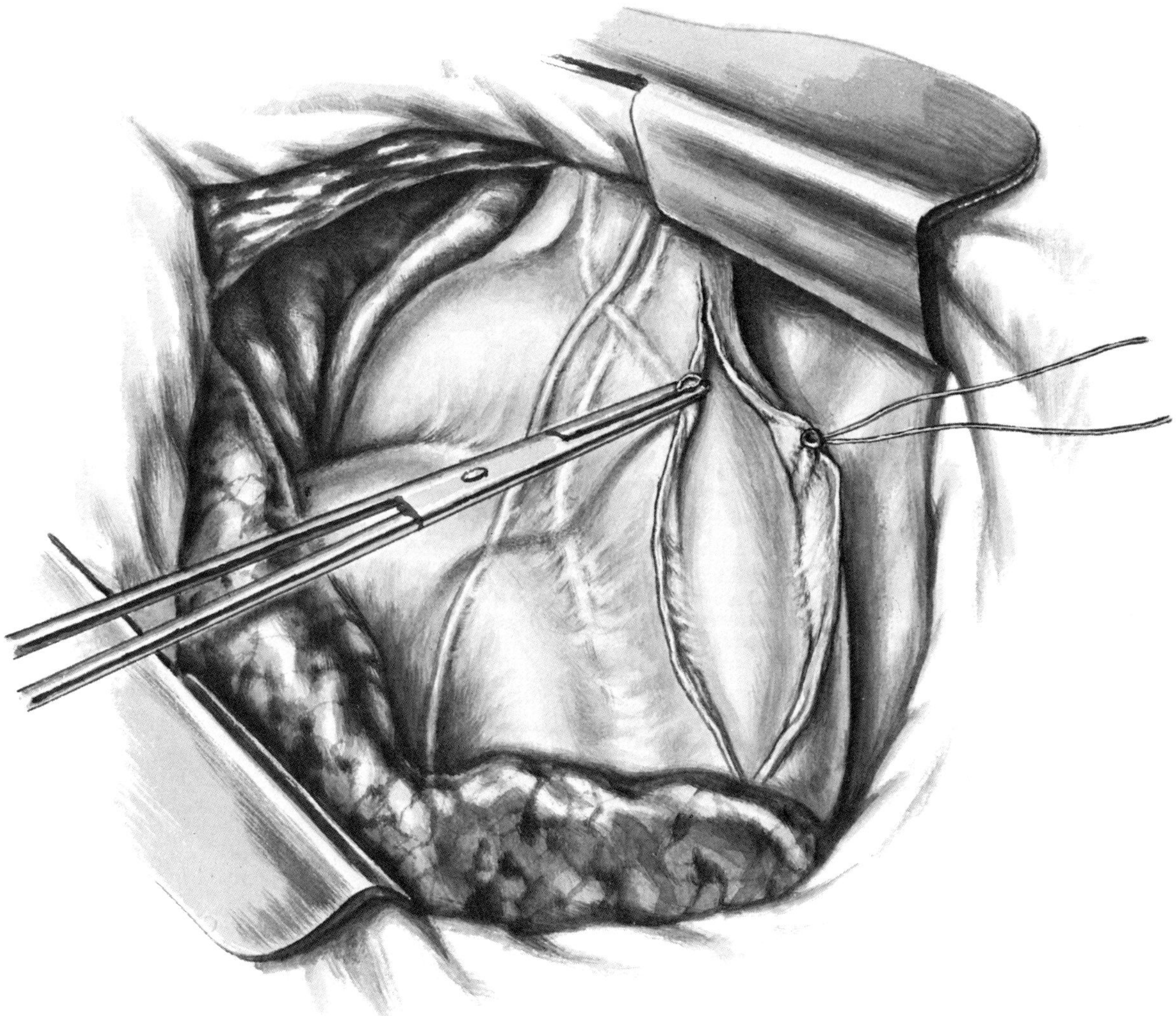

Fig. 284. Mediastinal pleura is incised over descending aorta.

severely sclerosed, its ligation may be hazardous because the threads may cut through the walls and recanalization of the duct may occur. In such cases the duct is transected, and its ends closed with sutures. The aorta is separated distal and proximal to the duct; rubber loops are passed around it with a large dissector; and then its dorsal wall is mobilized.

After these precautionary measures have been taken in the event of bleeding and trial clamping of the duct has been performed, two special clamps are applied to it between which the duct is transected (Fig. 288). To avoid damaging the recurrent laryngeal nerve when the clamps are applied, attention should be focussed on the position of this nerve, which passes caudally and dorsally around the patent ductus arteriosus. The ends of the duct are closed with a continuous suture, using an atraumatic needle (Figs. 289 and 290).

If the ductus arteriosus is short and wide, the pericardium is opened over the left pulmonary artery, and the pulmonary end of the duct is exposed intrapericardially for clamping it within the pericardium with partial clamping of the wall of the pulmonary artery.

When a patent ductus arteriosus is combined with other congenital anomalies that are corrected through a transsternal extrapleural approach, the duct is ligated intrapericardially, separating it in the region of the superior wall where the left pulmonary artery arises (Fig. 291). The pulmonary trunk should not be constricted during this manipulation; such an occurrence is fraught with sudden dilatation of the right ventricle.

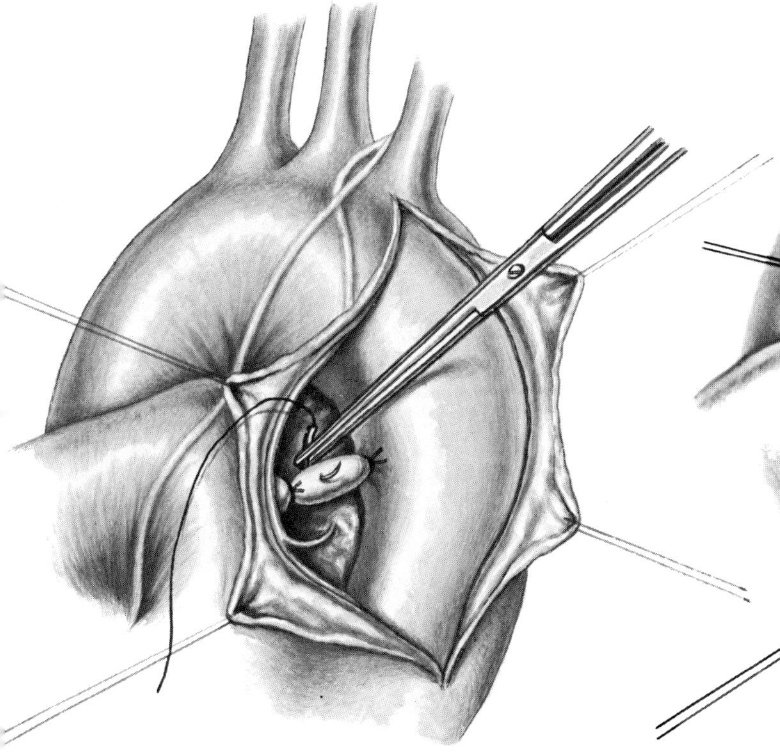

Fig. 285. Double ligation of duct, which is then stitched through.

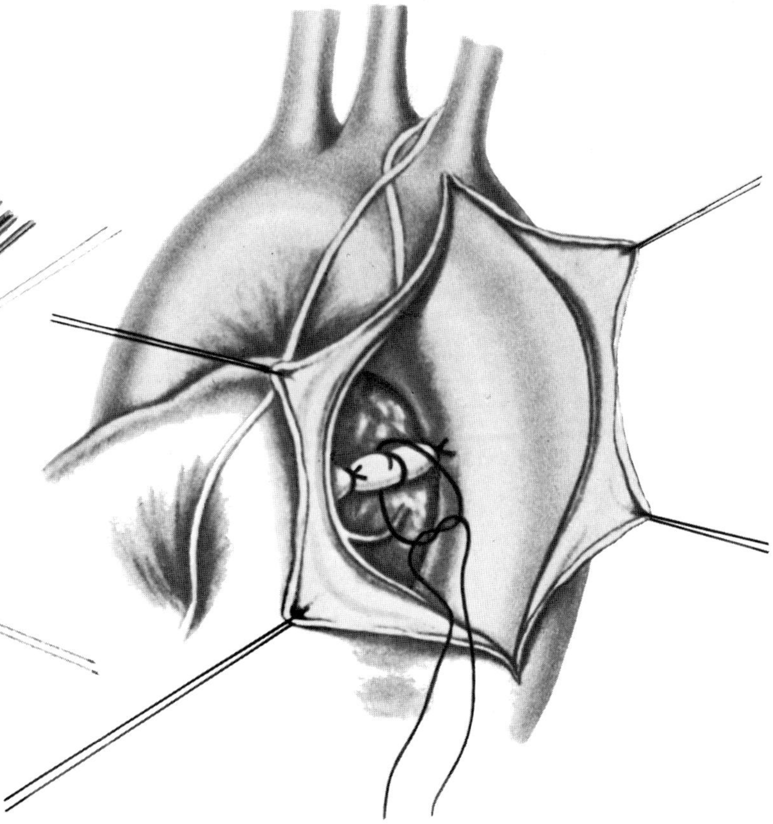

Fig. 286. Ductus arteriosus is tied with ligature that had been stitched through it.

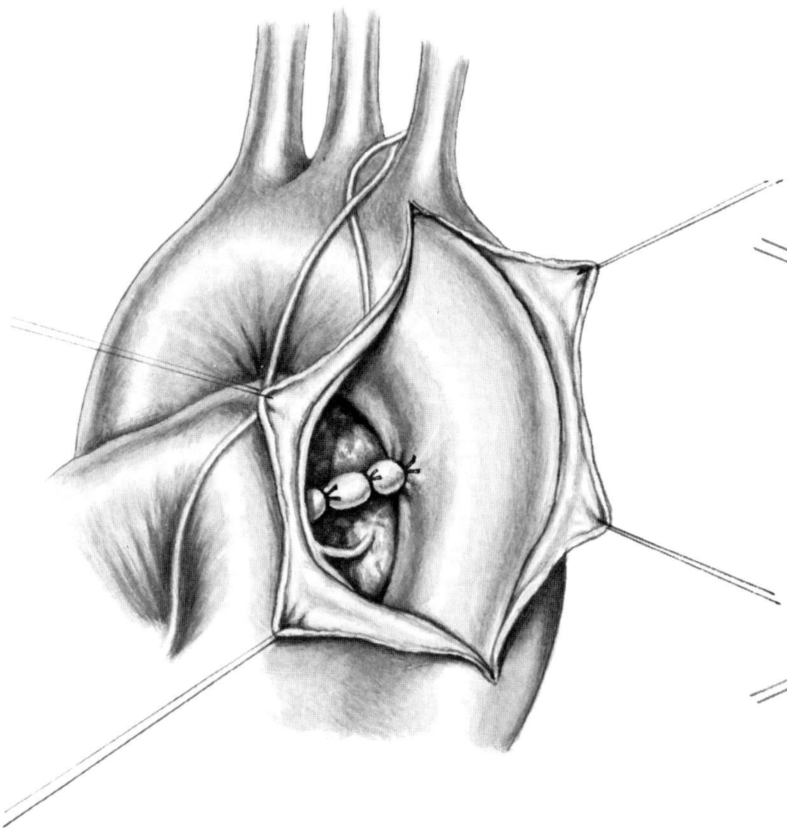

Fig. 287. Patent ductus arteriosus has been stitched through and ligated.

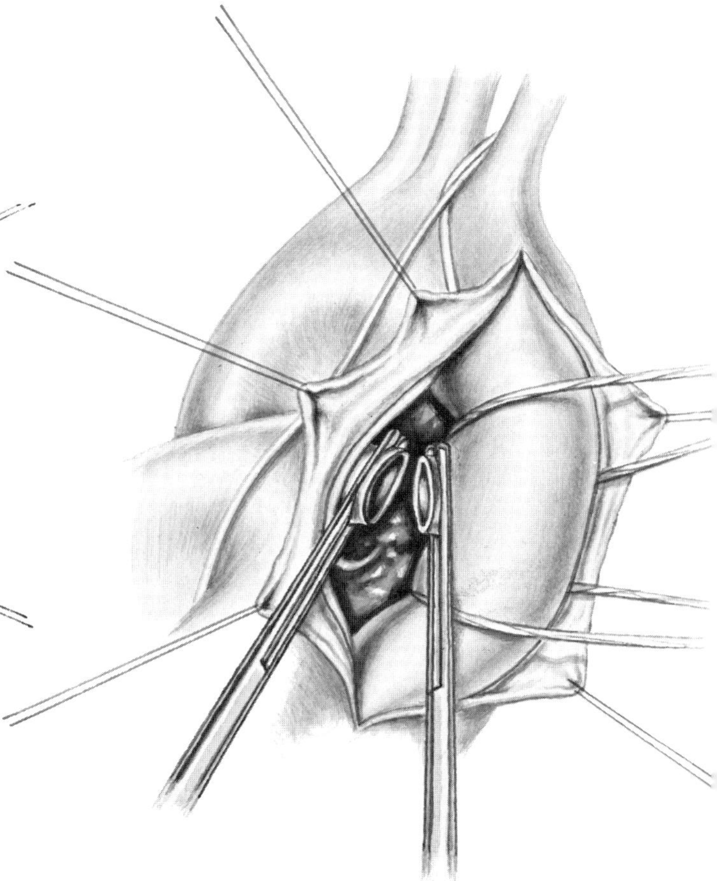

Fig. 288. Transection of wide ductus arteriosus between two clamps. Recurrent laryngeal nerve can be seen next to medial clamp.

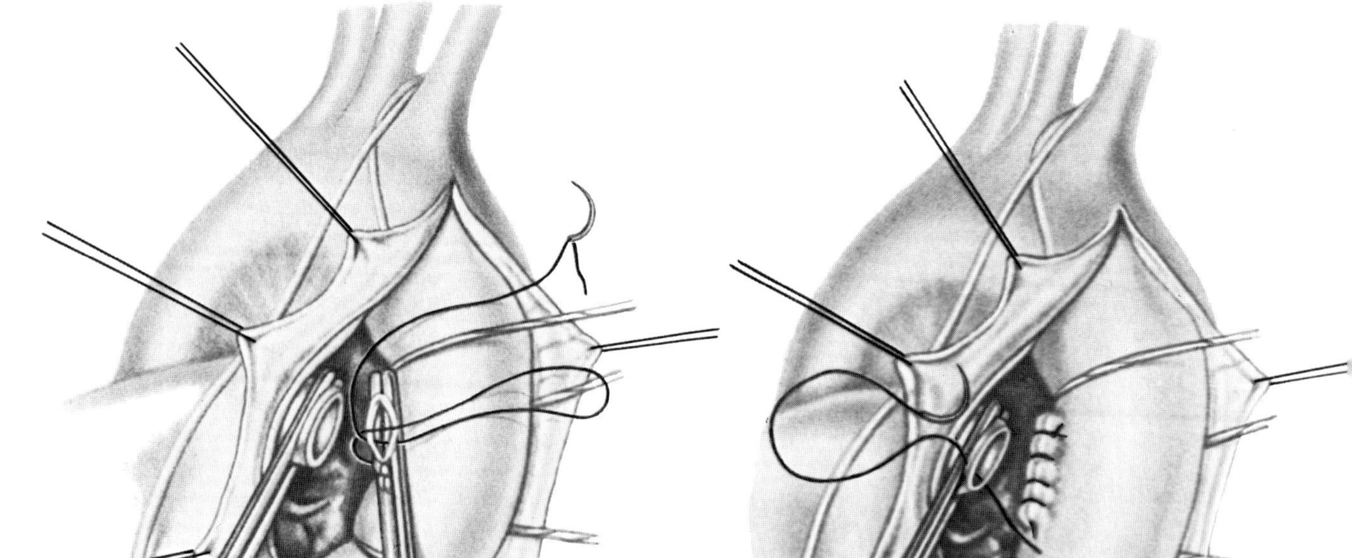

Fig. 289. Ends of transected ductus arteriosus are closed with sutures.

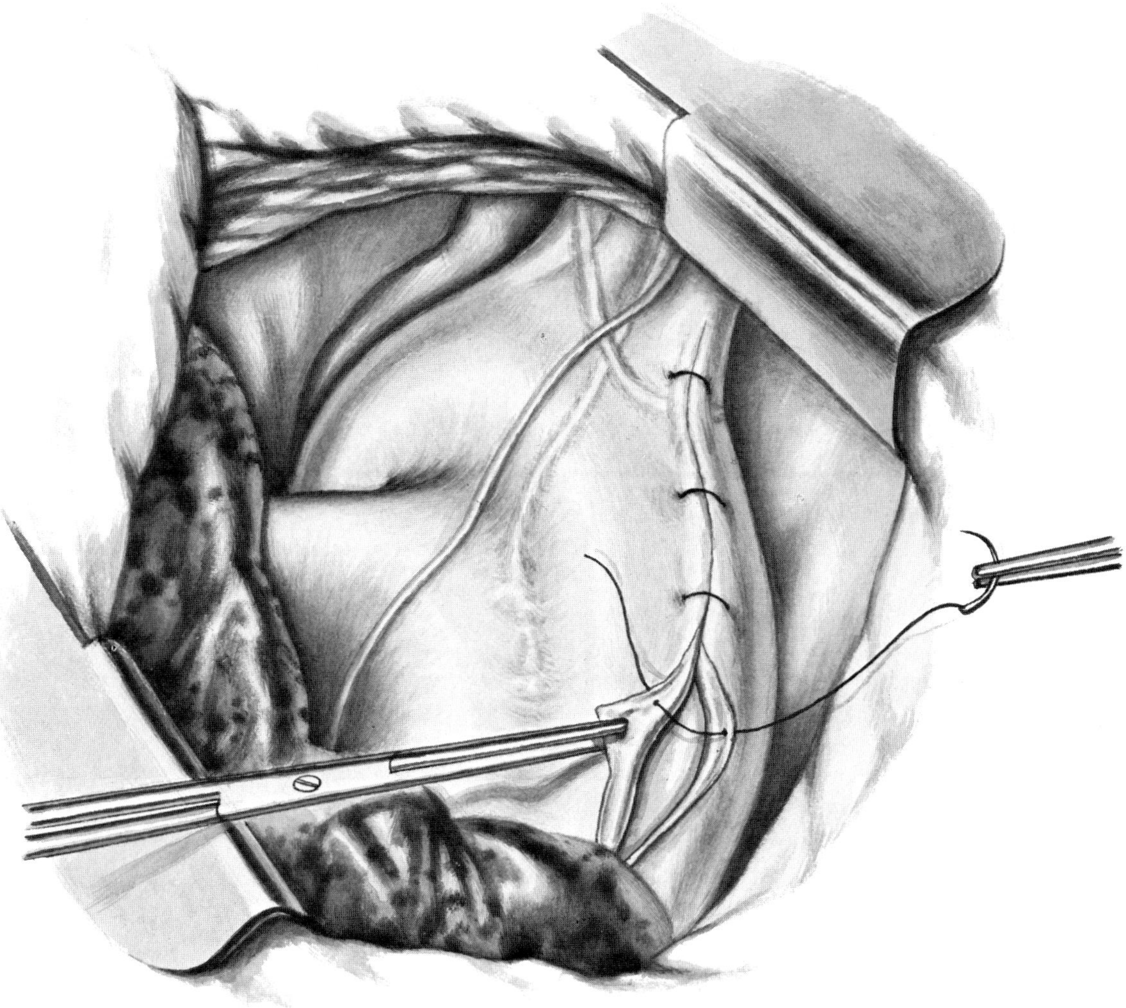

Fig. 290. Sutures are applied to mediastinal pleura.

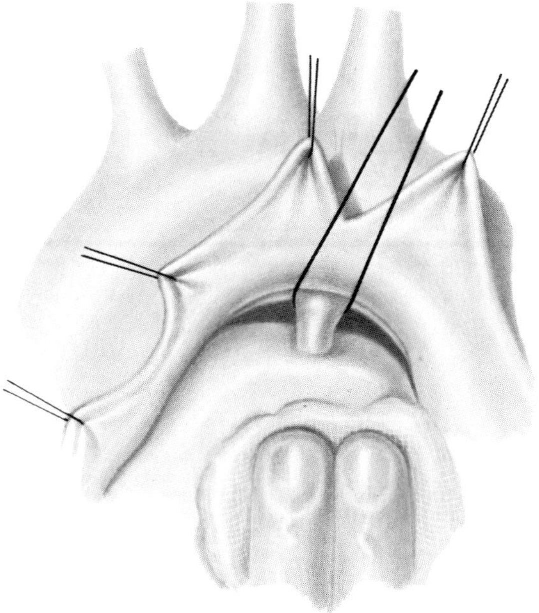

Fig. 291. Intrapericardial separation and ligation of patent ductus arteriosus.

CORRECTION OF COARCTATION OF AORTA

The approach in coarctation of the aorta is typical, left lateral thoracotomy with subperiosteal resection of the fourth or, less frequently, the fifth rib.

Thoracotomy is marked by peculiarities that are due to the presence of powerful arterial collaterals in the thoracic wall. Careful hemostasis with ligation of the vessels is necessary. Since the inferior border of the rib is eroded with the dilated and tortuous intercostal artery, resection of the rib is performed with careful separation of its periosteum using a straight raspatory. It is risky to use Doyen's rib raspatory, because the intercostal arteries may be easily injured.

In children, thoracotomy may be carried out without rib resection.

Two main types of coarctation of the aorta are distinguished: one of short length and with a normal aortic arch (adult type) and the other of considerable length and a hypoplastic arch (children's type). The coarctation may be combined with patent ductus arteriosus located cranially or caudally to the constriction (Fig. 292).

The lung is moved ventrally and caudally, exposing the posterior mediastinum and the arch of the aorta. After procaine hydrochloride solution is injected under the mediastinal pleura, it is opened wide beginning from the middle of the intrathoracic part of the left subclavian artery and ending 5 cm caudally to the constriction. Rubber loops are drawn under the aorta, proximal and caudal to the constriction (Fig. 293). The ligamentum arteriosum is cut (Fig. 294). If there is patent ductus arteriosus, its ends are sutured (Fig. 295). Transection of the ligamentum arteriosum is the ''key point'' of the operation, because as the result of this manipulation the aorta may be easily moved with rubber loops as it is mobilized. The left subclavian artery is separated, and then the dorsal surface of the arch of the aorta up to the origin of the left common carotid artery. One or two pairs of intercostal arteries are ligated last of all (Fig. 296).

The intercostal arteries in patients with coarctation of the aorta have thin walls and are particularly fragile; this is why they should not be skeletized.

After it is mobilized, the aorta is clamped distal and

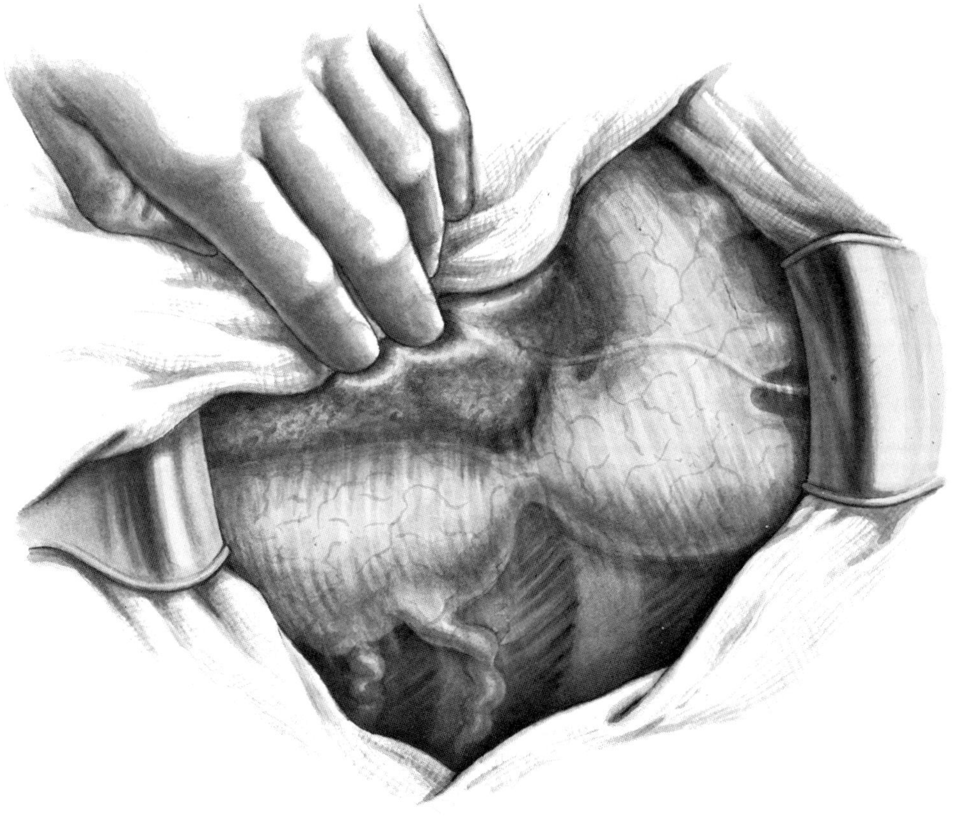

Fig. 292. General appearance of coarctation of aorta (adult type). Dilated and tortuous intercostal arteries are visible.

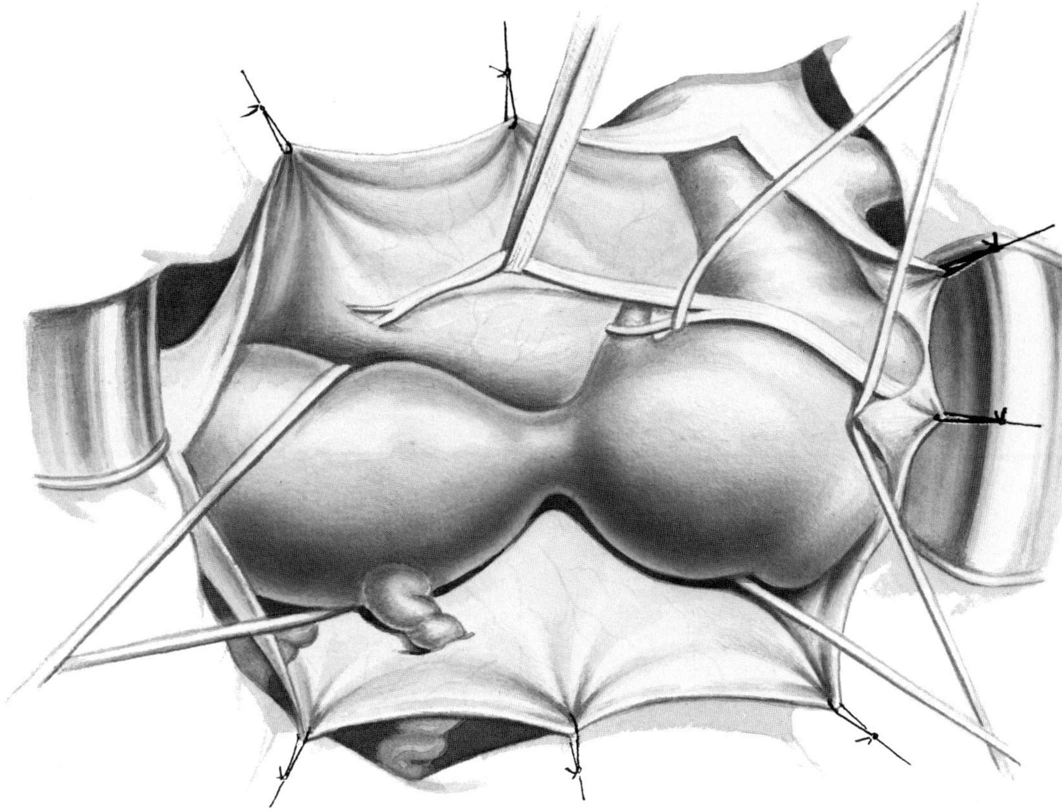

Fig. 293. Mediastinal pleura has been cut. Vagus nerve is moved medially. Loops have been brought under aorta above and below coarctation.

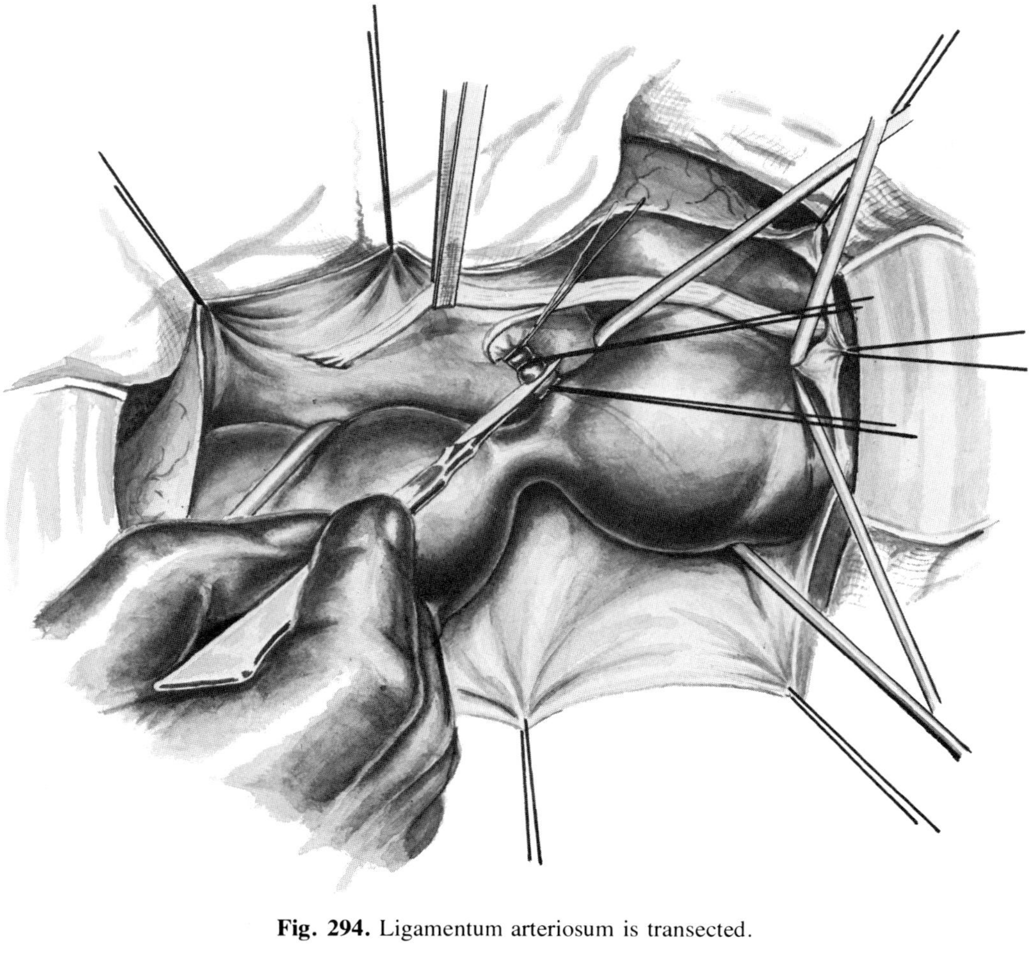

Fig. 294. Ligamentum arteriosum is transected.

proximal to the constriction so that the diameter of the transected ends left after resection of the constricted portion would be no less than 12 to 15 mm (Fig. 297).

Construction of the anastomosis is begun by applying a Halsted suture to the dorsal wall, although without tying it. The wall of the anastomosis is formed by pulling the thread after it has been stitched through the entire dorsal semicircumference of the aorta (Fig. 298). The ends of the continuous suture are tied with the ends of the previously applied lateral interrupted sutures. After that the anterior wall of the anastomosis is formed with a continuous Halsted or blanket suture, pulling every stitch tight (Fig. 299).

First the caudal and then the cranial clamps are removed from the aorta (Fig. 300). The bloodstream that escapes through the line of the anastomosis is stopped with additional interrupted sutures.

When the coarctation of the aorta is long, a plastic Teflon or Dacron crimp prosthesis is used. It is inexpedient to employ plastic prosthesis with a diameter less than 12 mm, because they fail to provide for the normal flow of blood in the aorta of an adult.

After the constricted portion of the aorta has been resected so as to provide anastomoses of maximum width, the caudal aortic segment is sutured with the prosthesis. The Halsted suture is tightened after each stitch or after stitching the entire semicircumference of the anastomosis (Fig. 301). The continuous suture is reinforced with interrupted sutures. Then the anterior wall of the anastomosis is formed (Fig. 302). The cranial anastomosis is formed in a similar mannner (Figs. 303 and 304). If the diameter of the prosthesis does not fit that of the cranial aortic segment, the latter is widened by cutting it lengthwise.

The prosthesis and the anastomoses are wrapped in napkins moistened with physiological saline solution

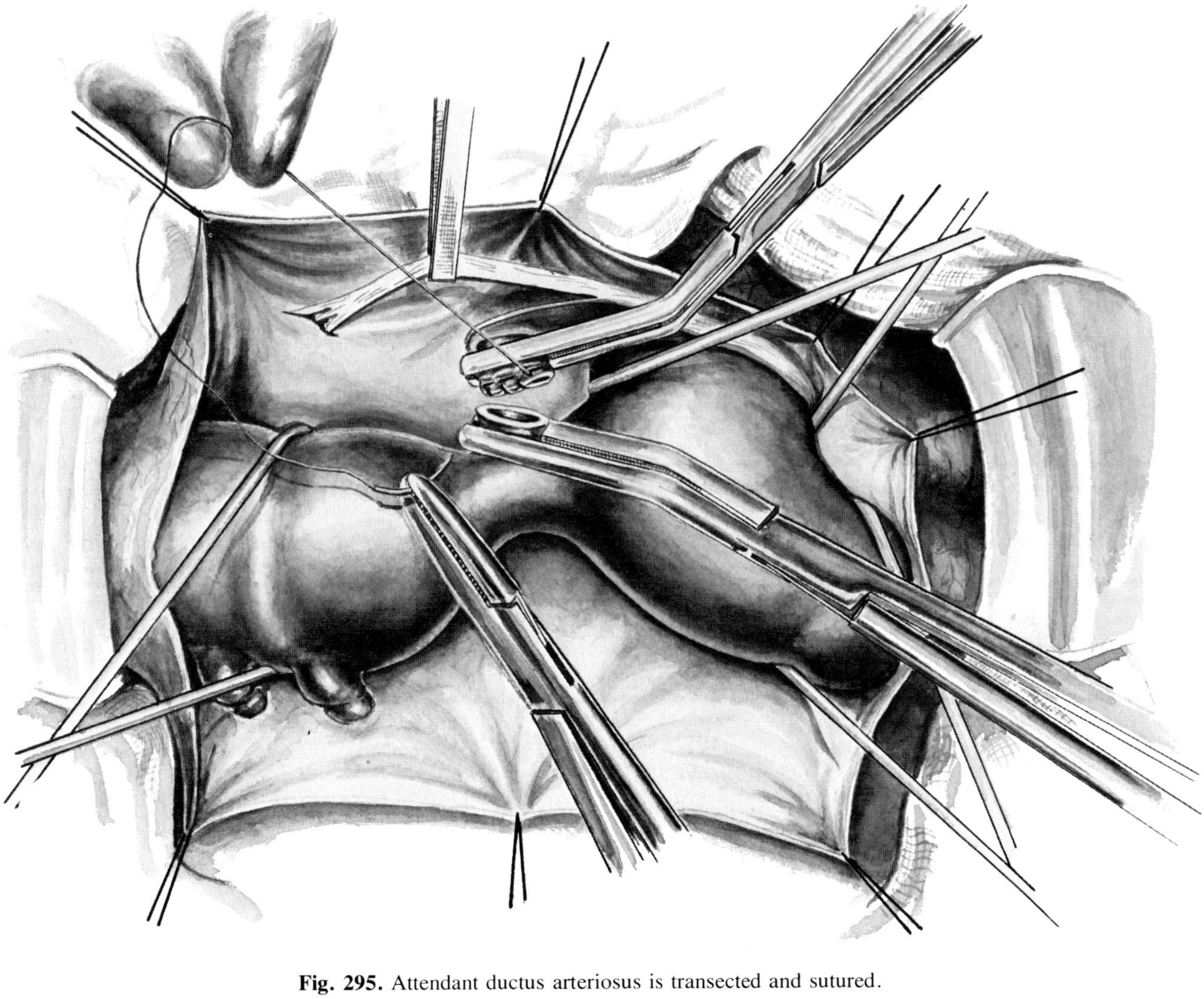

Fig. 295. Attendant ductus arteriosus is transected and sutured.

heated to a temperature of 55 to 60 C, which promotes rapid clotting of the blood. First the caudal and then the cranial clamps are taken off the aorta (Fig. 305).

If a considerable length of the aorta is constricted and its arch is hypoplastic, the portion of the descending aorta cranial to the constriction does not permit the creation of a sufficiently wide anastomosis. In such cases the prosthesis is stitched directly into the arch of the aorta. The caudal anastomosis with the prosthesis is formed. The aorta is clamped in the region of the coarctation. Before the cranial anastomosis is created, the constricted segment is resected with a clamp placed on the arch of the aorta between the left common carotid and subclavian arteries and another applied to the left subclavian artery. The opening for the anastomosis is formed on the ventral surface of the aortic arch, extending the incision to the base of the left subclavian artery. A wide subclavian artery may be used for bypassing the coarctation. The artery is transected, and its cranial end stitched into the lateral wall of the descending aorta (Fig. 306). Part of the aortic wall is clamped off in such cases for the creation of an end-to-side anastomosis (Figs. 307 and 308).

Mild coarctation of the aorta is corrected by direct or indirect isthmoplasty. In direct isthmoplasty the aorta is usually mobilized without ligation of the intercostal arteries. After the aorta is clamped proximal and distal to the constriction, the constricted segment is cut lengthwise, the inner diaphragm forming the constriction is excised, and the aorta is sutured transversely (Fig. 309). The possibility of performing such an operation, however, and the indications for it are limited.

Indirect isthmoplasty is undertaken more frequently. It consists in the stitching of a rhomboid plastic graft into a longitudinal incision made in the aorta at the level of the constriction (Figs. 310 and 311).

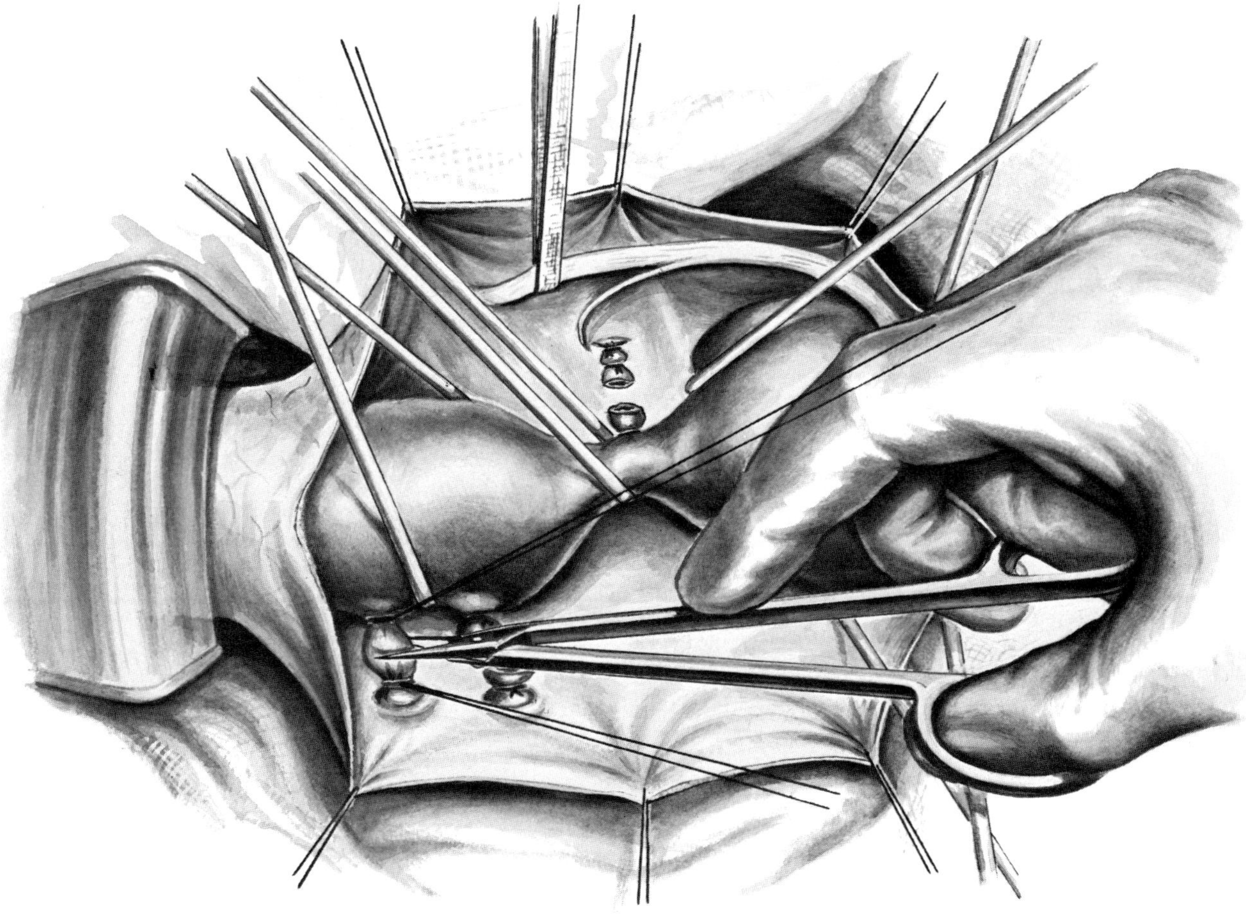

Fig. 296. Intercostal arteries are ligated and transected.

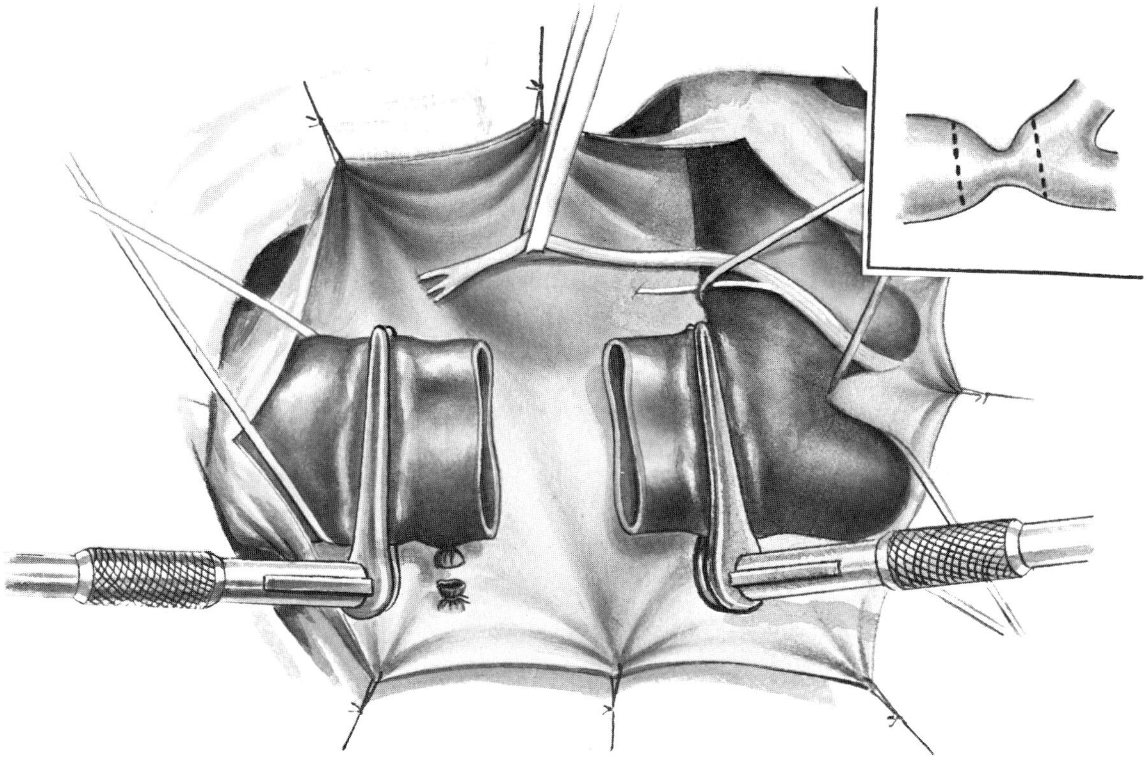

Fig. 297. Constricted segment of aorta is resected.

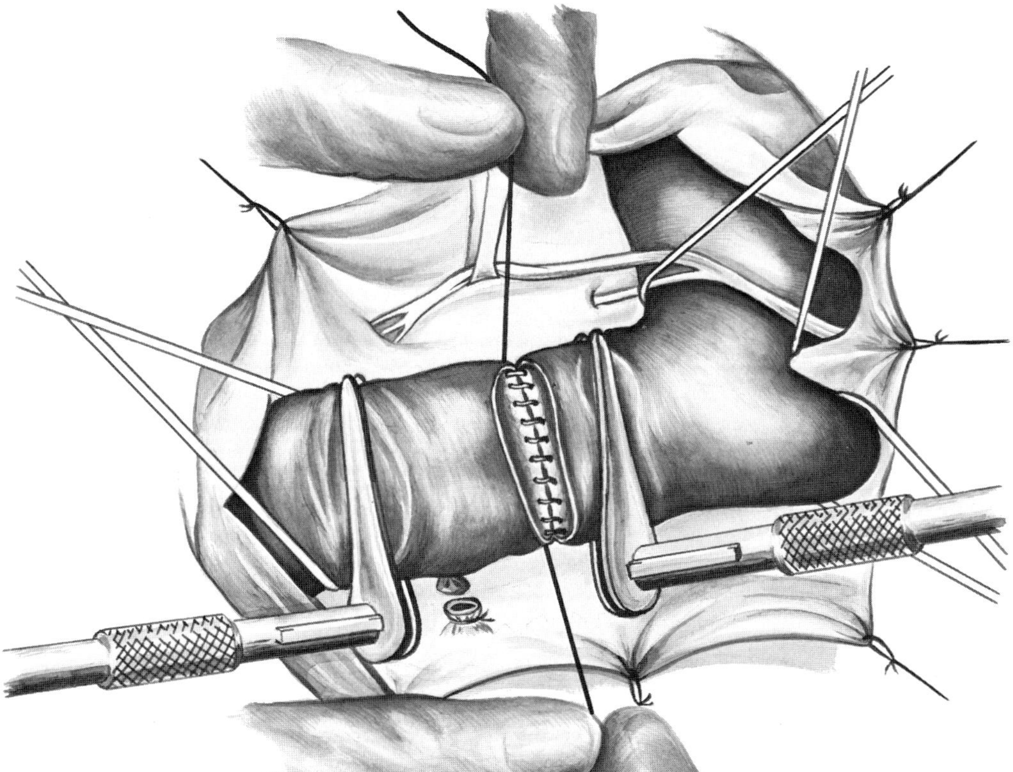

Fig. 298. Continuous Halsted suture is applied to dorsal wall of anastomosis.

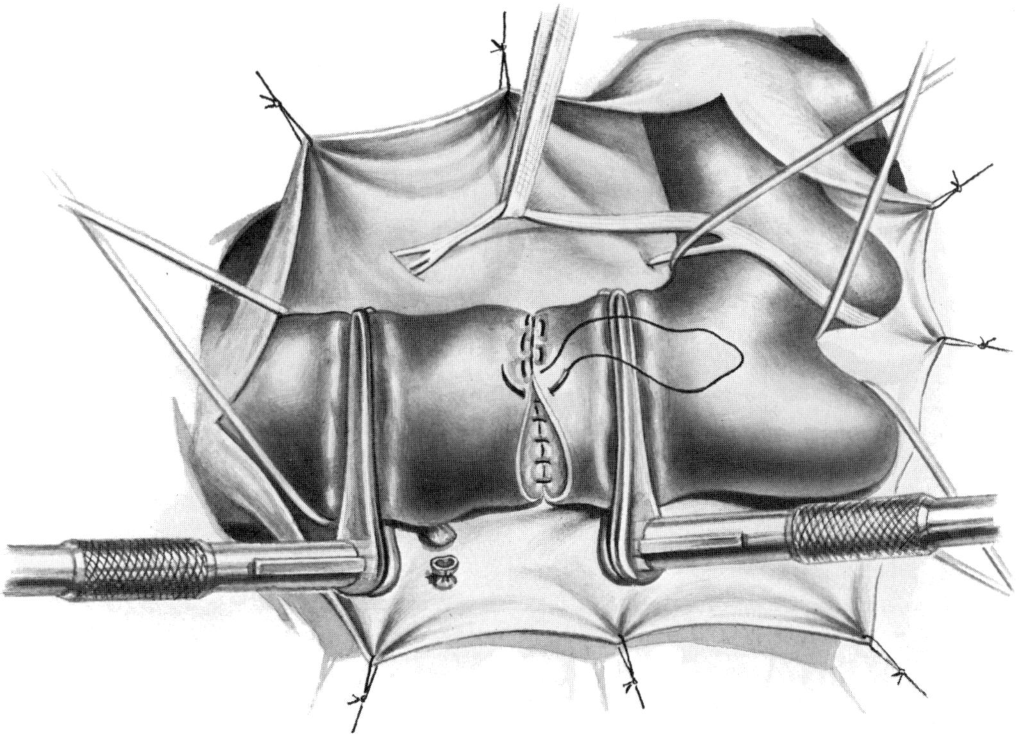

Fig. 299. Suture is applied to ventral wall of anastomosis.

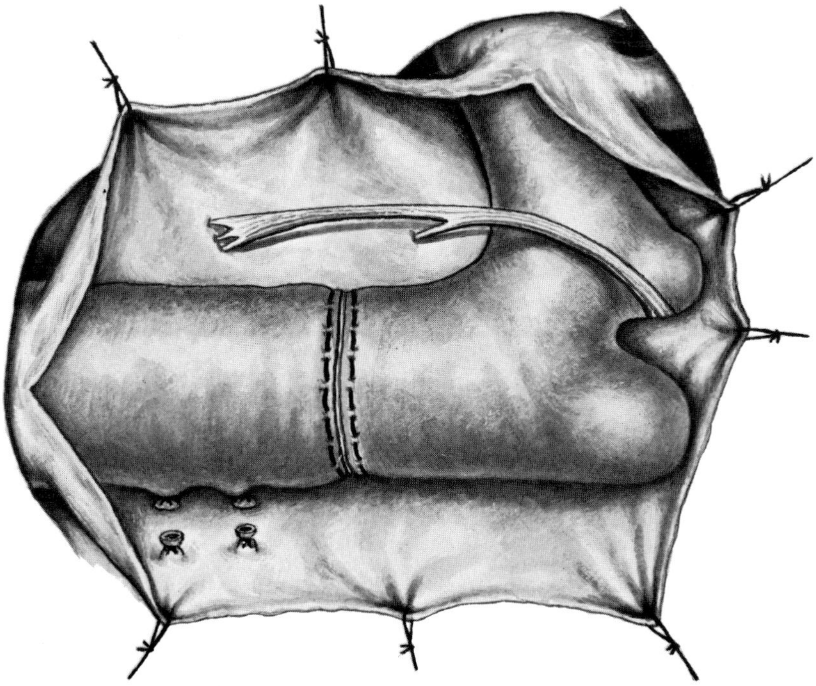

Fig. 300. Clamps have been removed from aorta. View of aorta after the anastomosis has been established and blood flow restored.

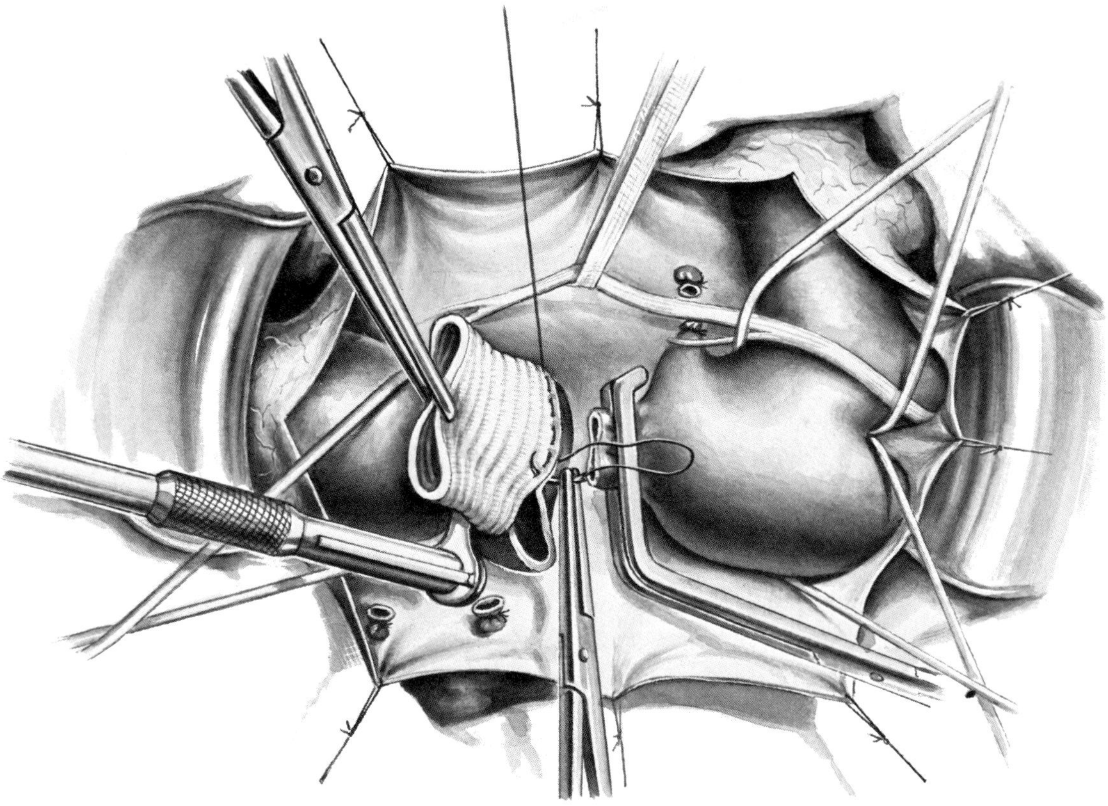

Fig. 301. Creation of anastomosis between caudal end of aorta and crimped prosthesis.

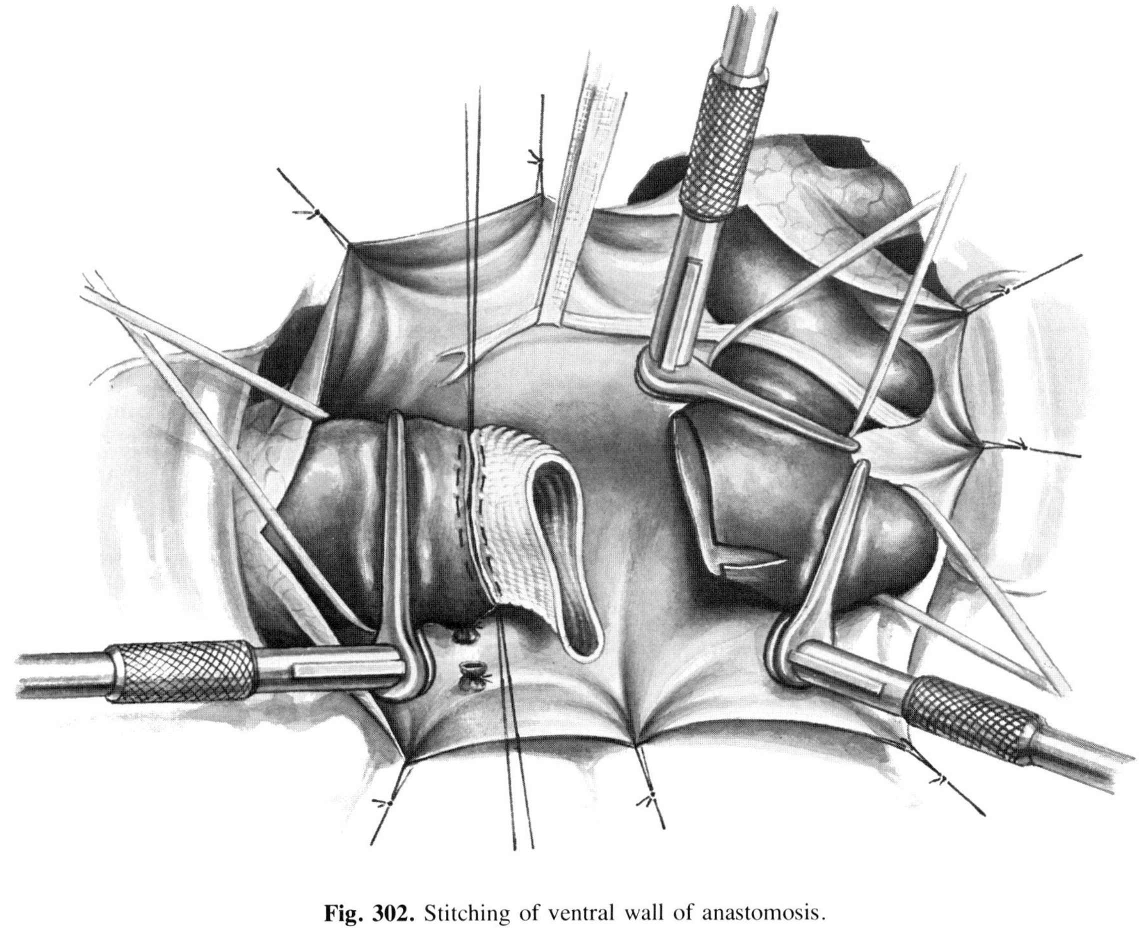

Fig. 302. Stitching of ventral wall of anastomosis.

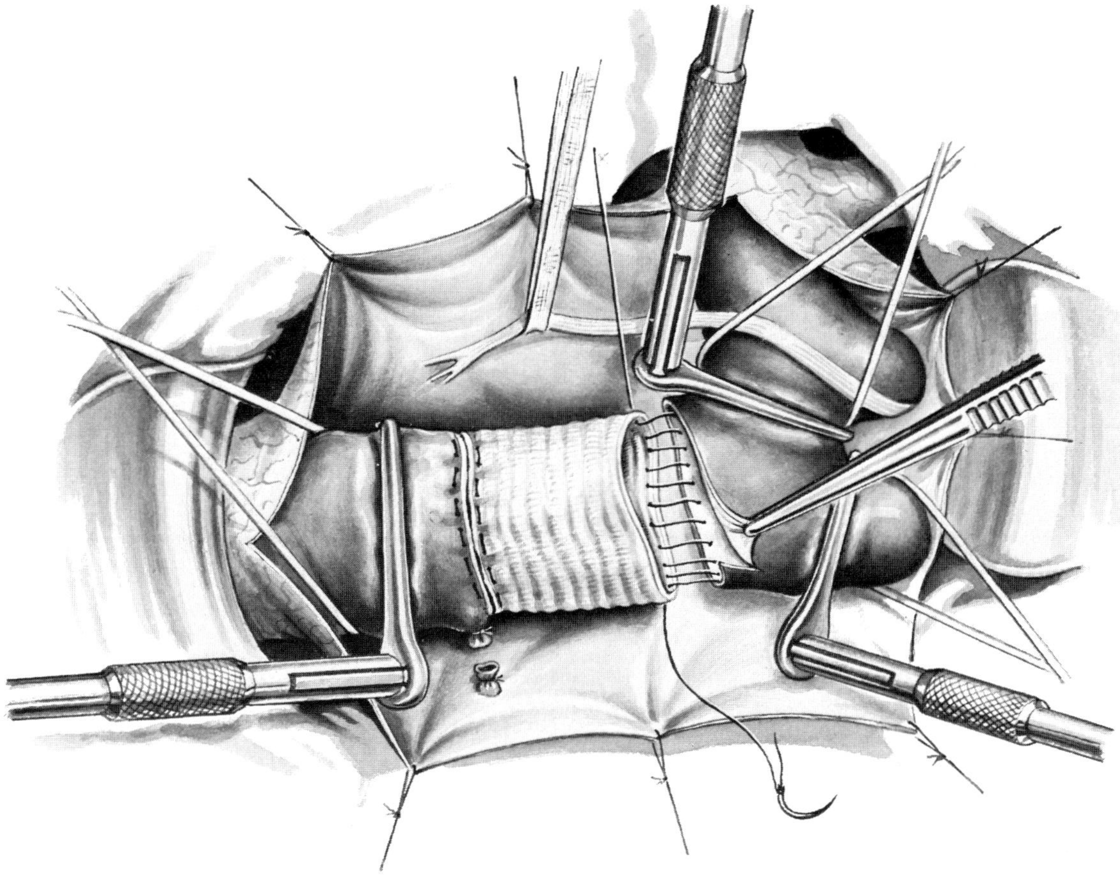

Fig. 303. Continuous Halsted suture is applied to dorsal wall of cranial anastomosis.

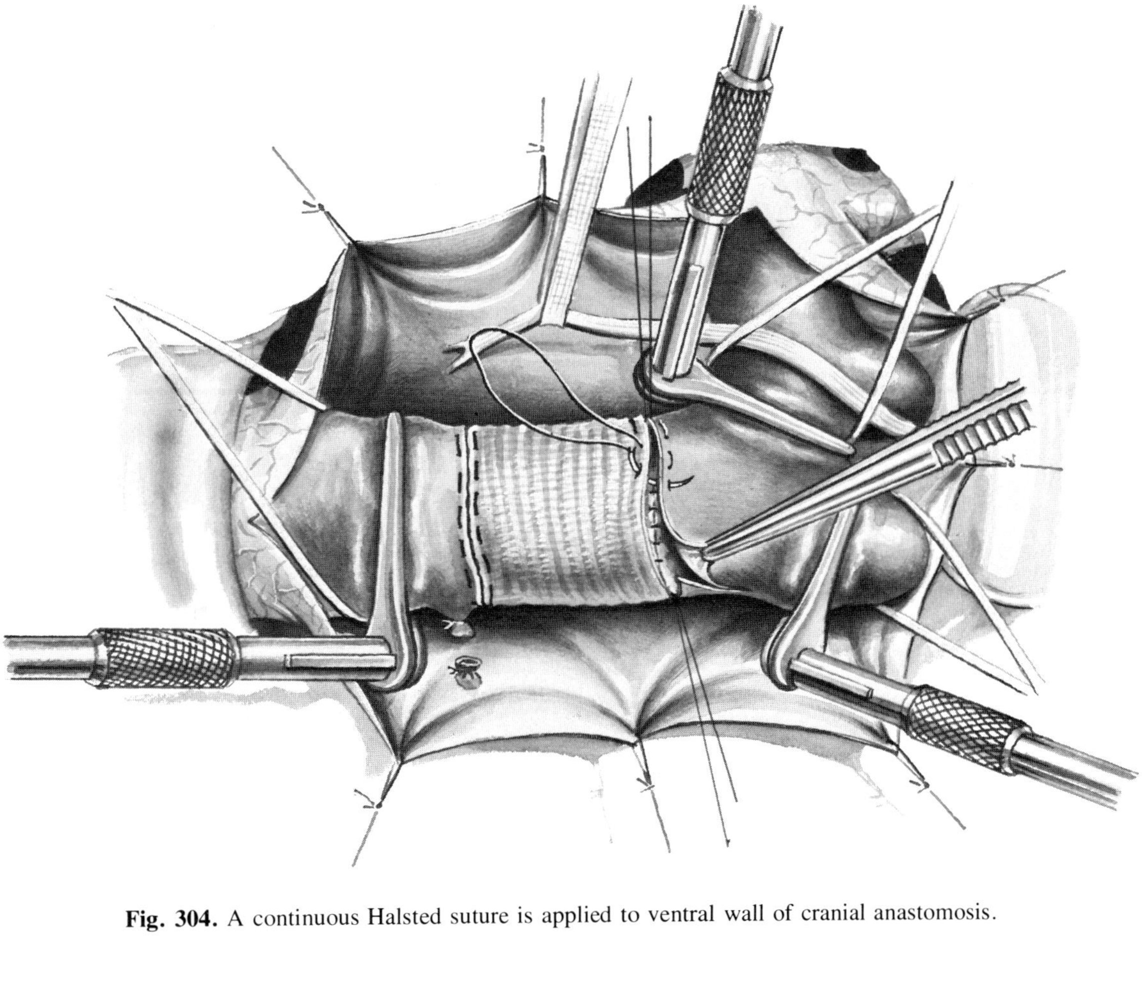

Fig. 304. A continuous Halsted suture is applied to ventral wall of cranial anastomosis.

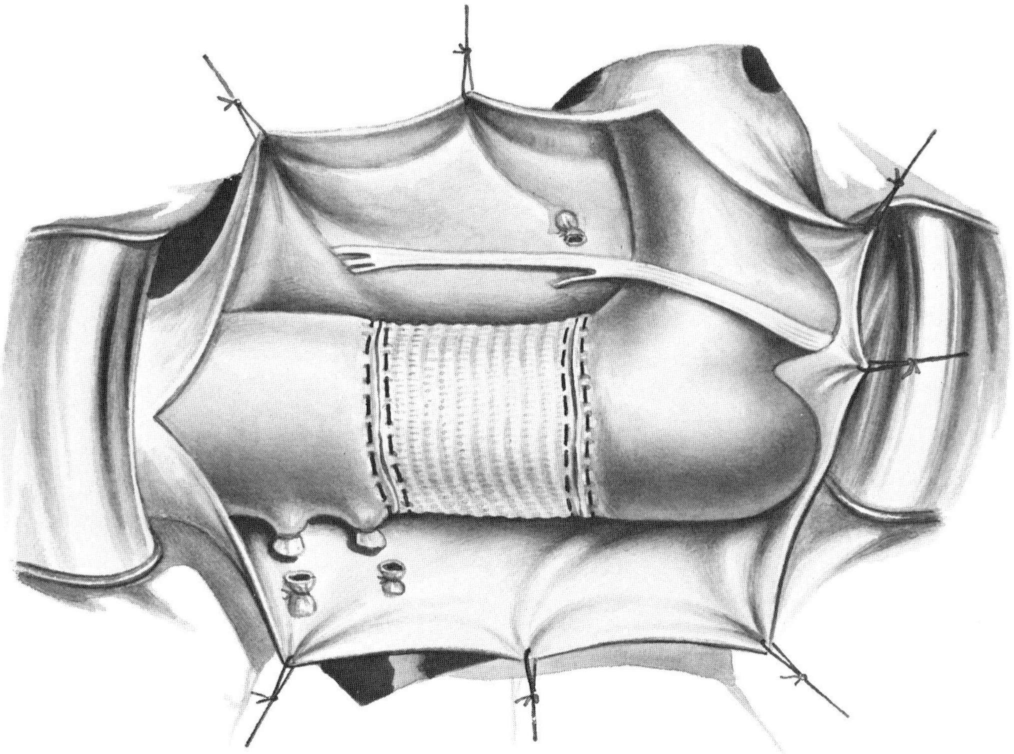

Fig. 305. View of aortic segment repaired with prosthesis after clamps had been removed and circulation restored.

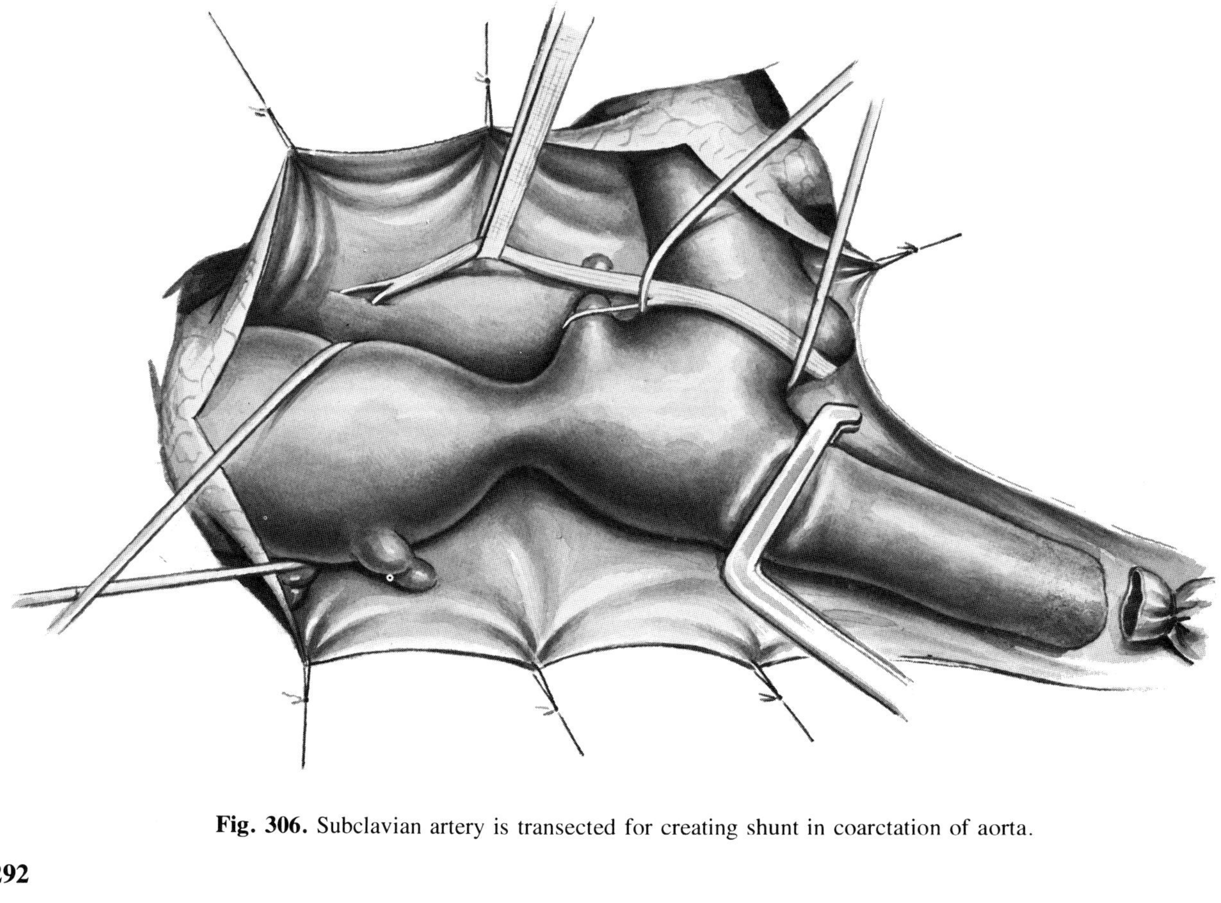

Fig. 306. Subclavian artery is transected for creating shunt in coarctation of aorta.

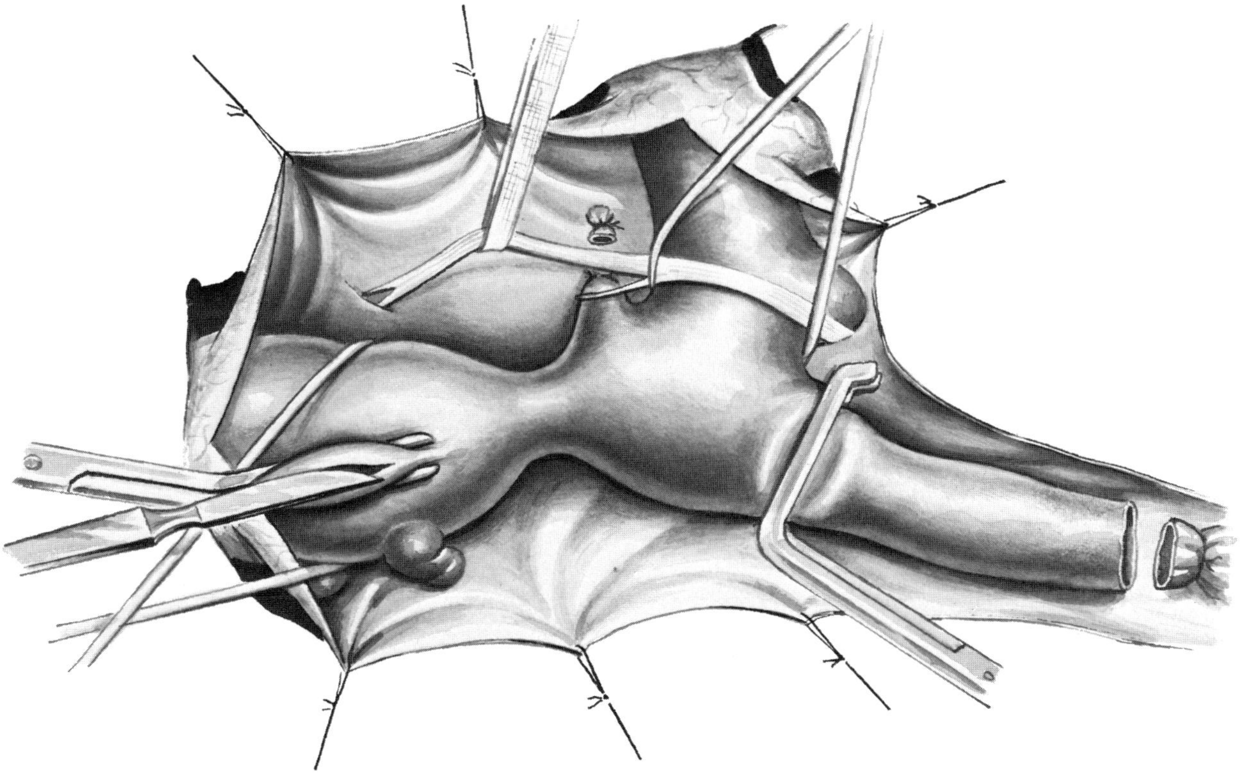

Fig. 307. Aortic wall is pressed off with clamp, and opening is formed for creating anastomosis with subclavian artery.

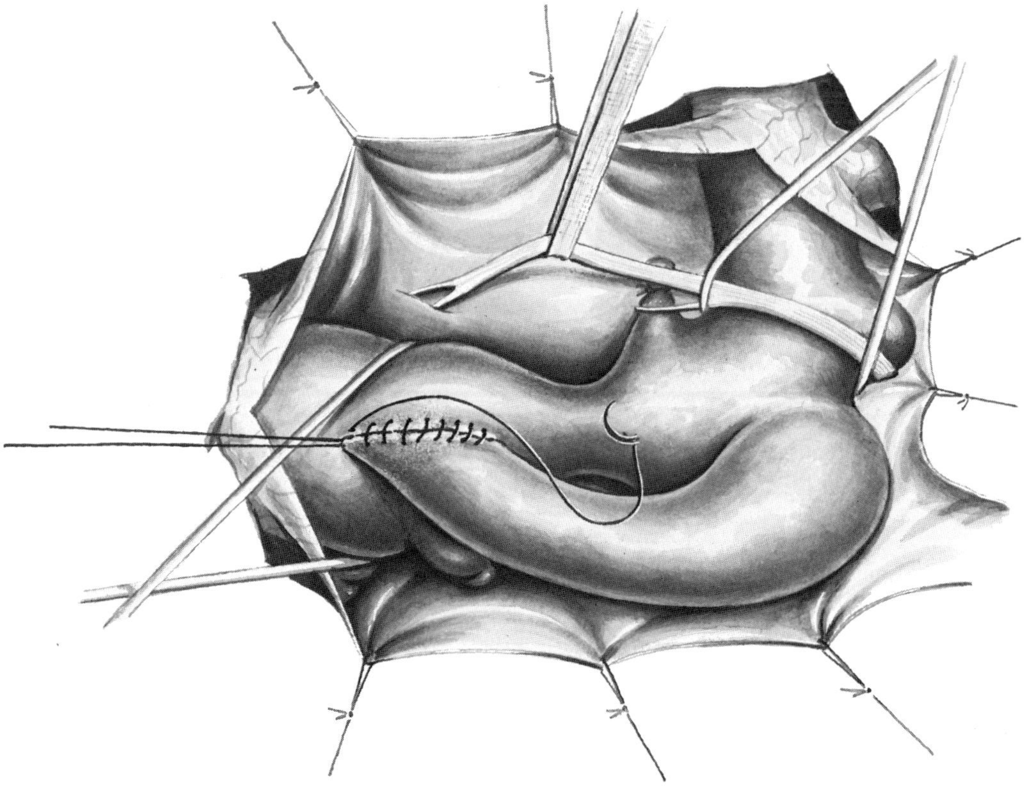

Fig. 308. End-to-side anastomosis has been formed between subclavian artery and descending aorta.

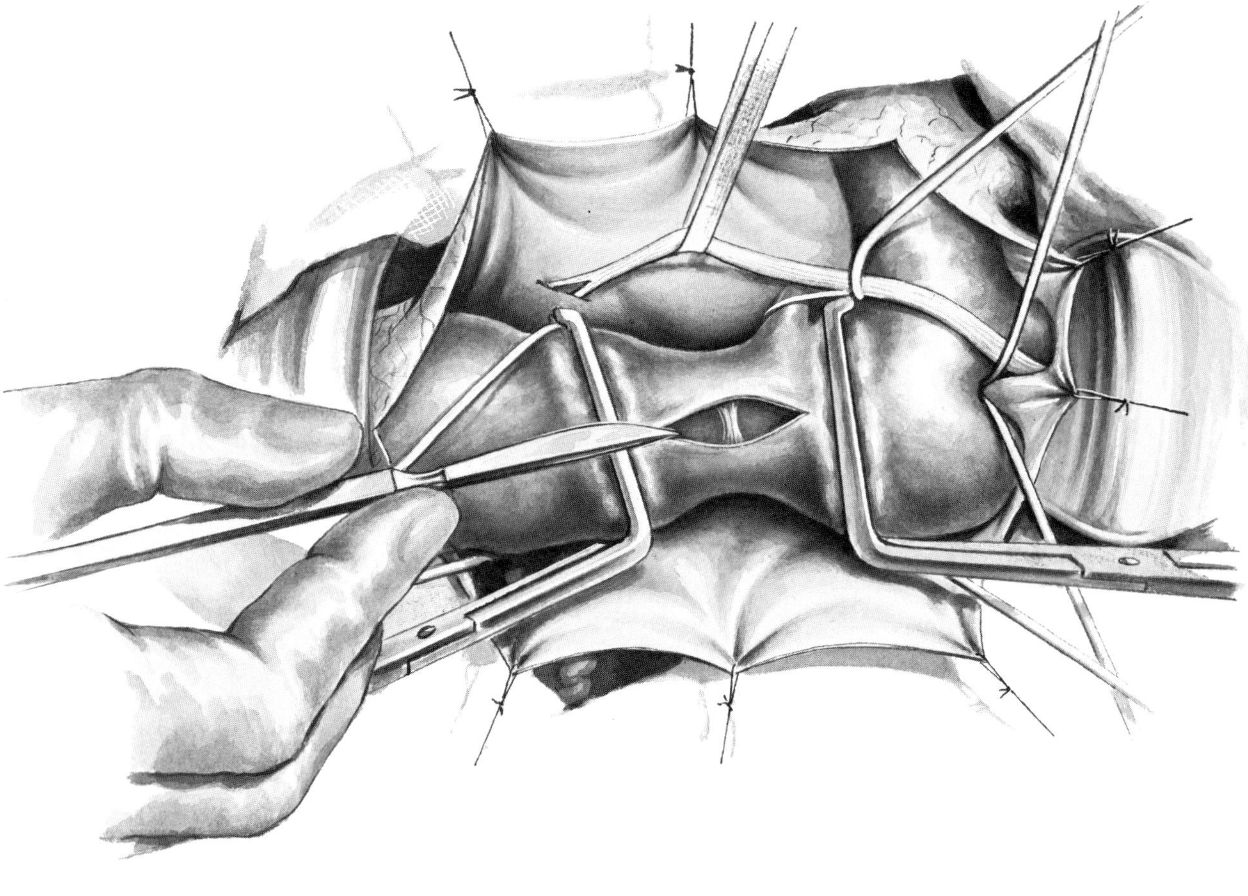

Fig. 309. Anterior wall of constricted part of aorta is incised for accomplishing isthmoplasty.

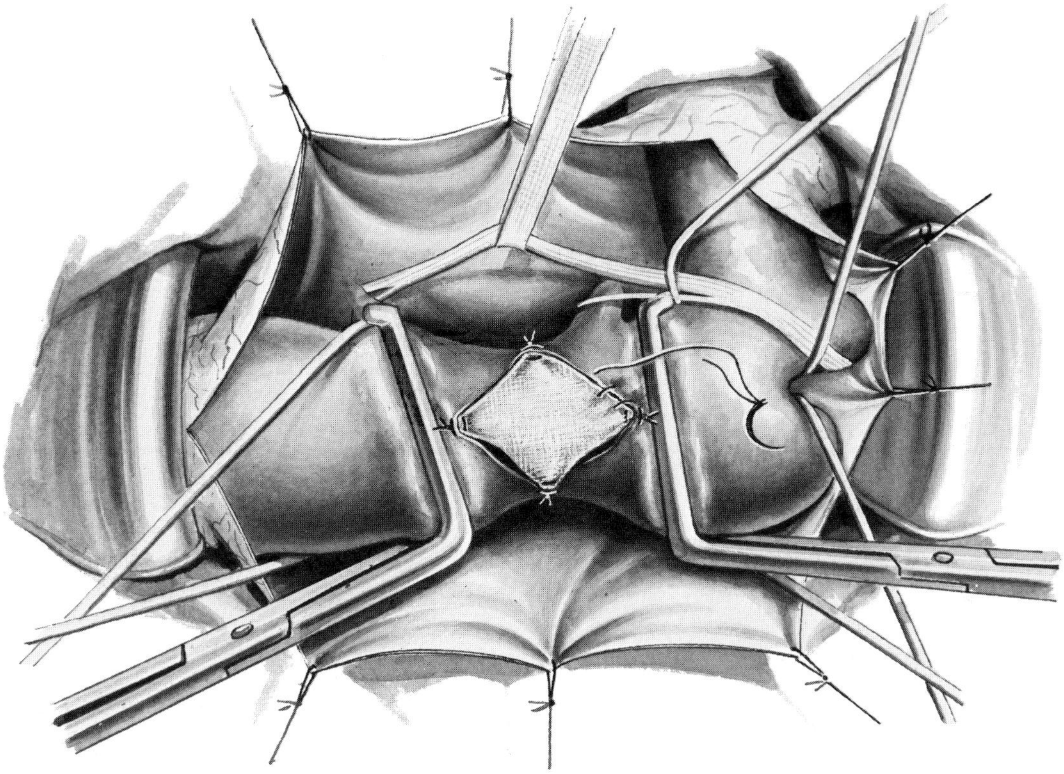

Fig. 310. Techniques of applying graft in isthmoplasty.

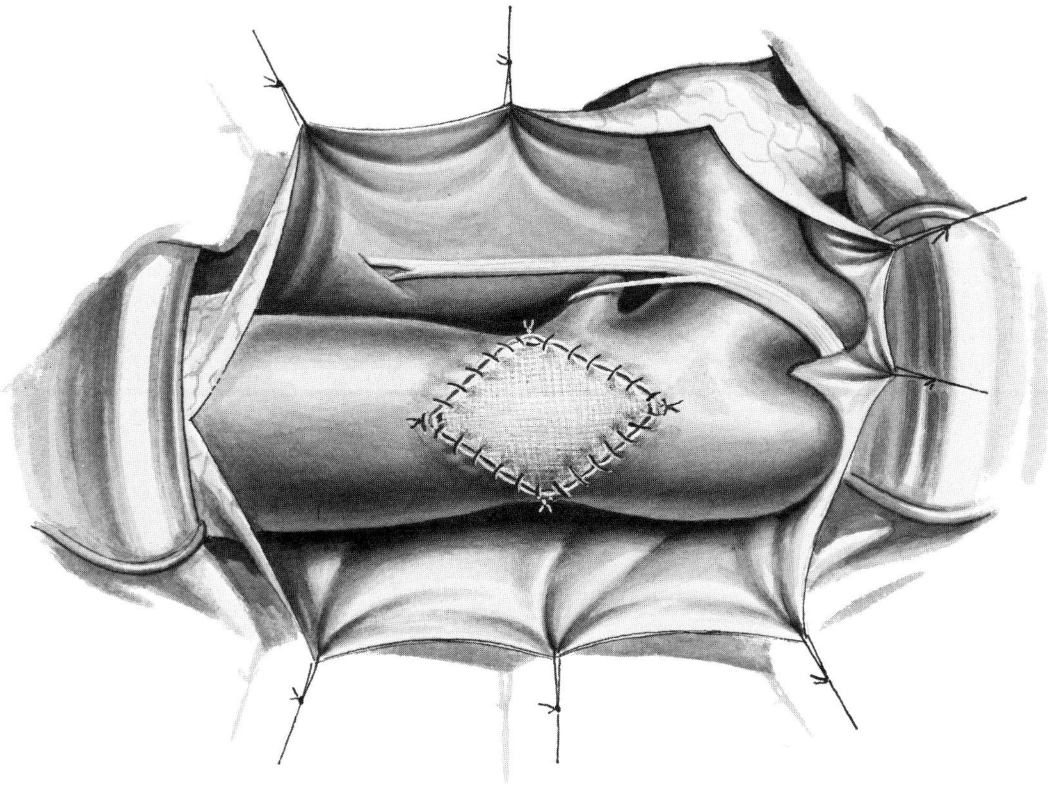

Fig. 311. General view of aorta after isthmoplasty has been accomplished and circulation restored.

INTERARTERIAL ANASTOMOSES IN TETRALOGY OF FALLOT

The purpose of these operations lies in connecting one of the arteries of the systemic circulation with one of the pulmonary arteries to intensify pulmonary circulation. They may be carried out through a left or right thoracotomy in the fourth intercostal space. The anastomosis between the ascending aorta and the right pulmonary artery may be created by a transsternal approach.

Blalock's subclavian-pulmonary anastomosis is created in the left pleural cavity. For this purpose the lung is pulled laterally and caudally. The left pulmonary artery is mobilized in the segment between the site of its division and the pericardium. During this procedure several small anastomoses with the bronchial artery, considerably developed in tetralogy of Fallot, have to be transected. Next, the intrathoracic segment of the left subclavian artery where the vertebral artery, internal thoracic artery, and the thyrocervical and costocervical trunks arise from it is separated (Fig. 312). The distal segments of these arteries are ligated one after the other. After this the left subclavian artery is clamped, and the ligated branches and main trunk of the subclavian artery are transected proximal to the ligatures. A rosette is

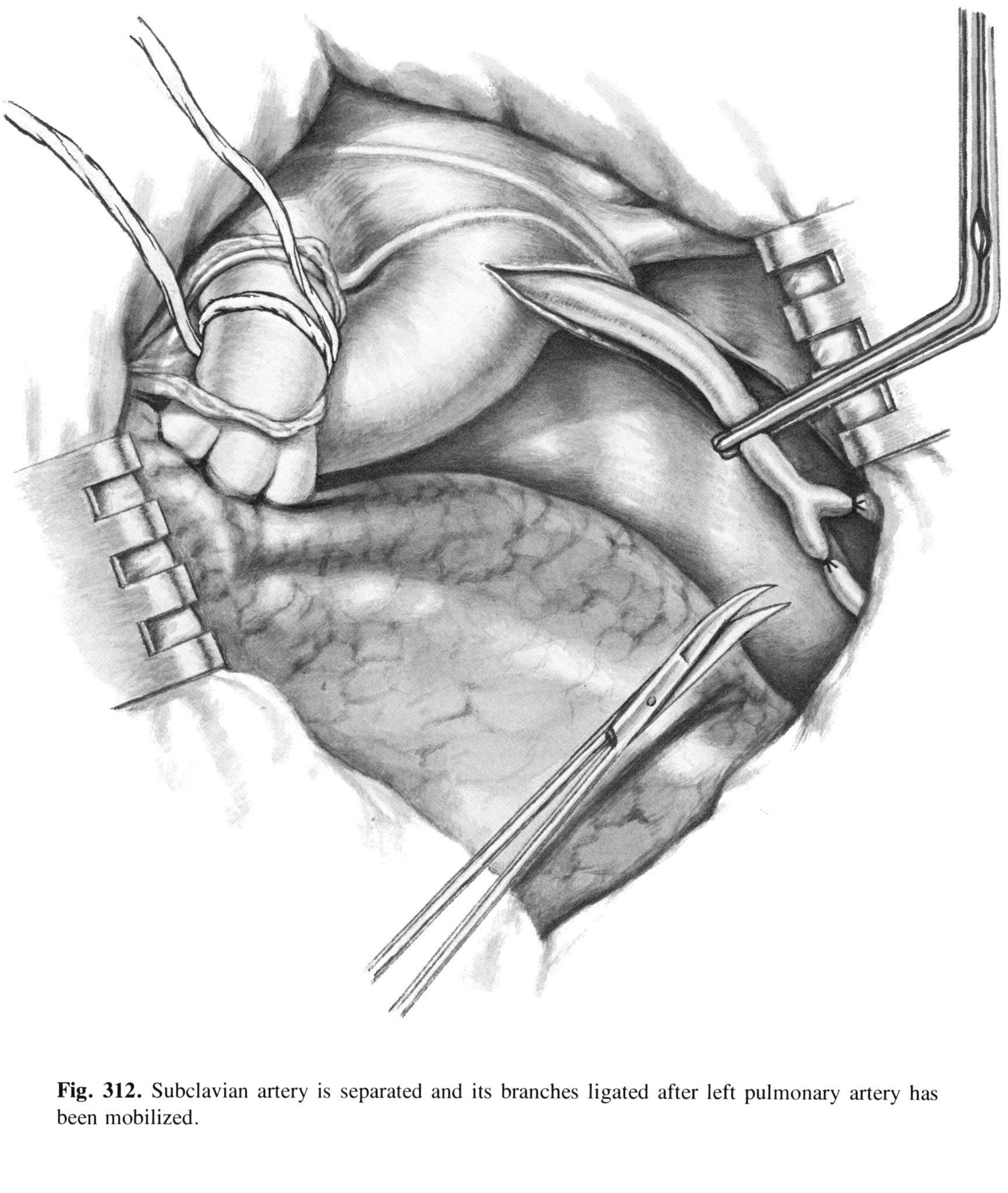

Fig. 312. Subclavian artery is separated and its branches ligated after left pulmonary artery has been mobilized.

formed out of the transected branches, depending on the level of their position and the level of the origin of the first lateral branch; this rosette is a scalloped dilatation of the transected end of the subclavian artery with the branches (Fig. 313).

The mobilized left pulmonary artery is ligated with looped ligatures, and its walls are stitched through between the ligatures with a thread on an atraumatic needle. This thread is used to pull out the wall in the shape of a cone, part of which is resected forming a round opening 7 mm in diameter. The posterior wall of the anastomosis is formed by means of a continuous Halsted suture stitched without tightening. The pulmonary and subclavian arteries are brought closer together by pulling the ends of the thread, causing the least strain on the anastomosis. The ends of the continuous suture are secured by tying them with the interrupted sutures.

The anterior wall of the anastomosis is formed with a blanket or Halsted suture. The finest possible needles and a thread steeped in vaseline oil are used for this operation. The blood flow in the pulmonary artery is restored by loosening the looped ligatures. The clamp is taken off the subclavian artery. The volumetric blood flow along the anastomosis depends greatly on the extent

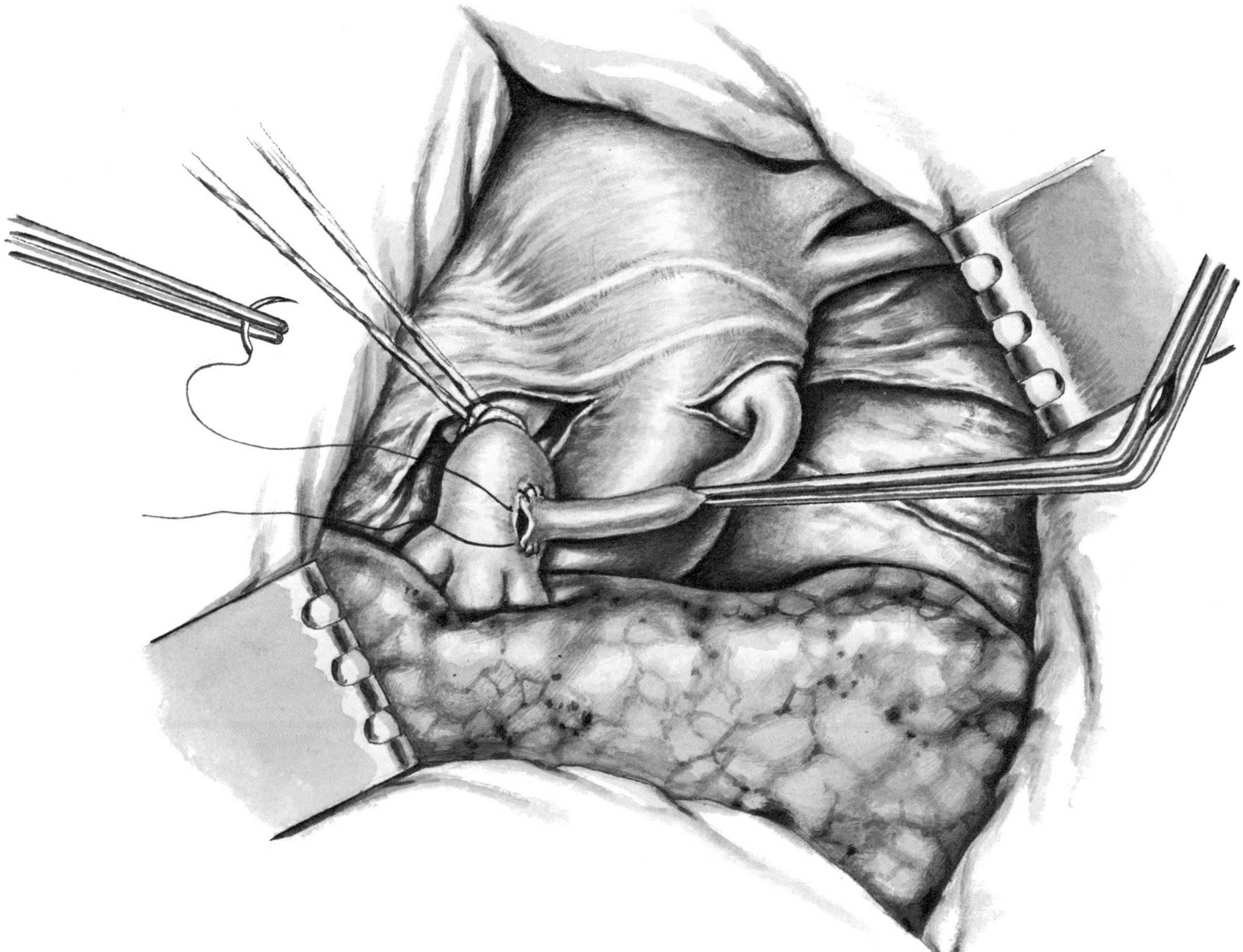

Fig. 313. Creation of subclavian-pulmonary anastomosis. Formation of ''rosette'' from branches of subclavian artery.

of the stretching of the subclavian artery and the degree to which it bends at its origin from the aorta. In unfavorable conditions the subclavian artery may be anastomosed end to end with one of the branches of the pulmonary artery (Fig. 314). To reduce stretching of the subclavian artery and trauma inflicted to the collaterals of the pulmonary root, the left pulmonary artery is mobilized intrapericardially, and an intrapericardial anastomosis is created (Figs. 315 and 316). The method of this operation differs only in the techniques of separating the left pulmonary artery after the pericardium is opened.

If the subclavian artery is not sufficiently long, the Vishnevsky-Donetsky operation may be conducted. It consists in side-to-side anastomosis of the subclavian

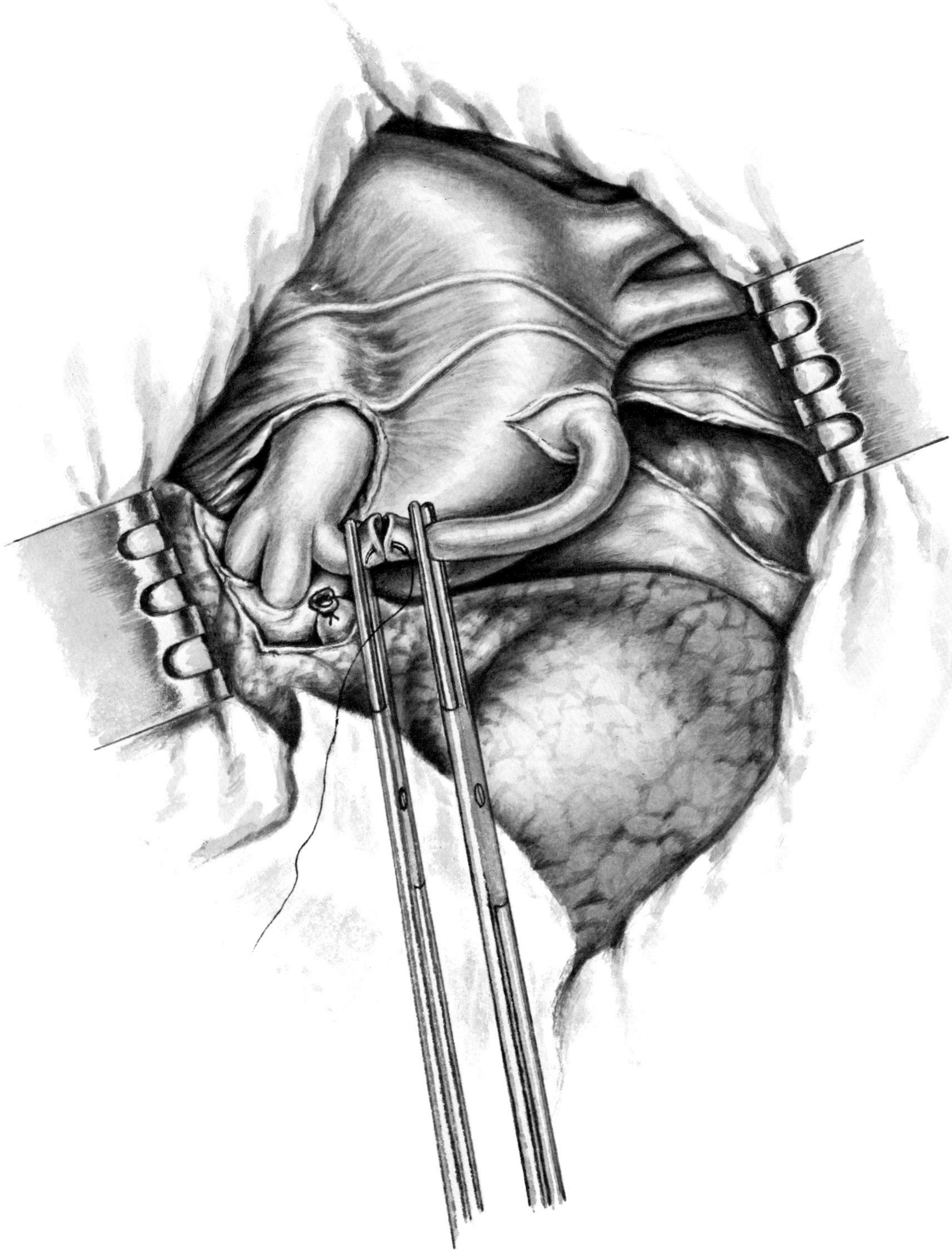

Fig. 314. Subclavian artery is connected to one branch of pulmonary artery.

and pulmonary arteries by means of a lyophilized arterial graft or a plastic prosthesis. The graft or the prosthesis is fastened by means of Donetsky's ring. Potts' aortico-pulmonary anastomosis between the descending aorta and the left pulmonary artery is accomplished by a lateral or posterolateral approach. The lung is moved ventrally and caudally, exposing the aorta and the root of the left lung. The aorta is mobilized directly distal to the isthmus with the ligation of three or four and sometimes five left intercostal arteries (Fig. 317). Rubber loops are placed around the aorta above and below the presumed site of the anastomosis. The pulmonary artery is separated from the root of the lung by the method described.

The aorta and pulmonary artery are clamped with the Vishnevsky-Doliotti clamp, which usually shuts off the pulmonary artery fully and the aorta partly along its wall with the external blade, bringing both vessels closer together. The clamped pulmonary artery and aorta are cut for a distance of 7 to 8 mm. The dorsal wall of the anastomosis is formed by applying a continuous blanket suture after the suture at the corners of the incision has been secured. The ventral wall of the anastomosis is created with a continuous blanket suture (Fig. 318).

The blood flow is restored along the pulmonary artery first, and the clamp is then taken off the aorta (Fig. 319).

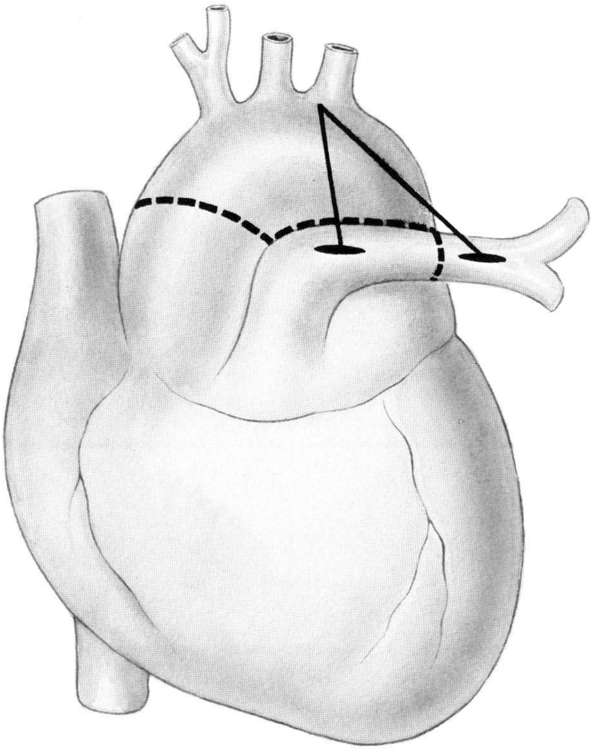

Fig. 315. Schema of correlations of required length of subclavian artery in intrapericardial and extrapericardial anastomosis.

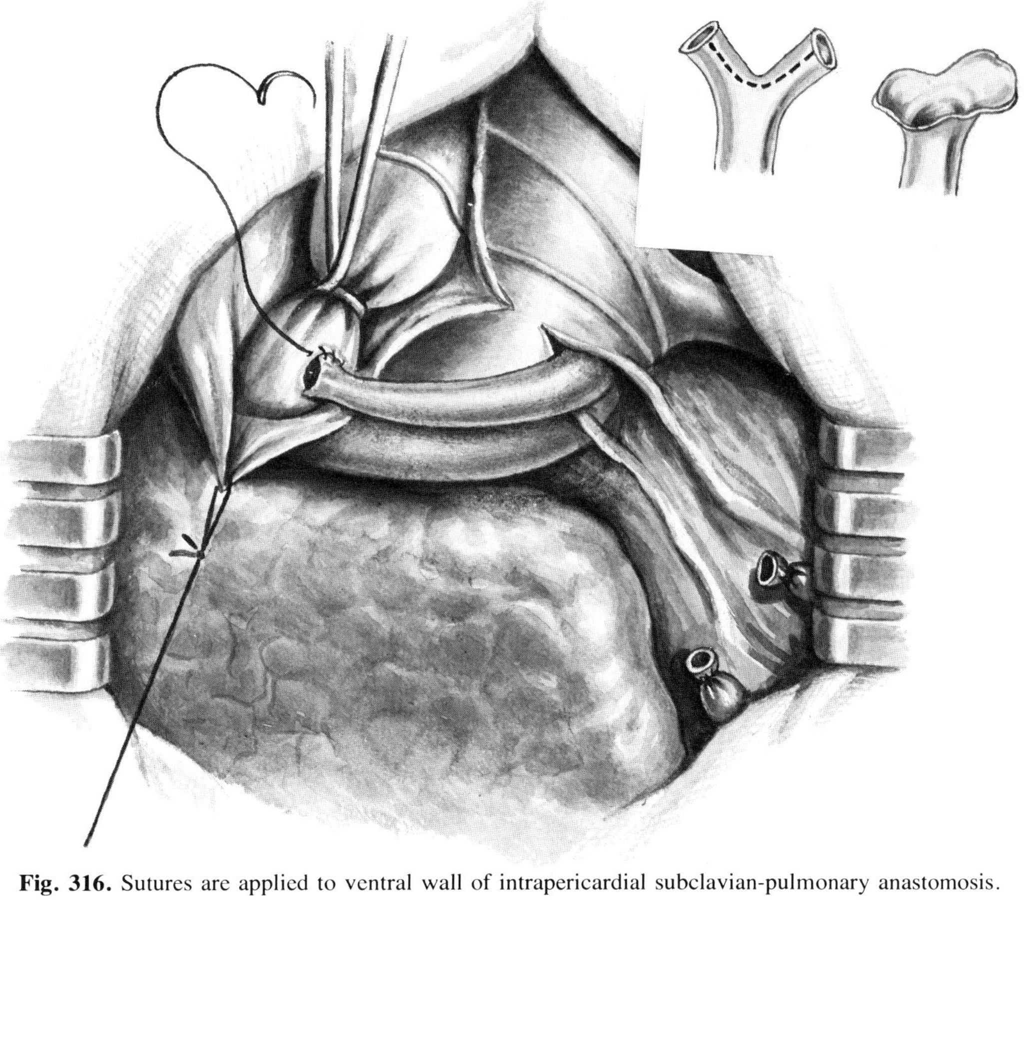

Fig. 316. Sutures are applied to ventral wall of intrapericardial subclavian-pulmonary anastomosis.

The efficient function of the vascular anastomoses is characterized by the occurrence of diffuse systolic-diastolic thrill on the pulmonary artery.

The interarterial anastomosis in the right pleural cavity is created through right anterolateral thoracotomy in the fourth intercostal space. The lung is moved dorsally and caudally. The azygos vein is ligated and transected. The superior vena cava is drawn away ventrally. The brachiocephalic trunk and the right subclavian artery are separated from the cellular tissue of the posterior mediastinum and the right pulmonary artery from the root of the lung. End-to-side anastomosis is formed between the

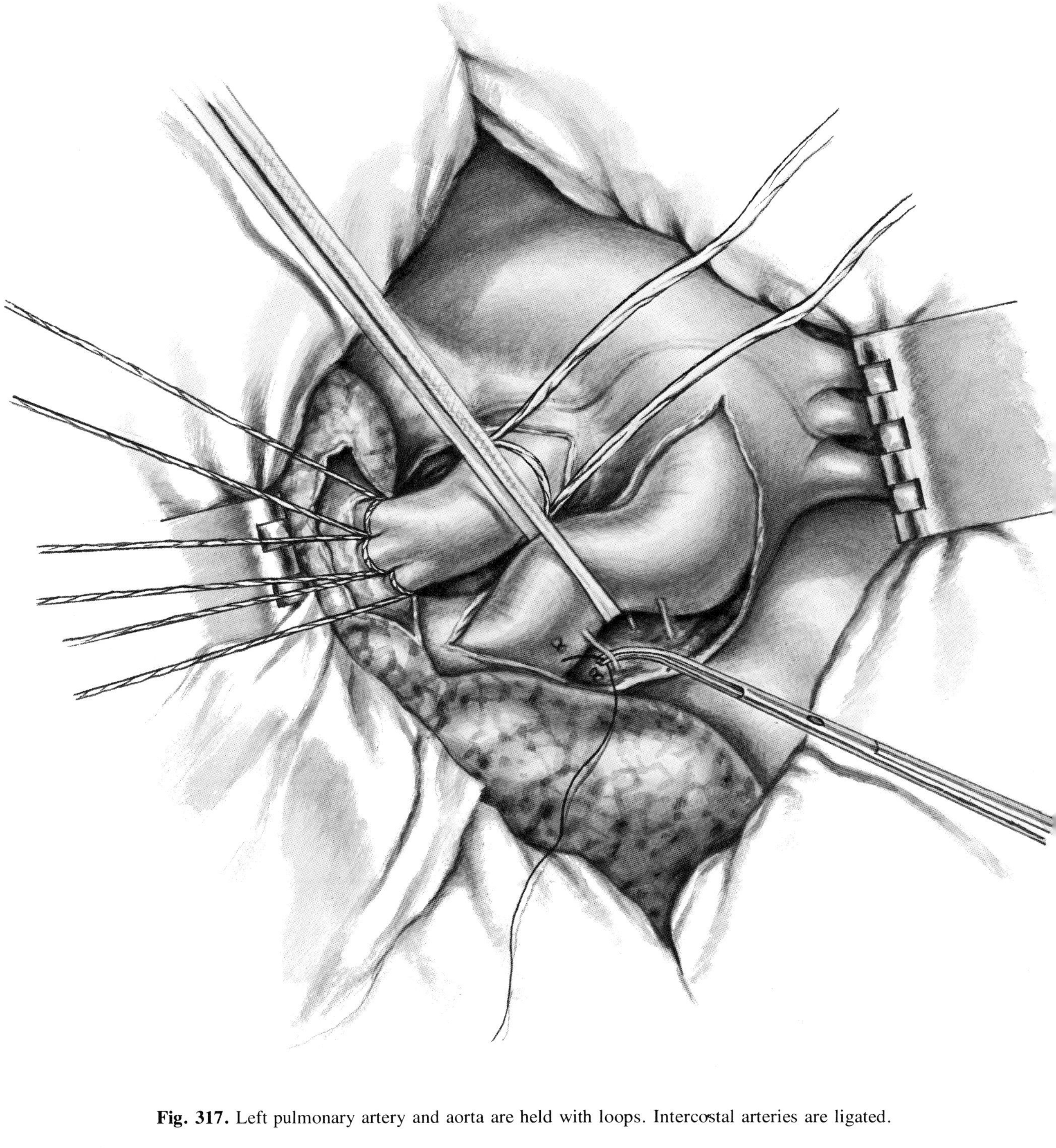

Fig. 317. Left pulmonary artery and aorta are held with loops. Intercostal arteries are ligated.

right subclavian and right pulmonary arteries by the method described. An insufficiently long subclavian artery is elongated with a plastic prosthesis or autologous vein.

In tetralogy of Fallot and in congenital atresia of the tricuspid valve, cavapulmonary anastomosis is formed. This may be done if the width of the right pulmonary artery is no less than half the diameter of the superior vena cava. The operation consists in the creation of end-to-end anastomosis between the superior vena cava and the right pulmonary artery. The operation is begun with the separation of the superior vena cava. The pericar-

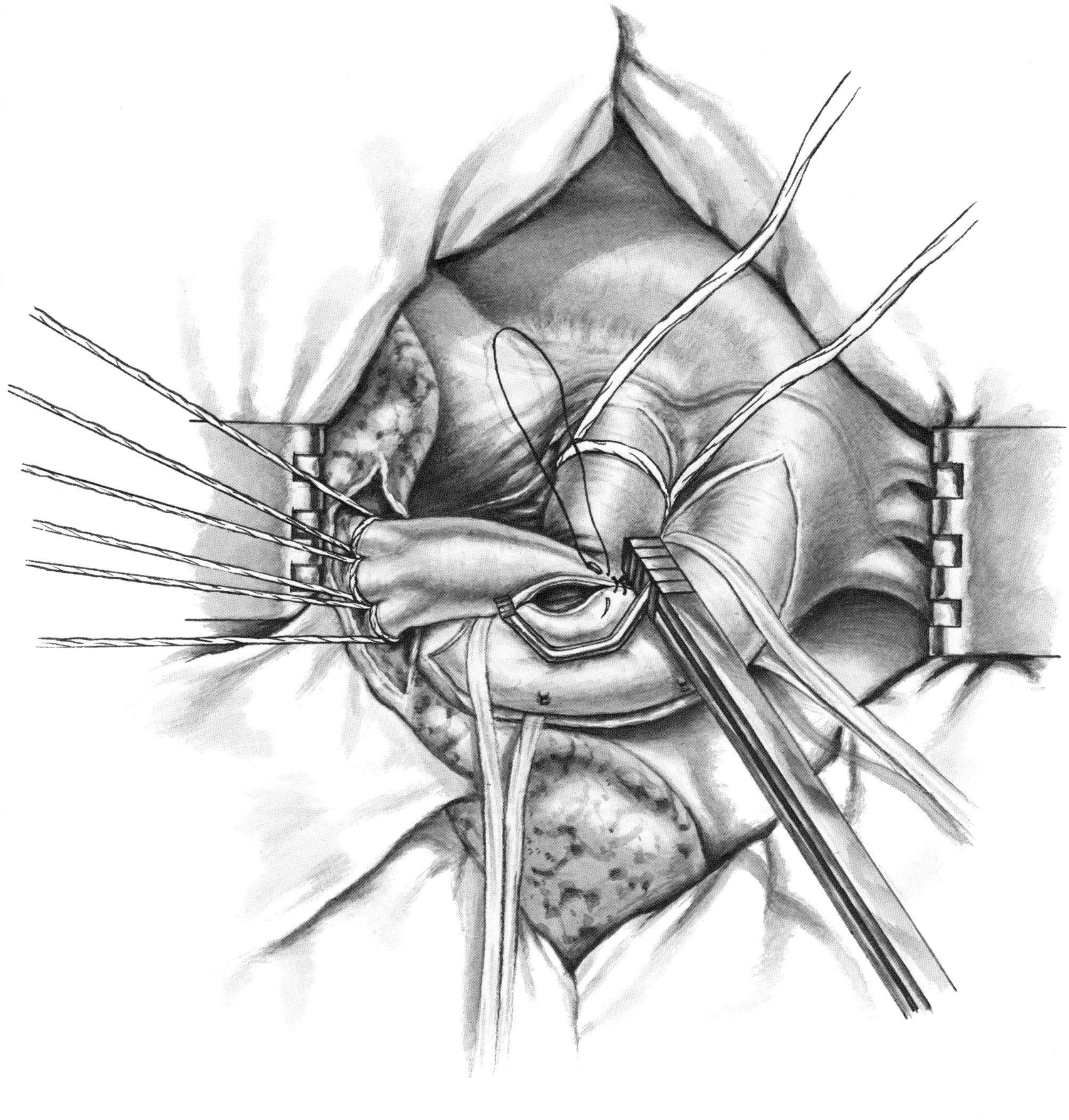

Fig. 318. Vishnevsky-Doliotti clamp is applied to walls of aorta and left pulmonary artery. Application of suture to anterior wall of anastomosis is shown.

dium is opened ventral to the phrenic nerve, and the right pulmonary artery is freed from the surrounding tissues (Fig. 320). After ligation and transection of the azygos vein, the superior vena cava is mobilized.

The central end of the pulmonary artery is ligated and stitched through; the peripheral end is compressed with artery forceps or loops.

The superior vena cava is stitched through with the УС instrument or ligated at the place where it drains into the right atrium (Fig. 321). An end-to-end anastomosis is rapidly created between the superior vena cava and the right pulmonary artery with a slight crimping of the vena cava (Fig. 322). After the anastomosis has been formed and the clamps removed, the cranial end of the superior vena cava is ligated or closed with sutures.

To relieve sharp hypertension in the system of the superior vena cava when it is clamped, several methods have been suggested for shunting the blood from this vein into the inferior vena cava (extracorporeal shunting, temporary internal shunt).

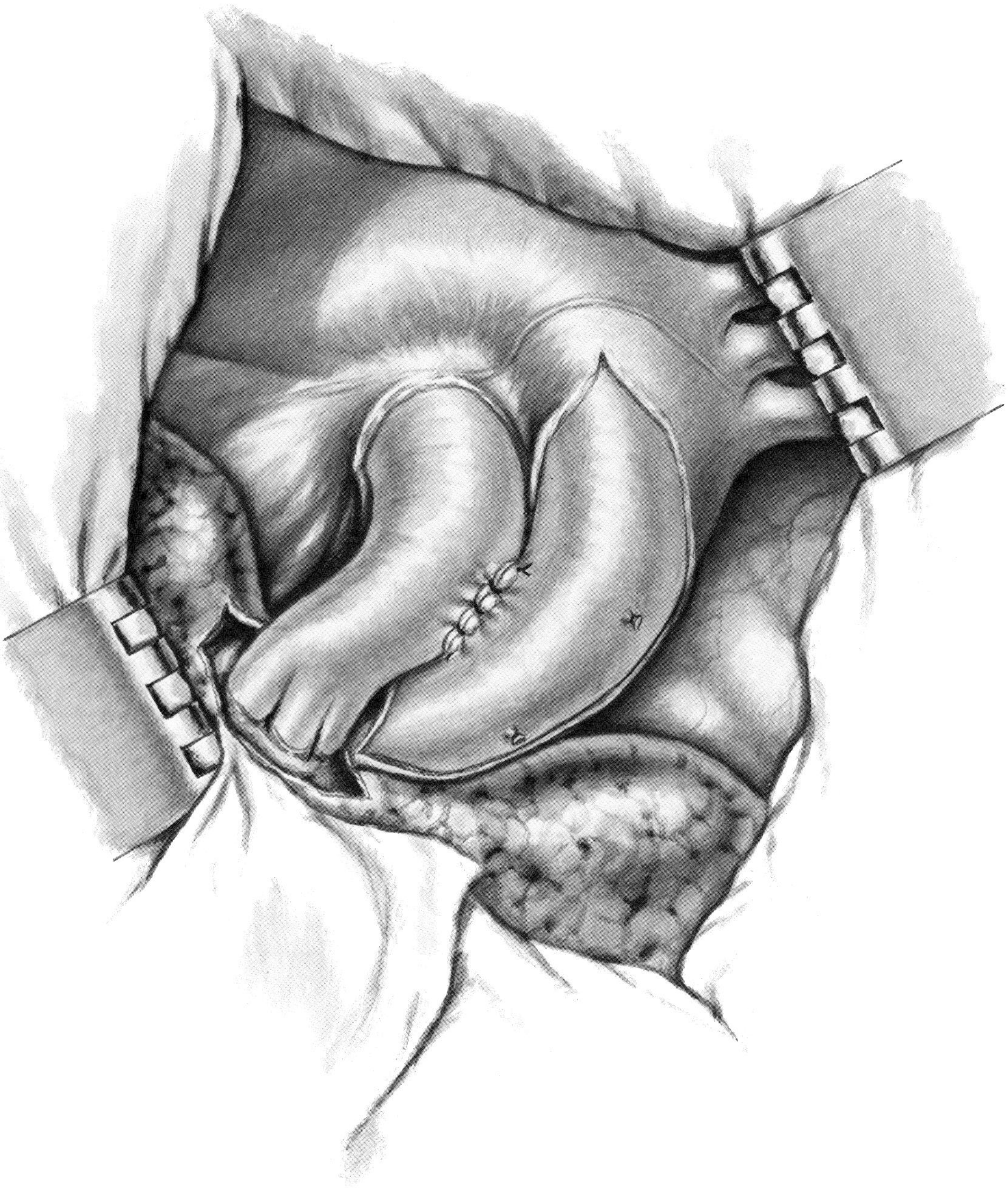

Fig. 319. Aorticopulmonary anastomosis according to Potts has been completed. Clamps have been removed and circulation restored.

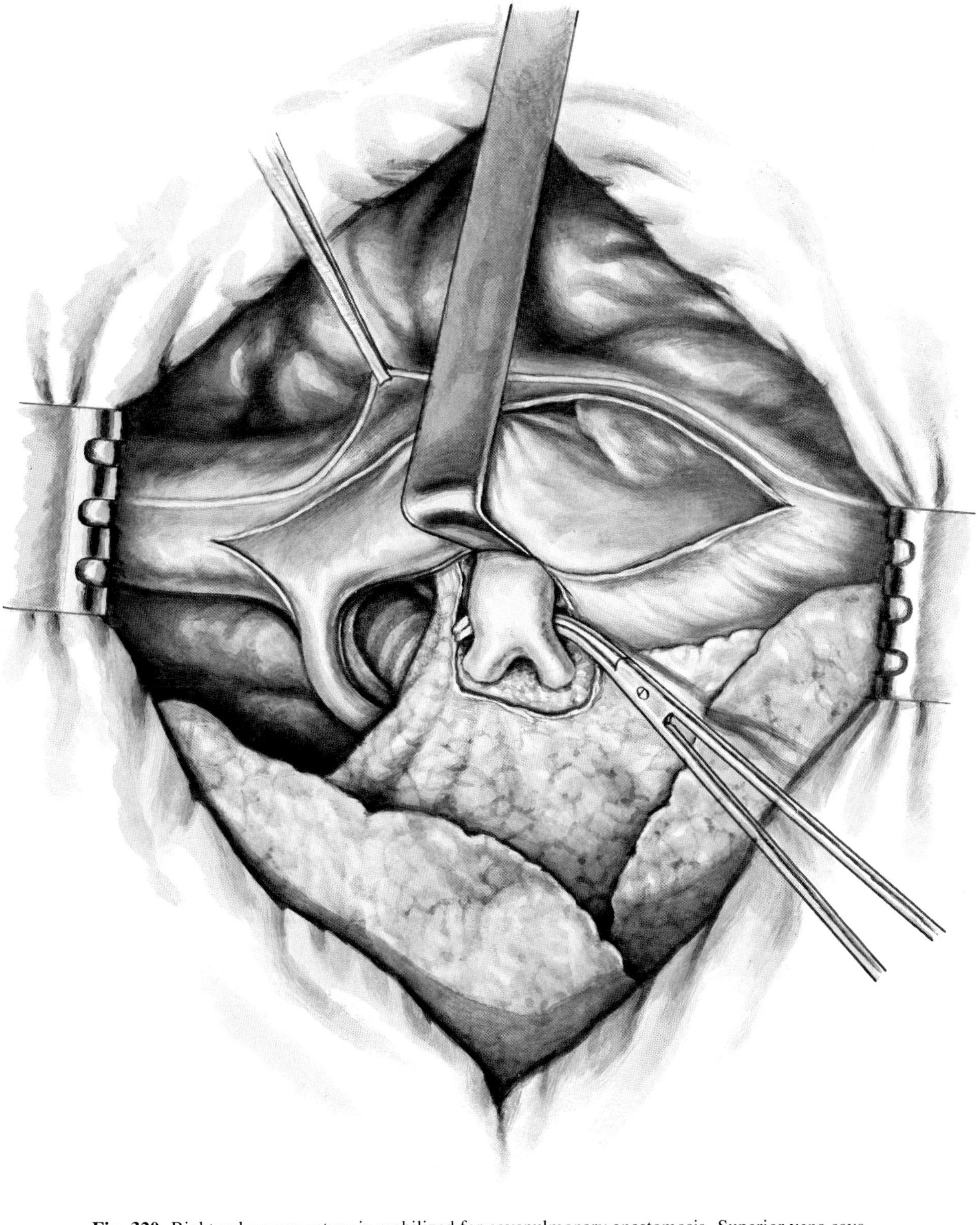

Fig. 320. Right pulmonary artery is mobilized for cavapulmonary anastomosis. Superior vena cava is moved medially.

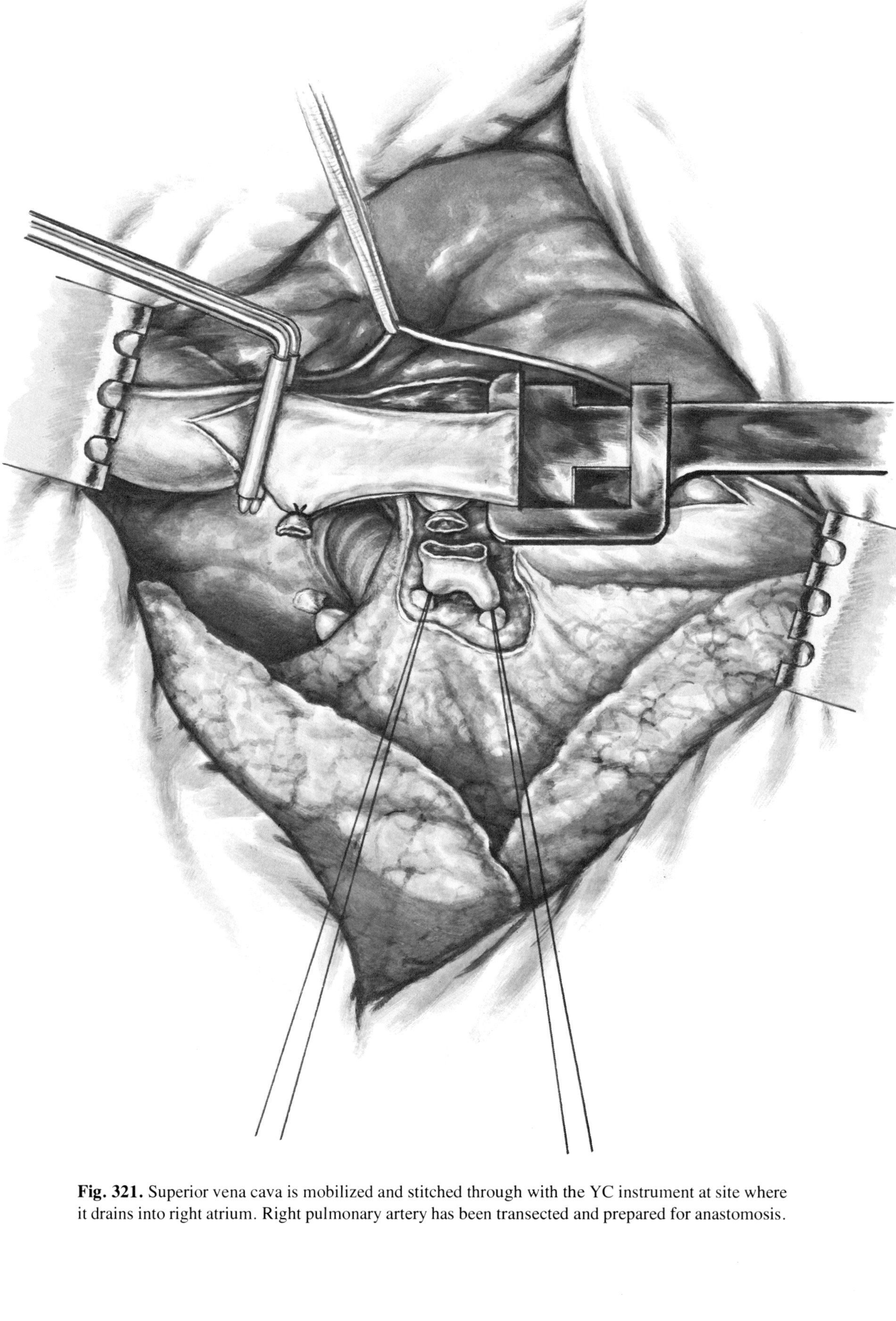

Fig. 321. Superior vena cava is mobilized and stitched through with the YC instrument at site where it drains into right atrium. Right pulmonary artery has been transected and prepared for anastomosis.

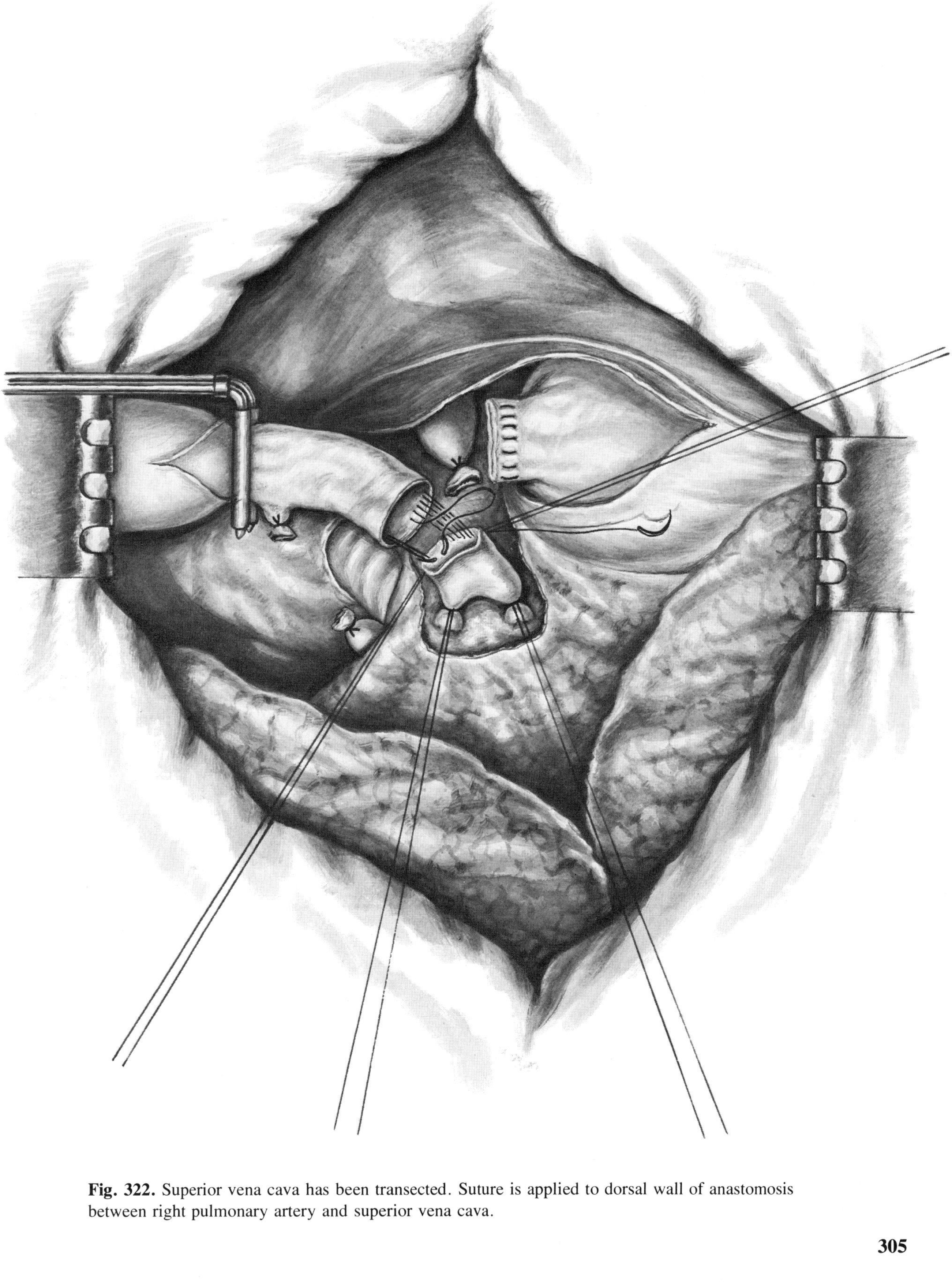

Fig. 322. Superior vena cava has been transected. Suture is applied to dorsal wall of anastomosis between right pulmonary artery and superior vena cava.

CORRECTION OF PULMONARY STENOSIS

Closed valvuloplasty of the pulmonary artery in stenosis of its valves is conducted through anterolateral thoracotomy in the left fourth intercostal space.

The pericardium is opened wide ventrally and parallel to the phrenic nerve.

The edges of the pericardial incision are held with traction sutures. Valvular stenosis of the pulmonary artery is usually attended with poststenotic dilatation of the pulmonary trunk and a coarse systolic thrill of its wall.

A Halsted or purse-string suture with two traction sutures are applied to an avascular area on the ventral wall of the right ventricle (Fig. 323). A stab wound is made in the wall with a narrow scalpel, and a double-blade vulvotome or a dilator is inserted into the pulmonary trunk through the cavity of the right ventricle (Fig. 324). The position of the end of the instrument is checked by palpation through the wall of the pulmonary artery before its blades are spread. The valvular stenosis is cut or dilated by pressing the handles of the valvulotome or dilator. The opening in the wall of the right ventricle is closed by tying the purse string or the Halsted suture (Fig. 325). The efficacy of the operation is determined by measuring the pressure gradient between the right ventricle and the pulmonary artery before and after the intervention.

In considerable dilatation of the left pulmonary artery the valvular stenosis may be corrected by introducing the dilator through it. The instrument is introduced in the retrograde direction toward the valves of the pulmonary trunk (Fig. 326). The end of the dilator is positioned below the level of the valve of the pulmonary trunk under control of the finger, and the stenosis is dilated by pressing on the handles of the instrument. With the blades closed, the instrument is withdrawn, a clamp is

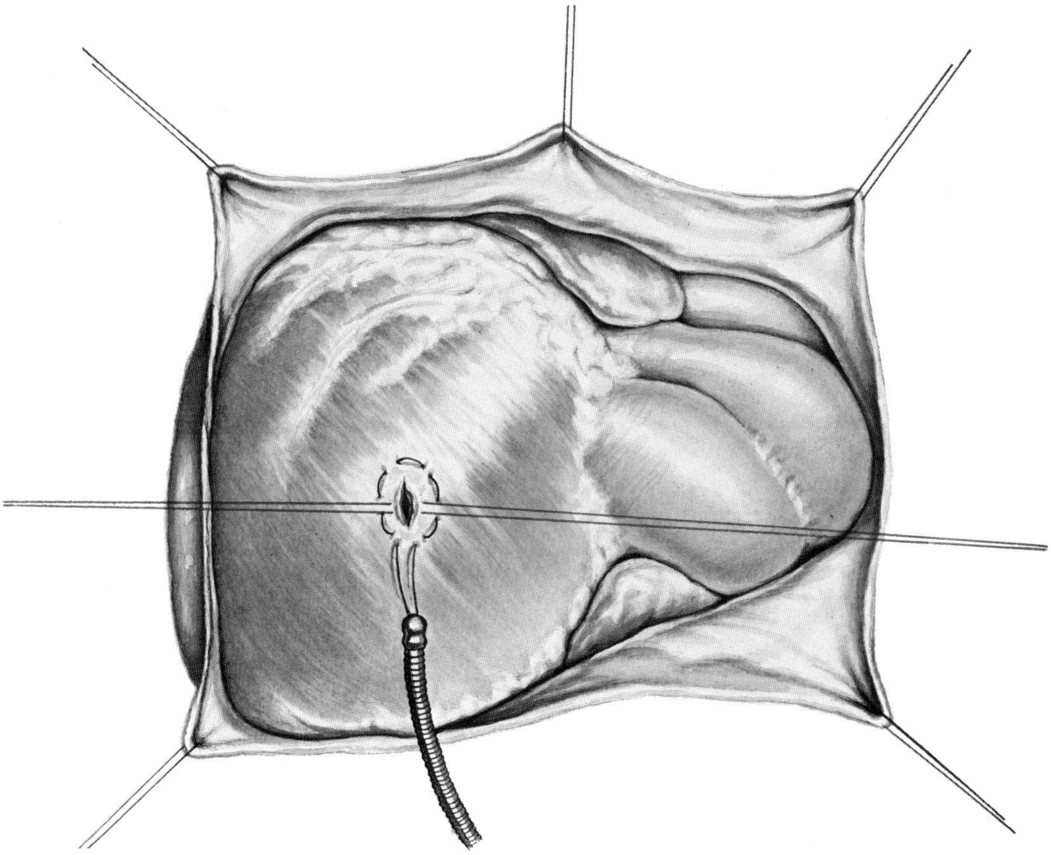

Fig. 323. Traction sutures and purse-string suture are applied to anterior wall of right ventricle.

applied to the side of the left pulmonary artery, and the opening is closed with a continuous suture.

Closed resection of the subvalvular (infundibular) stenosis of the pulmonary trunk is accomplished in a similar manner. The level of the stenosing swell or diaphragm in the right ventricular outflow tract is approximately determined by inspection and palpation of the anterior wall of the right ventricle. A purse-string suture is applied to this wall below the presumed level of the stenosis. Brock's resector is inserted to the level of the stenosing swell or diaphragm and opened, and the stenosing ring is resected (Fig. 327). The instrument is inserted into the right ventricle several times; the extent of the resection made is judged by the amount of muscular and fibrous tissues grasped and extracted. In some cases a dilator is introduced in place of Brock's resector after resection and dilation of the subvalvular stenosis is completed with it. The state of the orifice of the pulmonary trunk at the level of the valves is checked; if stenosed, the valves are dilated (Fig. 328). The efficacy of the operation is also judged by the changes in the pressure gradient between the cavities of the right and third ventricle and the pulmonary artery before and after the operation.

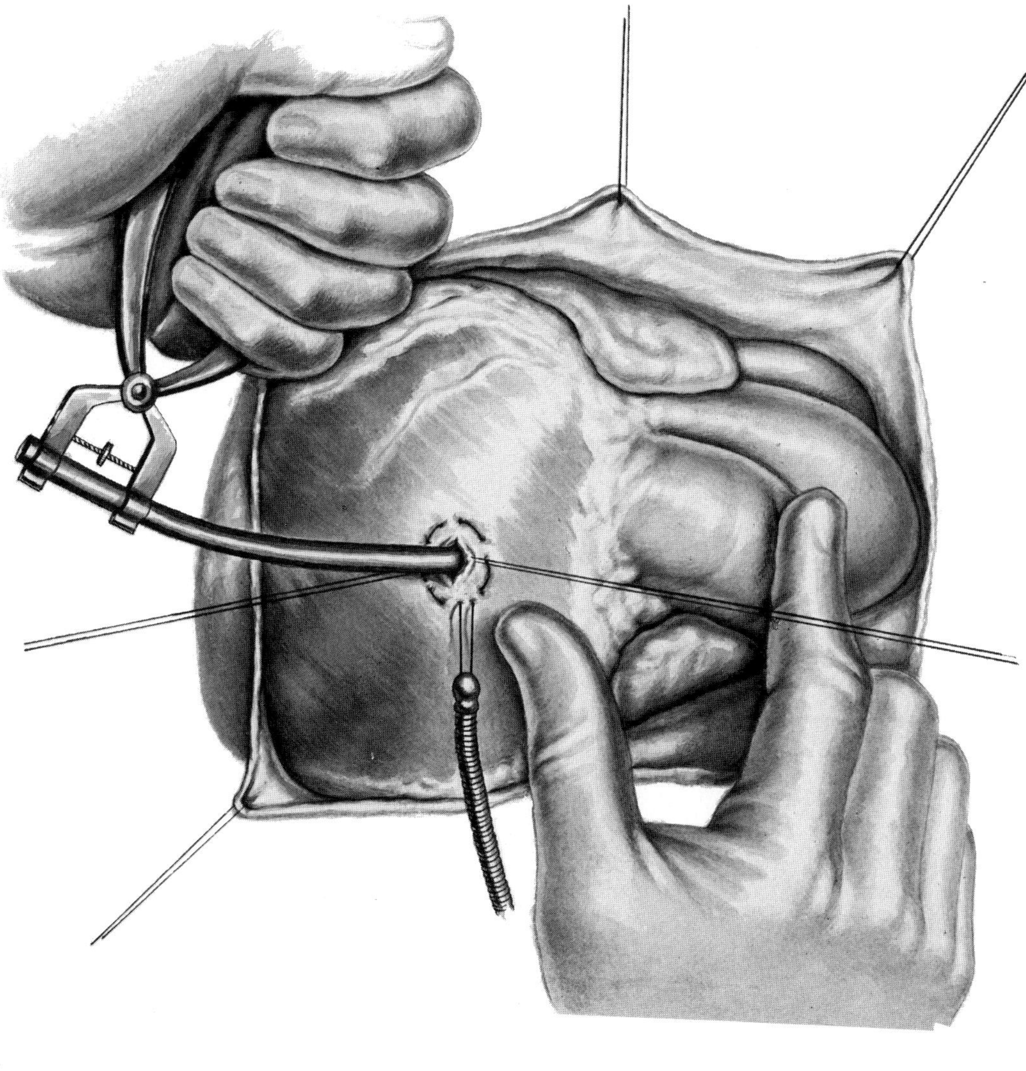

Fig. 324. Valvulotome is introduced into orifice of pulmonary artery under control of finger.

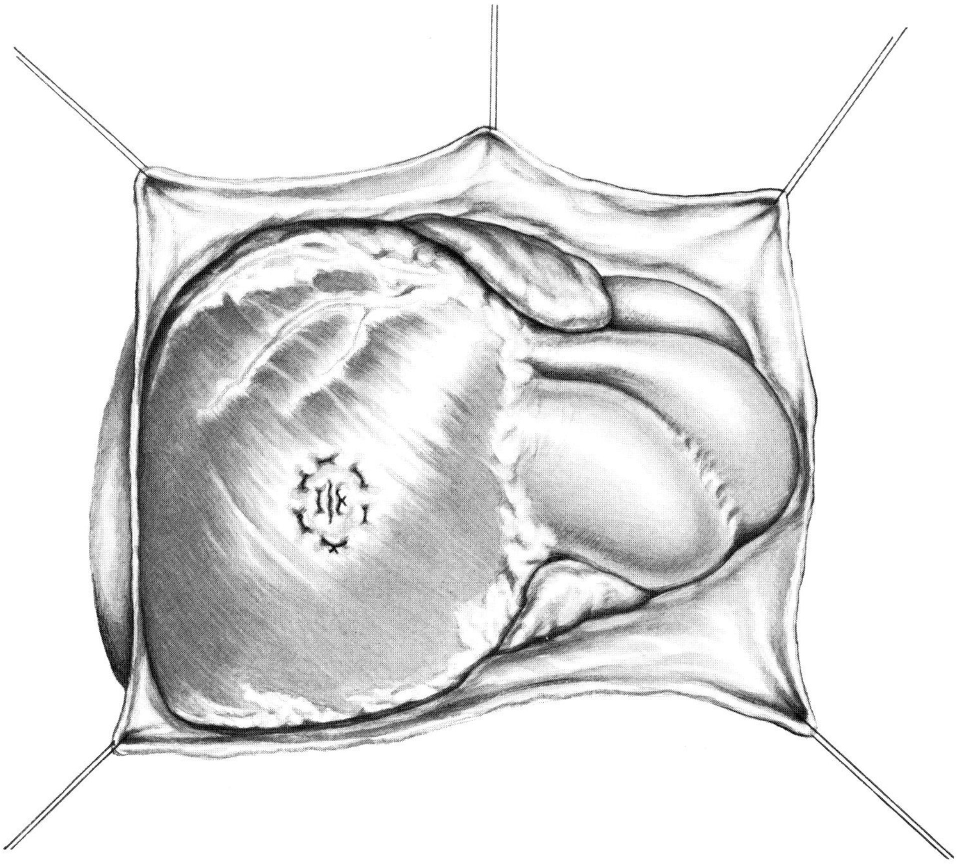

Fig. 325. Purse-string suture is tied after valvulotome has been removed.

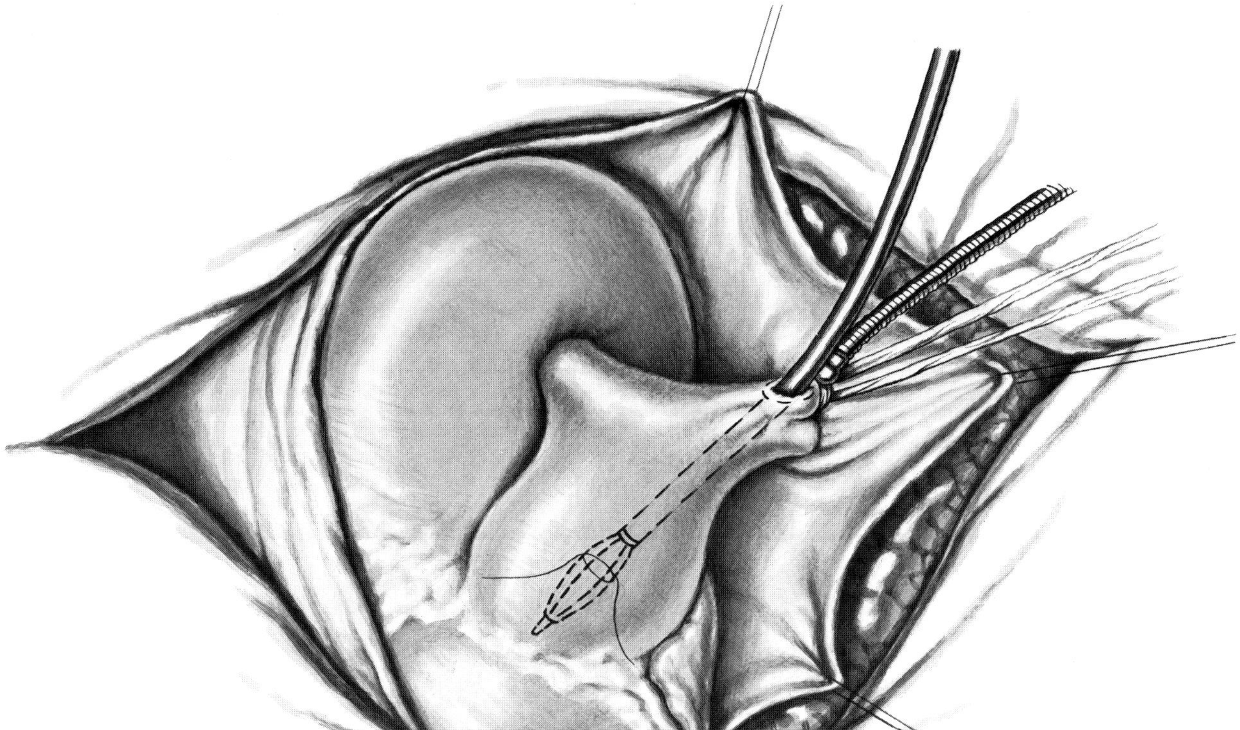

Fig. 326. Valvulotome is introduced into orifice of pulmonary trunk through left pulmonary artery.

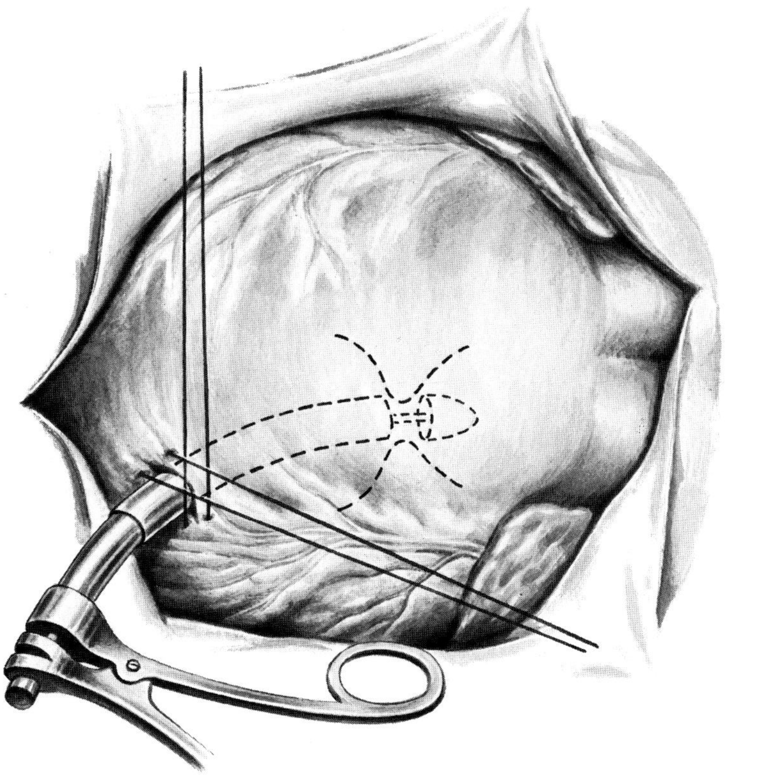

Fig. 327. Brock's resector is introduced through anterior wall of right ventricle.

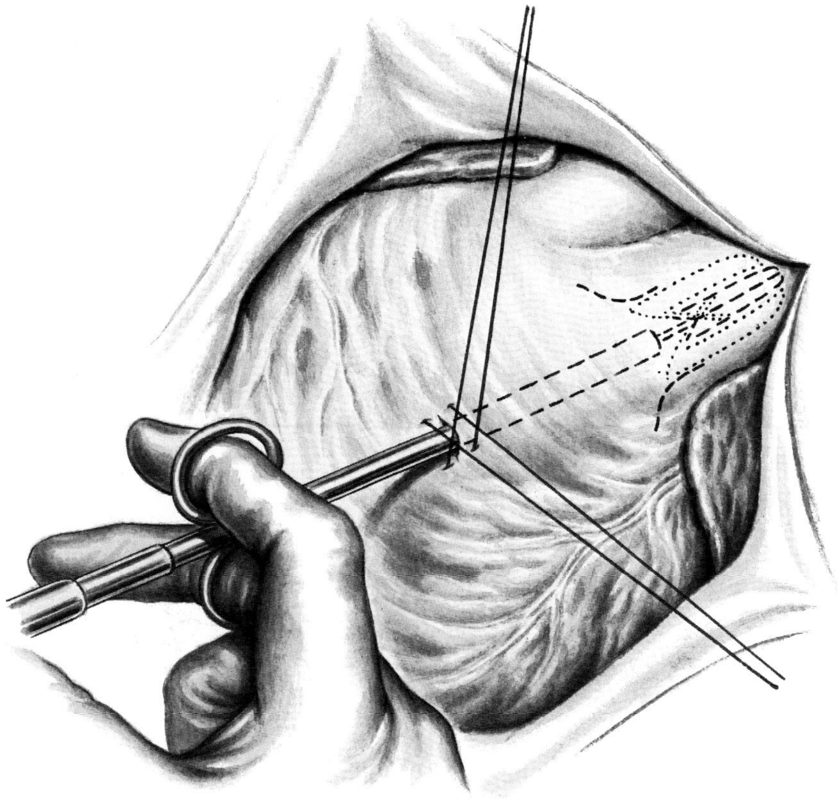

Fig. 328. Dilator is introduced into orifice of pulmonary artery after infundibular resection.

CORRECTION OF TRANSPOSITION OF MAJOR VESSELS AFTER BLALOCK-HANLON

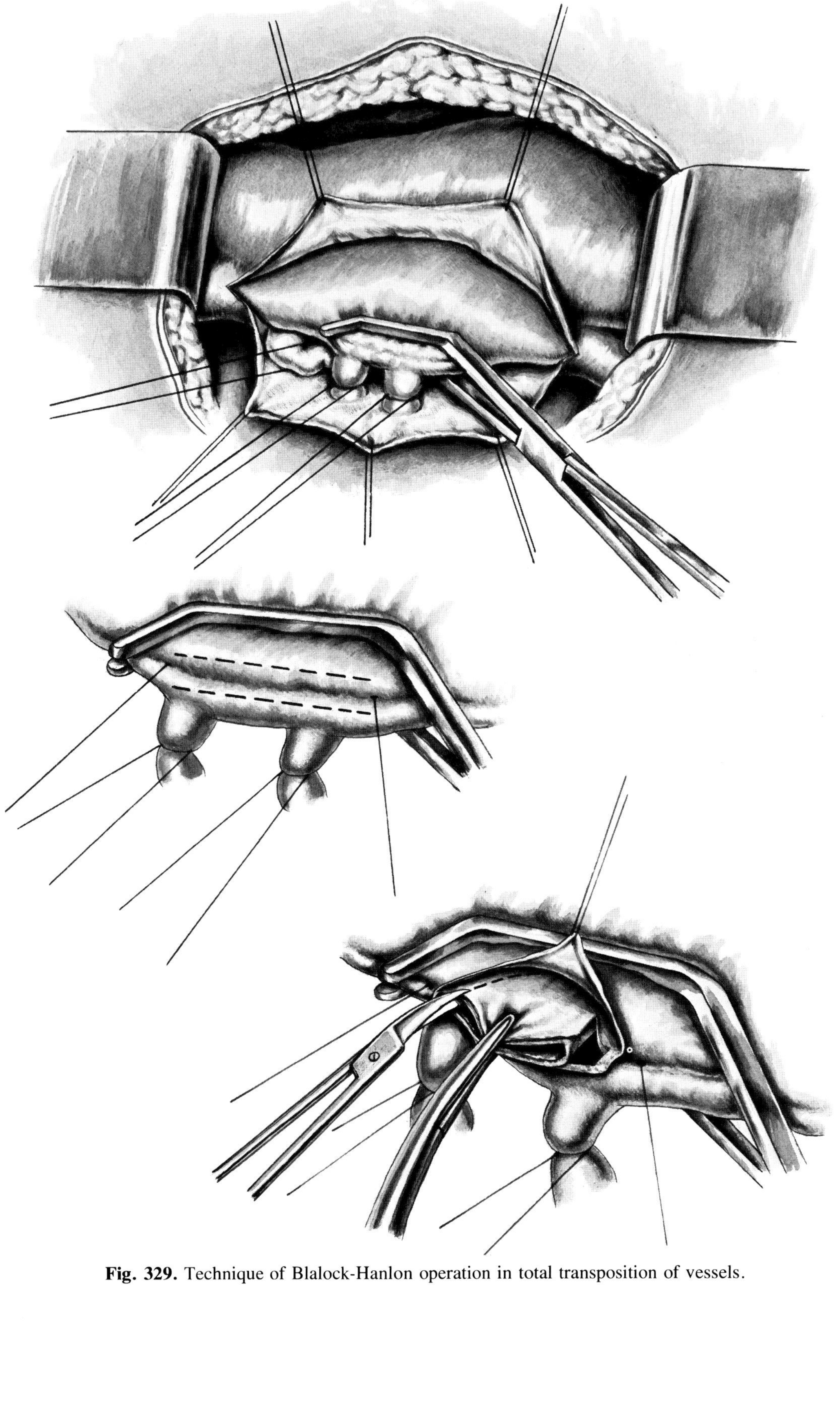

Fig. 329. Technique of Blalock-Hanlon operation in total transposition of vessels.

The operation is carried out by right thoracotomy in the fourth intercostal space, usually on infants and newborns, in the cyanotic form of transposition of the vessels.

With the pericardium opened wide, clamps are applied to the right pulmonary veins and to parts of the left and right atria and an area of the interatrial septum.

The right pulmonary veins are temporarily compressed with ligatures passed under them. The wall of the right atrium is cut longitudinally in the clamped area, and the interatrial septum is resected through its cavity. The incision in the wall of the right atrium is then sutured, the ligatures on the pulmonary veins loosened, the air removed from the atria and pulmonary veins, and the clamp taken off (Fig. 329). As the result of the operation a large interatrial defect is formed providing free drainage of venous blood to the mitral valve and arterial blood to the tricuspid valve (Fig. 330). The operation relieves cyanosis partly or completely.

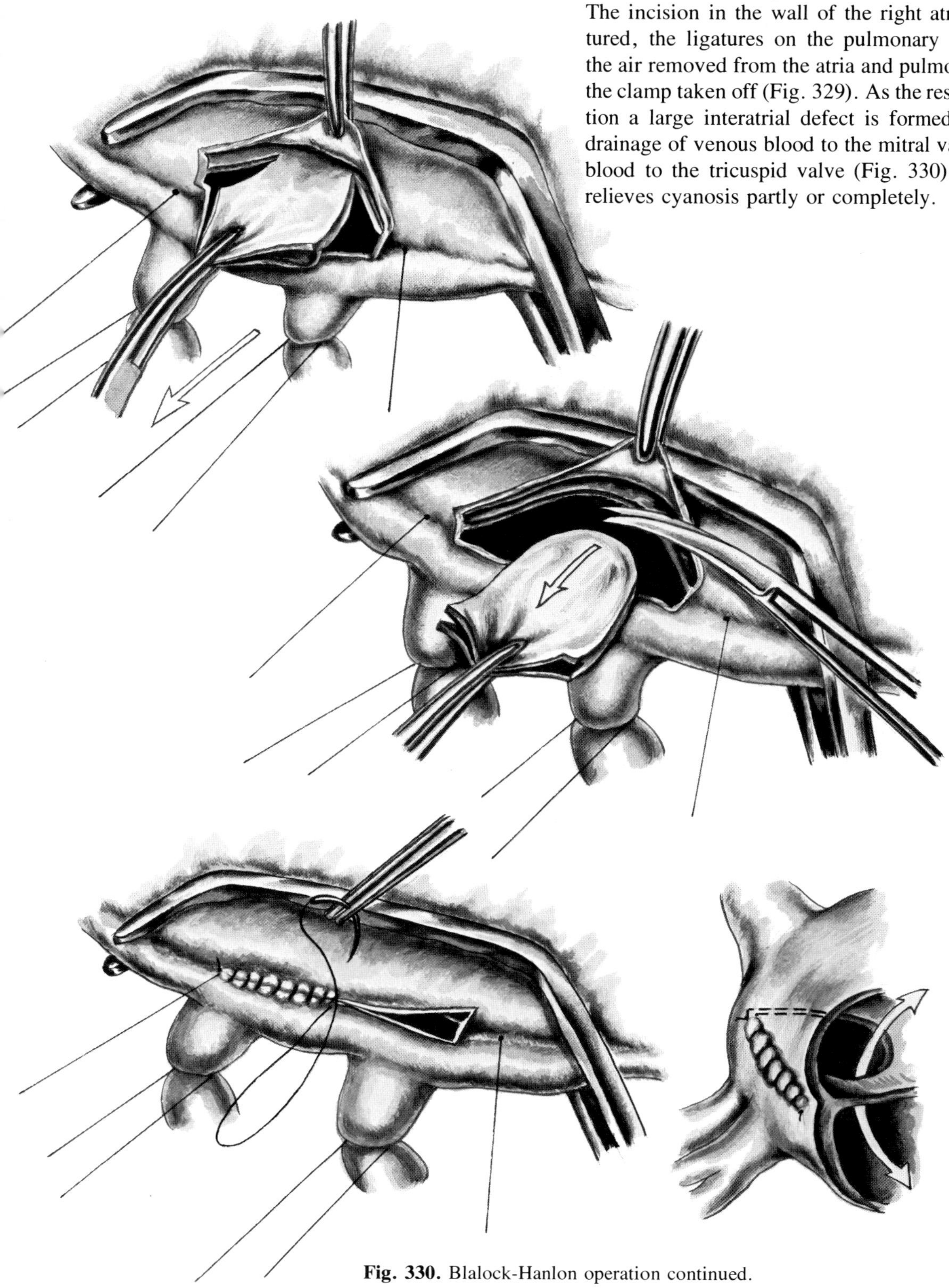

Fig. 330. Blalock-Hanlon operation continued.

Open heart surgery with extracorporeal circulation

METHOD FOR CONNECTING THE HEART-LUNG MACHINE

After the pericardium is opened, the superior vena cava is mobilized by means of a small dissector. To accomplish this, the apex of the right auricle and the ascending aorta are moved aside and the posterior wall of the transverse pericardial sinus is exposed. The dissector is most often advanced from the lateral wall of the superior vena cava, and the tissues are separated in the direction of the caudal border of the right pulmonary artery. It should be borne in mind that the superior vena cava is located mesopericardially with part of its dorsal wall not covered by the pericardium.

The perivascular cellular tissue is cut with scissors, and a tape is grasped with the end of the dissector and drawn around the vena cava (Fig. 331).

The inferior vena cava is separated with the largest dissector also after the pericardium has been opened. In drastic dilatation of the left atrium the inferior vena cava is spread wide over it. The dissector is usually passed from the medial side of the vena cava. The inferior vena cava is encircled with the thumb and index finger of the left hand from the side of the oblique sinus; they palpate the layer of the cellular tissue through which the dissector will be passed. This tissue is pushed out by the tip of the dissector laterally to the vena cava and then cut with scissors while the wall of the right atrum is moved aside a little. The end of the tape is grasped with a dissector and drawn around the vena cava (Fig. 332).

To insert the venous catheter into the superior vena cava, the apex of the right auricle is grasped with a triangular clamp. A purse-string suture is applied with an atraumatic needle at the base of the auricle (Fig. 333).

The catheter is introduced into the inferior vena cava through the wall of the right atrium close to the orifice of the vessel. A purse-string suture corresponding to the size of the venous cannula is applied. In some cases a Halsted suture is also added. The ends of the sutures for both venous cannulas are passed through tourniquets. To insert the catheter into the superior vena cava, the apex of the right auricle is clamped with Satinsky's clamp and opened with scissors, and traction sutures are applied to the edges of the incision. Before the venous cannula is introduced, the cavity of the right atrium is explored with the finger (Fig. 334). The venous cannula is introduced into the right atrium and advanced into the superior vena cava while Satinsky's clamp is removed (Fig. 335). The tourniquet purse-string suture is tightened around the cannula. The firm position of the cannula is ensured with a ligature tied around the apex of the right auricle and the cannula. To introduce the catheter into the inferior vena cava, part of the right atrial wall is pulled out by the purse-string and Halsted sutures (Fig. 336). Satinsky's clamp is applied to part of the wall with the purse-string suture. The atrial wall is cut with a scalpel in the center of the purse-string suture, and traction sutures are placed on the edges of the incision (Fig. 337). The venous cannula is introduced into the inferior vena cava with the simultaneous removal of Satinsky's clamp. The purse-string suture is tightened. The cannula is held fast with a circular ligature passed through the atrial wall (Fig. 338).

In operations on the aortic valve the ascending aorta is separated from the pulmonary trunk through a longitudinal transsternal approach and encircled with a tape by means of a dissector (Fig. 339). These two large vessels are separated with scissors; careful electrocoagulation of the vessels in the cellular tissue between them is performed. Whenever necessary the pulmonary trunk is encircled with a tape through this incision and the transverse pericardial sinus (Fig. 340).

In left thoracotomy (mitral valve prosthetics) the venous cannula of the machine is introduced into the right ventricle. For this purpose a wide Halsted suture with Teflon bolsters is applied to the outflow tract of the right ventricle. Two traction sutures are applied between the bolsters (Fig. 341). A longitudinal incision is made with a scalpel between the traction sutures; the incision is compressed with the left index finger, and then the venous cannula of the heart-lung machine is advanced into the cavity of the right ventricle. The Halsted suture is tied around the inserted cannula (Fig. 342). The cannula is additionally tied to the wall of the right ventricle. After the operation is completed, the cannula is taken out and bleeding is first temporarily arrested by crossing the traction sutures and compressing the line of the incision with the finger and then by applying a continuous blanket suture.

The arterial cannula of the machine is connected through the common femoral artery. To expose the artery, the overlying tissues are cut immediately caudal to the inguinal ligament (Fig. 343). Blanket traction sutures

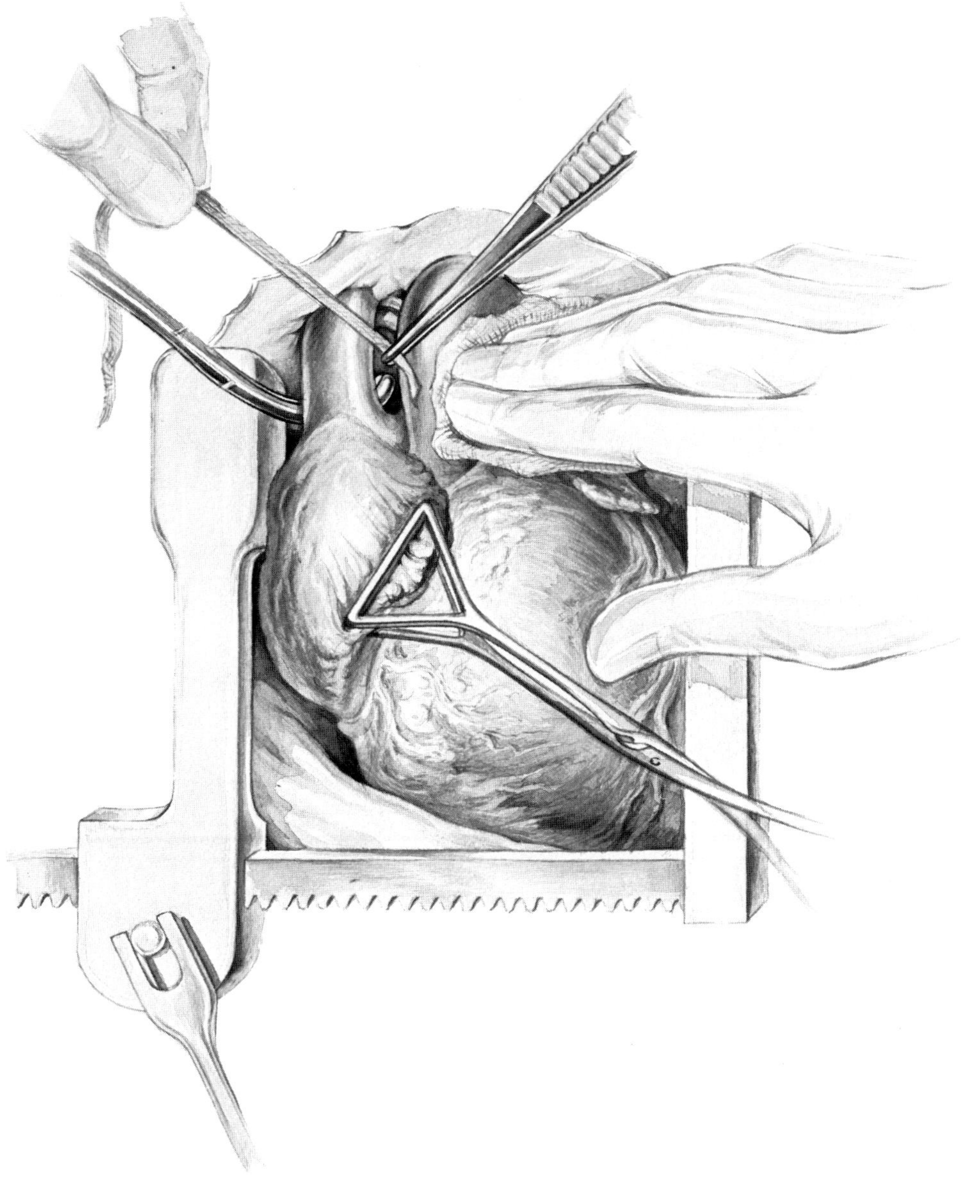

Fig. 331. Superior vena cava is mobilized. Apex of right auricle and descending aorta are moved medially.

are placed around the lateral branches of the artery cranial to the origin of the deep femoral artery for temporary arrest of blood flow in the artery after the cannula is connected. The common femoral artery is encircled with a tape, clamped with two pairs of artery forceps, and opened longitudinally cranial to the deep femoral artery.

The arterial cannula of the machine is advanced cranially into the femoral artery, while the artery forceps are removed (Fig. 344). The encircling tape is tightened around the artery with the cannula inside. After the operation is ended and the cannula is removed, a lateral vascular suture is placed on the artery with an atraumatic needle.

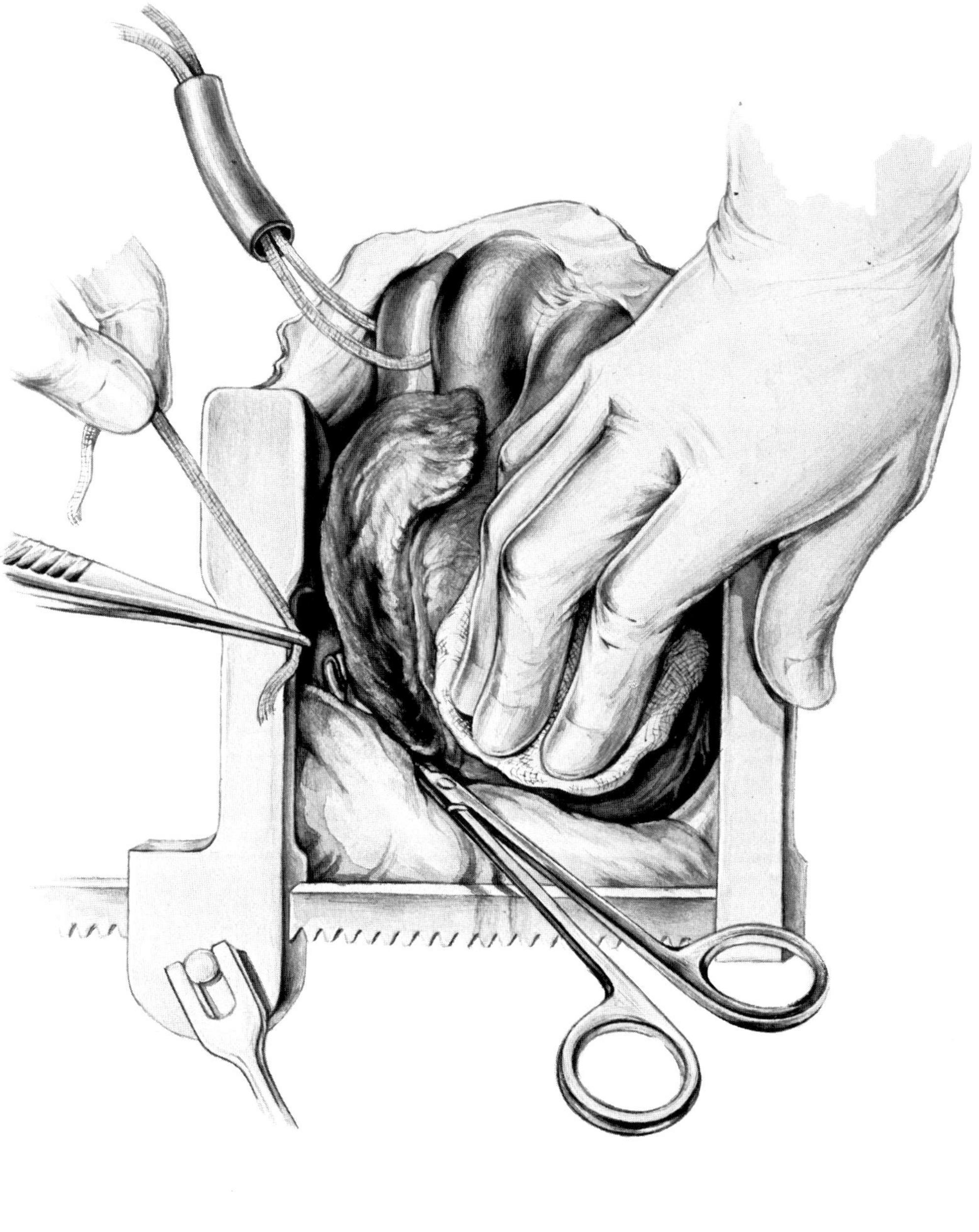

Fig. 332. Inferior vena cava is mobilized. Dissector is brought under vein from medial side.

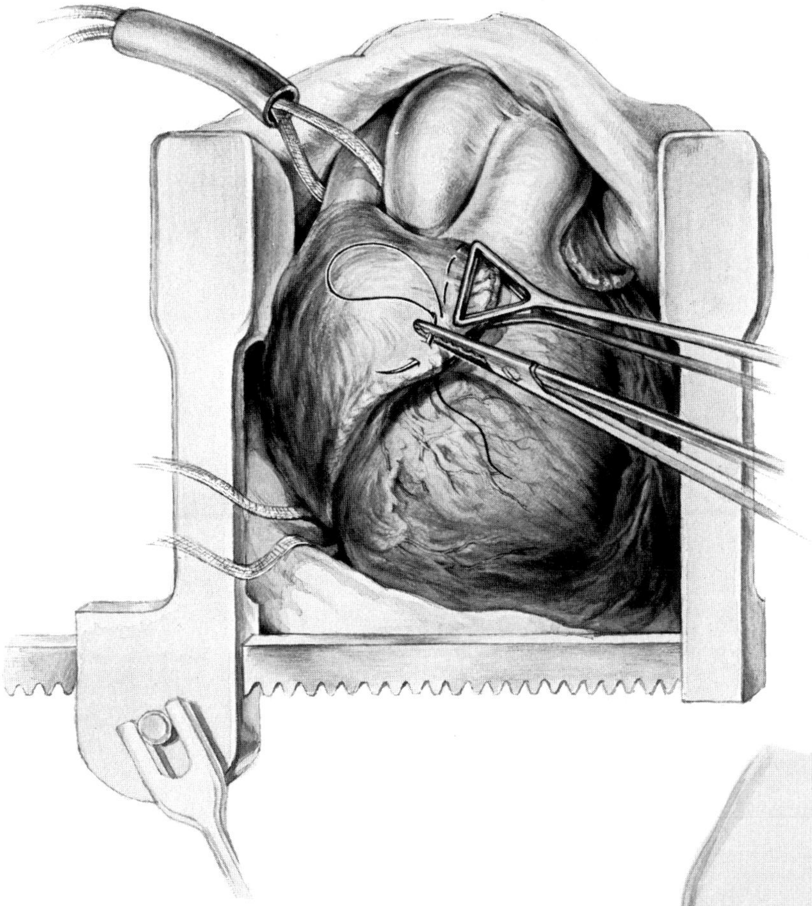

Fig. 333. Purse-string suture is applied to base of right atrial auricle.

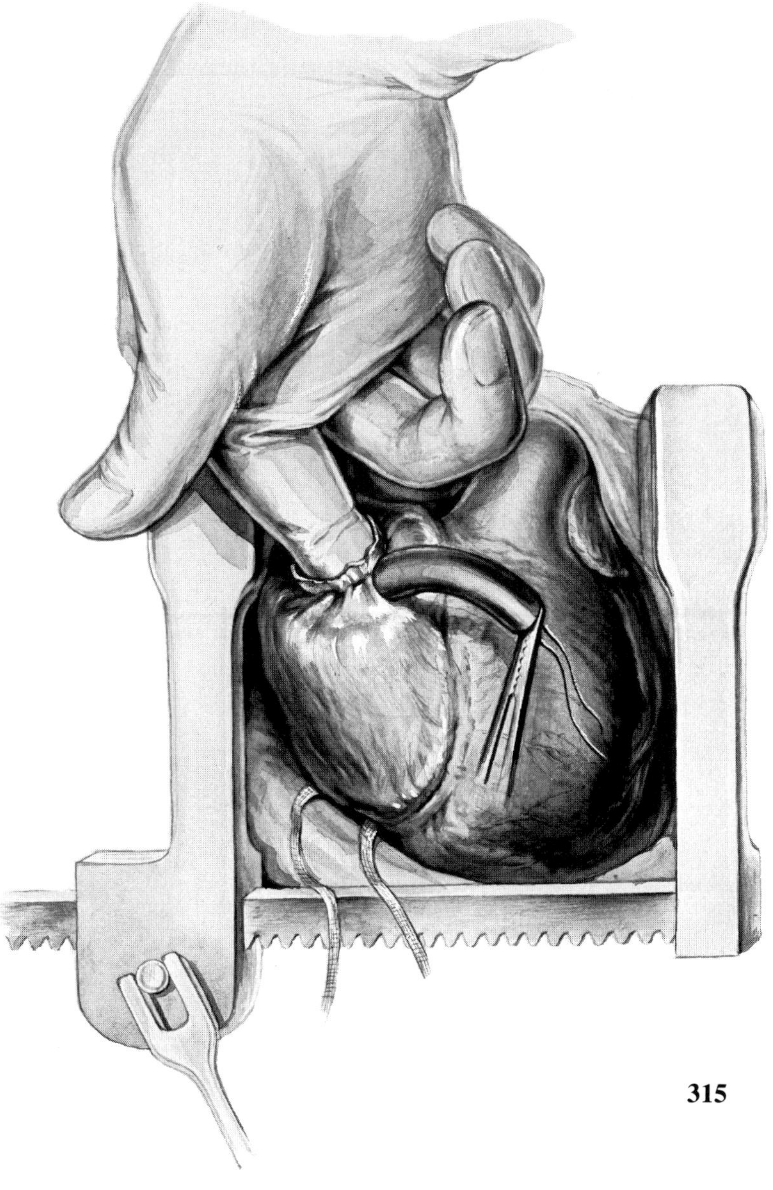

Fig. 334. Right atrium is explored with finger through right auricle. Purse-string suture is tightened around finger by means of tourniquet.

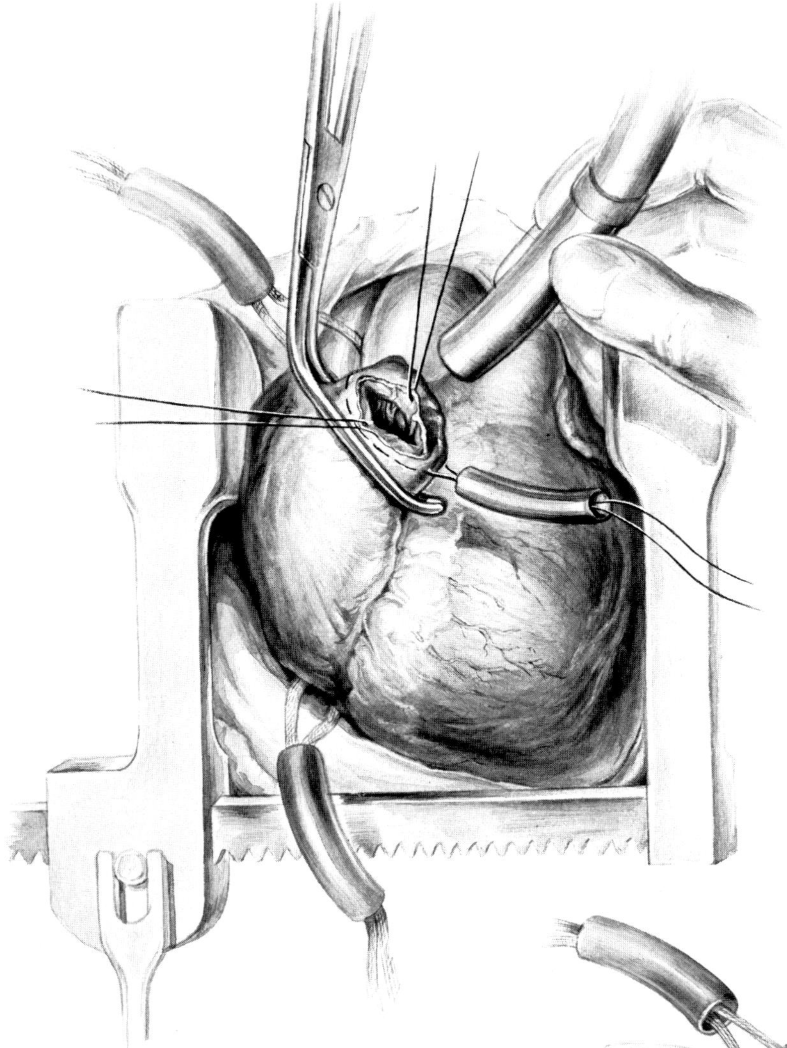

Fig. 335. Introduction of cannula into superior vena cava. Auricle of right atrium has been clamped with Satinsky's clamp and opened. Two traction sutures have been applied to edges of incision.

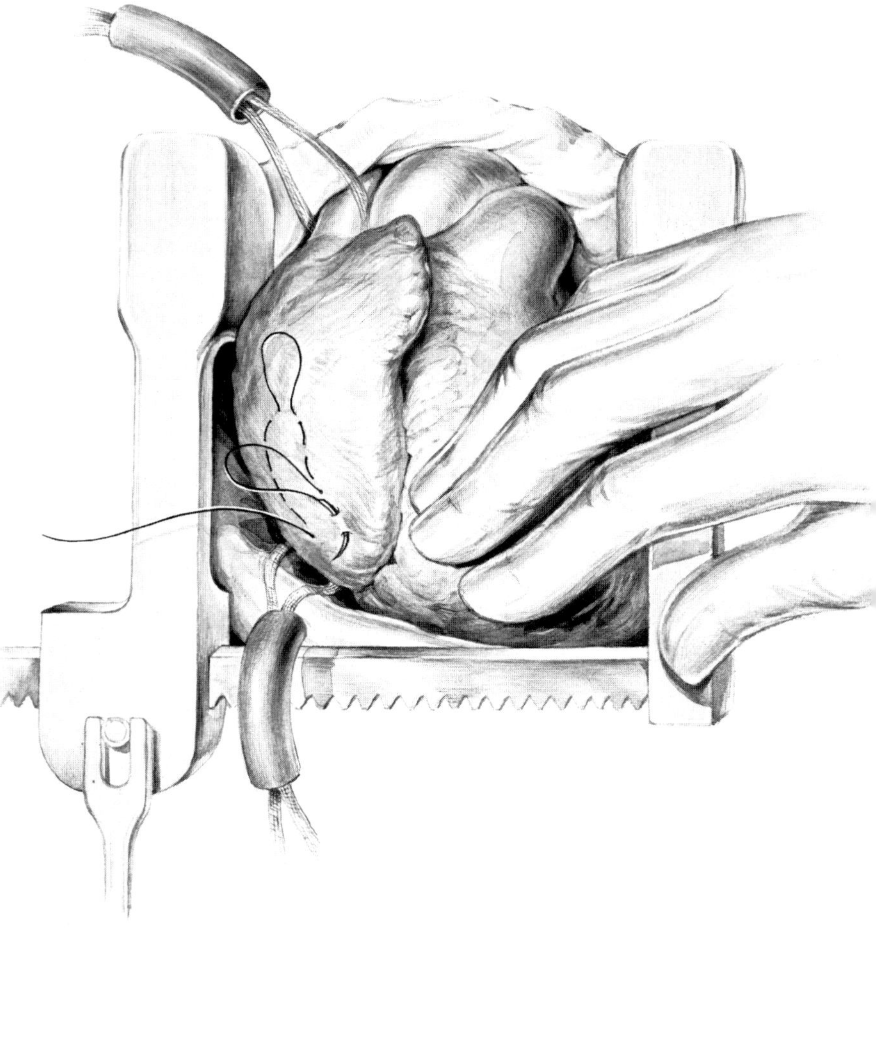

Fig. 336. Purse-string suture is applied to wall of right atrium for cannulation of inferior vena cava.

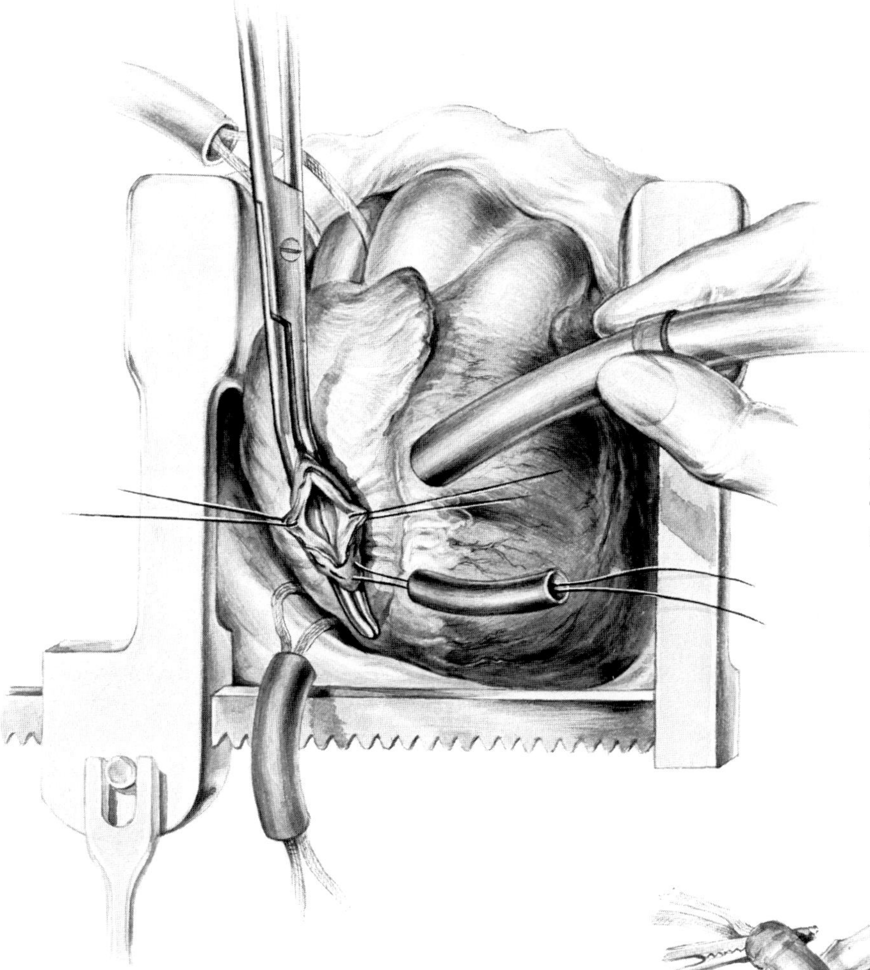

Fig. 337. Introduction of cannula into inferior vena cava. Wall of right atrium is clamped with Satinsky's clamp and cut. Traction sutures are applied to edges of incision.

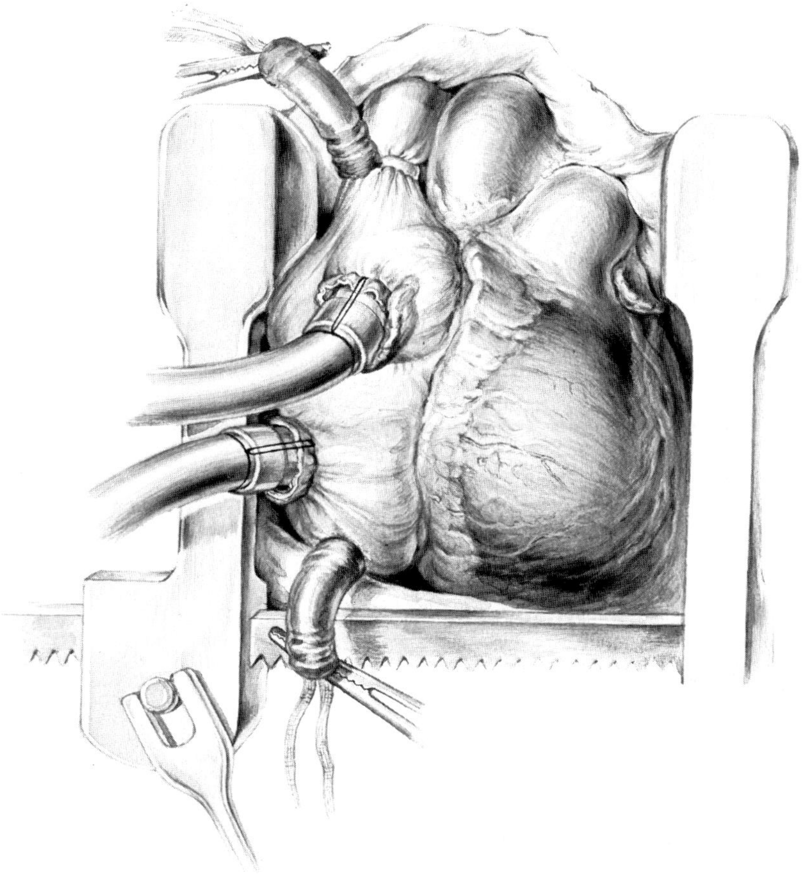

Fig. 338. View of heart after cannulation of superior and inferior venae cavae.

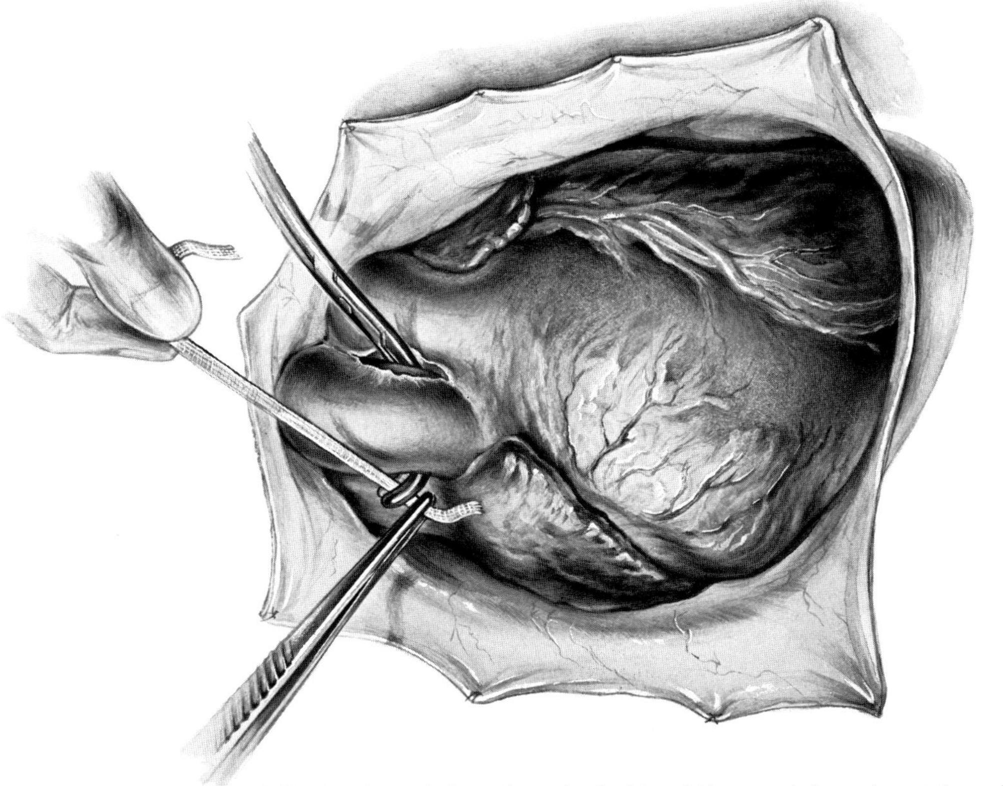

Fig. 339. Aorta is mobilized and tape is brought under it. Tip of dissector is brought out through transverse pericardial sinus.

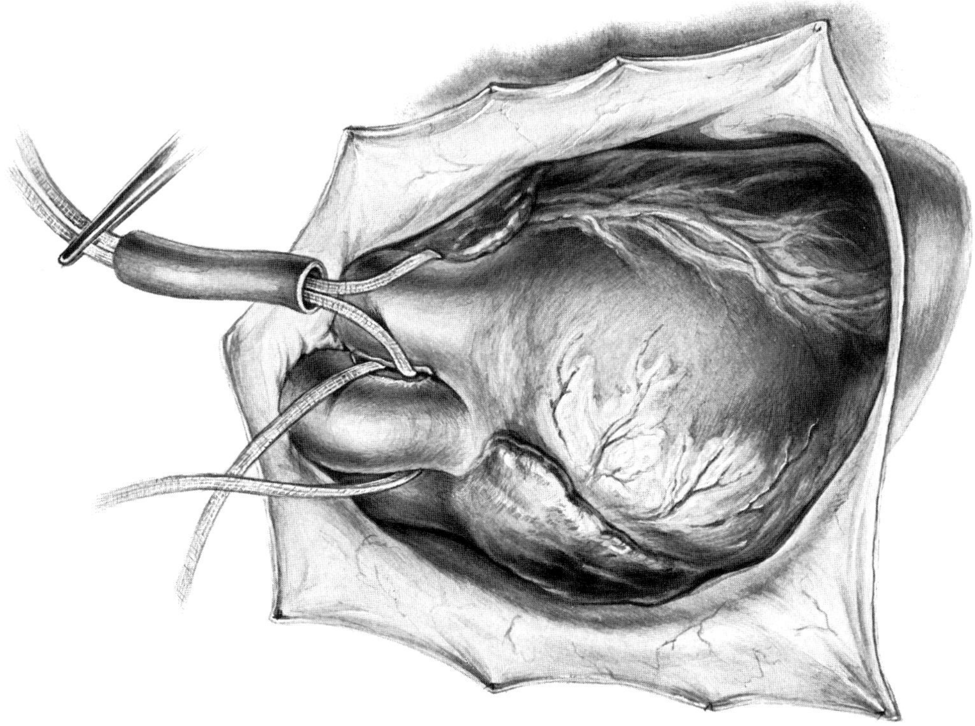

Fig. 340. Aorta and pulmonary trunk are encircled with tapes.

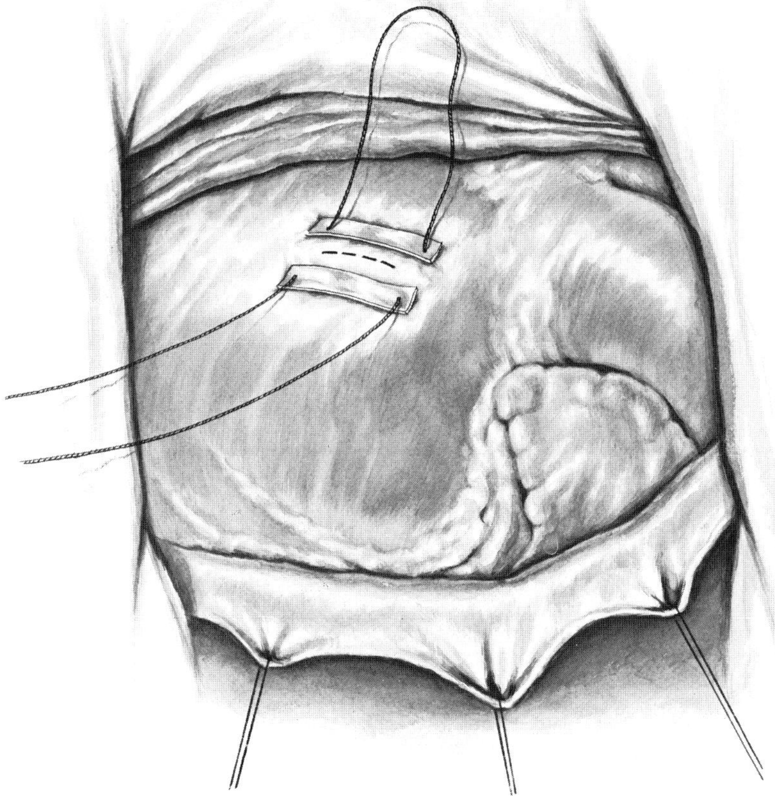

Fig. 341. Application of Halsted suture with use of plastic bolsters to region of right ventricular outflow tract.

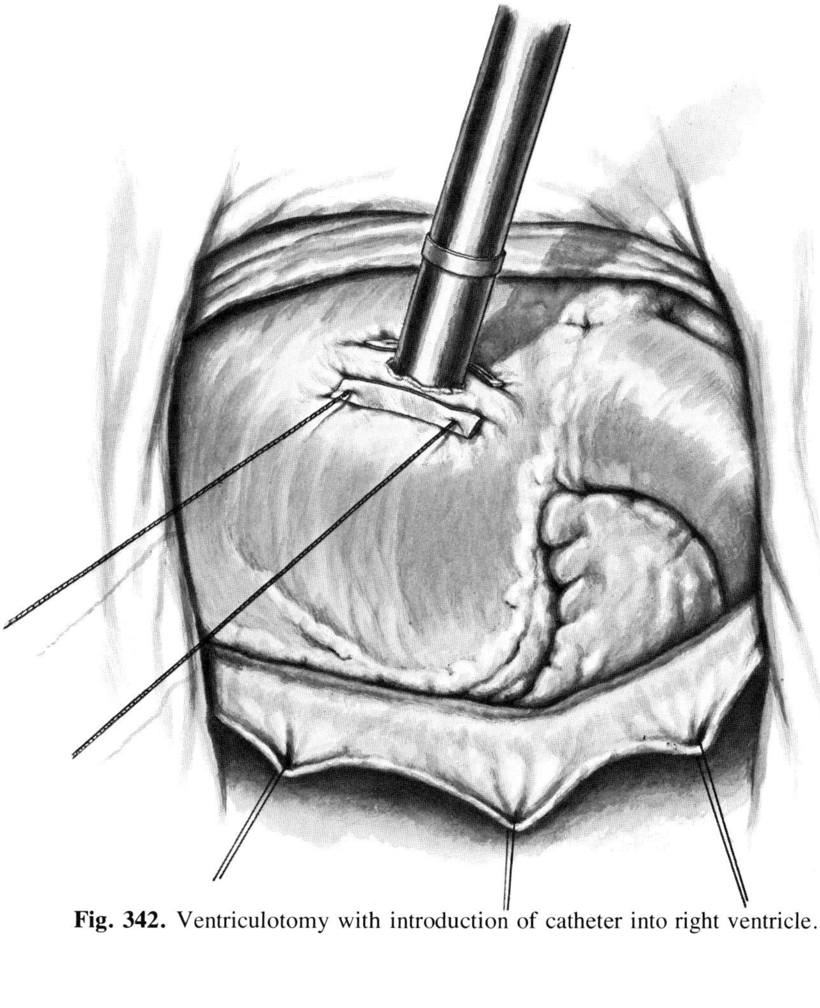

Fig. 342. Ventriculotomy with introduction of catheter into right ventricle.

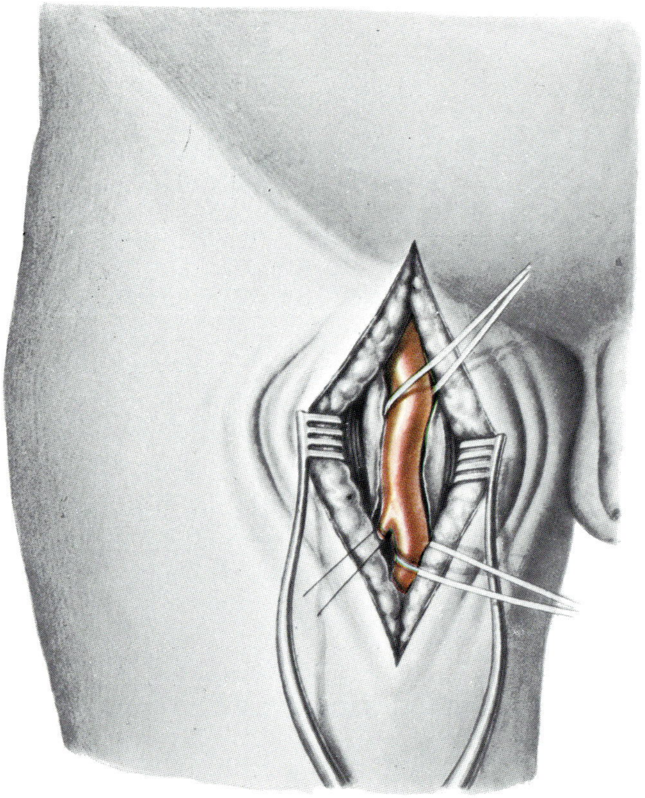

Fig. 343. Femoral artery is mobilized and loops brought under its branches.

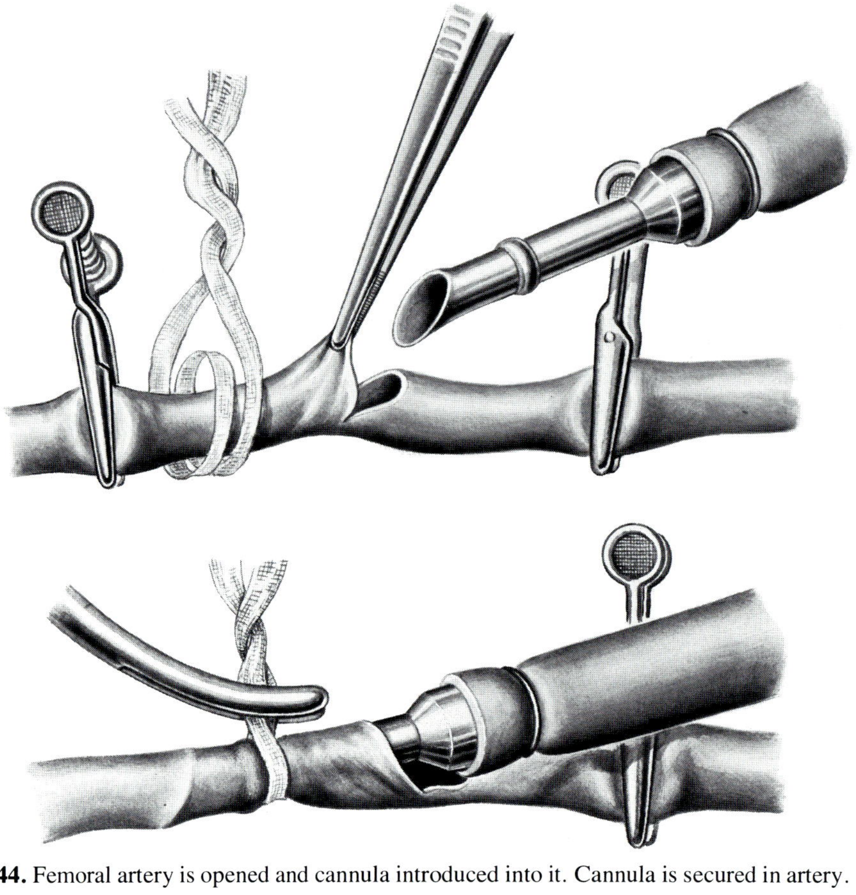

Fig. 344. Femoral artery is opened and cannula introduced into it. Cannula is secured in artery.

CORRECTION OF INTERATRIAL SEPTAL DEFECTS

CLOSURE AND PLASTIC SURGERY OF SECONDARY DEFECTS

Secondary defects in the interatrial septum are repaired with the heart disconnected from circulation under conditions of both moderate artificial hypothermia and extracorporeal circulation.

The operation is performed by right thoracotomy in the fourth intercostal space or by longitudinal transsternal approach. Intraoperative diagnosis of secondary interatrial defects with left-to-right shunt includes inspection of the heart, its palpation, and intracardiac probing with the finger.

In secondary interatrial defects with left-to-right shunt the right atrium and right ventricle are enlarged, and the walls of the right atrium are pink (Fig. 345). The defect may be determined by palpation by inverting the outer wall of the right atrium. For intraatrial examination of the defect the index finger is introduced through the right auricle.

The degree of pulmonary hypertension is determined by puncture of the right cardiac cavities and pulmonary artery. When there is a large arteriovenous shunt due to

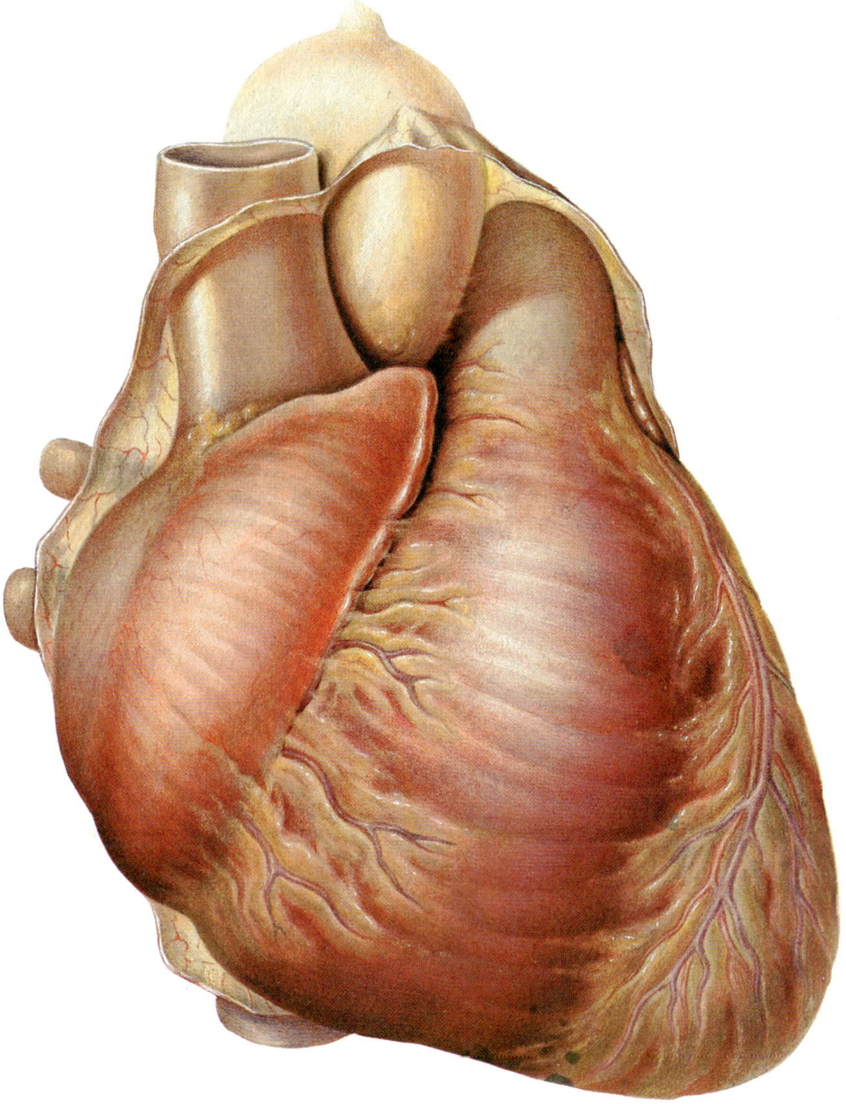

Fig. 345. View of heart in interatrial septal defect with left-to-right shunt. Right atrium is enlarged and pink. Right ventricle and pulmonary trunk are enlarged. Venae cavae are somewhat constricted.

muscular hypertrophy of the right ventricular outflow tract, a pressure gradient between the right ventricle and the pulmonary artery may be determined during systole without the presence of organic stenoses. In operations conducted under artificial hypothermia, after the venae cavae have been clamped the right atrium is opened with an incision stretching from the superior to the inferior vena cava. After the defect has been sutured, the edges of the incision to which traction sutures have been previously applied are clamped with Derra's or Satinsky's clamp. As the clamp is applied the cavity of the right atrium is filled with physiological saline solution and the anesthetist inflates the patient's lungs. The incision in the clamped part of the right atrial is closed with a double row of Halsted sutures and a blanket suture.

In operations under conditions of extracorporeal circulation the right atrium is opened with an incision made between catheters introduced into the inferior and superior venae cavae through the wall of the right atrium and the auricle.

A central secondary defect in the interatrial septum is located in the region of the oval foramen. Its lower border is usually formed by a thin endocardial fold, which is actually a deficiently developed eustachian valve (Fig. 346).

Closure of the defect is begun with the application of extreme sutures in the cranial and caudal parts of the defect. In the caudal part the sutures are placed on the muscular edges of the defect and the thin endocardial fold mentioned. After the sutures are tied, the caudal

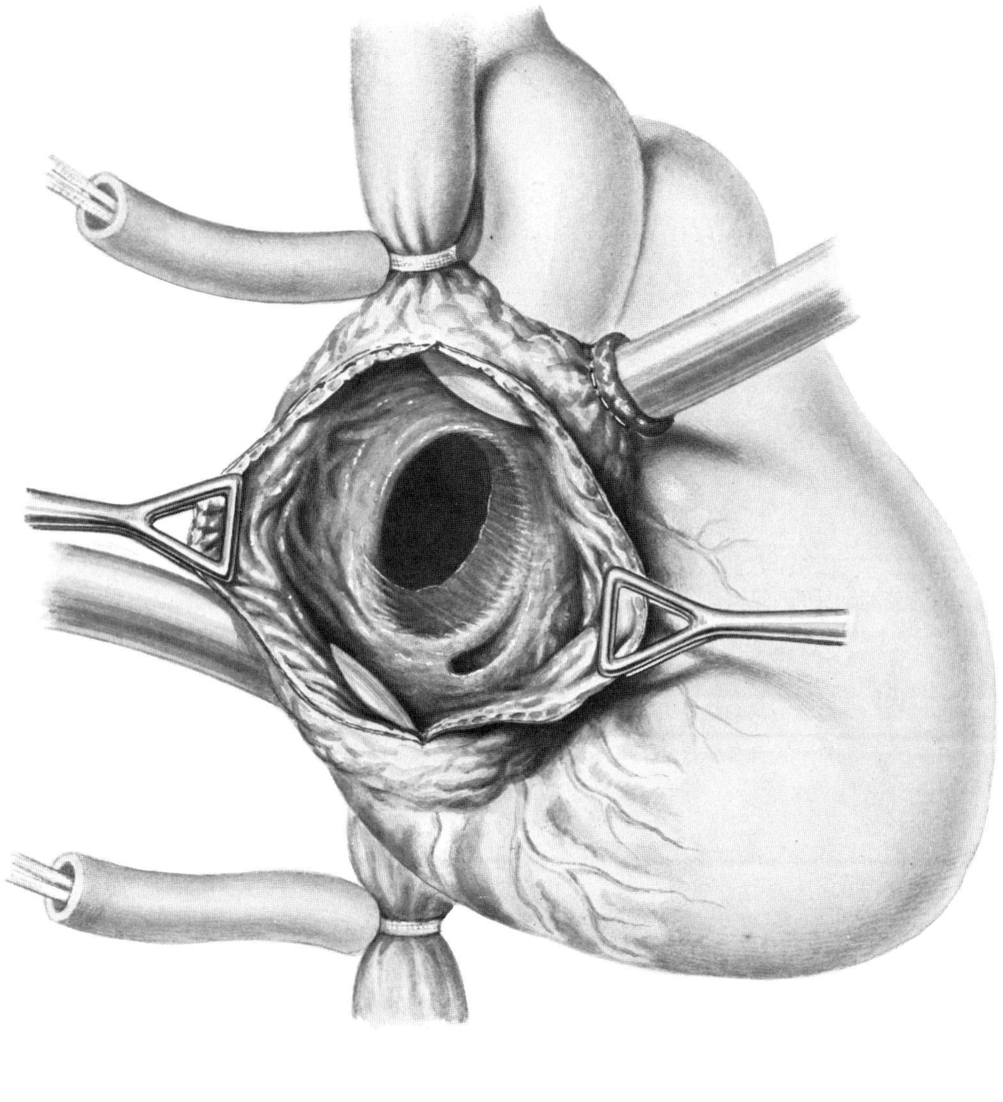

Fig. 346. Central secondary defect in interatrial septum viewed from opened right atrium. Cannulas have been introduced into both venae cavae.

thread is used for placing the continuous suture on the remaining part of the defect (Fig. 347). When the last suture in the cranial part of the defect is being tightened, the anesthetist inflates the patient's lungs, removing the air from the left atrium. Under conditions of extracorporeal circulation it is possible to apply a second row of blanket sutures, because of which the interatrial septum is made reliably airtight.

A central secondary defect in the region of the oval foramen is quite often latticed because of development of an anomaly of the secondary septum of the heart (Fig. 348). The technique of closure under such conditions follows the pattern described. The sutures are applied to the muscular edges of the oval foramen; the latticed membrane is ignored. Large secondary defects in the interatrial septum giving the appearance of the total absence of the septum are closed with a plastic graft. A pericardial graft is sometimes used for the purpose.

Interrupted Halsted sutures are applied to the edges of the defect. The same threads are stitched through the edges of the graft, which is then lowered on the septum, and all the sutures are tied one by one (Figs. 349 and 350).

Another technique may be used. Two Halsted sutures are applied to the cranial and caudal corners of the defect with which the graft is stitched through. The sutures are tied. The same threads are used to stitch the edges of the defect to the graft by means of continuous sutures (Fig. 351).

In a secondary interatrial defect the endocardial fold

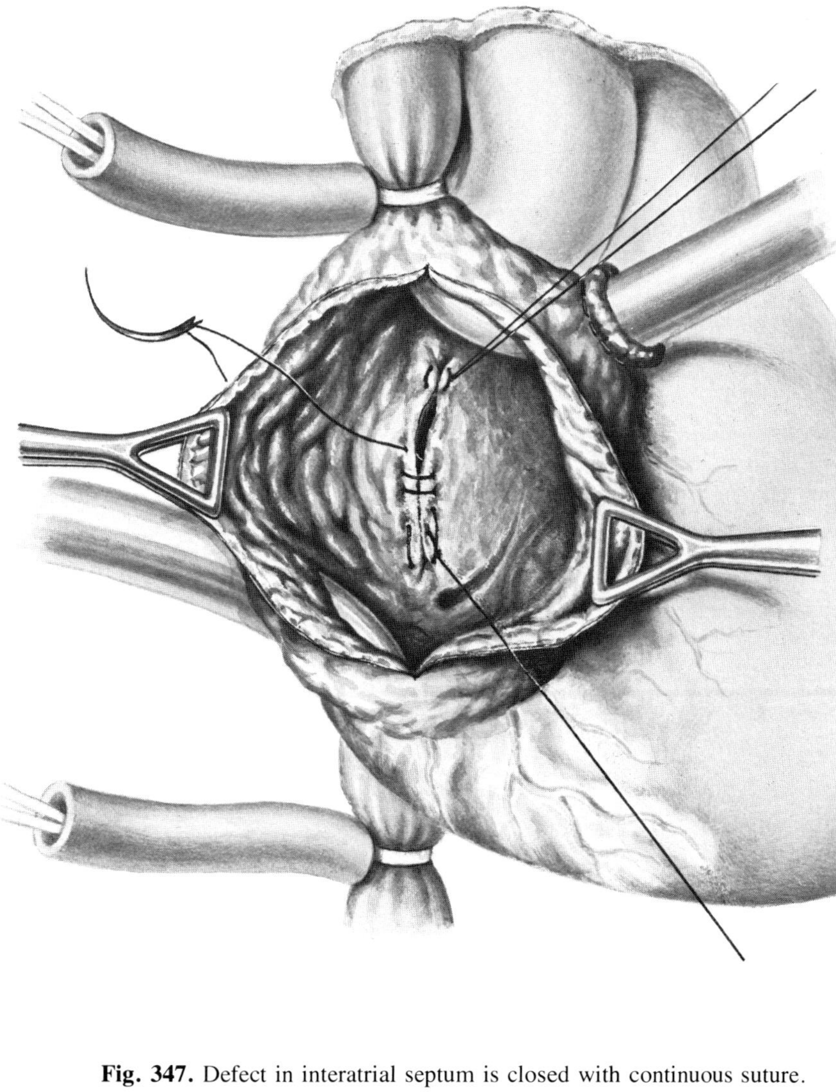

Fig. 347. Defect in interatrial septum is closed with continuous suture.

forming its lower border is inconspicuous, and in the region of the defect the inferior vena cava drains the inferior simultaneously into the right and left atria. In such cases the defect is sutured using Lewis's method. Its peculiarities consist in the techniques of the closure of the caudal margin of the defect. A semi-purse-string suture is stitched beginning from the muscular edge of the defect, then passing the needle through the dorsal wall of the left atrium where the inferior vena cava drains into it, and ending on the muscular part of the outer edge of the defect. In tightening of this suture the wall of the left atrium in the region of the inferior vena cava is crimped, while the inferior vena cava is isolated from the cavity of the left atrium. This suture forms the caudal margin of the interatrial defect, which is sutured by one of the methods described above (Figs. 352 to 354).

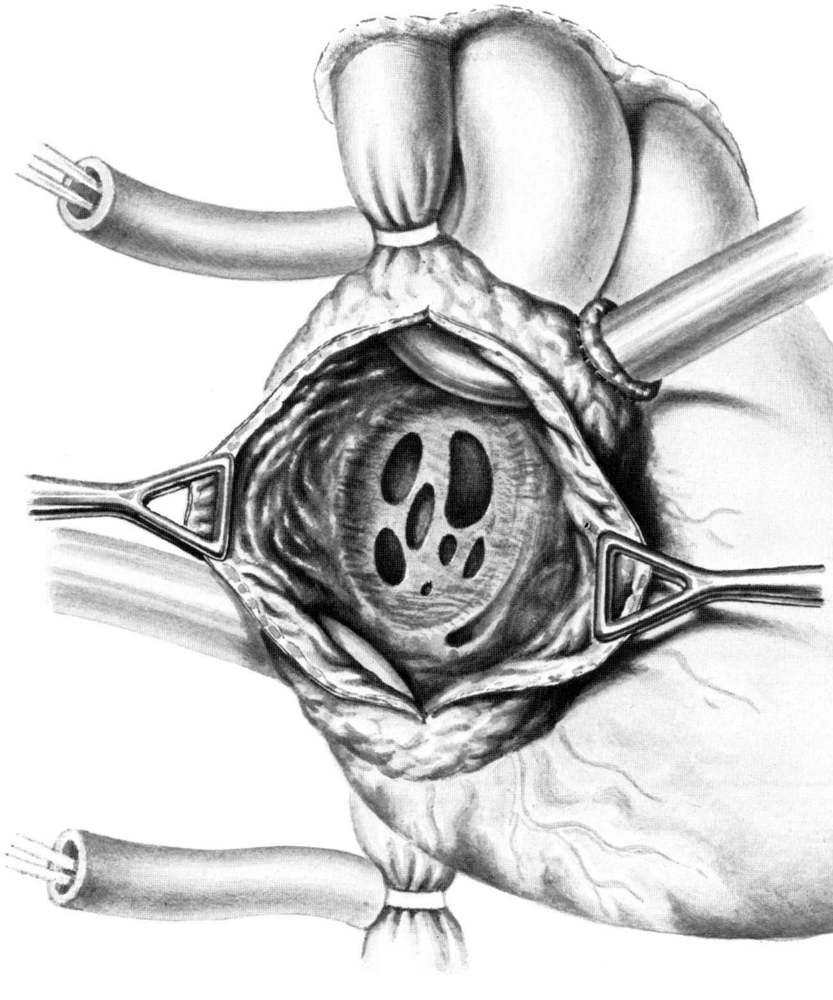

Fig. 348. Latticed form of secondary interatrial septal defect.

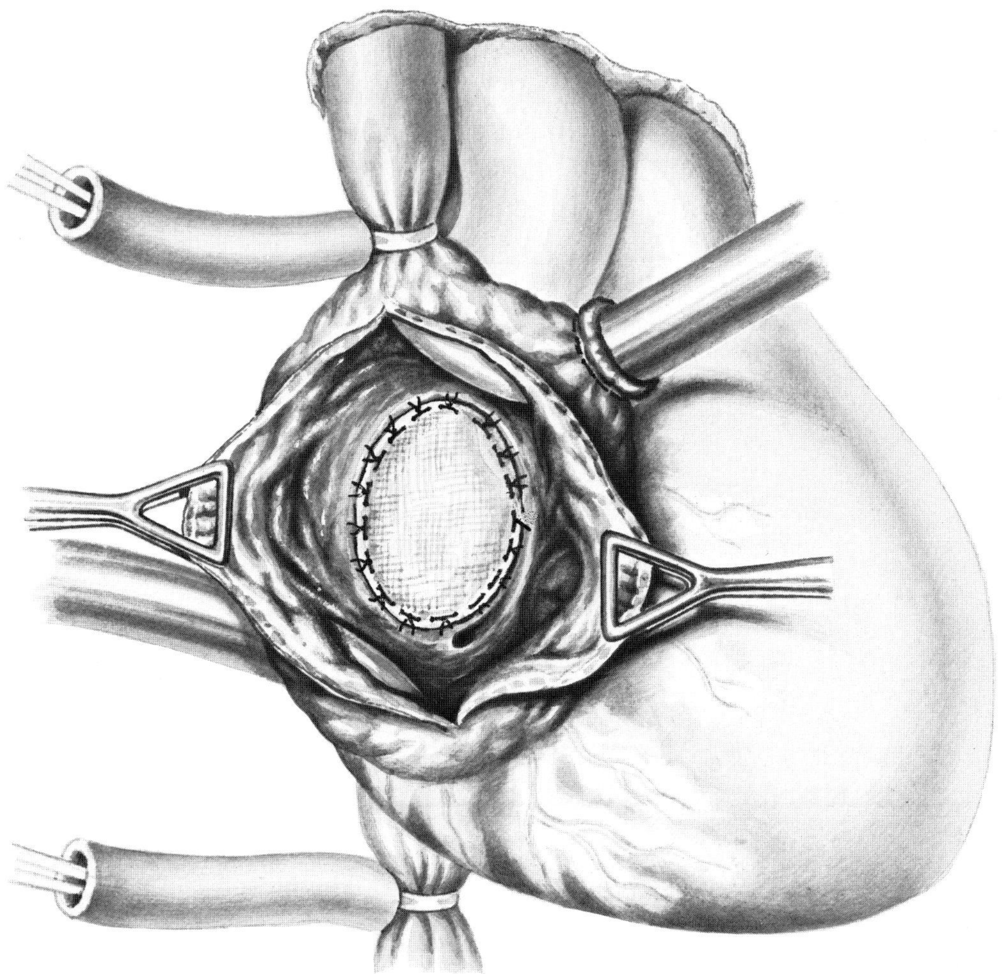

Fig. 349. Repair of interatrial septal defect with plastic graft and application of Halsted sutures to edge of defect.

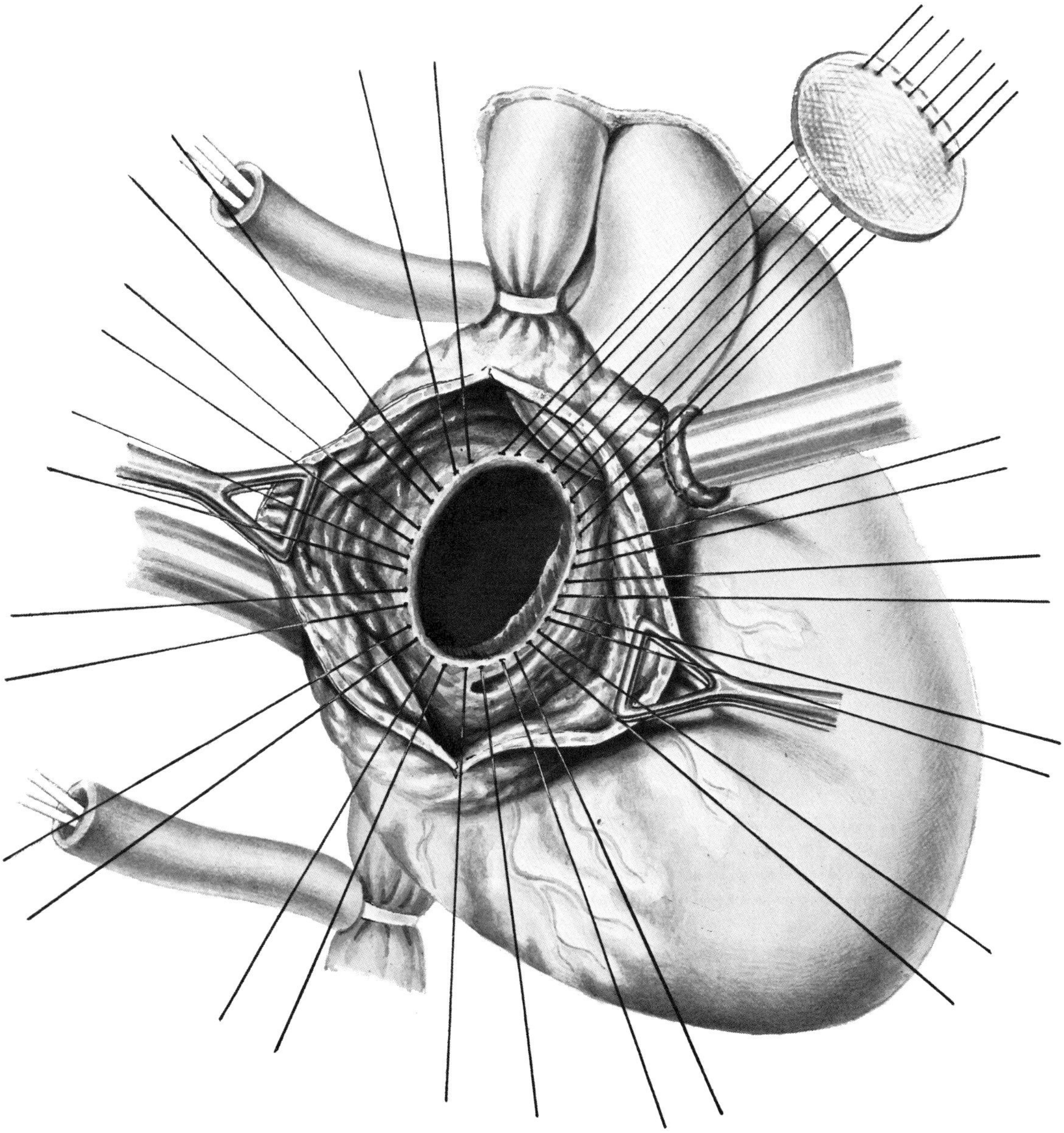

Fig. 350. Interatrial septal defect is closed with graft.

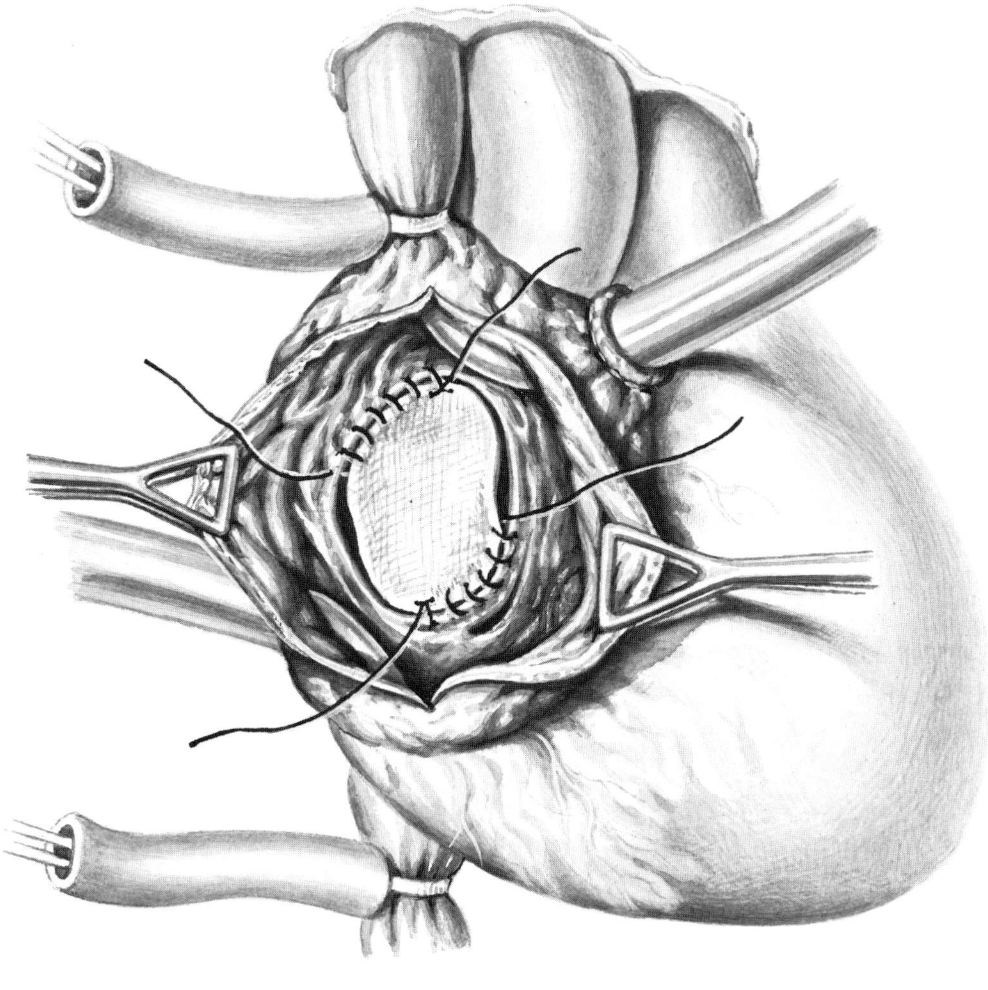

Fig. 351. Repair of secondary defect in interatrial septum with graft by means of continuous blanket suture.

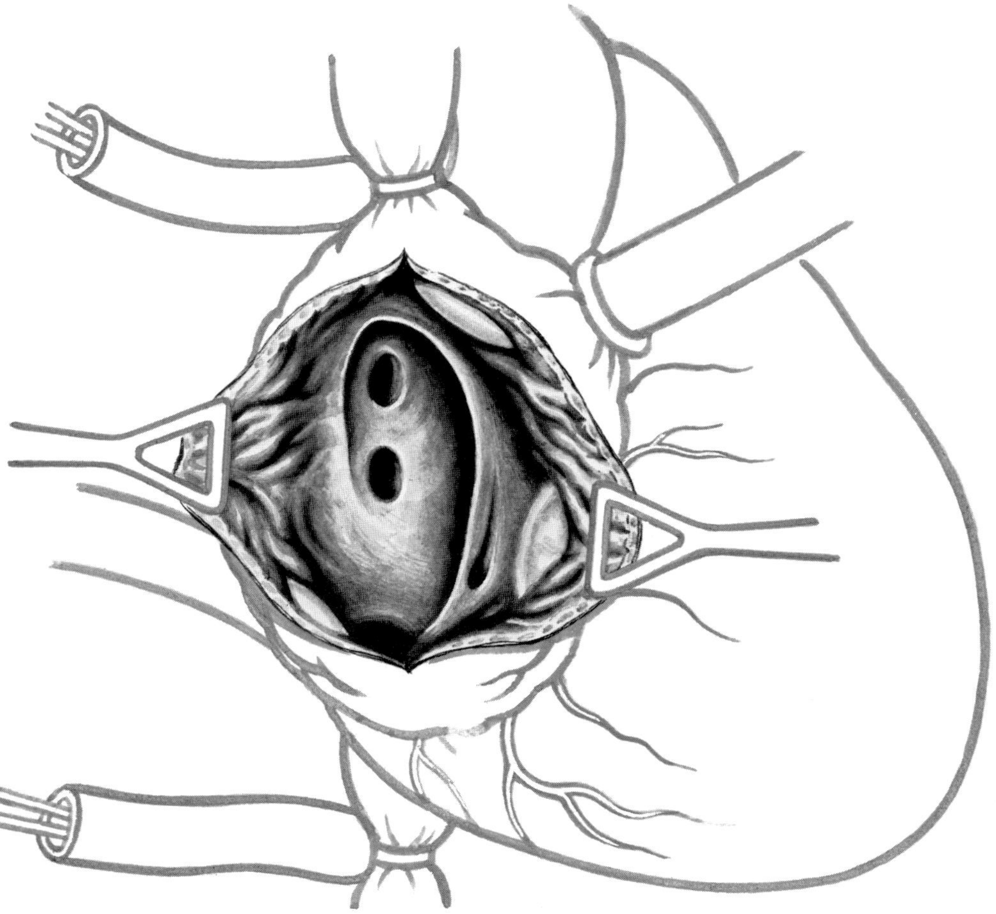

Fig. 352. Lewis method for repairing large secondary defect in interatrial septum when inferior vena cava drains into both atria.

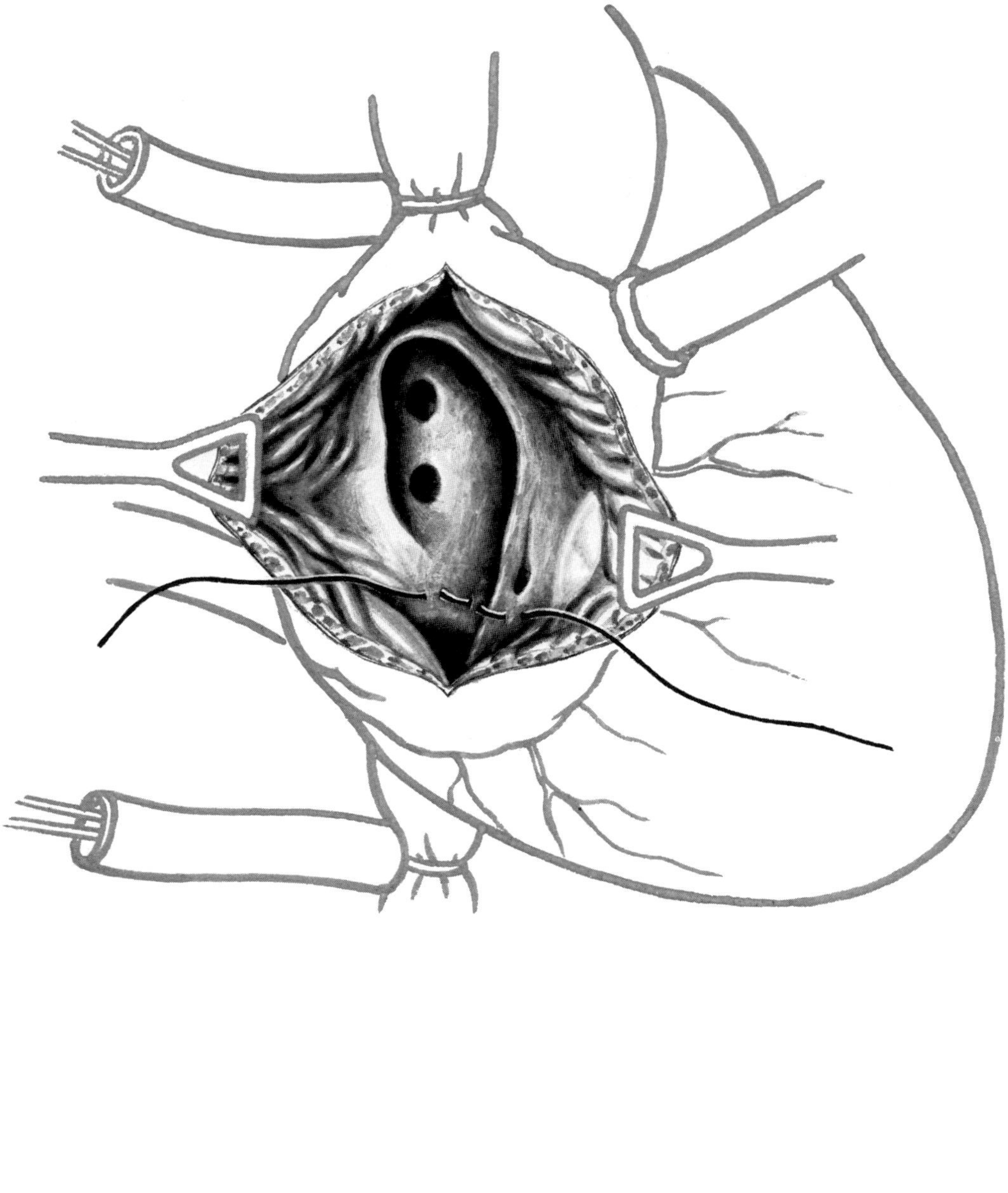

Fig. 353. Semi-purse-string suture is applied to edges of defect and dorsal wall of left atrium.

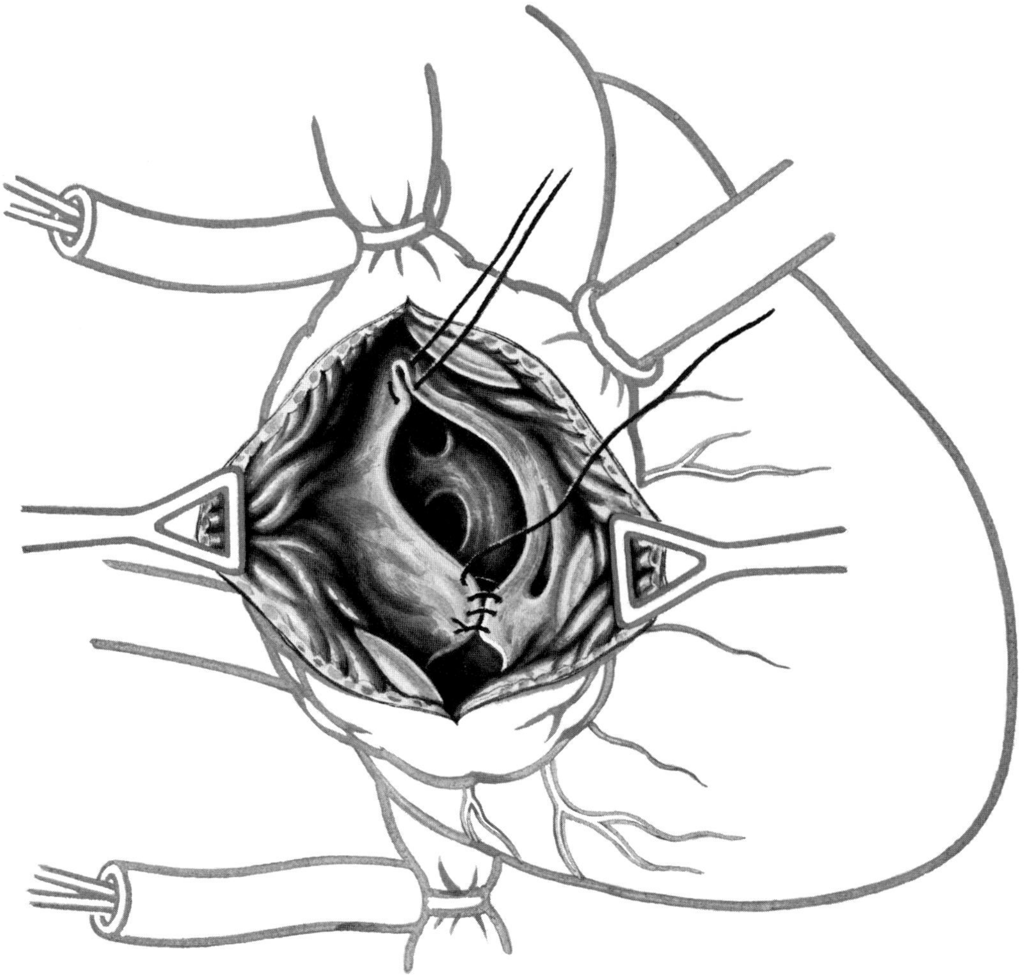

Fig. 354. Tying of suture and repair of secondary defect with channeling of inferior vena cava drainage into right atrium.

PLASTIC SURGERY OF PRIMARY DEFECT

A primary defect in the interatrial septum is located above the junction of the fibrous rings of the right and left atrioventricular orifices. It is semielliptoid, with the upper border formed by the muscular margin of the interatrial septum. The orifice of the venous coronary sinus of the heart, with the bundle of His encircling it, is in the vicinity of the inferolateral corner of the defect (Fig. 355).

In primary interatrial defect the orifice of the venous coronary sinus is always located lateral to the defect. The defect is repaired with a graft (Fig. 356). Halsted sutures are applied to the edges of the defect with an atraumatic needle. When the sutures are being applied in the region of the heart's conduction tracts, it is essential to check the cardiac rhythm by electrocardiography. If total atrioventricular block occurs, the needle is immediately removed.

The operation is completed by stitching the wall of the right atrium with double-row Halsted and blanket sutures. With the first row of the sutures applied, the tourniquets over the venae cavae are loosened, and the venous cannula is moved into the right atrial cavity. Air is removed from the right atrium through this cannula.

The wound in the right atrium may be closed by the staple-glue method. This is accomplished with a stitching instrument that approximates the edges of the atrial wound and with polymerizing MK-2 cyacrine glue.

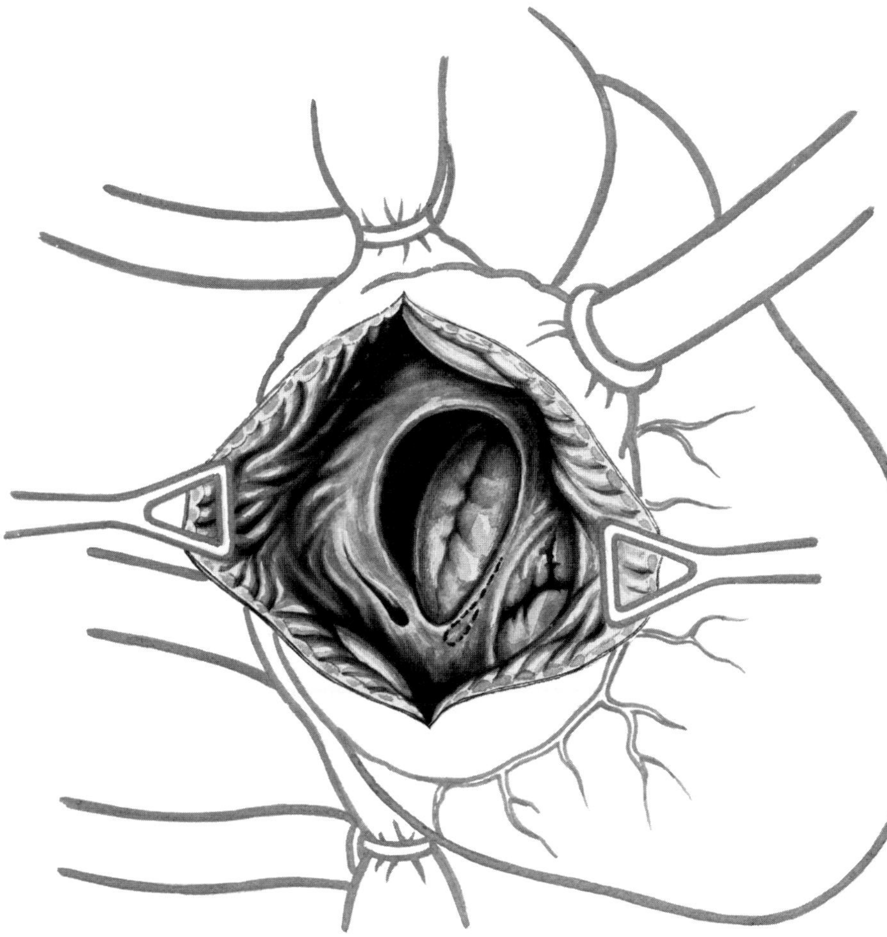

Fig. 355. Primary interatrial septal defect viewed through opened cavity of right atrium. Dashed line shows projection of atrioventricular node.

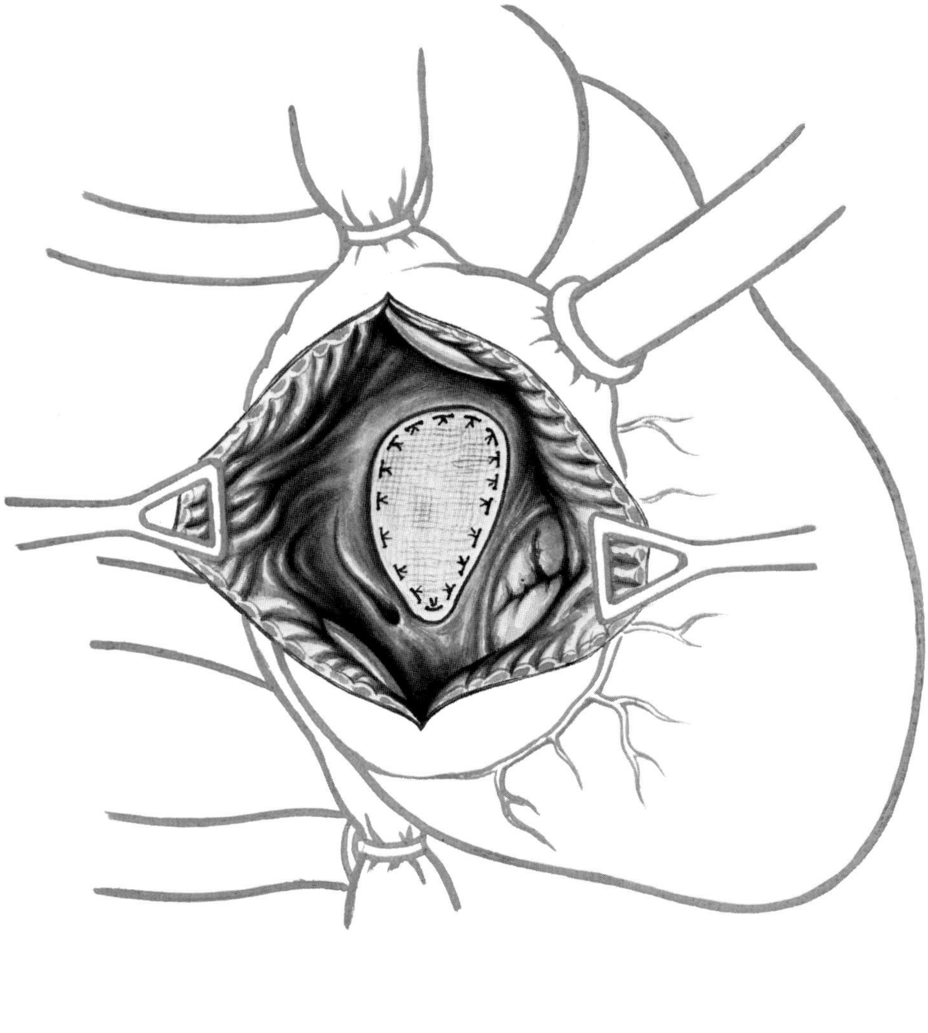

Fig. 356. Repair of primary defect with graft and Halsted sutures. Defect is closed.

PLASTIC SURGERY OF DEFECT IN THE VENOUS SINUS SEPTUM

The "septum of the cardiac venous sinus" is an embryologic conception. It forms the part of the interatrial septum located caudal to the place where the superior vena cava drains into the atrium. This defect does not have a superior border. The superior vena cava as if "saddles" it, simultaneously draining into the right and left atria.

This defect is always combined with anomalous drainage of the right pulmonary veins, which may enter the right atrium in the region of the defect or into the dilated superior vena cava, the wall of which in such cases is thickened and includes muscular fibers stretching from the right atrium.

The intraoperative diagnosis of a defect in the septum of the venous sinus may be made on the grounds of the appearance of the superior vena cava and the location of the right pulmonary veins in relation to it.

The defect is usually closed with a graft, which simultaneously shifts the orifices of the pulmonary veins into the left atrium. To provide for the sufficiently free flow of blood from the pulmonary veins into the left atrium, it is expedient in some cases to resect the lower border of the interatrial septum before the graft is applied (Figs. 357 and 358). Depending on the position of the orifices of the abnormally draining pulmonary veins, the upper edge of the graft is attached with a Halsted suture to the dorsal wall of the superior vena cava or to the left atrium (Fig. 359). The lower edge of the graft is stitched to the caudal border of the defect, and the medial and lateral edges to the sides of the defect, so that the orifices of the right pulmonary veins would be under the graft and directed into the left atrium, while the superior vena cava would be directed into the right atrium.

The defect in the venous sinus septum may be repaired

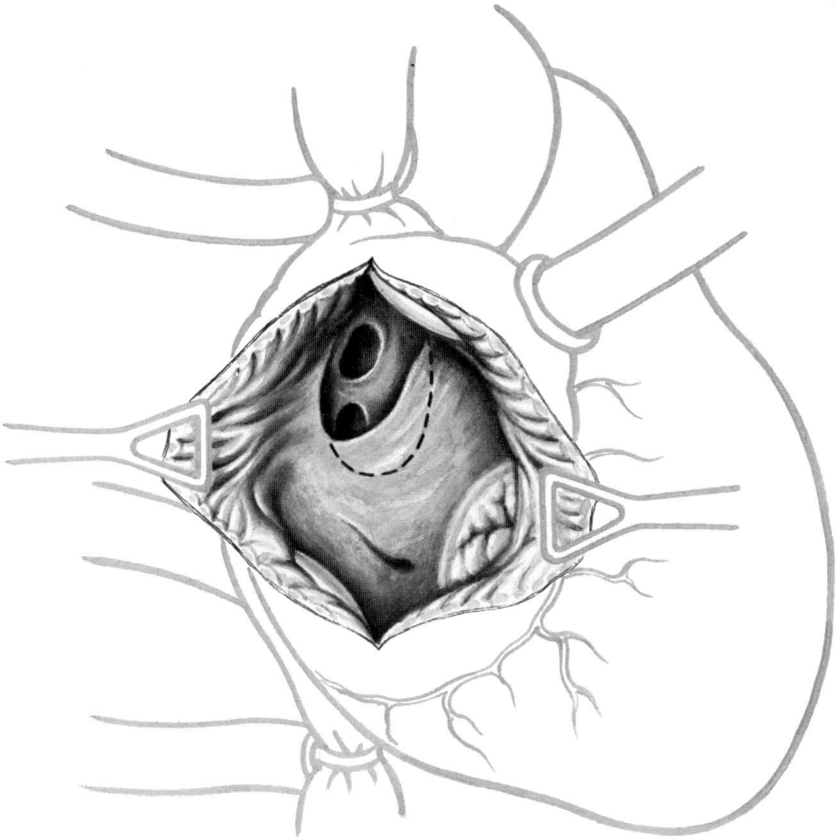

Fig. 357. Defect in septum of venous sinus with right superior pulmonary vein draining into superior vena cava. Dashed line shows boundaries of resection of interatrial septum.

with a graft of the interatrial septum itself, formed by parallel incisions continuous with the edges of the defect (Fig. 360). The Π-shaped graft thus formed is moved cranially and, just as the plastic graft, is attached to the dorsal wall of the superior vena cava or to the dorsal wall of the left atrium (Fig. 361).

A large secondary interatrial defect is often attended with abnormal drainage of the right pulmonary veins into the right atrium. Simple suturation or plastic surgery with a graft may close this defect and correct the drainage of the pulmonary veins (Figs. 362 and 363).

The sutures are applied to the conspicuous muscular border of the inner part of the defect and the wall of the right atrium ventral to the orifices of the pulmonary veins draining abnormally into the right atrium. The graft is sutured ventral to the orifices of these veins.

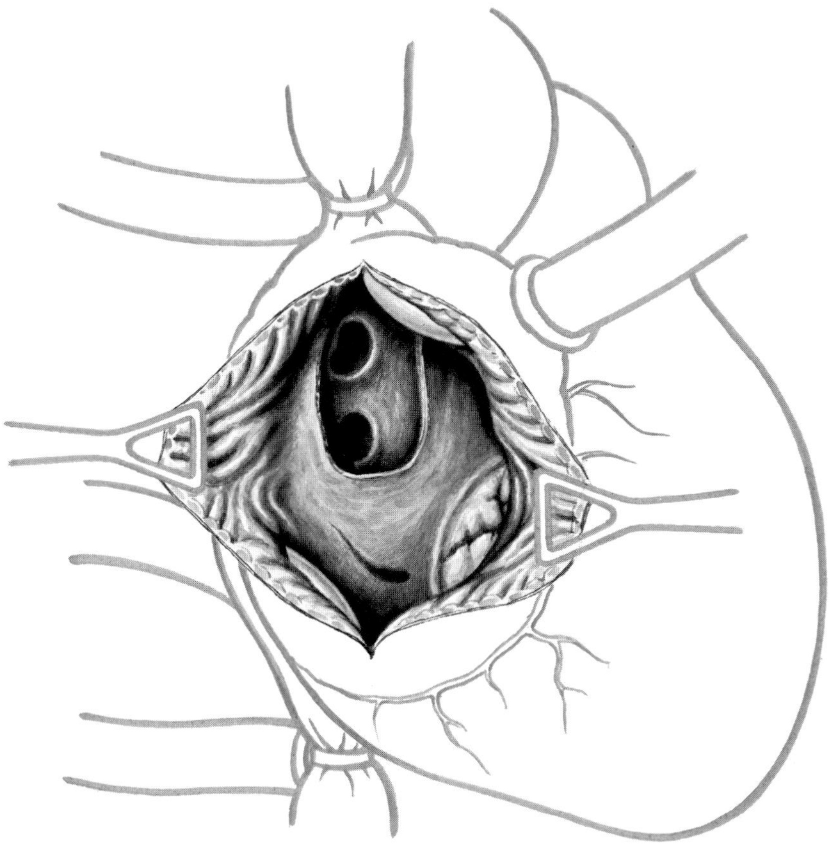

Fig. 358. View of defect in septum of venous sinus after part of interatrial septum has been resected.

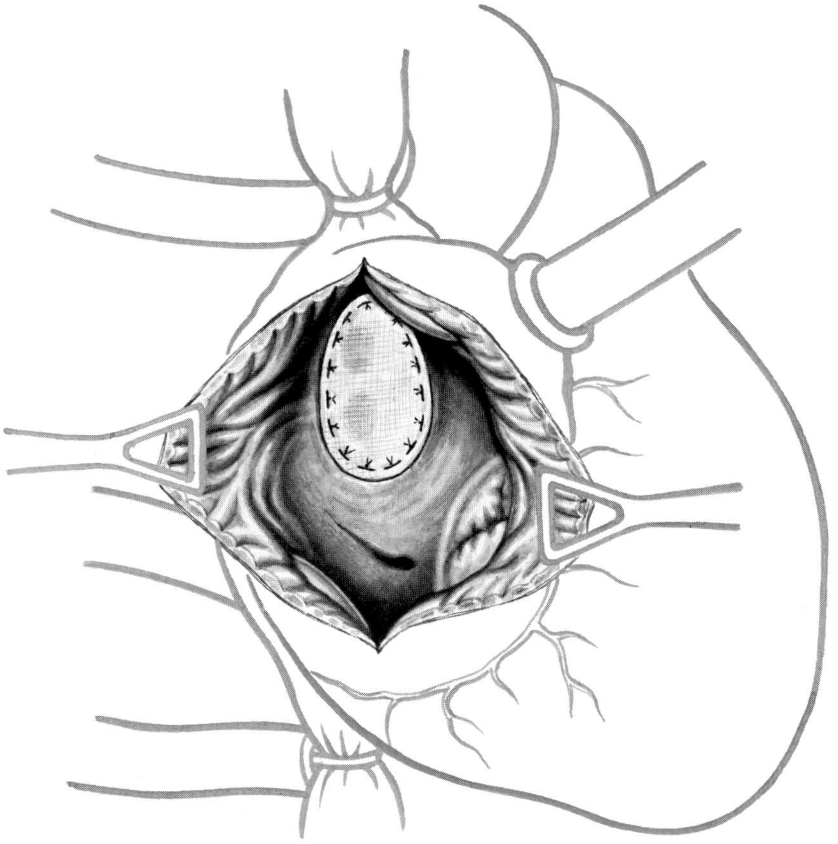

Fig. 359. Repair of defect in septum of venous sinus by means of plastic graft.

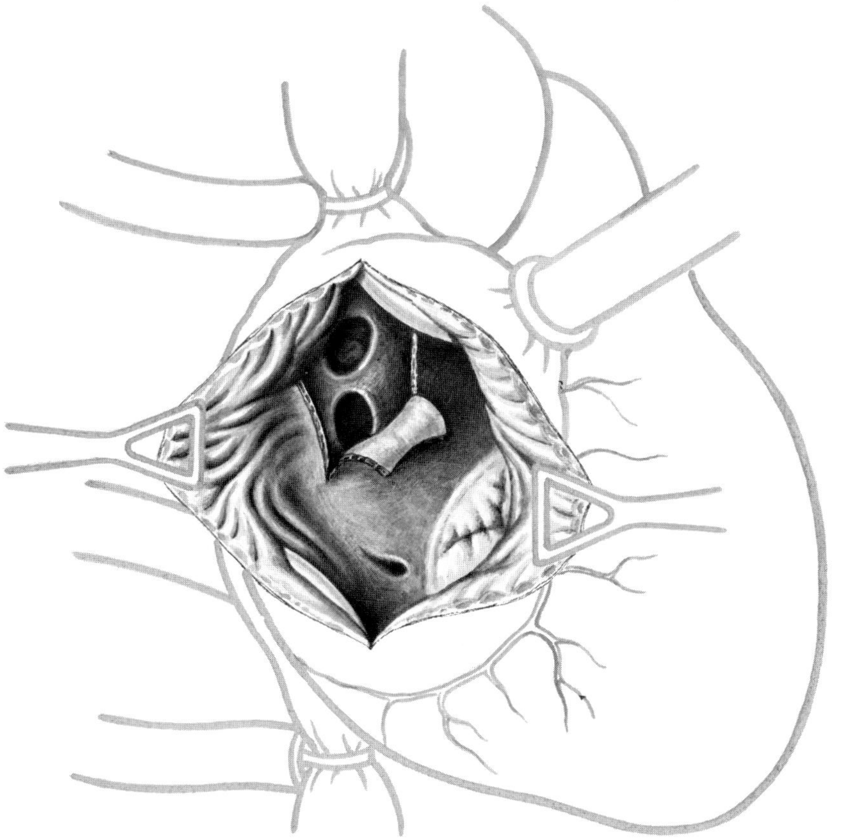

Fig. 360. Graft is formed from interatrial septum for plastic surgery of defect.

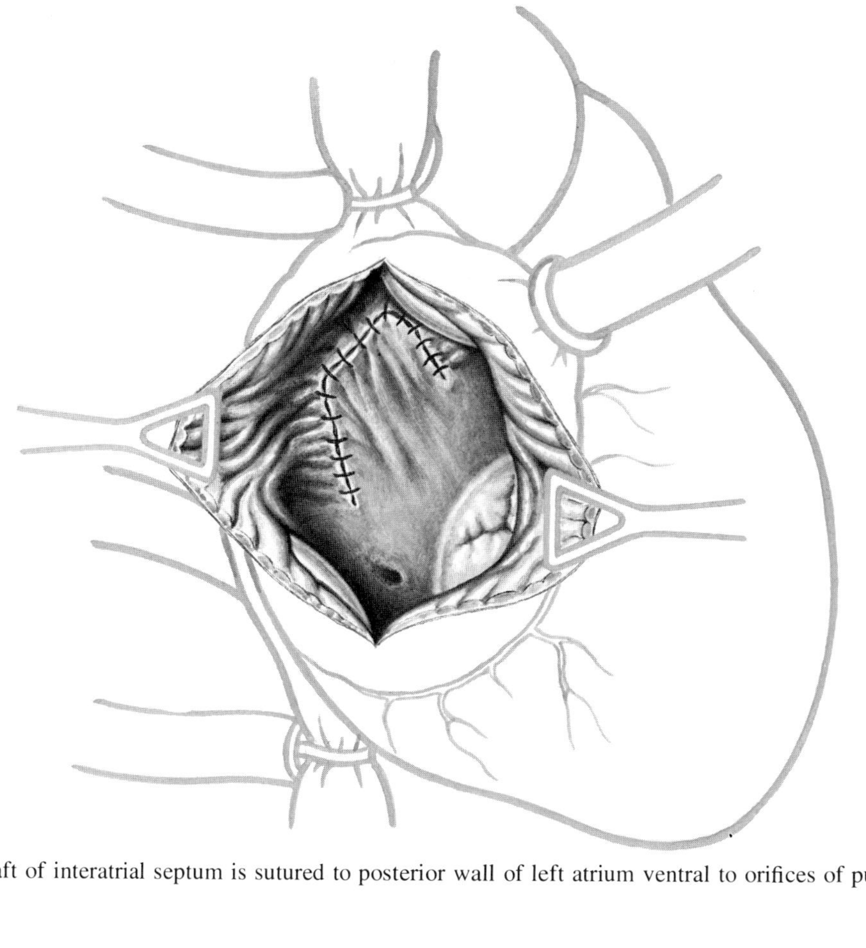

Fig. 361. Graft of interatrial septum is sutured to posterior wall of left atrium ventral to orifices of pulmonary veins.

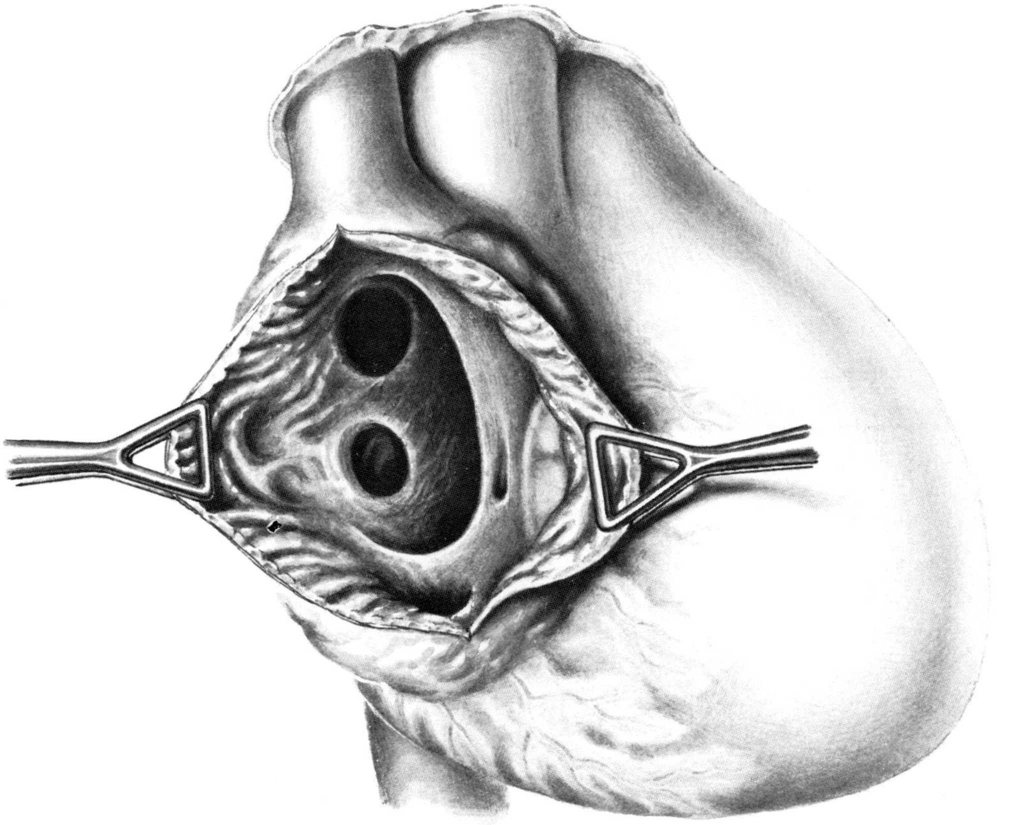

Fig. 362. Combination of large secondary interatrial defect with abnormal drainage of pulmonary veins.

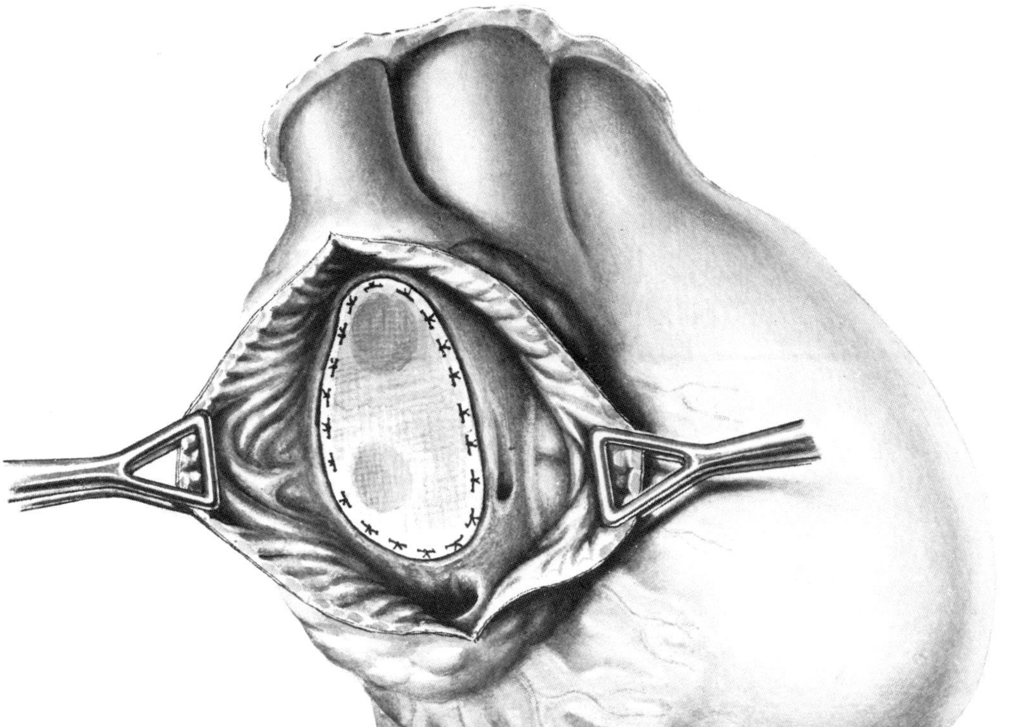

Fig. 363. Repair of large secondary interatrial defect and abnormal drainage of pulmonary veins with plastic graft.
with plastic graft.

PLASTIC SURGERY OF ATRIOVENTRICULAR COMMUNICATION WITH CLEFT CUSPS OF THE MITRAL AND TRICUSPID VALVES

The atrioventricular canal may be complete or incomplete. An incomplete atrioventricular canal is a primary interatrial defect with a cleft medial cusp of the tricuspid or mitral valve (Fig. 364). In a complete atrioventricular canal there are clefts in the cusps of both valves and an interventricular septal defect corresponding to these clefts. The repair of an incomplete atrioventricular canal is begun with closure of the defect in the cusp of the mitral or tricuspid valve. Sutures are first applied to the free margin of the medial cusp where there are sclerosed, thickened chordae and callous margins of the valve (Fig. 365). It should be borne in mind that the closure function of the valve is ensured because it turns under, and suturation therefore is begun with the chordae. After one interrupted suture is applied, the cusps are stitched with a continuous blanket suture. The primary interatrial defect is then repaired (Fig. 366).

To avoid injuring the conduction tracts, the graft is stitched to the base of the medial cusp of the tricuspid valve and not to the fibrous ring of the right venous orifice (Fig. 367). To determine the shape and size of a complete atrioventricular communication, it is convenient to apply temporary traction sutures to the cleft edges of the medial cusps in the region of the fibrous ring, by means of which a better view is provided of the complex intracardiac anomaly (Fig. 368). Repair of the atrioventricular communication is begun with closure of the interventricular defect, semicircular in shape. A graft of thick felt Teflon of the corresponding shape is stitched to the free border of the interventricular septum by means of Halsted sutures. The upper edge of this graft is placed between the chordae of the mitral and tricuspid valves and attached to the ventricular surface of the medial cusp of the tricuspid valve; the ends of the threads are brought out to the atrial surface of the cusp. After that the clefts in the mitral and tricuspid valves are sutured. The primary defect in the interatrial septum is closed last of all with a graft by the method described above (Fig. 369).

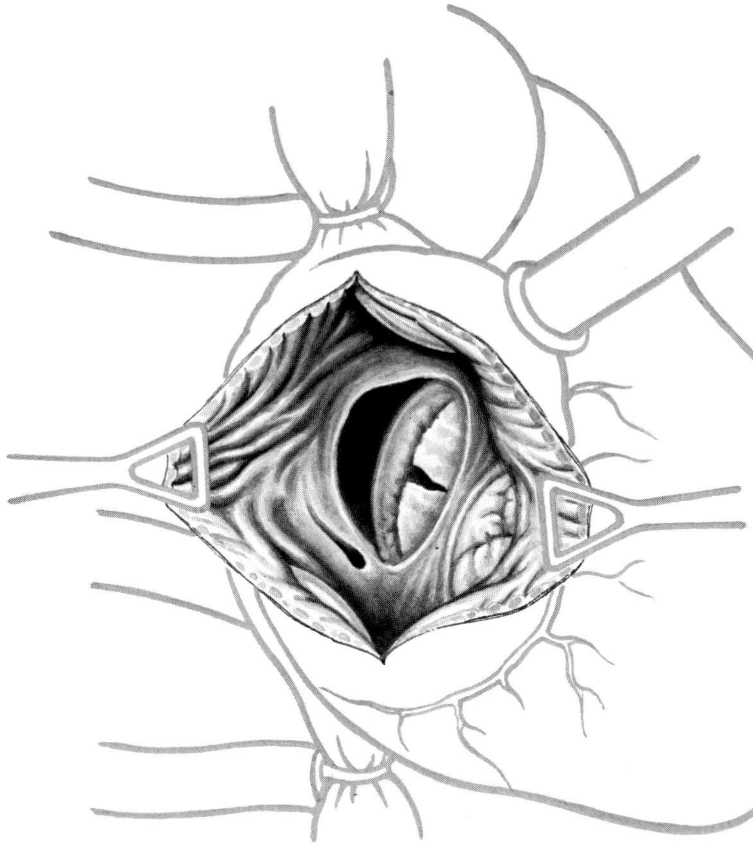

Fig. 364. General view of incomplete atrioventricular canal with cleft in cusp of mitral valve.

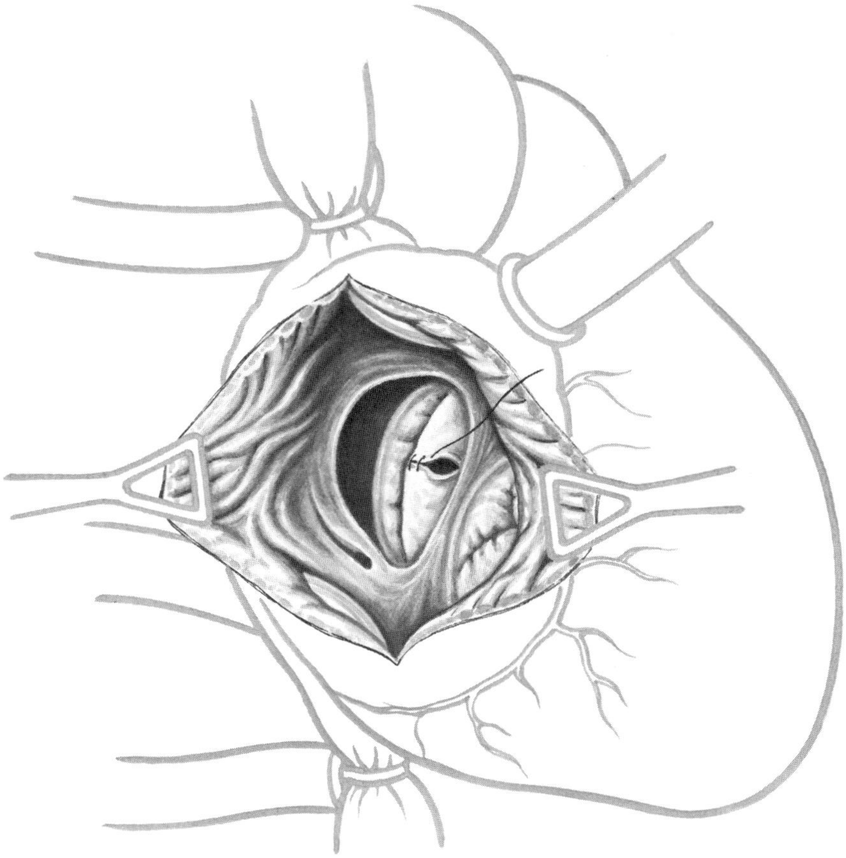

Fig. 365. Medial cusp of mitral valve is sutured.

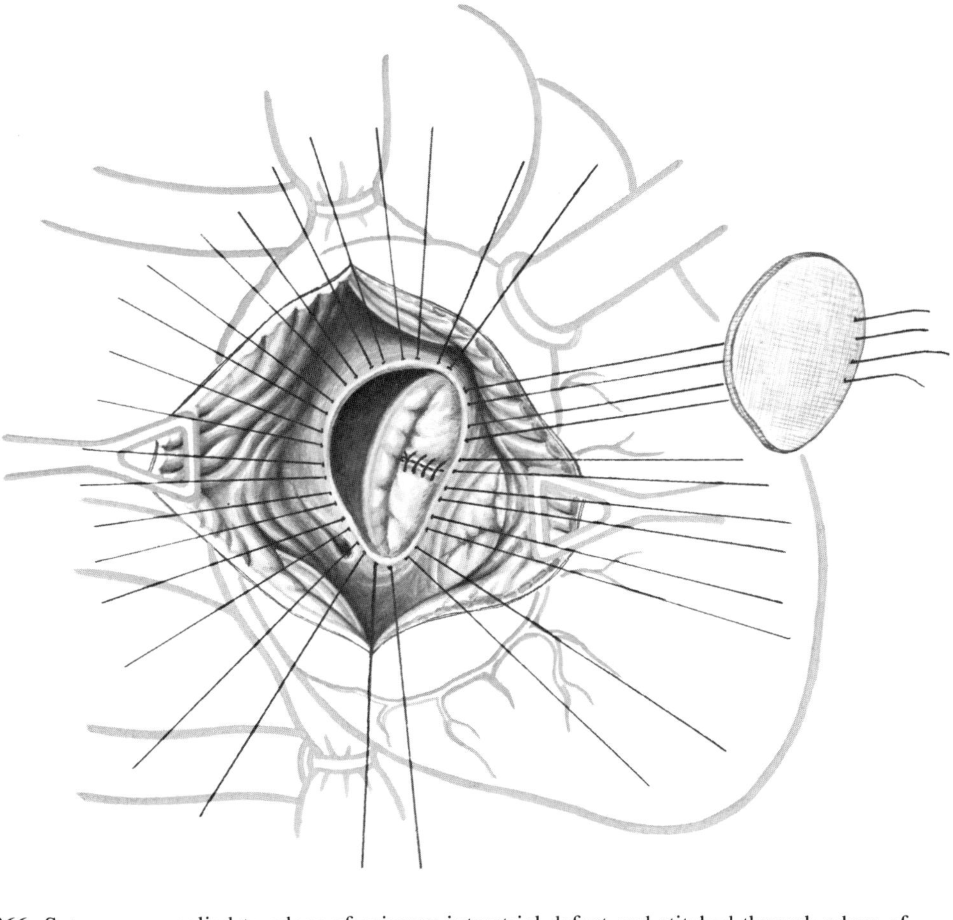

Fig. 366. Sutures are applied to edges of primary interatrial defect and stitched through edges of plastic graft.

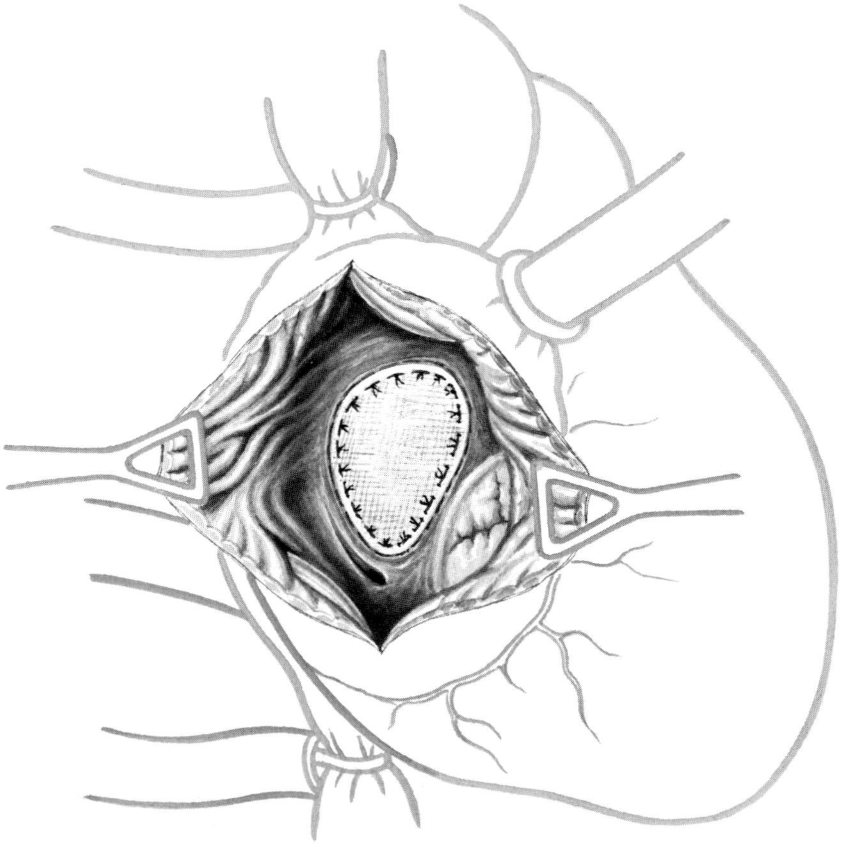

Fig. 367. Defect is closed with graft.

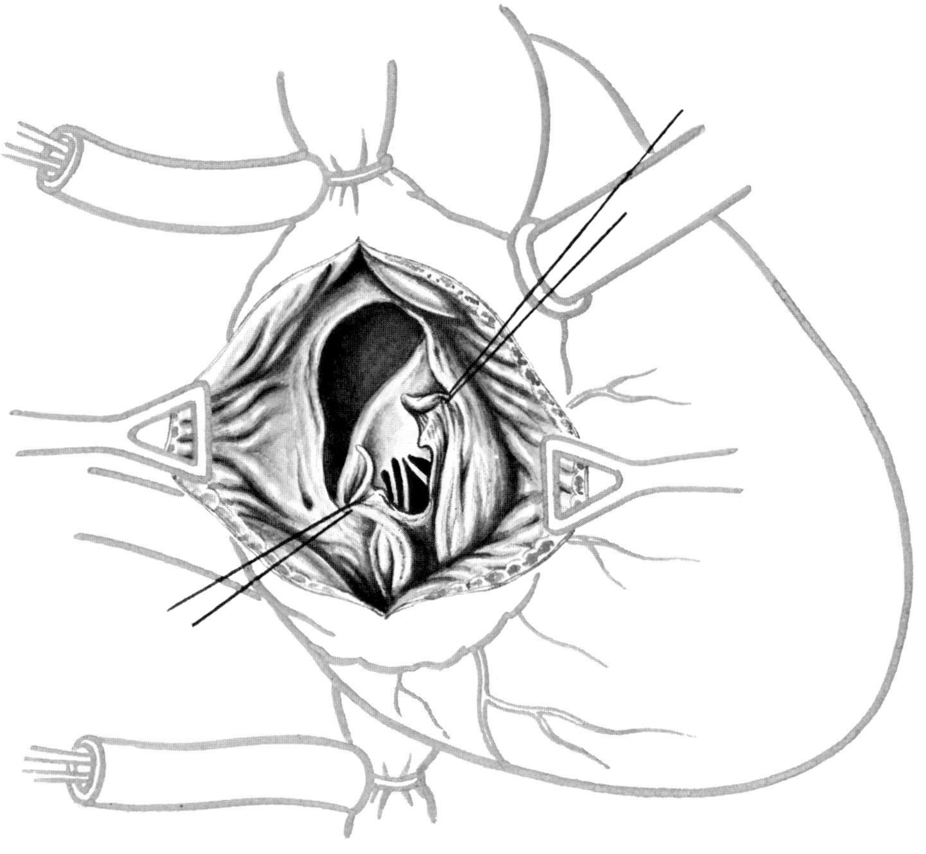

Fig. 368. General view of total atrioventricular communication. Cusps of valves are drawn apart. Defect in interatrial and interventricular septa can be seen.

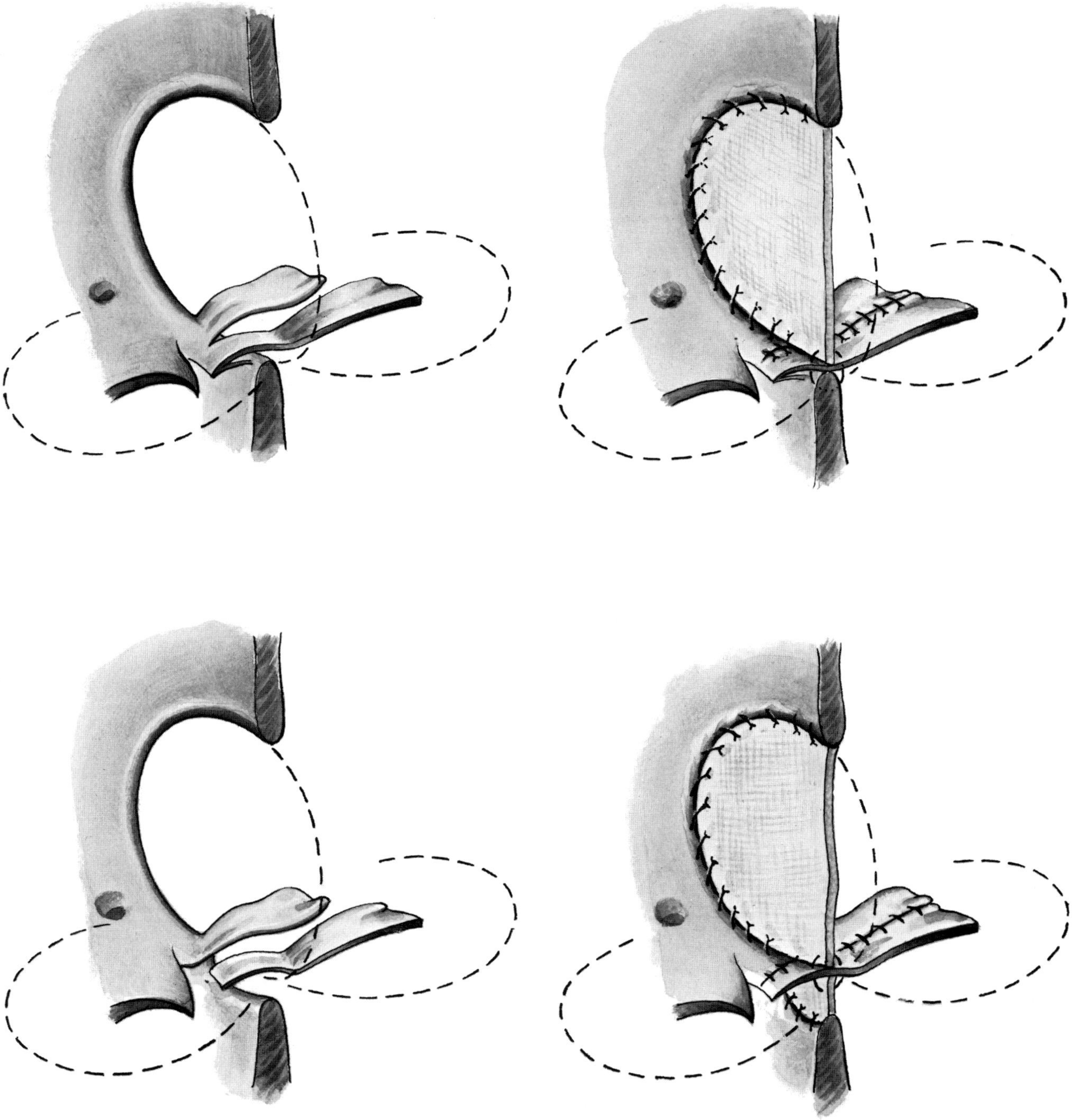

Fig. 369. Correction of total and incomplete atrioventricular communication.

CORRECTION OF INTERVENTRICULAR SEPTAL DEFECTS

PLASTIC SURGERY OF DEFECT BY APPROACH THROUGH RIGHT VENTRICLE

Defects in the interventricular septum are repaired through longitudinal sternotomy or a bipleural approach with transection of the sternum. Longitudinal sternotomy is most commonly used.

Four types of interventricular septal defects are distinguished (Fig. 370). The most commonly encountered is the posterior supraventricular defect below the supraventricular crest in the dorsal part of the septum. This defect may be partly or completely covered by the medial cusp of the tricuspid valve.

The anterior infracristal and supracristal defects occur less frequently. A defect in the inferior part of the septum, a cleft in the muscle, is the rarest form of all. Large defects, more than 1 cm in diameter, are posterior infracristal defects as a rule.

After the heart-lung machine has been connected, a longitudinal or transverse incision is made in the avascular zone of the anterior wall of the right ventricle. A transverse incision is preferable, since it impairs myocardial contractions less. The edges of the wound in the right ventricle are stretched apart with hooks, and the localization of the defect is determined by the blood gush-

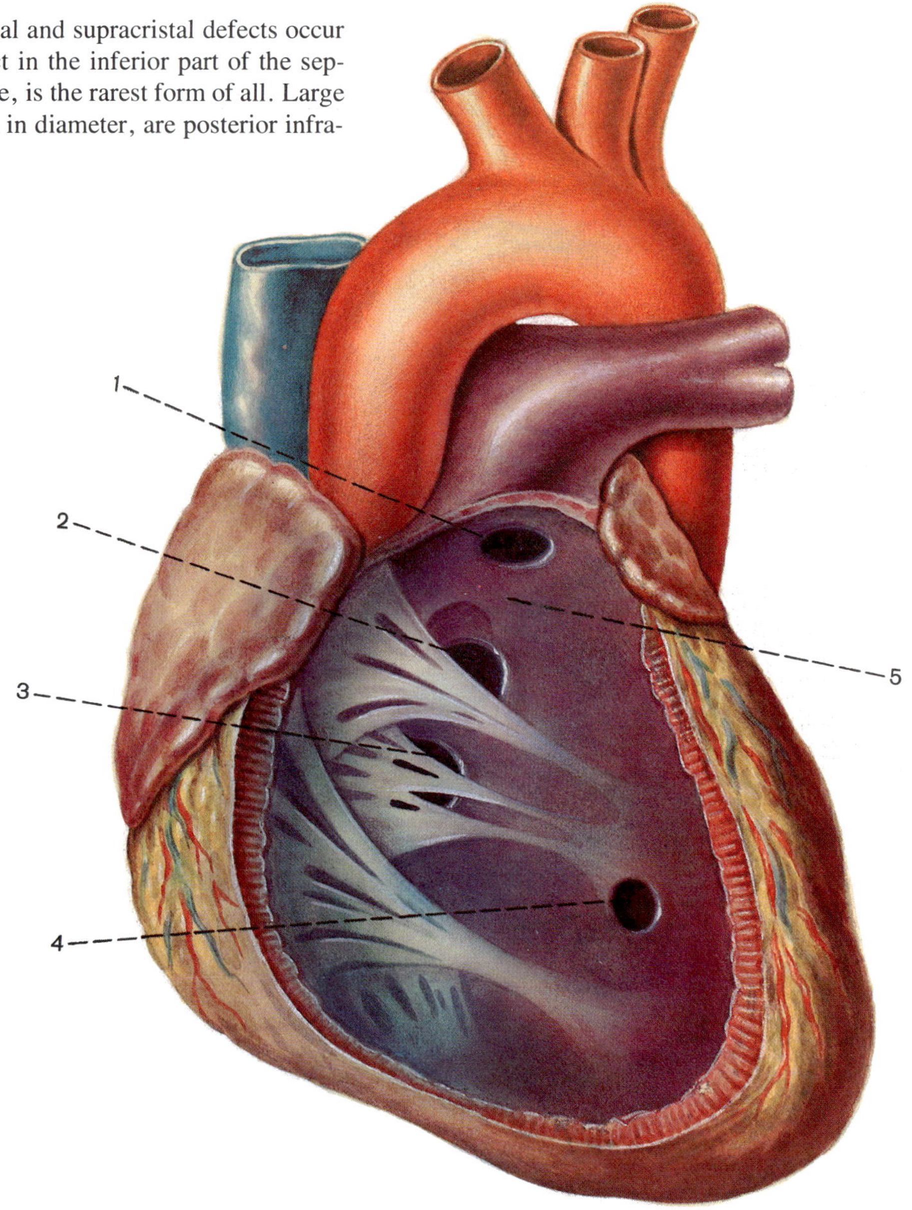

Fig. 370. Schema of location of defects in interventricular septum. **1,** Above crista supraventricularis. **2,** Below crista supraventricularis. **3,** Below crista supraventricularis in posterior part of septum. **4,** In muscular part of septum. **5,** Crista supraventricularis.

ing from it. When there are no cardiac contractions (fibrillation), the edges of a small septal defect are recognized by a thickening of the endocardium (Fig. 371).

Cleft defects in the interventricular septum are closed with Halsted sutures. The fibrous margins of the defect with the thickened endocardium usually prevent these sutures from cutting through later. If the margins of the defect are muscular tissue, however, plastic bolsters are used (Fig. 372).

Since the interventricular septum is contracting all the time and resisting the systolic pressure of the left ventricle, there is always the risk that the sutures applied for closing a defect in it may cut through. This is why the defect in such cases is repaired with a plastic graft of Teflon felt. Halsted sutures are passed through the edges of the defect and the graft. A graft of the same size as the defect is fitted in place and the sutures tied (Fig. 373). In some cases with a sclerosed myocardium and a large defect, the Halsted sutures are applied with bolsters, which remain on the side facing the left ventricle.

When posterior infracristal defects covered with the medial cusps of the tricuspid valve are repaired, electrocardiographic control is needed in suturing the posterolateral edge of the defect because the bundle of His may be injured. To prevent such injury, Gerbode suggested applying two or three sutures to the base of the medial cusp of the tricuspid valve that adjoins the margin of the defect.

The incision in the right ventricle is closed with a double-row widely-spaced blanket suture. Severe sclerosis of the myocardium requires extreme caution in tightening the stitches of the suture.

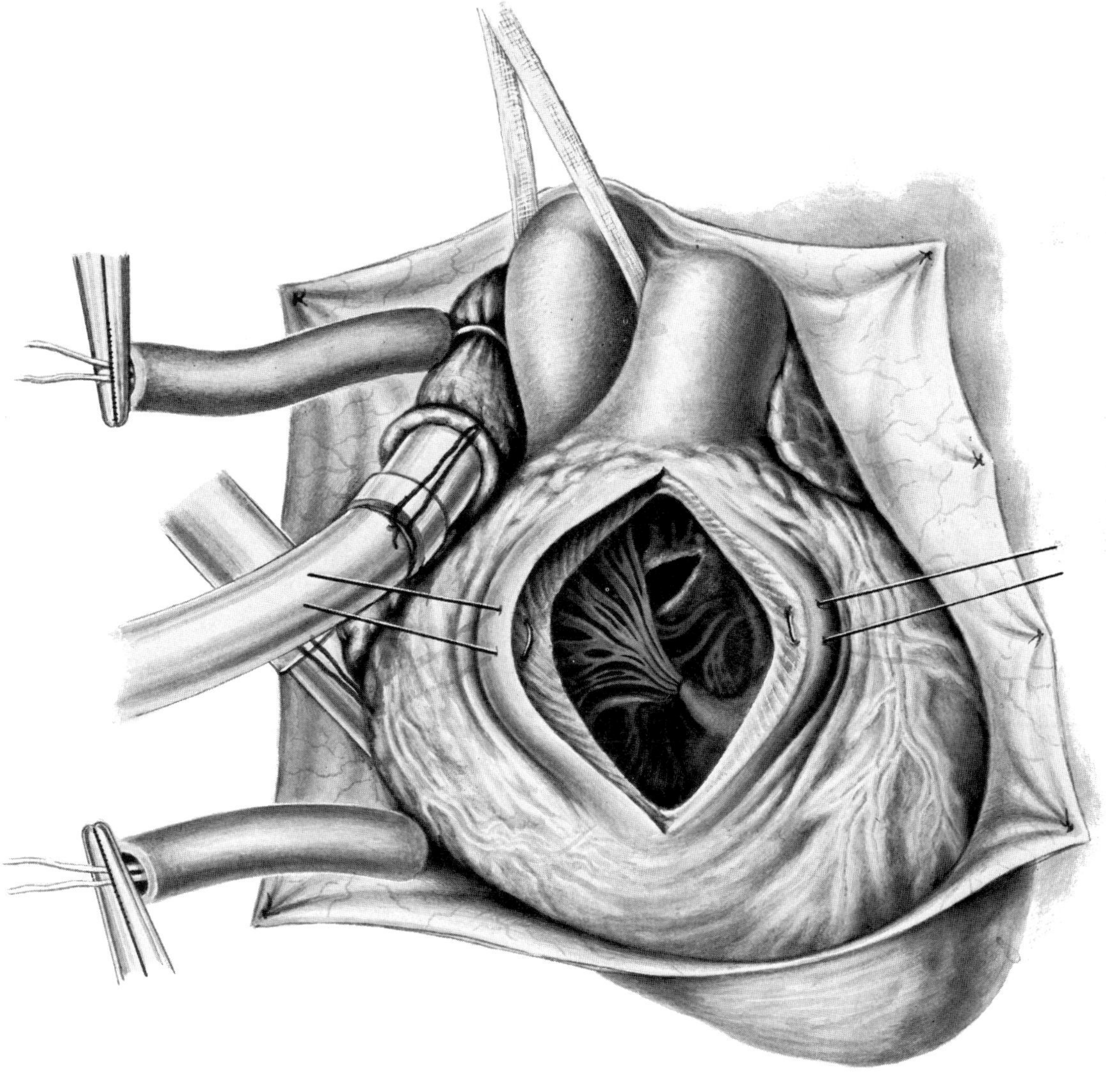

Fig. 371. Wall of right ventricle has been cut and edges drawn apart. Posterior infracristal defect covered with medial cusp of tricuspid valve can be seen.

A

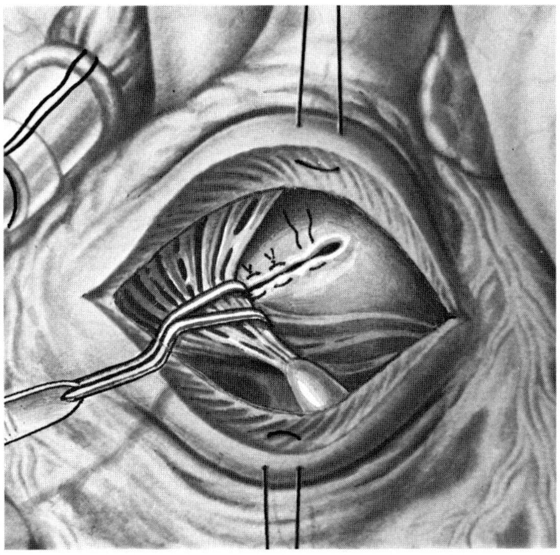

B

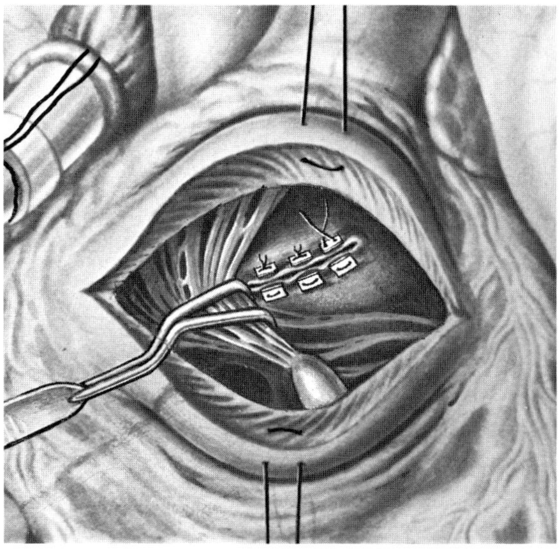

C

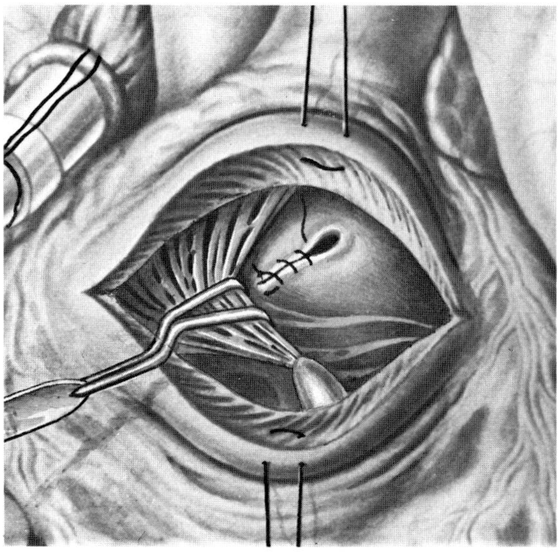

Fig. 372. Transverse ventriculotomy in closure of interventricular defect. **A,** Closure of defect with interrupted Halsted sutures. **B,** Closure of defect with interrupted sutures using plastic bolsters. **C,** Closure of defect with continuous suture.

A

B

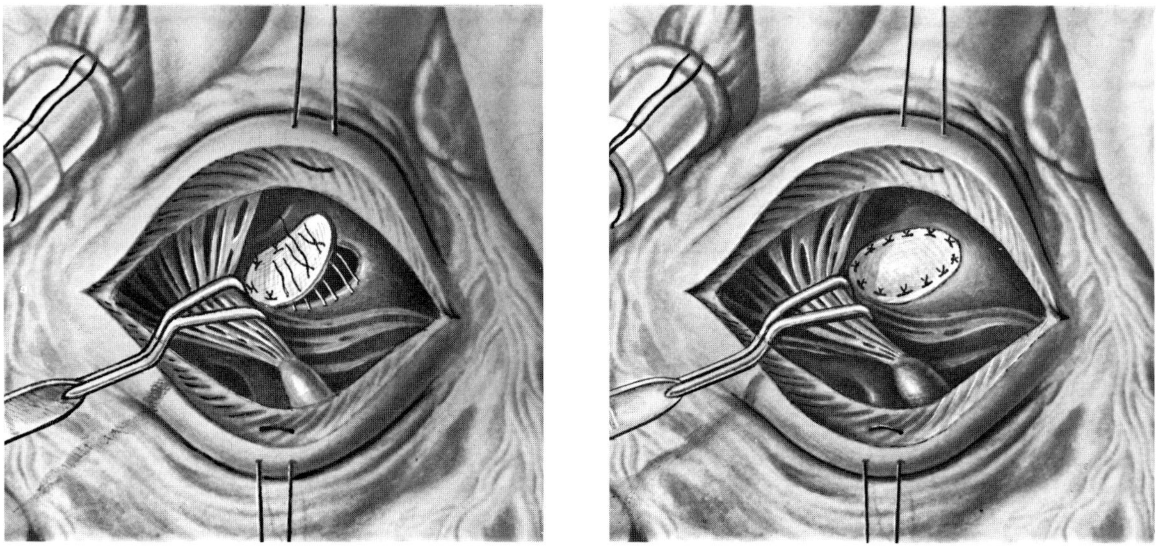

Fig. 373. Plastic surgery of interventricular defect by means of graft. **A,** Techniques of applying sutures. **B,** Procedure is completed.

PLASTIC SURGERY OF DEFECT BY APPROACH THROUGH RIGHT ATRIUM*

The operation is carried out through a right approach in the fourth intercostal space or by an incision made on the midline.

The venous cannula is introduced into the inferior vena cava through the wall of the right atrium and into the superior vena cava through the apex of the right auricle.

The right atrium is opened 1 to 1.5 cm above and parallel to the atrioventricular sulcus. The incision is continued to the right auricle, into which the venous cannula for the superior vena cava had been introduced (Figs. 374 and 375).

A large interventricular defect may be inspected with the cusps of the tricuspid valve drawn apart with hooks. Cleft defects in contractions of the left ventricle are identified by the jet of blood or found by means of a small dissector. This dissector is advanced through the left ventricular cavity into the aorta where its tip is felt through the wall (Fig. 376).

Most anterior infracristal cleft defects may be sutured from the side of the right atrial cavity when the cusps of the tricuspid valve are drawn apart (Fig. 377). With this end in view a holder suture is applied to the distant corner of the cleft, by means of which the defect is pulled into the right atrioventricular orifice. Two or three Halsted sutures are applied in succession. Teflon bolsters are used if necessary.

Large posterior infracristal defects covered with the medial cusp of the tricuspid valve are closed while this cusp is temporarily cut off along the fibrous ring. In some cases the cusp may be cut away with transection of the commissures between the medial and anterior cusps of the tricuspid valve (Fig. 378).

A traction suture is applied with an atraumatic needle to the detached cusp, which is then drawn aside medially. Halsted sutures are applied to the margins of the defect. The same threads are stitched in succession through the Teflon graft. After this the graft is lowered in place

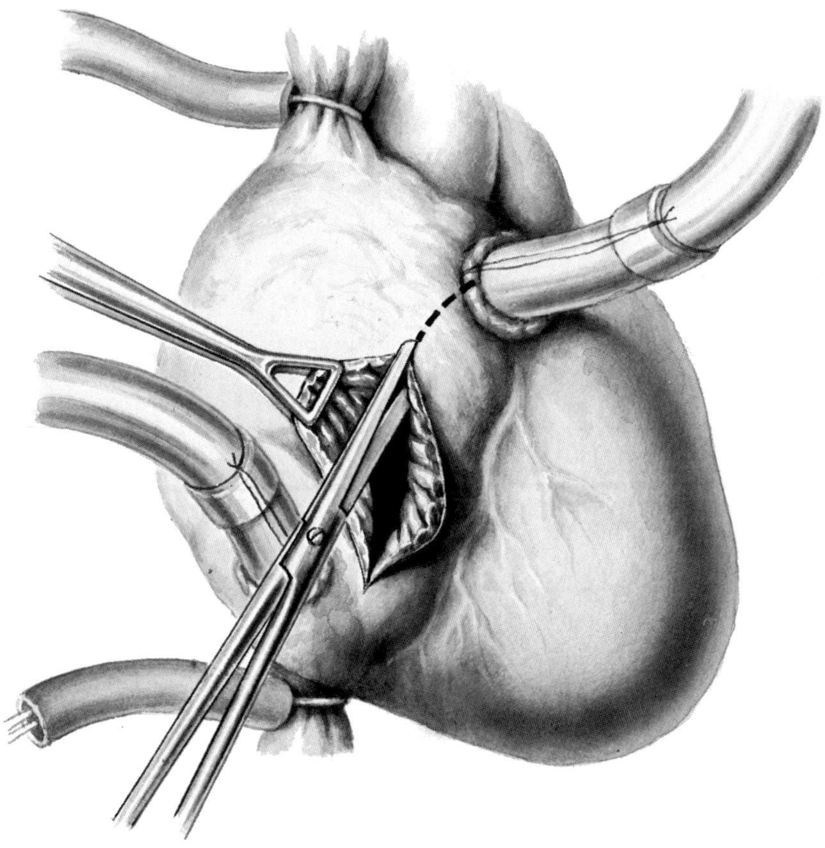

Fig. 374. Cut is made in right atrium along atrioventricular sulcus and extended to include opening for catheter in superior vena cava.

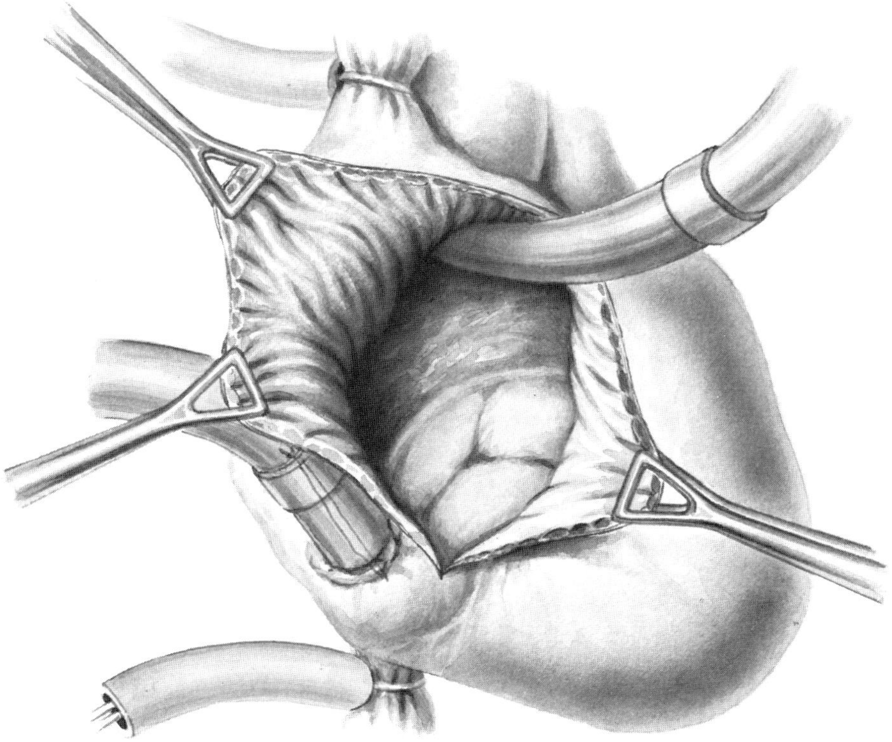

Fig. 375. Cavity of right atrium has been opened. Right atrioventricular orifice is visible.

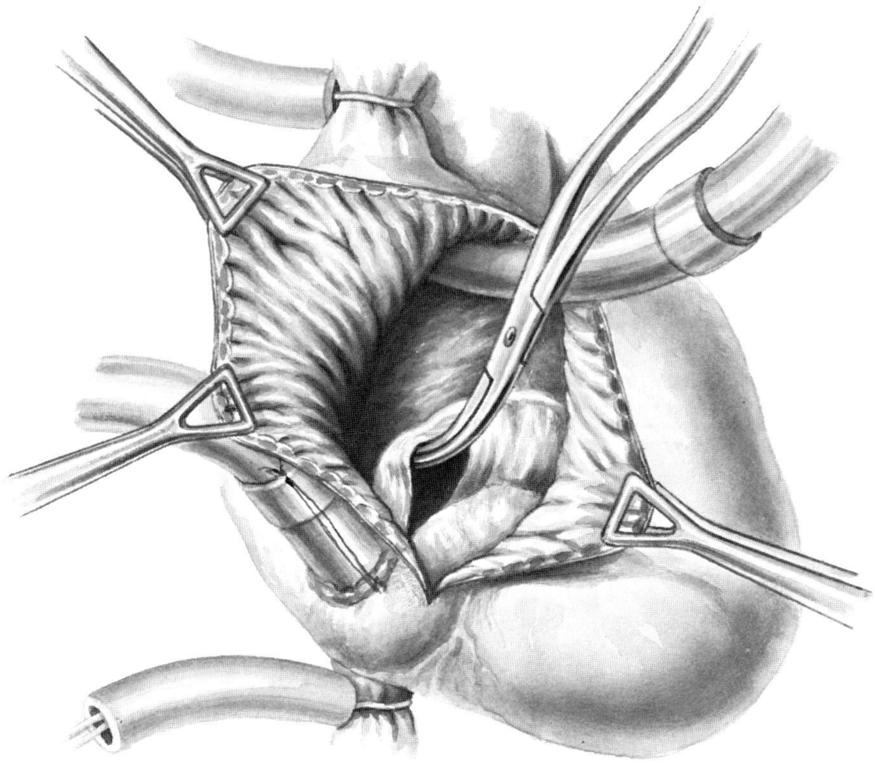

Fig. 376. Interventricular septal defect is inspected by means of dissector.

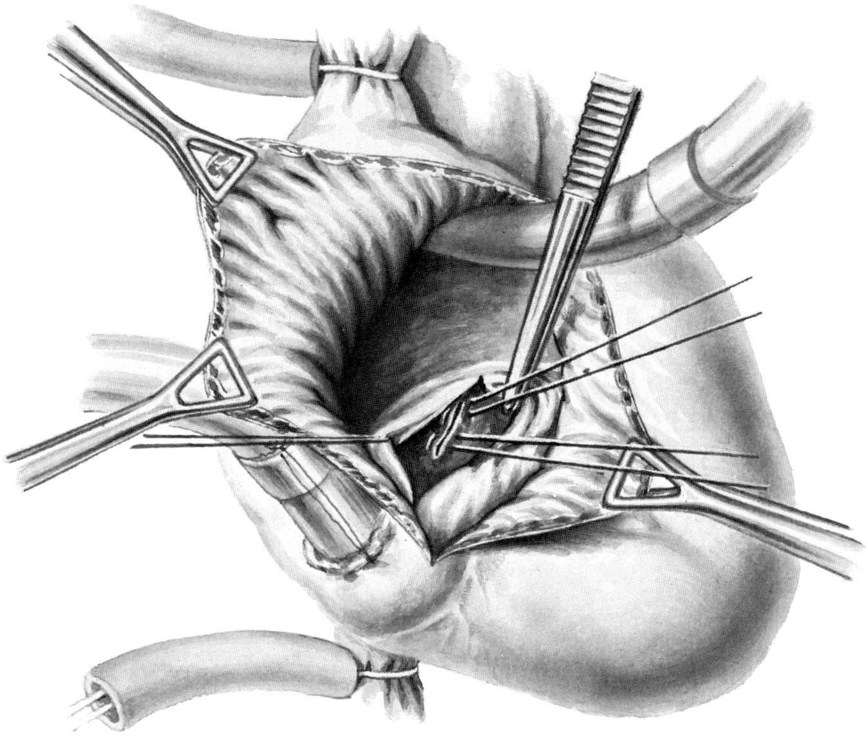

Fig. 377. Cusps of tricuspid valve are drawn apart, and anterior infracristal cleft is sutured.

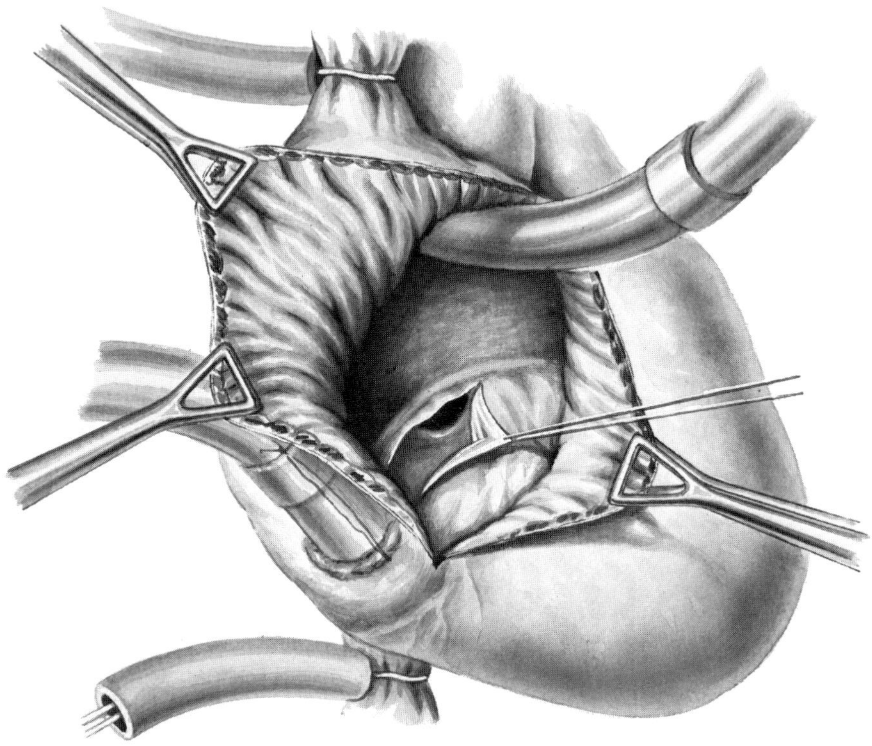

Fig. 378. Medial cusp is stitched through and drawn aside. Margin of large posterior infracristal defect in interventricular septum is visible.

and the sutures tied (Fig. 379). The incision in the medial cusp of the tricuspid valve is sutured with a continuous blanket suture on an atraumatic needle (Fig. 380). In some cases the sutures to the posterior margin of the defect may be applied from the side of the right atrium with the ends of the Halsted suture brought out through the edge of the defect.

A right atrium is closed with double-row Halsted and continuous blanket sutures. After the first row of sutures has been applied, the tourniquets on the venae cavae are loosened, and the cannula is moved from the superior vena cava into the atrium.

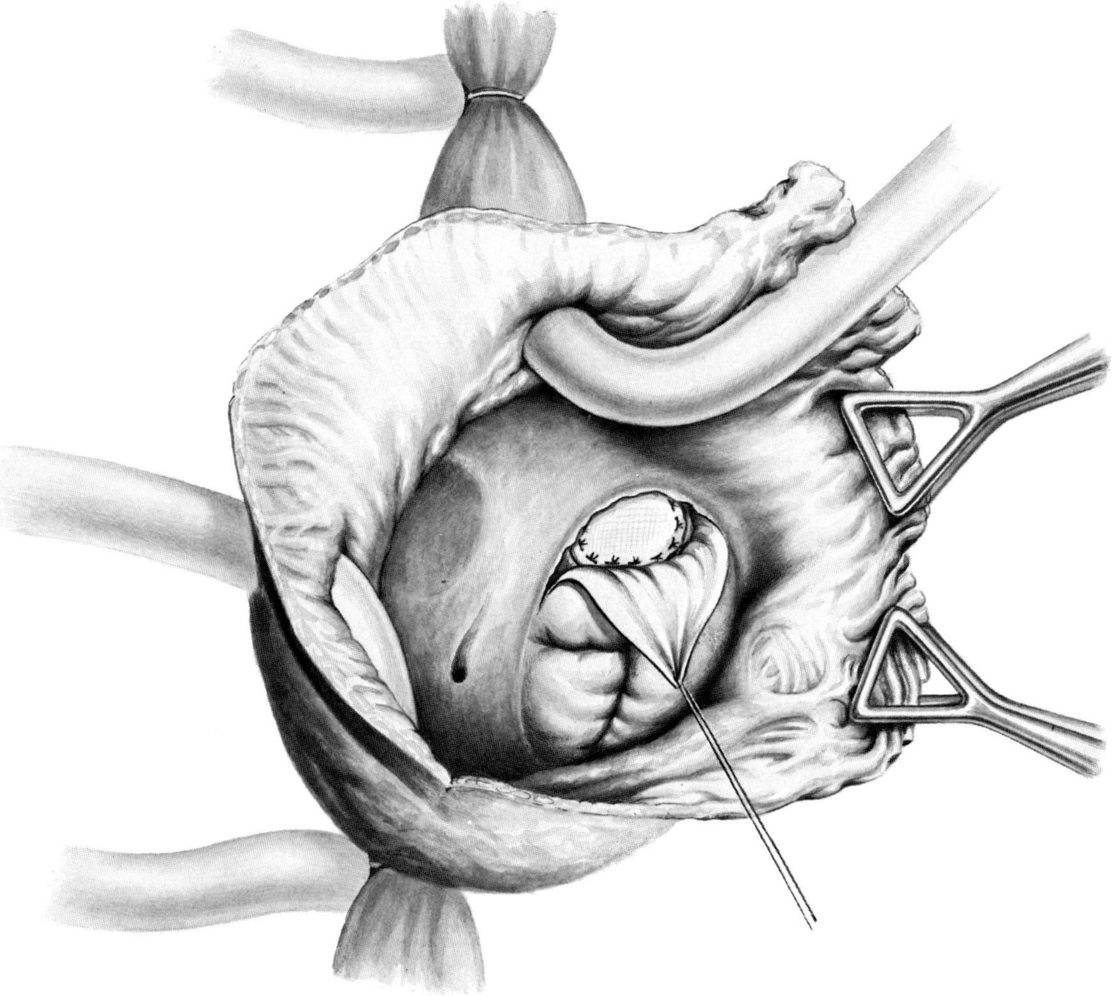

Fig. 379. Interventricular septal defect is closed with graft.

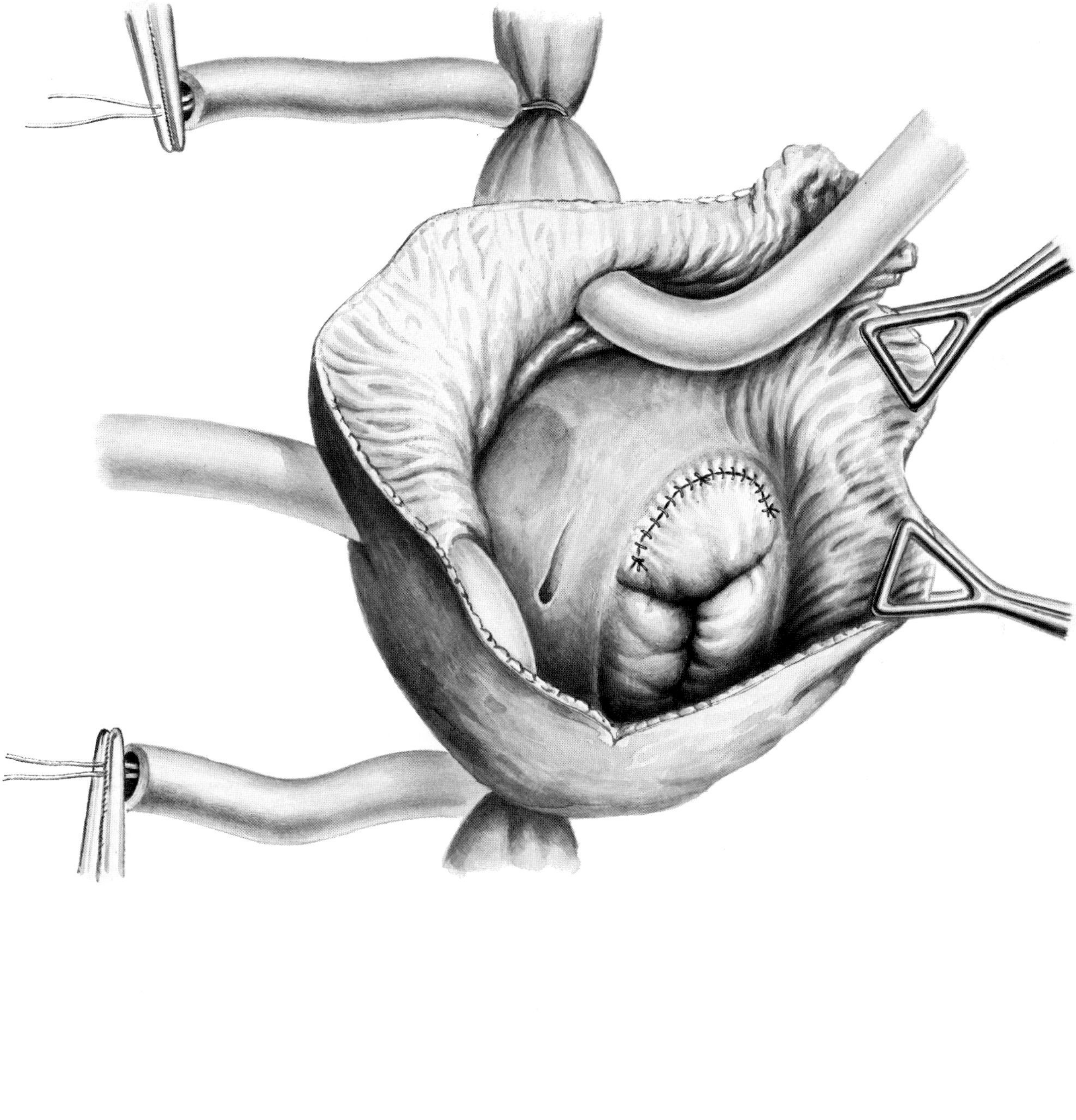

Fig. 380. Incision in medial cusp of tricuspid valve has been sutured.

CORRECTION OF PULMONARY STENOSIS

Open heart surgery is conducted by means of longitudinal sternotomy.

Valvular stenosis is usually attended by poststenotic dilatation of the pulmonary trunk (Fig. 381). The thrill of its walls is easily determined during the operation.

The heart is disconnected from circulation, and extracorporeal circulation is begun. The pulmonary trunk is cut longitudinally. The valvular stenosis has the appearance of a cone formed by the fused semilunar valves of the pulmonary trunk. A fine coronary aspirator is introduced into the cavity of the right ventricle through the stenosed opening. The commissures of the valve are pulled out with two pairs of forceps and cut with a scalpel. The wall of the pulmonary trunk is closed with double-layer Halsted and blanket sutures (Fig. 382).

In cases with subvalvular infundibular stenosis and valvular stenosis of the pulmonary trunk, transverse ventriculotomy is performed in the right ventricular outflow tract. Infundibular resection by excising muscles of the anterior wall of the right ventricle and medial half of the height of the supraventricular crest is carried out first (Fig. 383).

The trabecular muscles narrowing the right ventricular outflow tract are resected, pulling them out of the ventricular wound with a dissector. Infundibular resection is carried out by the sharp technique, using scissors, a scalpel, and cutting instruments of the type of conchotomes and Brock's resector. The cone of the fused semilunar valves of the pulmonary artery are grasped with forceps and everted through the wound in the ventricle into its cavity. The commissures are then transected with the scalpel. In the event of an error in the diagnosis, in a

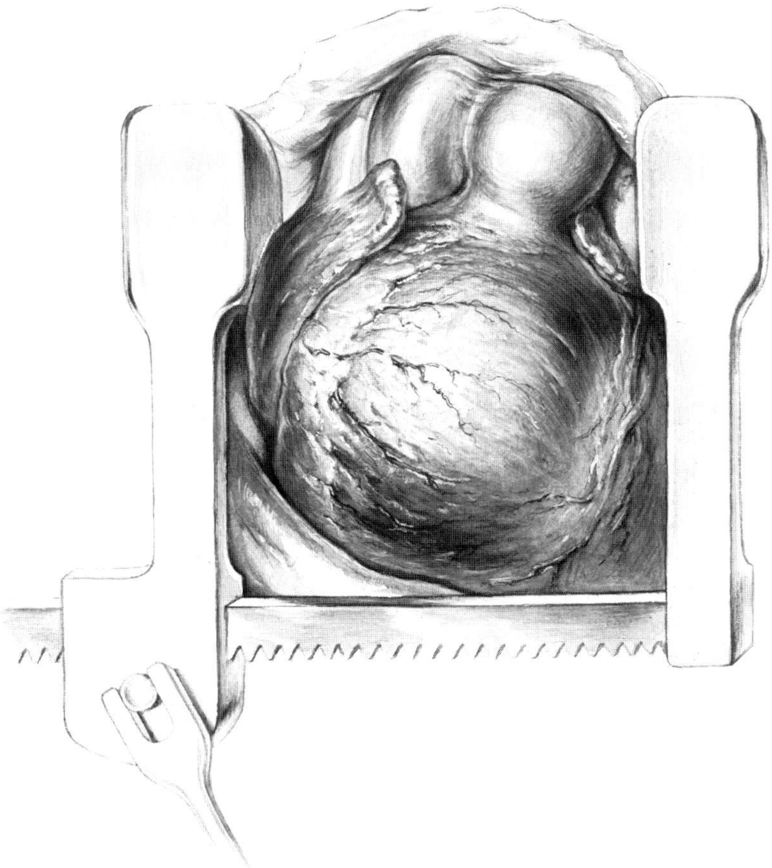

Fig. 381. View of heart exposed by means of longitudinal sternotomy in valvular stenosis of pulmonary trunk.

right approach to the heart, valvular stenosis of the pulmonary artery may be corrected through the right atrium. After the right atrium is opened, the cusps of the tricuspid valves are drawn apart with hooks. Stenosis of the pulmonary valve is determined with a finger introduced into the right ventricular outflow tract. A dilator is advanced along the finger, and the valvular stenosis is dilated with it. The result of the operation is also checked with the finger. The right atrium is sutured by the routine technique.

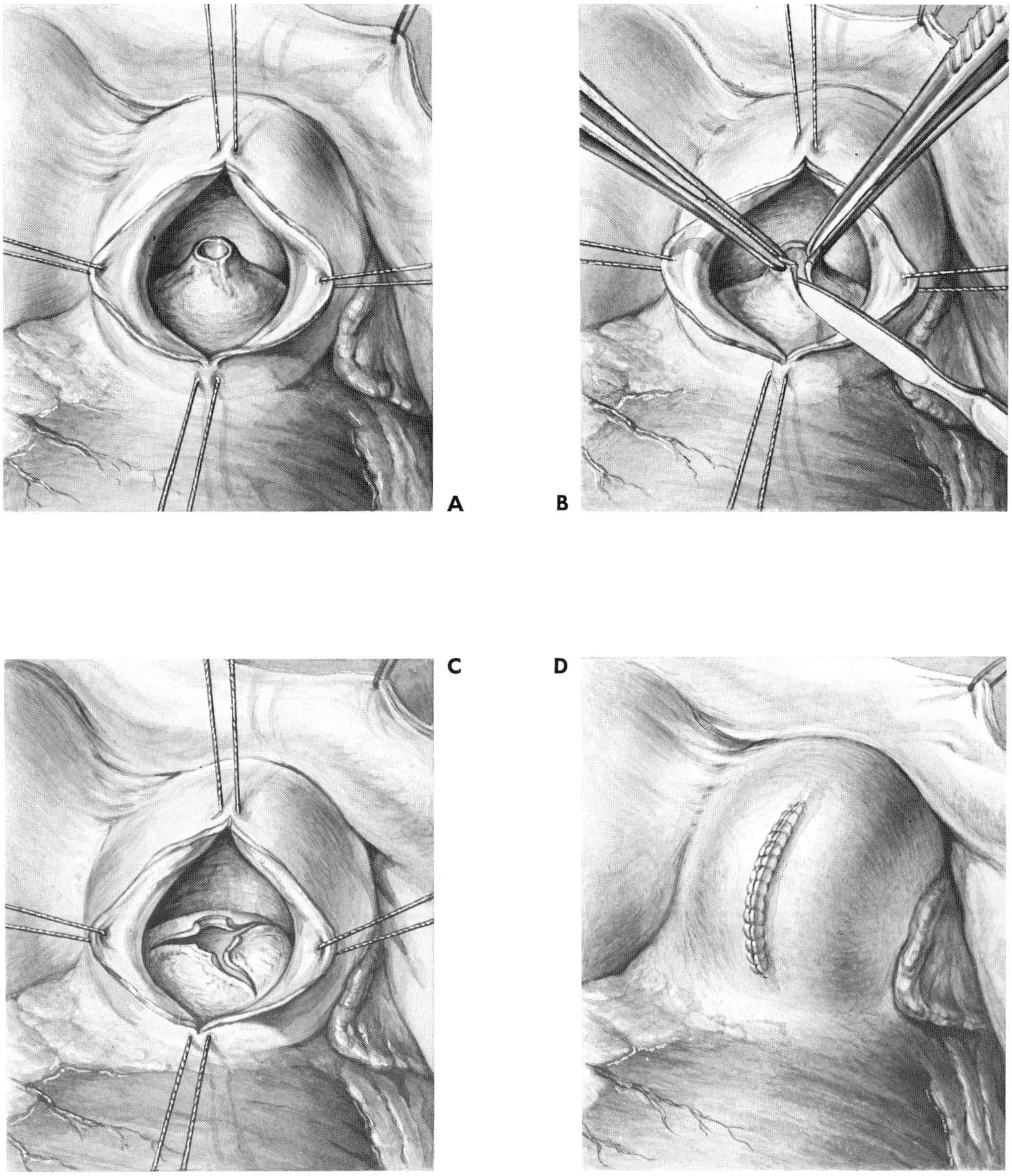

Fig. 382. Anterior wall of pulmonary trunk is cut after heart-lung machine is connected. **A,** Cone of fused semilunar valves of pulmonary trunk is seen. **B,** Narrowing is cut along commissures. **C,** Commissures have been cut. **D,** Incision in pulmonary trunk has been sutured.

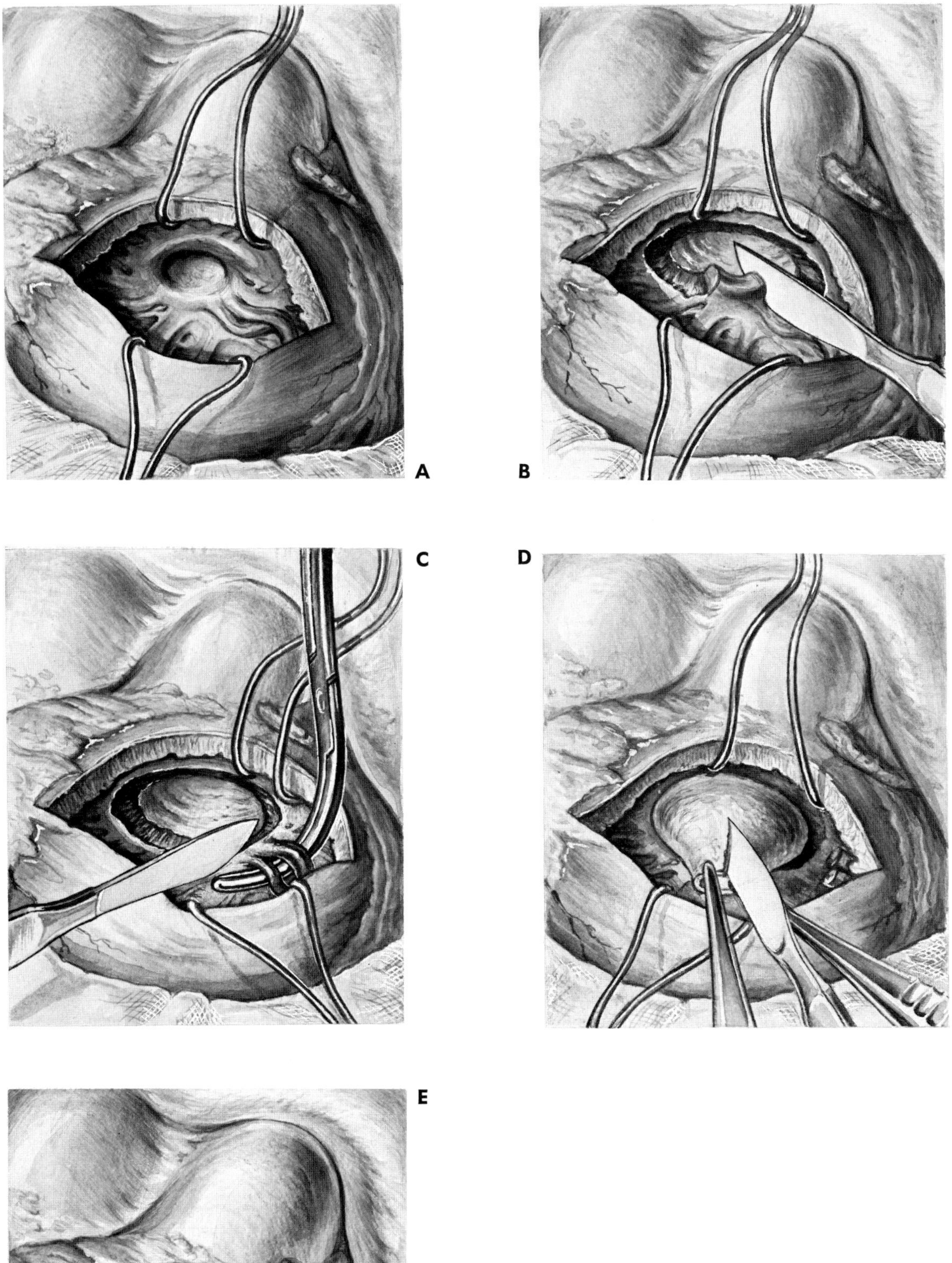

Fig. 383. A, Transverse ventriculotomy in infundibular and valvular stenosis of pulmonary trunk. **B,** Infundibular resection of thickened right atrial wall. **C,** Trabecular muscles are resected. **D,** Valvular cone of pulmonary trunk is everted into cavity of right ventricle and commissurotomy is performed. **E,** Wound of transverse ventriculotomy is closed with blanket suture.

OPERATIONS IN TETRALOGY OF FALLOT

RADICAL CORRECTION BY APPROACH THROUGH RIGHT VENTRICLE

Longitudinal sternotomy is performed. The pericardium is opened wide (Fig. 384).

With the heart disconnected from circulation, wide longitudinal ventriculotomy is carried out on the anterior wall of the right ventricle in an avascular zone whenever possible. The incision is also continued to the wall of the third ventricle and the region of the infundibular stenosis, as a result of which the cavity of the right ventricle is opened wide (Fig. 385).

Infundibular resection is carried out. The stenosing muscular swell is cut out with scissors and a scalpel. The right ventricular outflow tract is widened mainly by resecting the anterior wall of the right ventricle and the inner half of the hypertrophied supraventricular crest (Fig. 386). Resection of the deep layers of this crest is fraught with the hazard of inflicting injury to the right branch of the bundle of His.

In tetralogy of Fallot, because of the displacement of its root, the aorta itself arises simultaneously from the right and left ventricles, overriding the posterior interventricular defect, which is partly covered with the medial cusp of the tricuspid valve. The closed semilunar

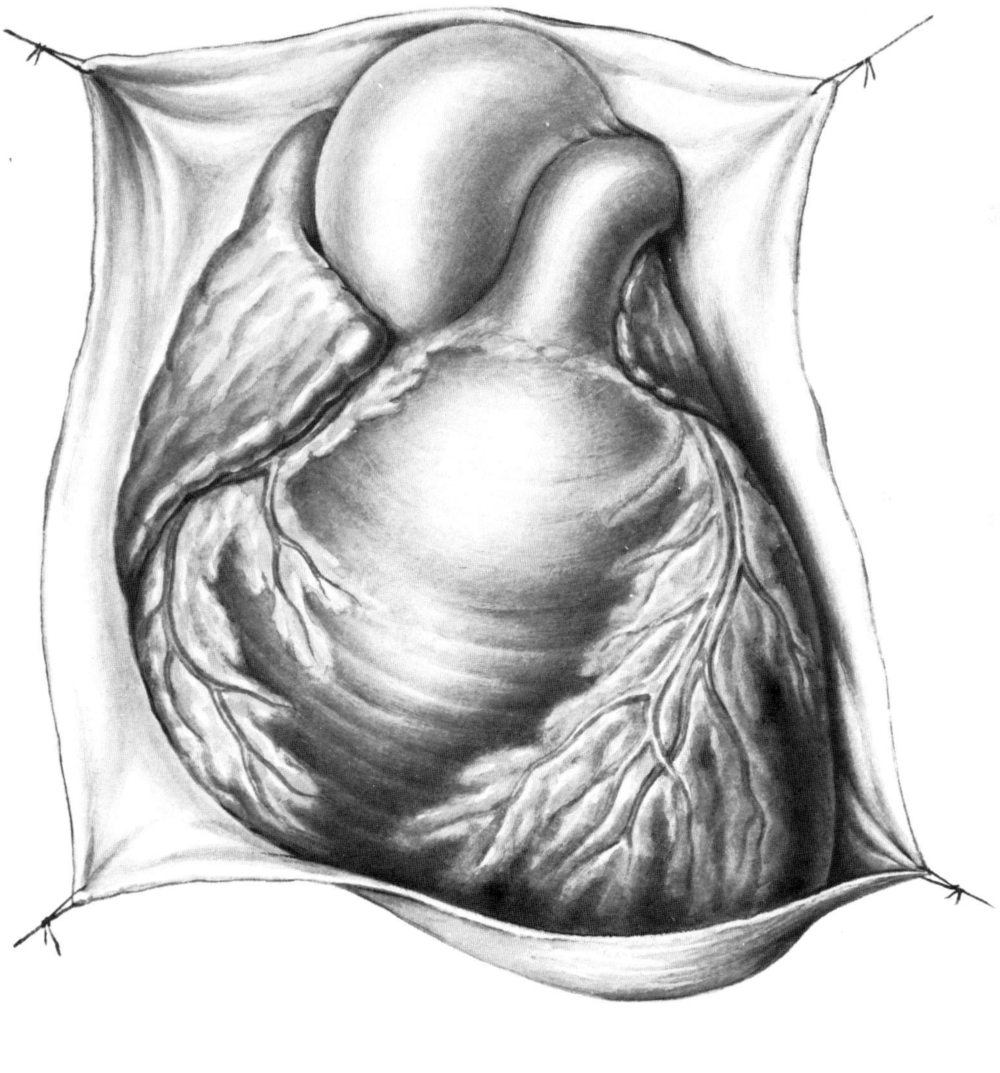

Fig. 384. View of heart exposed through longitudinal sternotomy in tetralogy of Fallot.

aortic valves are distinctly seen. When the edges of the incision in the right ventricle are shifted with hooks, regurgitation through the cusps of the aortic valves occurs. In some cases regurgitation is also observed when the walls of the heart and the aorta are not moved. In marked regurgitation the ascending aorta has to be clamped from time to time, due to which anoxic bradycardia develops. As the result of strong bronchial blood flow the cardiac cavity is constantly flooded with blood during the operation, which hampers the surgeon's work. To make the

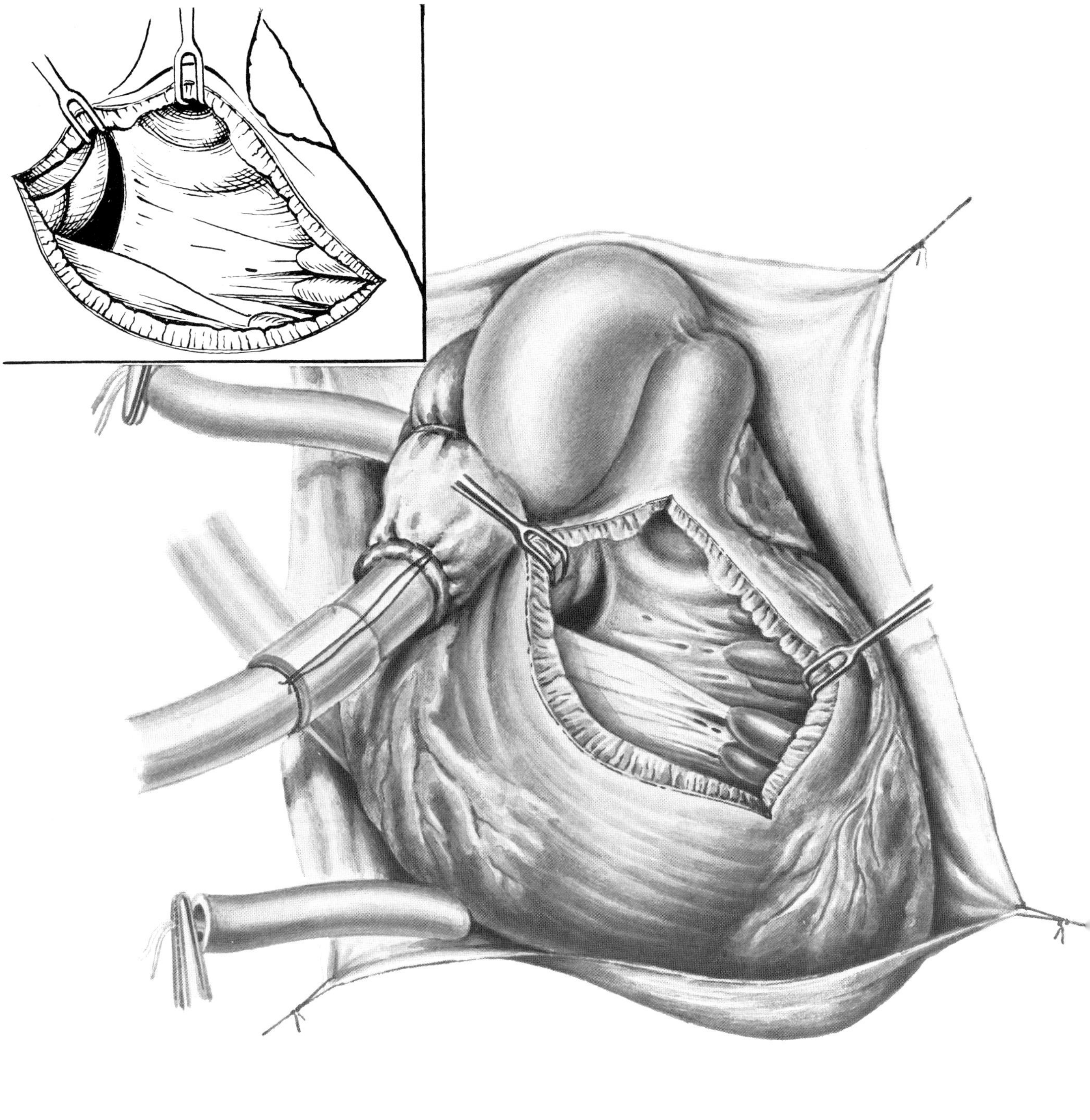

Fig. 385. Longitudinal ventriculotomy carried out after heart is disconnected from circulation. *Inset,* schema of transverse ventriculotomy.

manipulations easier, the cardiac cavity is additionally drained through a system of coronary drainage of the left atrium.

The interventricular septal defect and the transposition of the aorta are always corrected by means of a felt Teflon graft attached with Halsted sutures. In some cases Teflon bolsters are arranged from the side of the left ventricular cavity (Fig. 387).

The right ventricle is closed with a double-row continuous blanket suture with careful ligation of the small branches of the right coronary artery (Fig. 388).

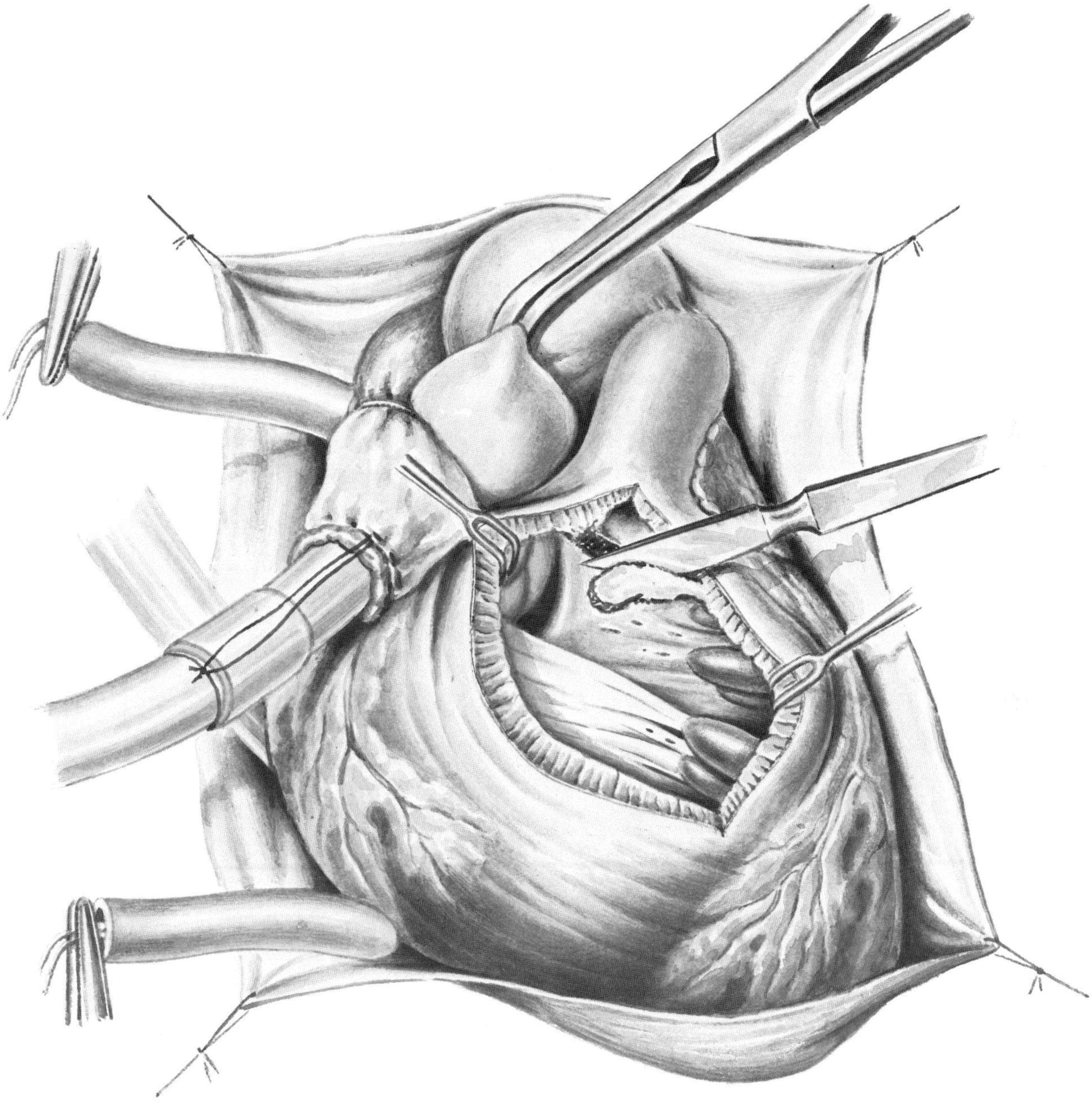

Fig. 386. Techniques of infundibular resection in region of anterior wall of right ventricle.

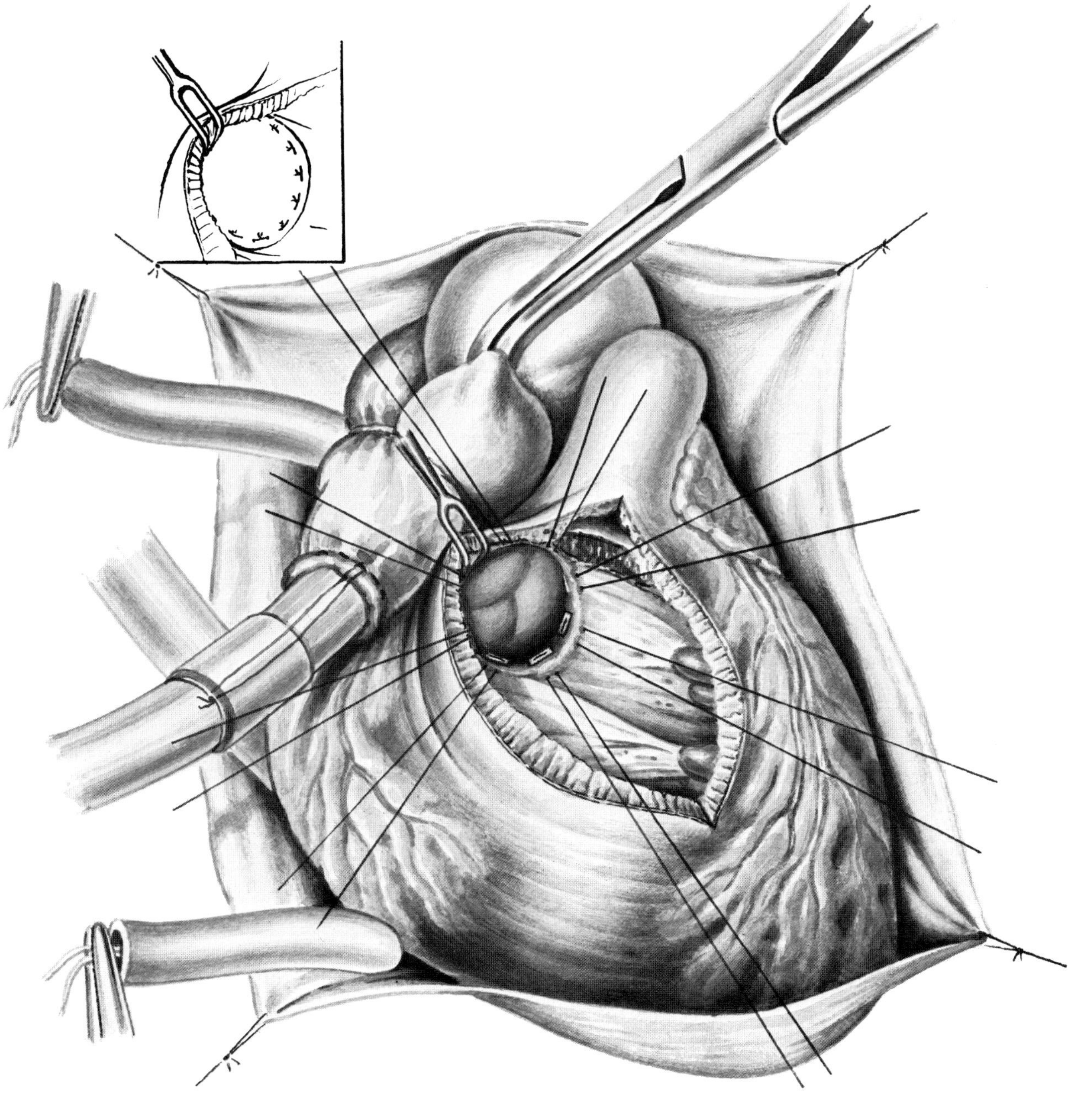

Fig. 387. Interventricular septal defect and displaced orifice of aorta viewed from cavity of right ventricle. Application of sutures to edges of defect with use of Teflon bolsters.

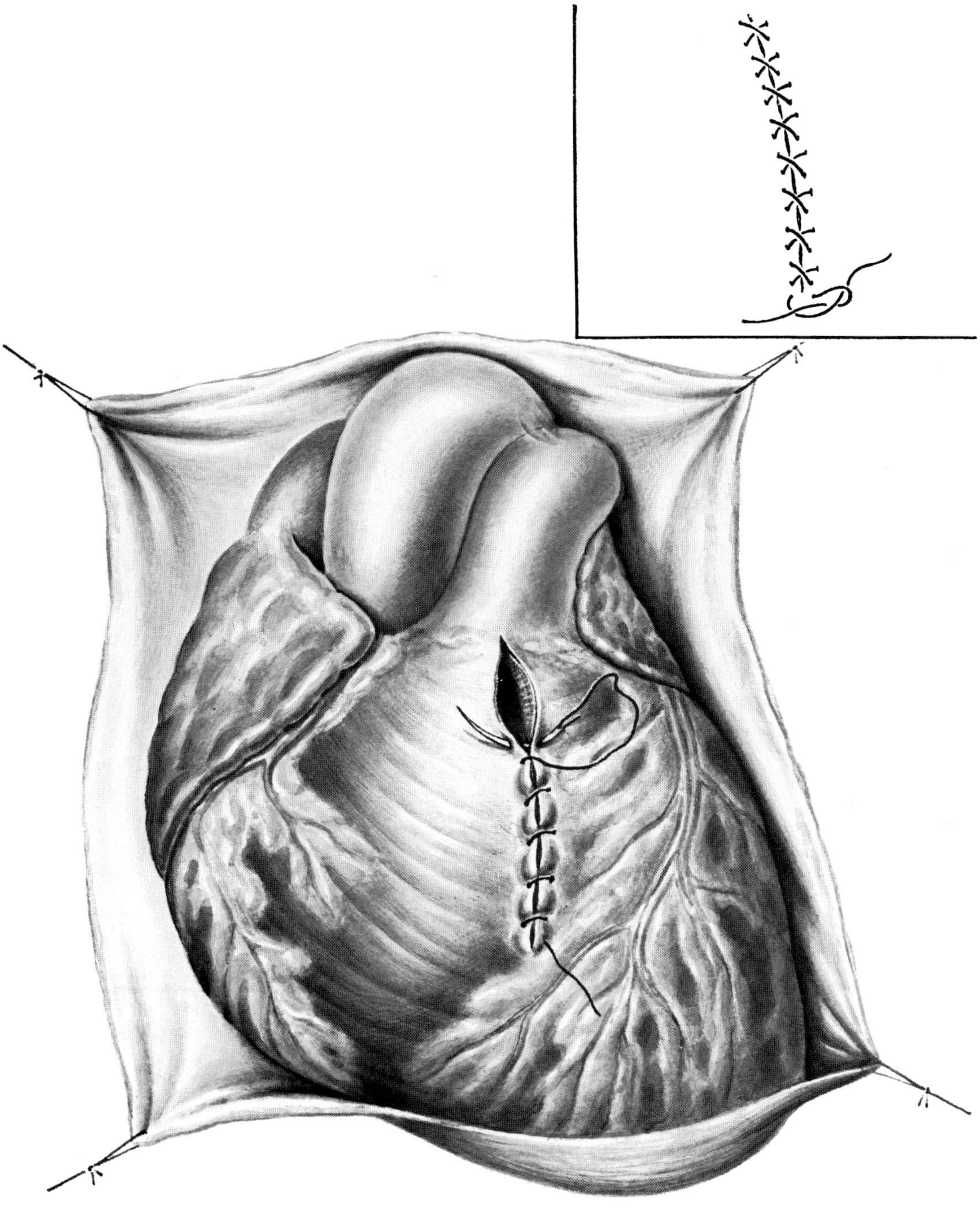

Fig. 388. Wound in wall of right ventricle is closed with sutures.

*PLASTIC SURGERY OF INTERVENTRICULAR SEPTAL DEFECTS BY APPROACH THROUGH RIGHT ATRIUM

The right atrium is opened wide by an incision made parallel to the atrioventricular sulcus and continued through the apex of the right auricle, accommodating the venous cannula for the superior vena cava. The edges of the incision are grasped with triangular forceps, and the cavity of the right ventricle is explored with the finger inserted through the tricuspid valve. The medial cusp of the tricuspid valve is temporarily cut off along the fibrous ring (Fig. 389). For easier access to the defect, traction sutures are stitched through the cusp (Fig. 390). The lower muscular part of the defect is stitched with Halsted sutures, each of which serves as a traction thread when the next sutures are applied (Fig. 391).

Sutures separating the aorta from the cavity of the right heart are applied from the side of the right atrium with the ends of the threads brought out close to the noncoronary cusp of the aortic valve. The caudal-lateral edge of the defect is the most dangerous place with regard to possible injury to the right branch of the bundle of His. The sutures here are placed tangentially to the right-ventricular side of the septum. The same threads are stitched through the Teflon felt graft made to fit the defect (Fig. 392). The graft is lowered through the cusp incision to the septum, and the sutures are carefully tied successively with due consideration for the character of the defect margins.

The cusp of the tricuspid valve is secured in place with a continuous suture (Fig. 393).

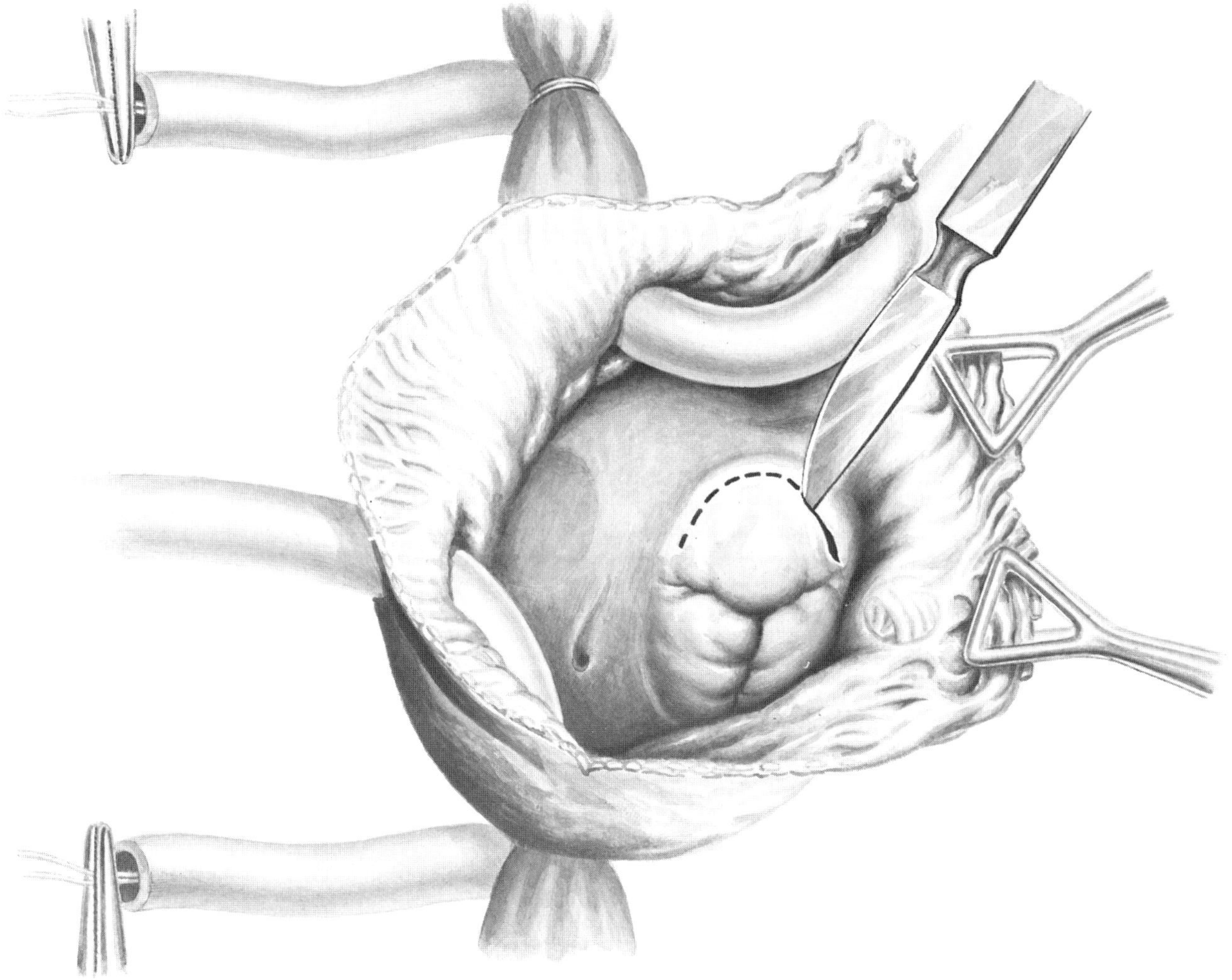

Fig. 389. Medial cusp of tricuspid valve is cut away.

Infundibular resection is performed by longitudinal or transverse ventriculotomy over the third ventricle (Fig. 394). The incision is stretched with hooks, and circular resection of the infundibular stenosis is performed from the third ventricle (Fig. 395).

Ventriculotomy over the third ventricle makes it possible to inspect the condition of the valves of the pulmonary artery. In the event of a valvular stenosis it is dilated with a dilatator or separated along the commissures with eversion of the valve into the right ventricular cavity (Fig. 396).

The incision in the right ventricle is closed with a double-row blanket suture (Fig. 397), and last of all the wound in the wall of the right atrium is closed by the method described above.

The infundibular stenosis may be extended over a considerable distance in the form of a canal with a hardly noticeable third ventricle. A wide infundibular resection is traumatic in such cases. It is preferable to follow longitudinal infundibular ventriculotomy and partial infundibular resection with plastic surgery of the right ventricular outflow tract by means of a spindle-shaped plastic graft. The ends of the graft are stitched into the edges of the incision with Halsted sutures. Plastic surgery is completed by applying a continuous blanket suture (Fig. 398).

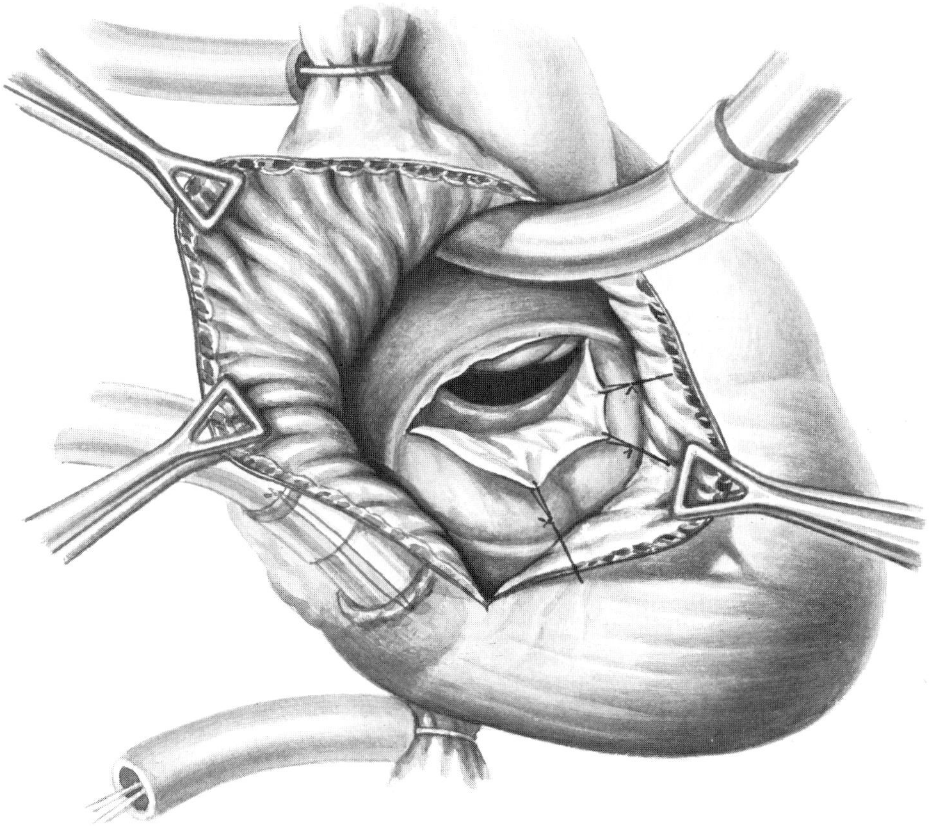

Fig. 390. Medial cusp of tricuspid valve has been cut and drawn away caudally. Defect in interventricular septum is visible.

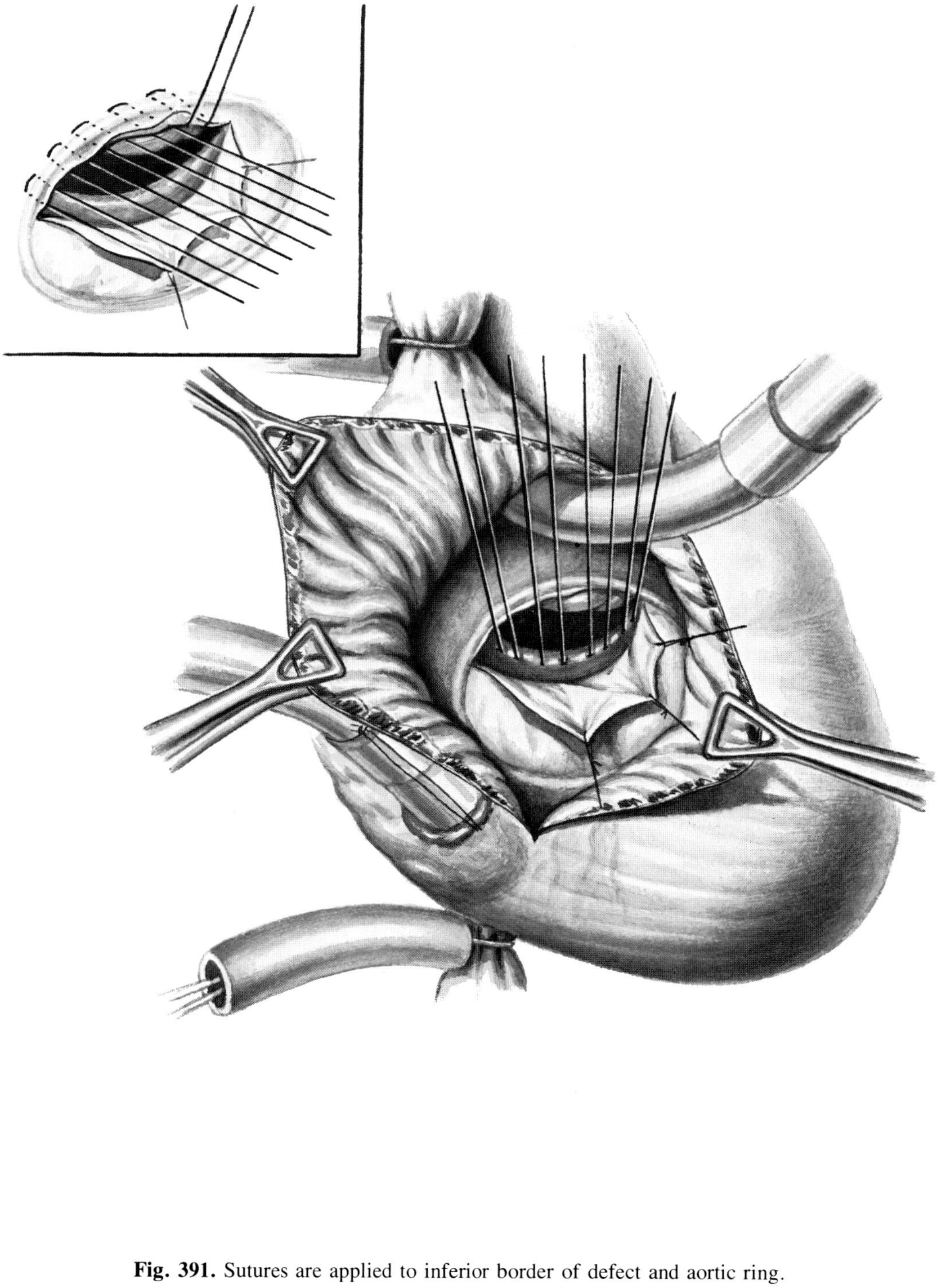

Fig. 391. Sutures are applied to inferior border of defect and aortic ring.

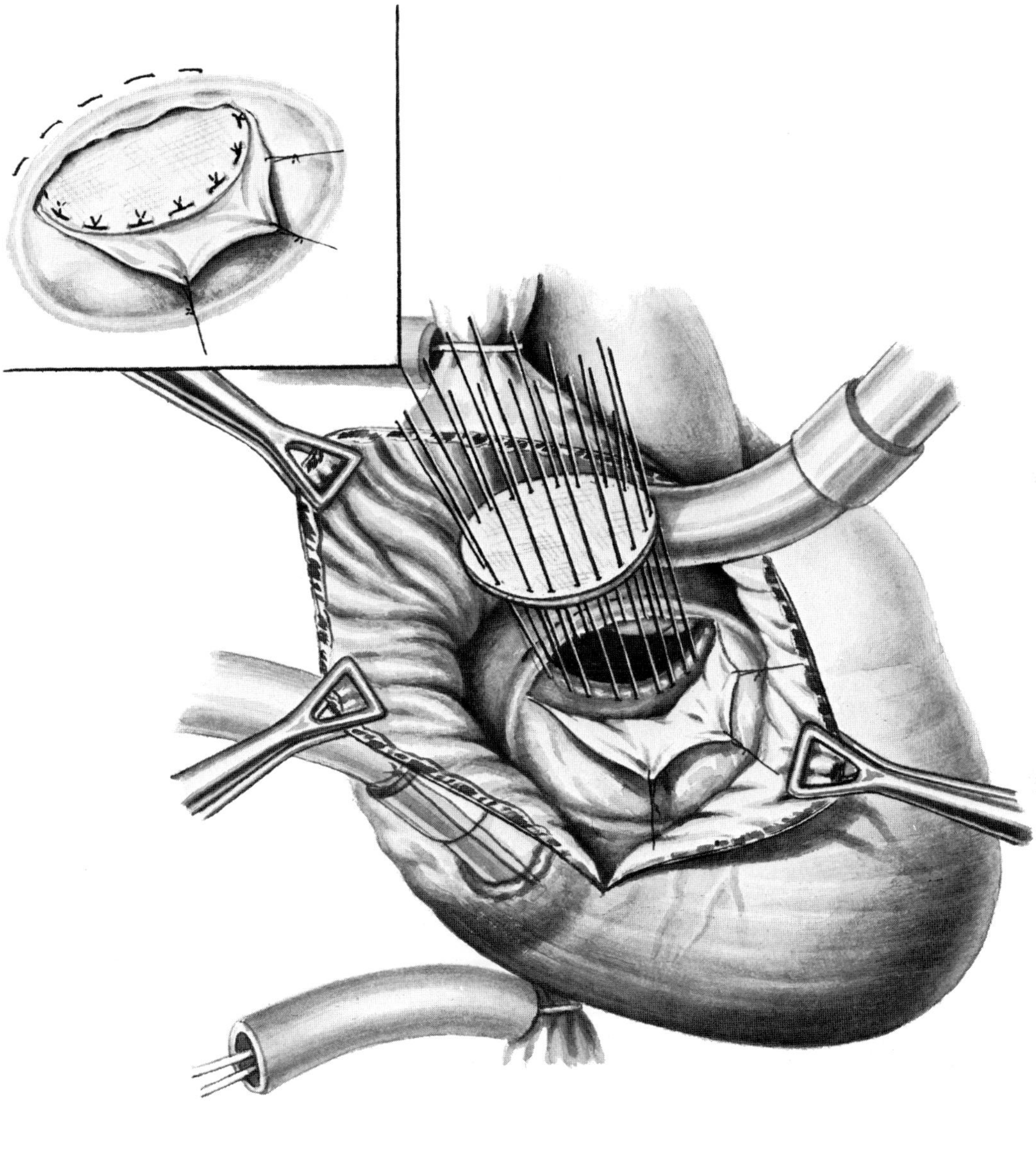

Fig. 392. Sutures are passed through edges of graft. *Inset,* graft closing interventricular defect.

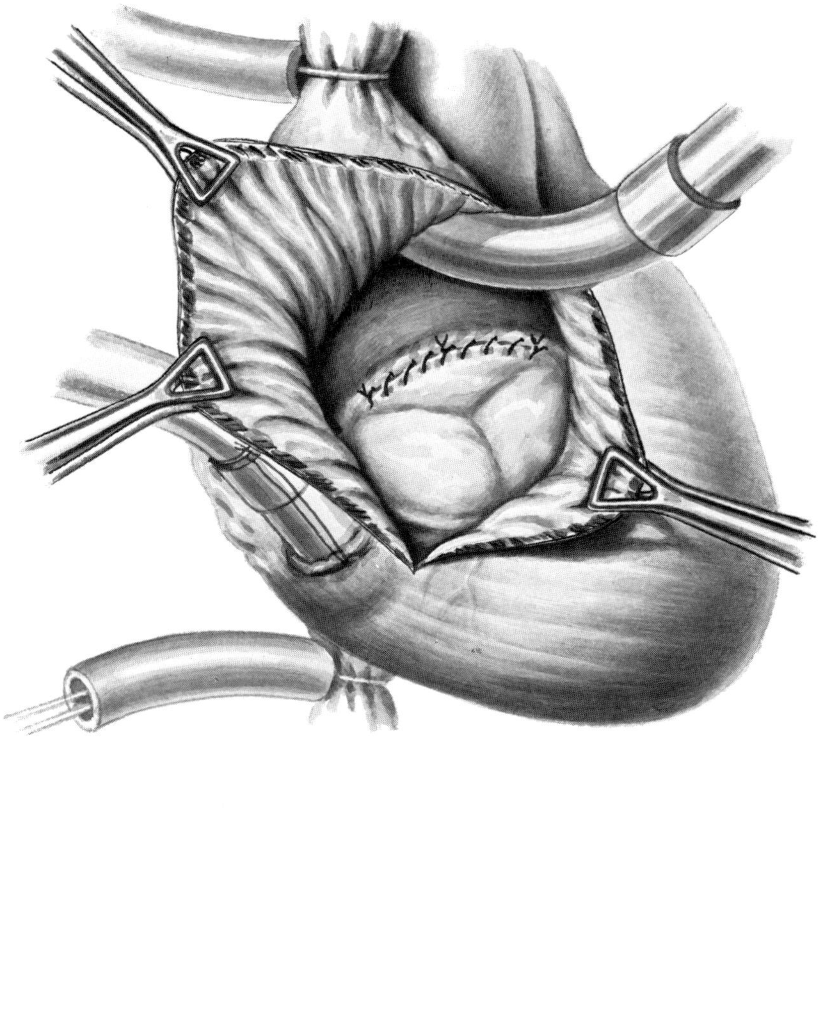

Fig. 393. Incision in cusp of tricuspid valve is closed with sutures.

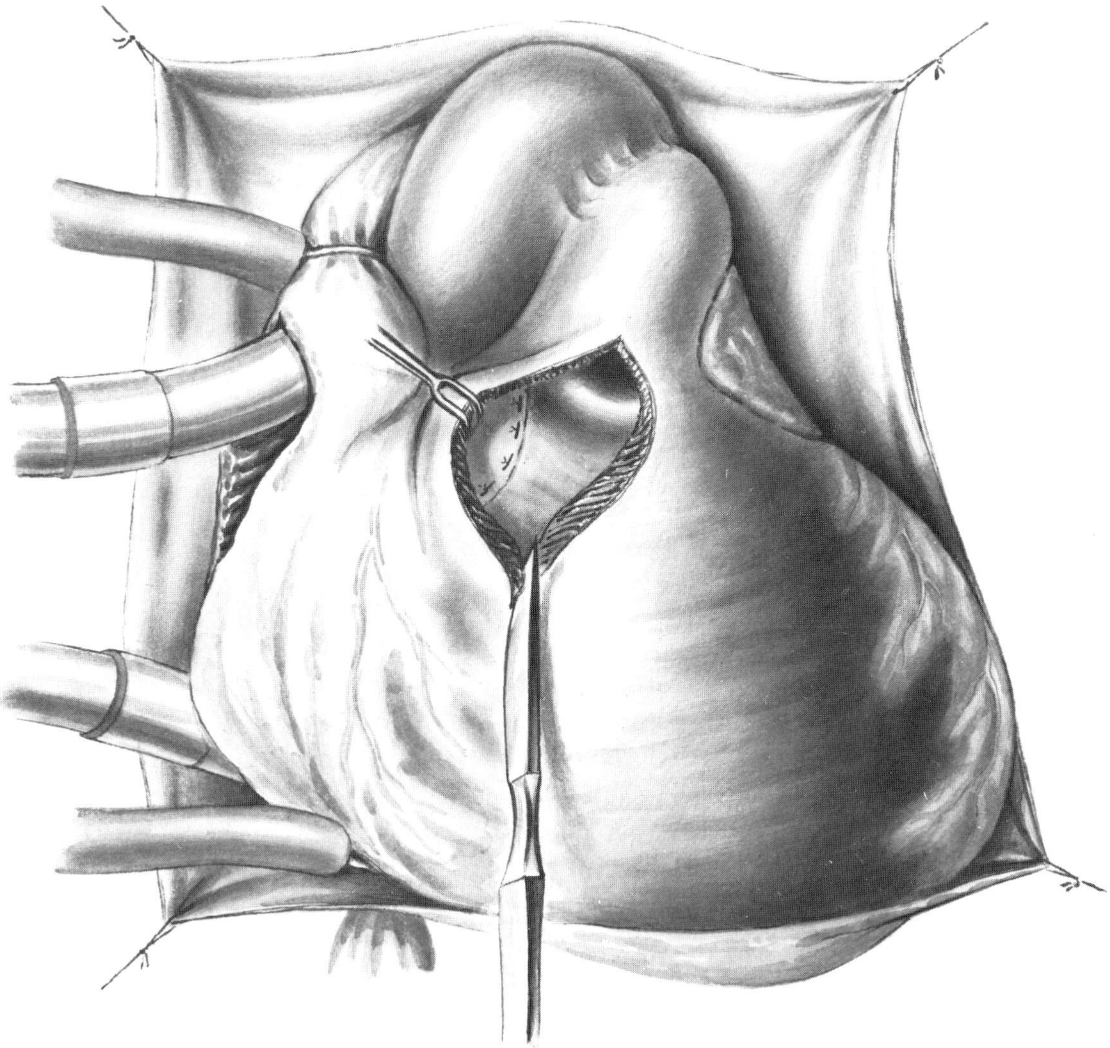

Fig. 394. Longitudinal ventriculotomy over third ventricle of heart.

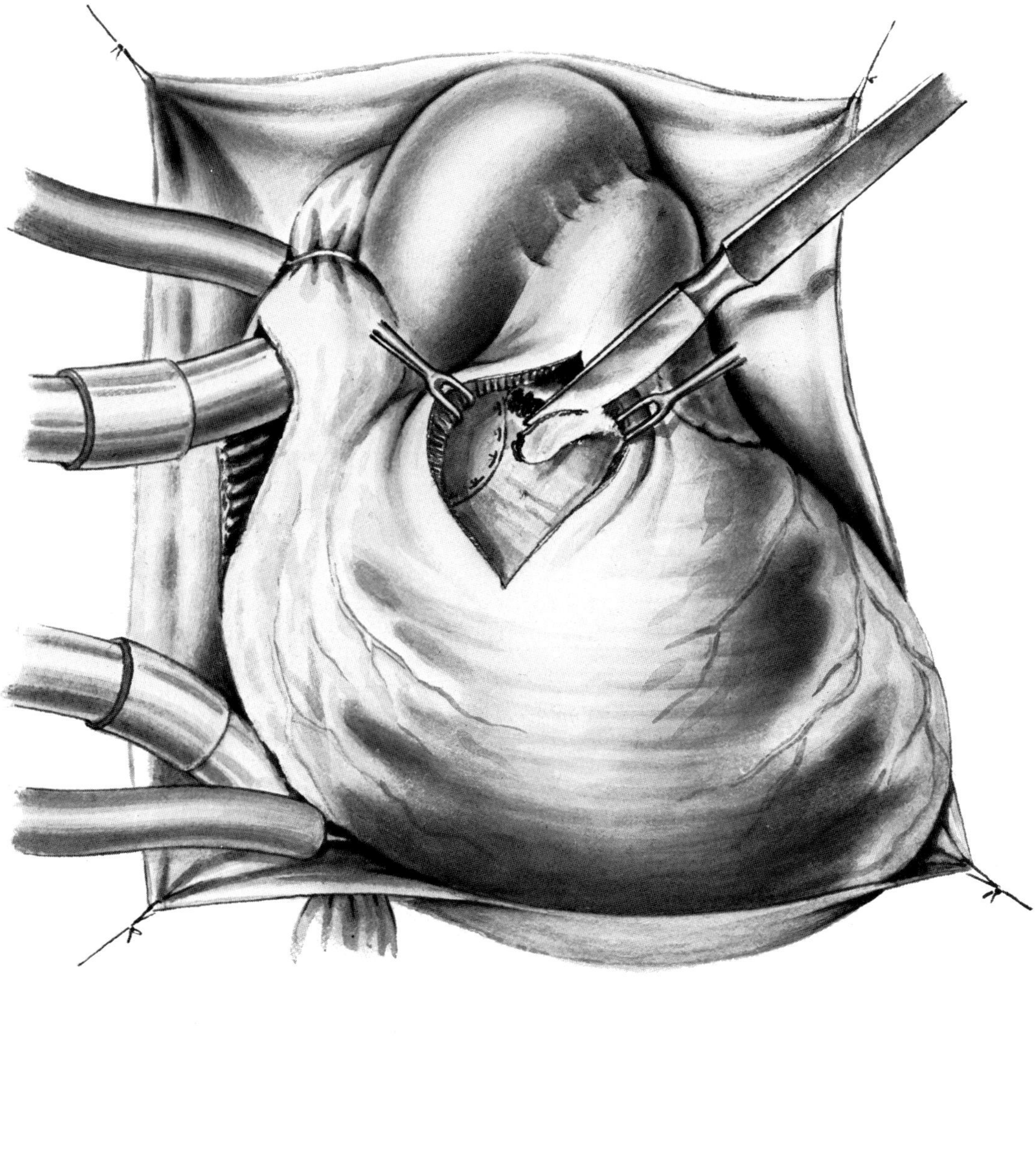

Fig. 395. Circular infundibular resection from side of third ventricle of heart.

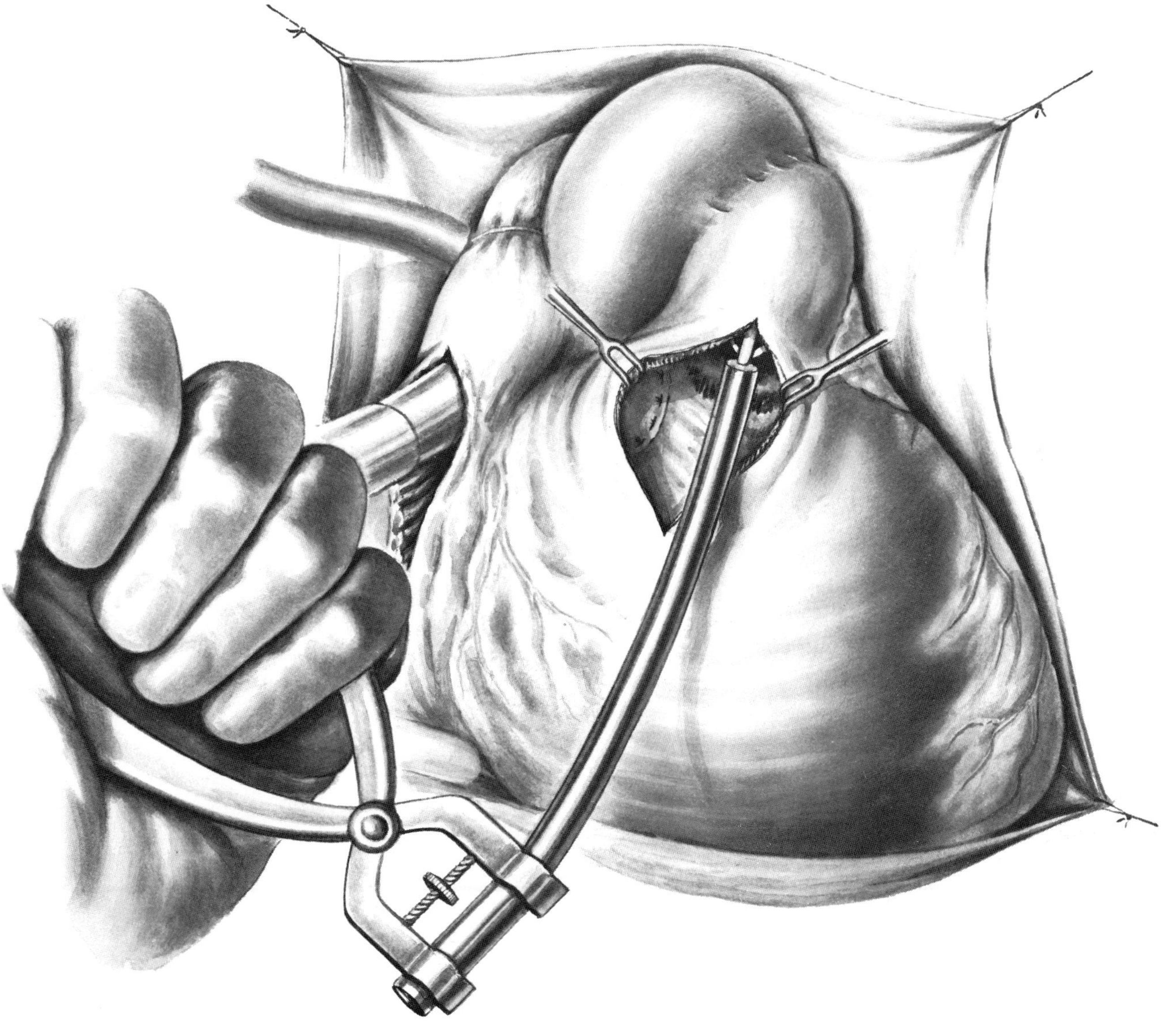

Fig. 396. Dilatation of valvular stenosis of pulmonary trunk with dilator.

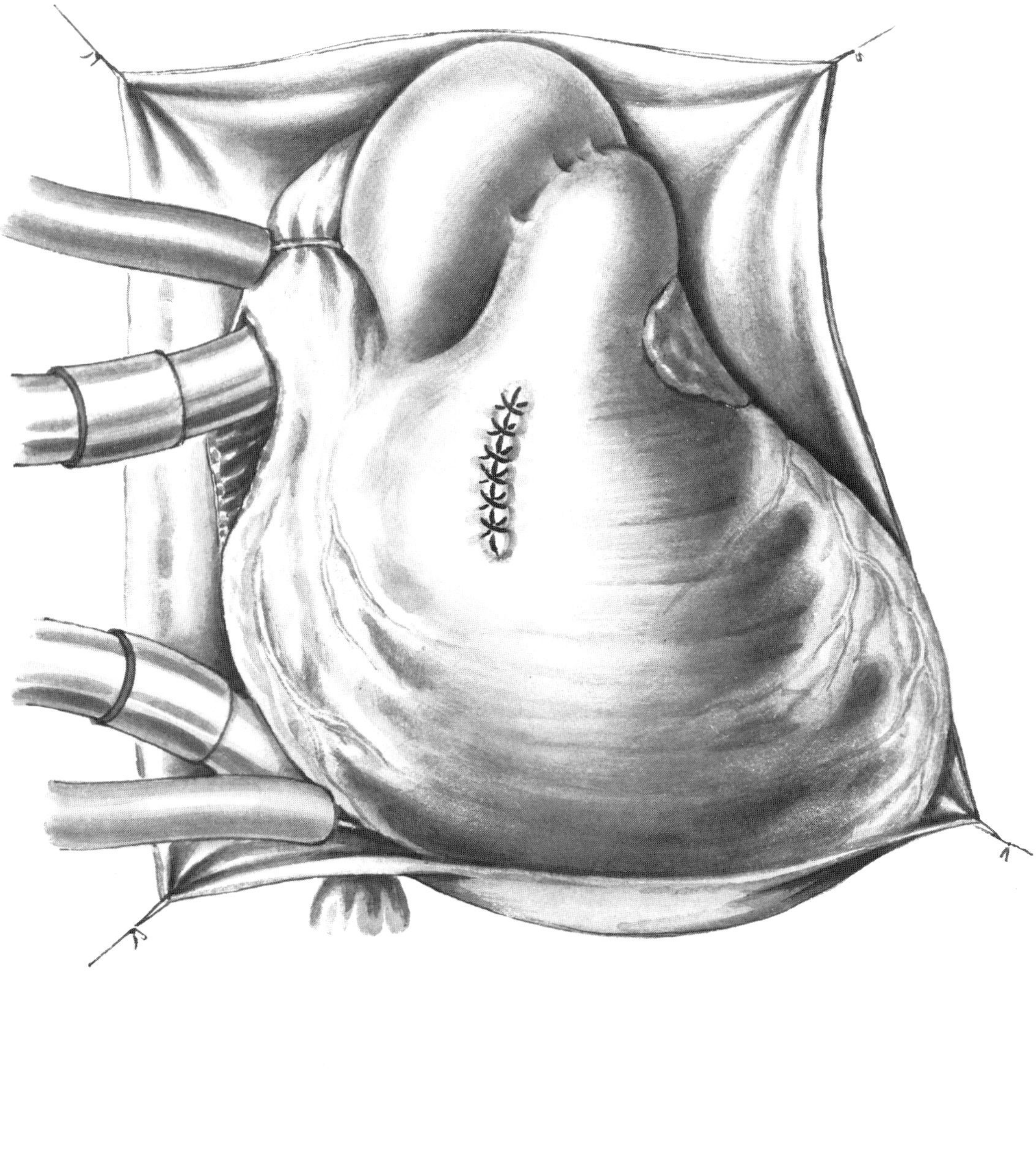

Fig. 397. Wound after longitudinal ventriculotomy of right ventricle is sutured.

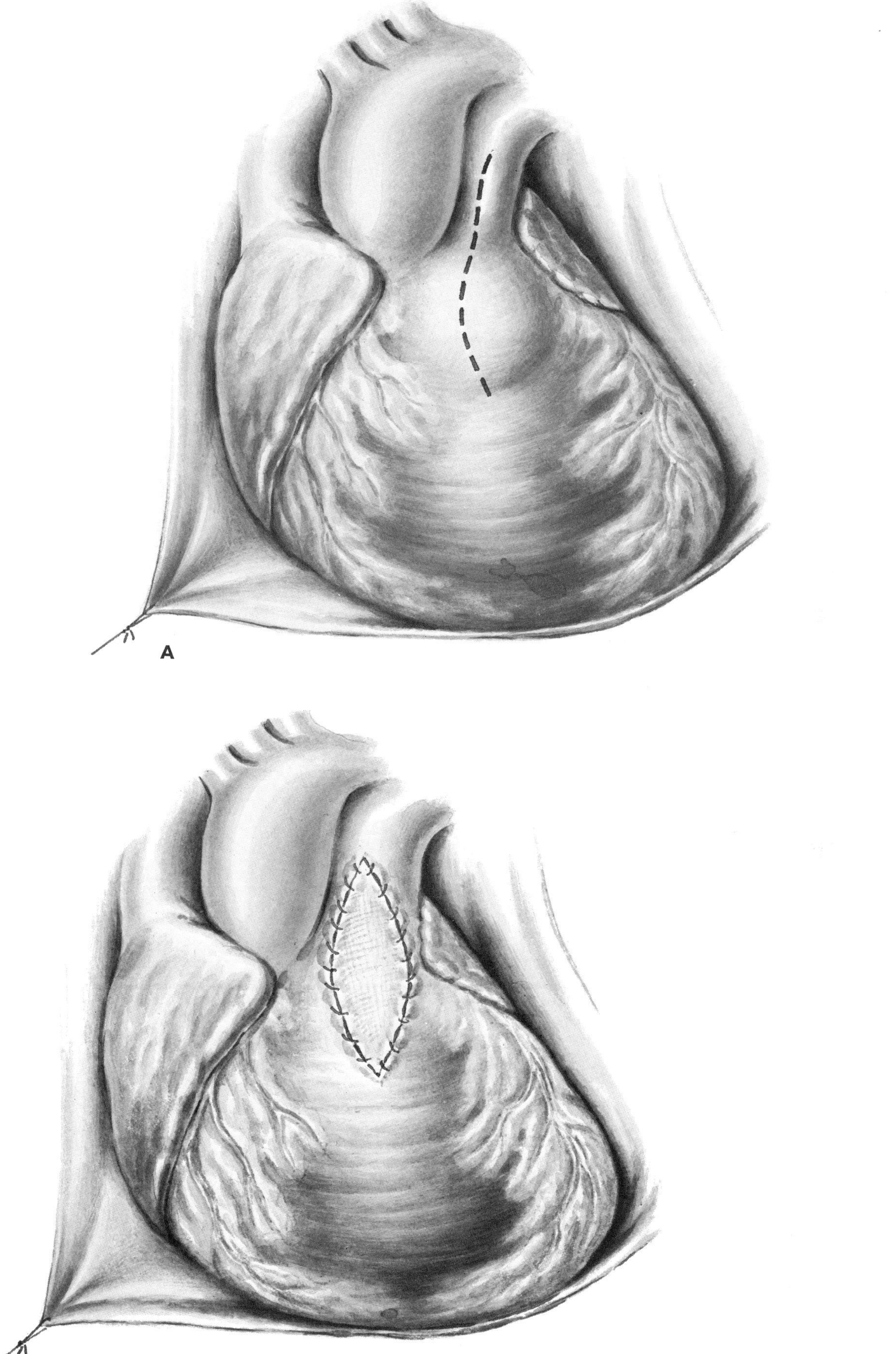

Fig. 398. A, Line of incision of right ventricle and pulmonary trunk for plastic surgery with spindle-shaped plastic graft. **B,** General view of heart after right ventricular outflow tract has been widened and graft sutured.

*RADICAL CORRECTION BY APPROACH THROUGH RIGHT ATRIUM

To inflict less injury to the right ventricle and in cases in which large branches of the right coronary artery may be transected when incisions are made in the anterior wall of the right ventricle in the region of its outflow tract, all manipulations for correction of tetralogy of Fallot may be performed from the right ventricular cavity; the medial cusp of the tricuspid valve is temporarily detached along the fibrous ring, and in the region of the medial commissure between the medial and anterior cusps (Fig. 399).

When the right atrioventricular orifice is stretched through this incision, the beginning of the stenosed infundibular canal becomes accessible. The stenosed infundibular part is resected, with the stenosing swell on the anterior wall of the right ventricle removed first (Fig. 400).

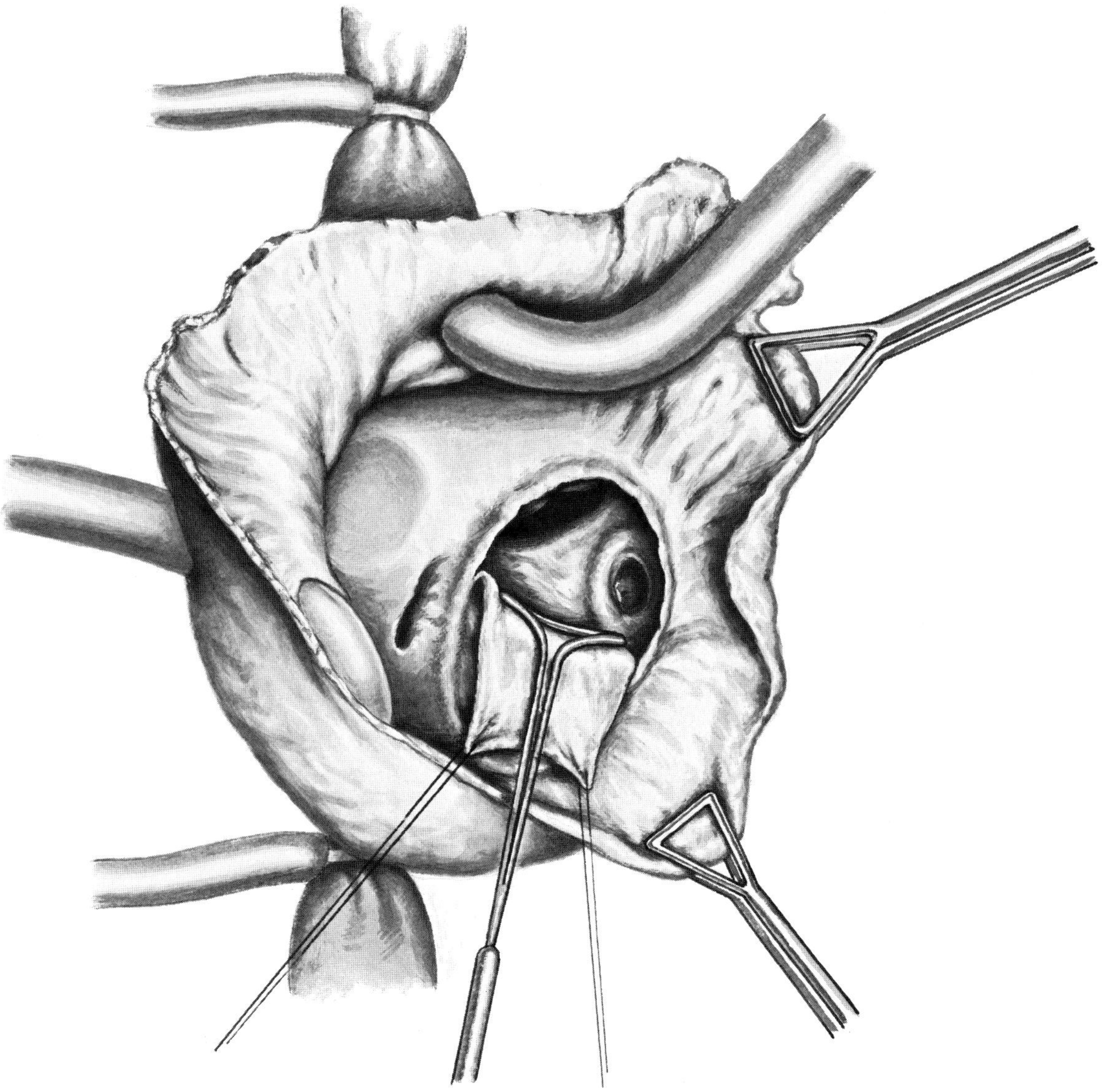

Fig. 399. Medial cusp of tricuspid valve is detached with transection of medial commissure in infundibular resection from cavity of right ventricle.

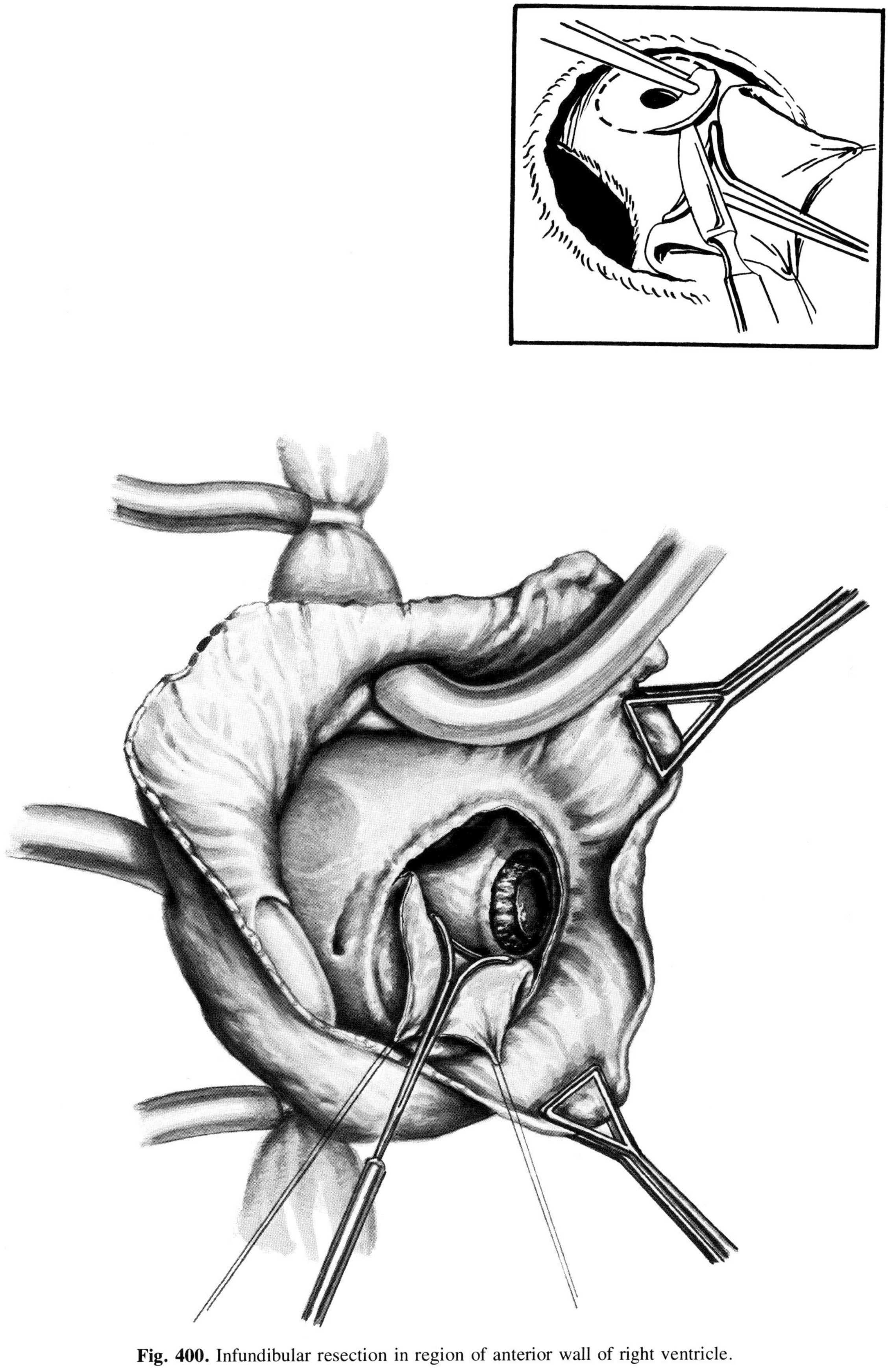

Fig. 400. Infundibular resection in region of anterior wall of right ventricle.

In estimating the radical character of the resection, it is expedient to have the heart contracting, since in fibrillation of the ventricles the finger may stretch the dilated infundibular canal, and its dimensions cannot be judged during the ventricular systole.

The defect is repaired with a graft after the infundibular resection is completed (Fig. 401). The medial cusp of the tricuspid valve is restored next, and the chordae of the medial and anterior cusps of the tricuspid valve are sutured with a separate suture in the region of the medial commissure (Fig. 402).

The right atrium is sutured. The wall in the right ventricle appears intact from the outside.

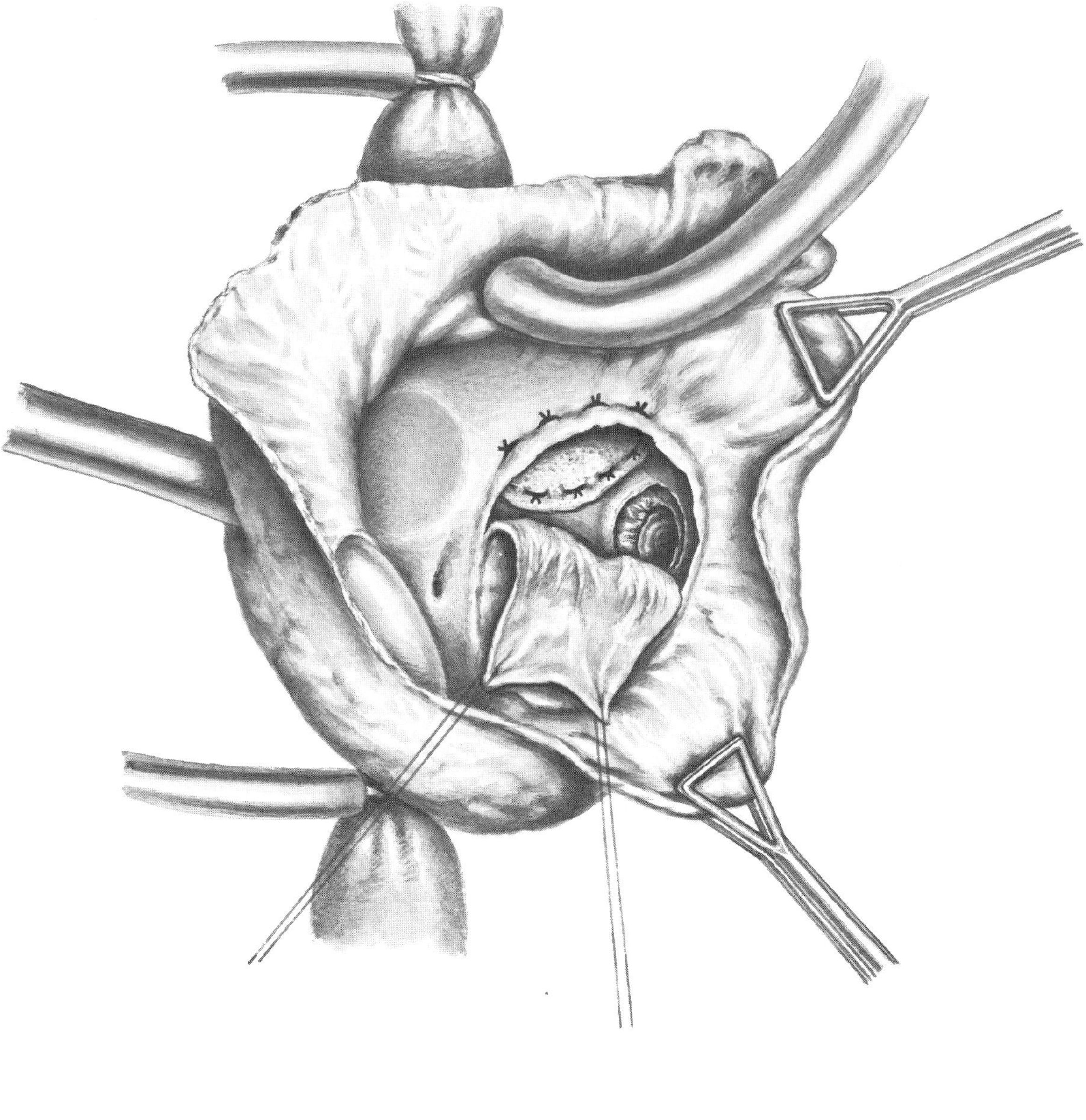

Fig. 401. View of graft on interventricular septal defect after infundibular resection.

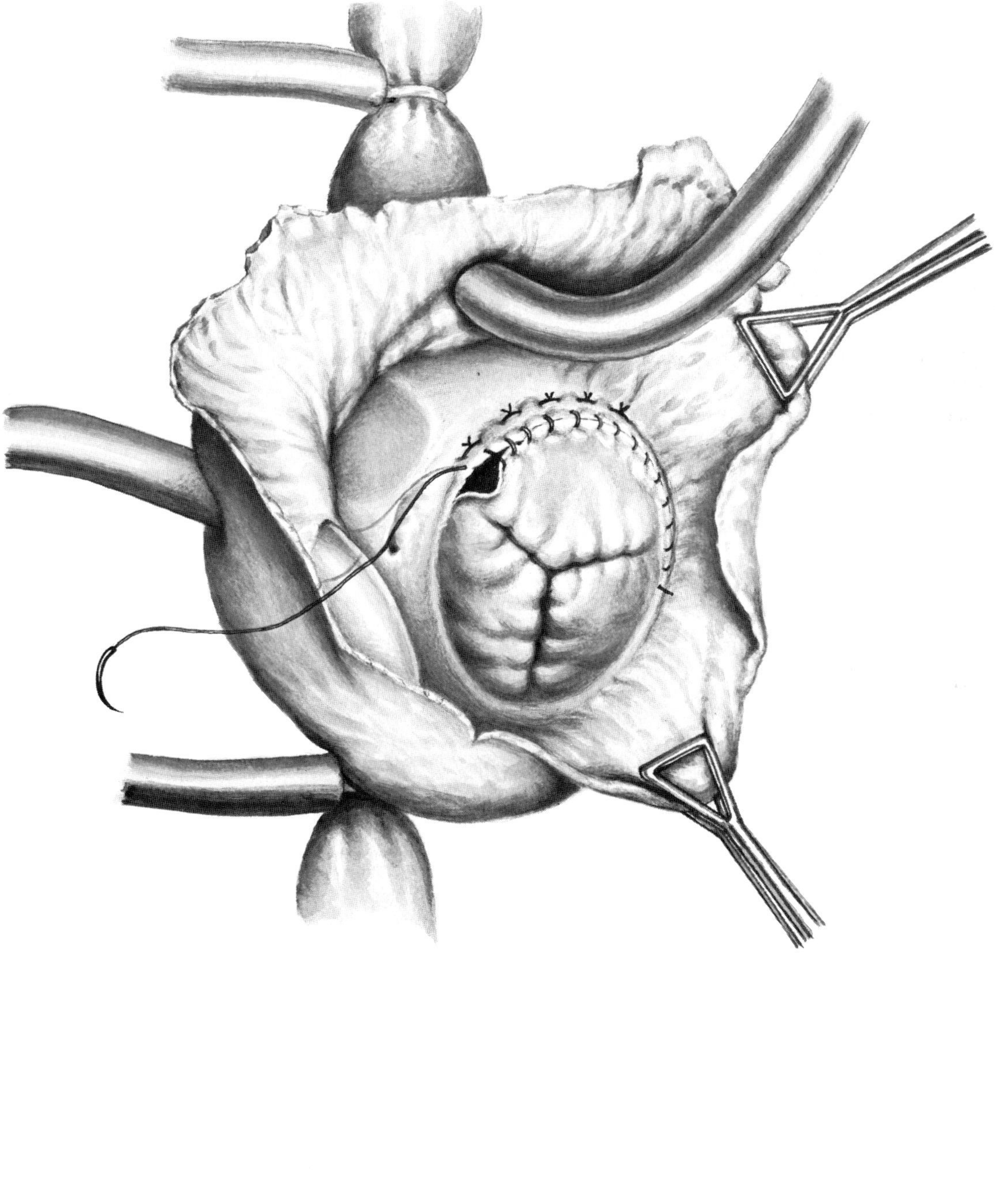

Fig. 402. Repair of cusp of tricuspid valve and medial commissure with sutures.

*RADICAL CORRECTION BY APPROACH THROUGH RIGHT ATRIUM WITH PLASTIC SURGERY AND PROSTHETICS OF VALVE OF PULMONARY TRUNK

In the cyanotic form of tetralogy of Fallot, when the pulmonary trunk is drastically narrowed and its diameter is less than one third of the aortic diameter, its stenosed part cannot allow passage into the pulmonary circulation of the entire minute volume of blood (Fig. 403). This is why radical correction of the anomaly is possible only with the simultaneous dilatation of the pulmonary trunk.

In adhesion the valves of the pulmonary trunk are fused not only to each other but with the wall of the trunk, forming blind sacs instead of the normal Valsalva sinuses. Simple transection of the commissures, which are short in such cases, does not correct the stenosis at the root of the pulmonary trunk. Its orifice may be widened only after total removal of the distorted cusps. Replacement of the valves of the pulmonary trunk with prostheses is indicated in such cases.

When the interventricular septal defect has been closed and the transposition of the aorta corrected, the pulmonary trunk and the wall of the third ventricle are cut longitudinally from the right atrium. The cusps of the valves of the pulmonary artery are excised (Fig.

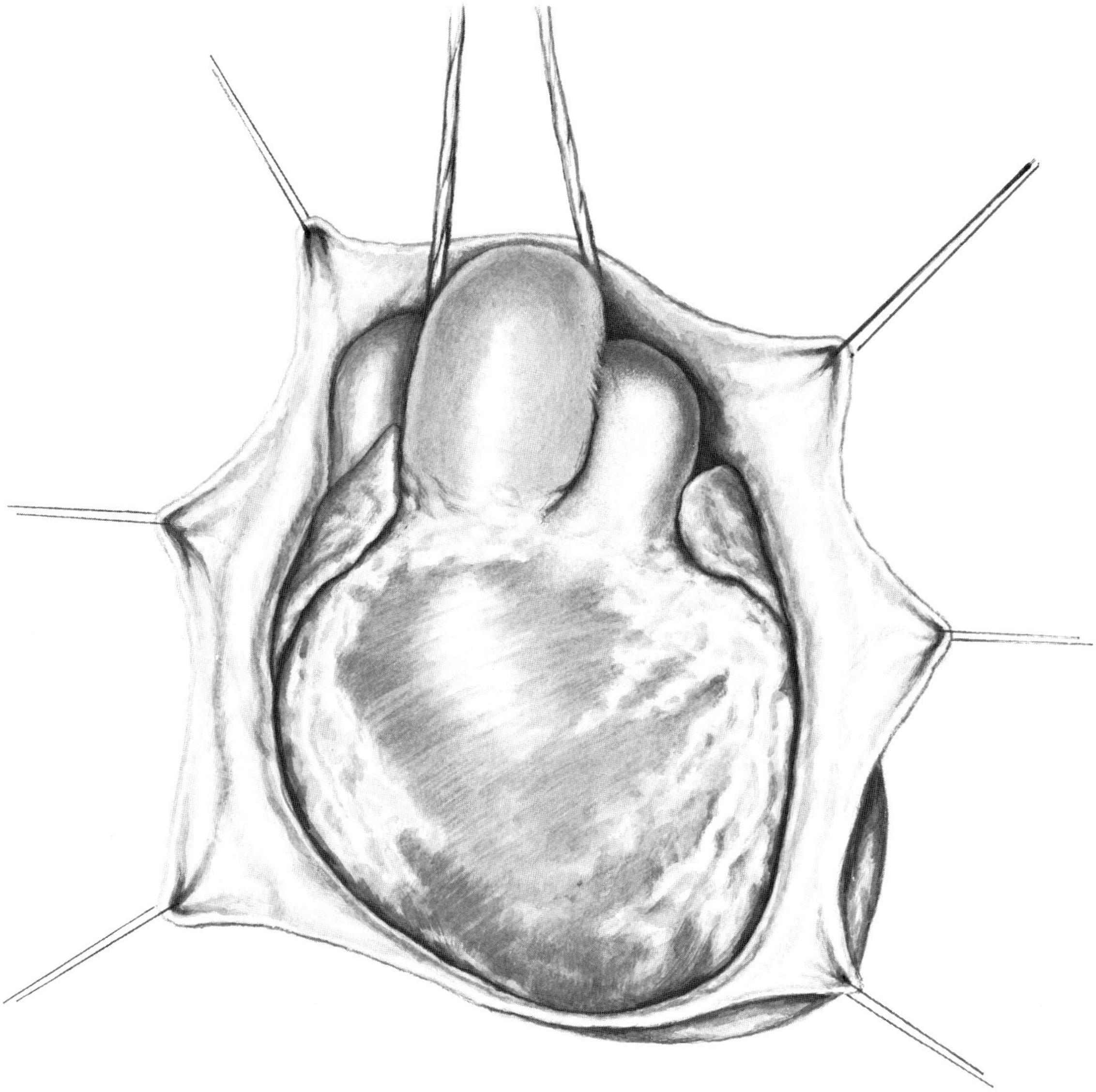

Fig. 403. View of heart in tetralogy of Fallot with drastic stenosis of pulmonary trunk.

404). The infundibular stenosis is corrected by resection from the third ventricle. Halsted sutures are applied along the line of the base of the cusps of the pulmonary artery valves. The ends of the threads are passed through the edges of two thirds of the circumference of an aortic ball prosthesis. The prosthesis is lowered in position, and the sutures are tied. The free part of the circumference of the prosthesis is used for subsequent plastics (Fig. 405).

A spindle-shaped graft fitting the incision in the pulmonary trunk and the right ventricular outflow tract is formed from the pericardium and Teflon fabric. These grafts are stitched together so that the inner surface of the pericardium becomes the inner surface of the graft. The graft is fitted in place with its pericardial surface in the lumen of the pulmonary trunk and attached with a Halsted suture to the corner of the incision in the region of the bifurcation. Then it is stitched into the incision in the pulmonary trunk to the level of the ball prosthesis with Halsted and blanket sutures (Fig. 406). The graft is attached to the free third of the circumference of the ball prosthesis with Halsted sutures. The remaining part of the graft is used to widen the outflow tract of the right ventricle (Figs. 407 and 408).

A short pulmonary trunk is sometimes an obstacle to the application of a ball prosthesis, and a homologous or heterologous aortic valve may be implanted in such cases.

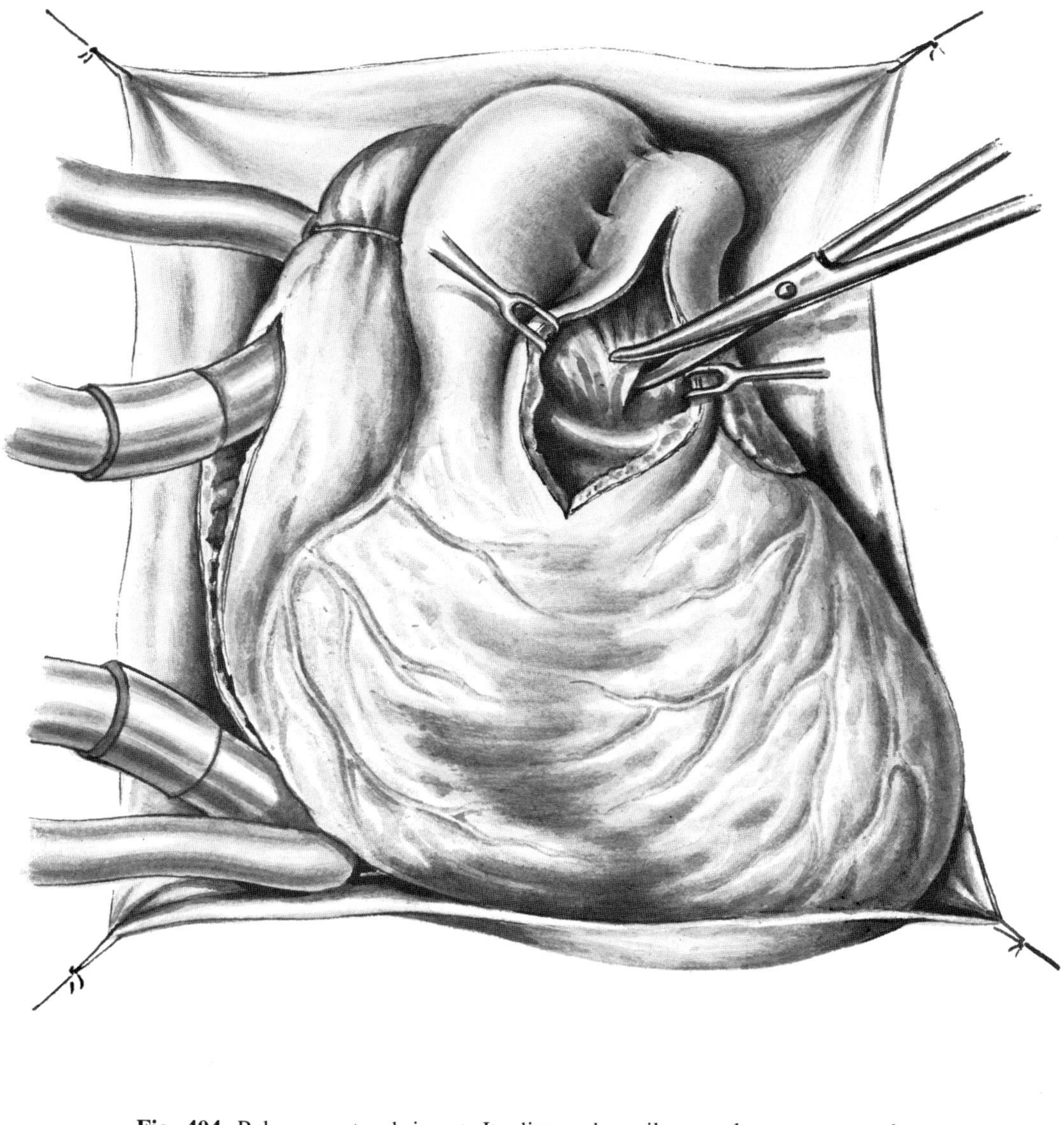

Fig. 404. Pulmonary trunk is cut. Its distorted semilunar valves are resected.

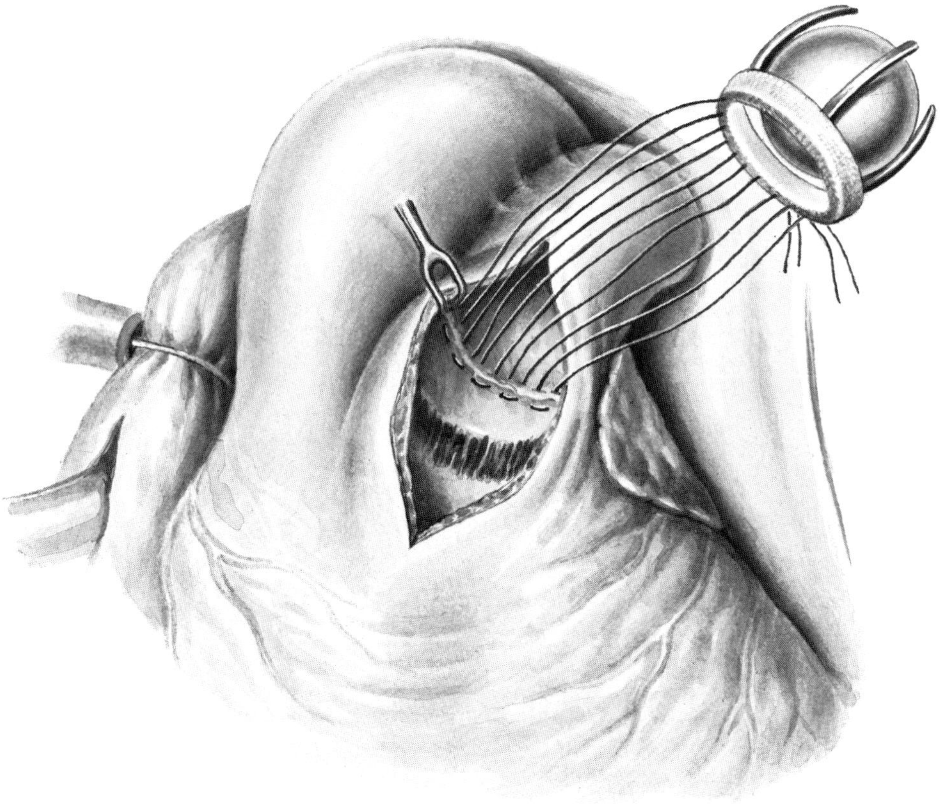

Fig. 405. Application of Halsted sutures along line of the fibrous ring of the pulmonary trunk after infundibular resection. Sutures are passed through base of ball prosthesis.

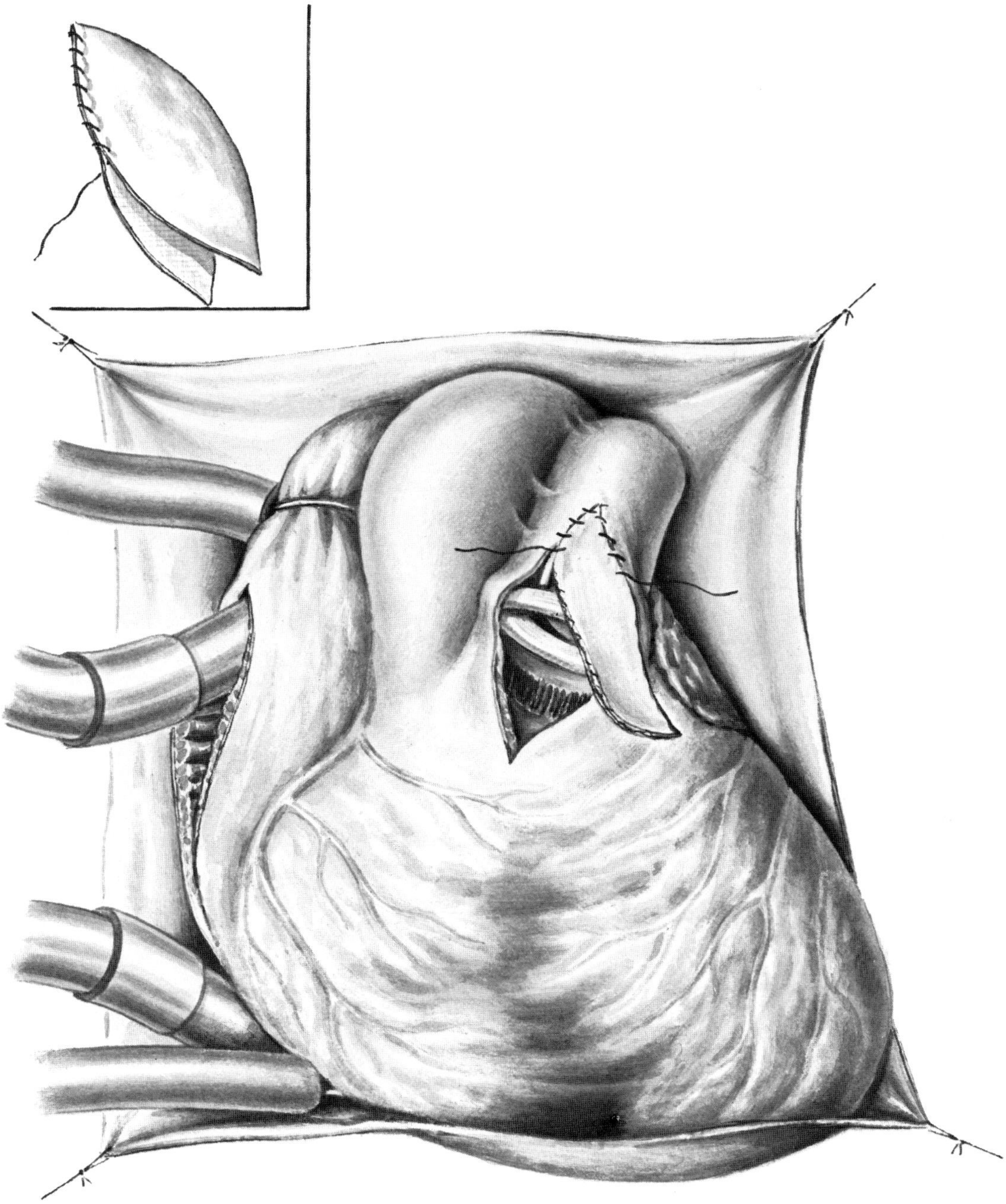

Fig. 406. Spindle-shaped graft is formed from pericardium and plastic material and sutured to edges of pulmonary trunk to level of prosthesis.

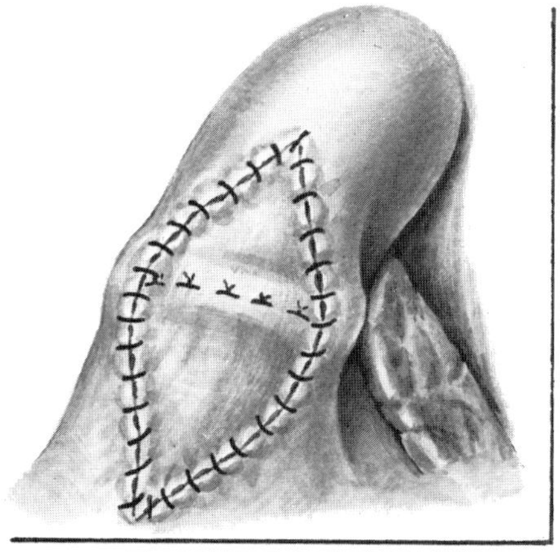

407

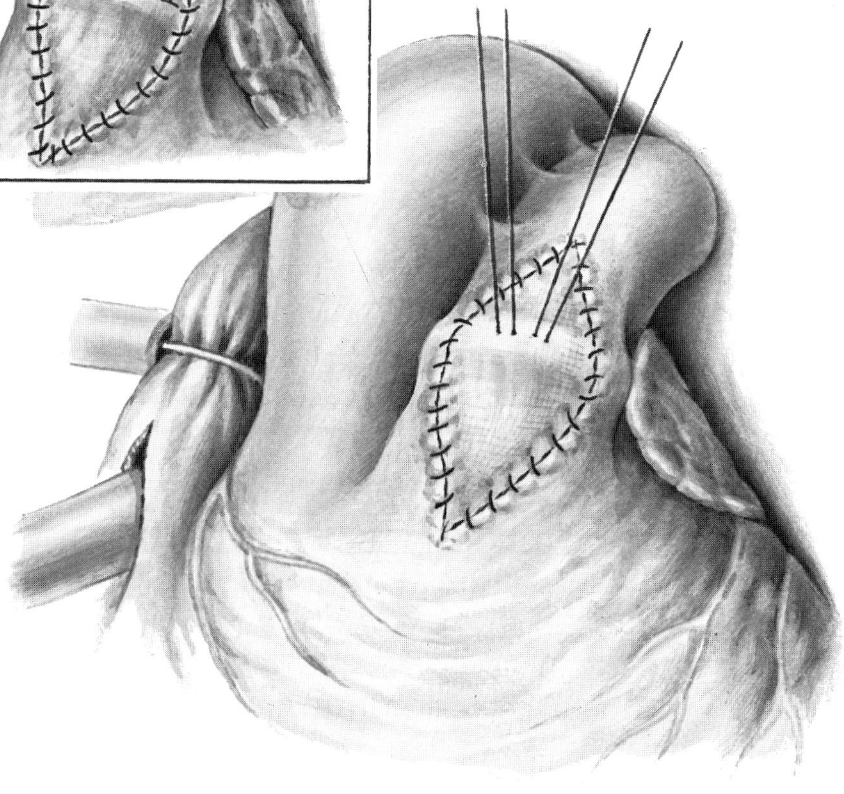

408

Fig. 407. General view of heart after radical correction of tetralogy of Fallot through right atrial cavity with plastic surgery of pulmonary trunk and replacement of its valves with ball prosthesis.
Fig. 408. Application of Halsted sutures through graft to outer part of prosthesis.

CORRECTION OF MITRAL DEFECT

OPEN-HEART CORRECTION OF STENOSIS

The operation is performed by left or right thoracotomy in the fourth intercostal space. In combined correction, access may be gained by means of longitudinal sternotomy with the left atrium opened by a longitudinal incision ventral to the right pulmonary veins or by incision of the right atrial wall and interatrial septum. In left thoracotomy the venous cannula of the heart-lung machine is introduced through the right auricle or, less frequently, through the outflow tract of the right ventricle (Fig. 409). After the heart-lung machine has been connected, the pulmonary trunk is clamped and the left atrium opened along the atrioventricular sulcus (Fig. 410). If any thrombi are found in the left atrium they are removed by detaching their organized part from the endocardium with a spade. The stenosed mitral valve in the region of the commissures is held with forceps and pulled out into the left atrial cavity. The commissures are cut with sharp scissors or a scalpel (Figs. 411 and 412). The left atrium is repaired with double-row Halsted and blanket sutures (Fig. 413). At the end of the operation the left ventricle and left atrium are punctured with DuFeau's needle to remove air from the left parts of the heart. During application of sutures to the left atrium the clamp is removed from the pulmonary trunk; as the heart is punctured, the anesthetist inflates the lungs.

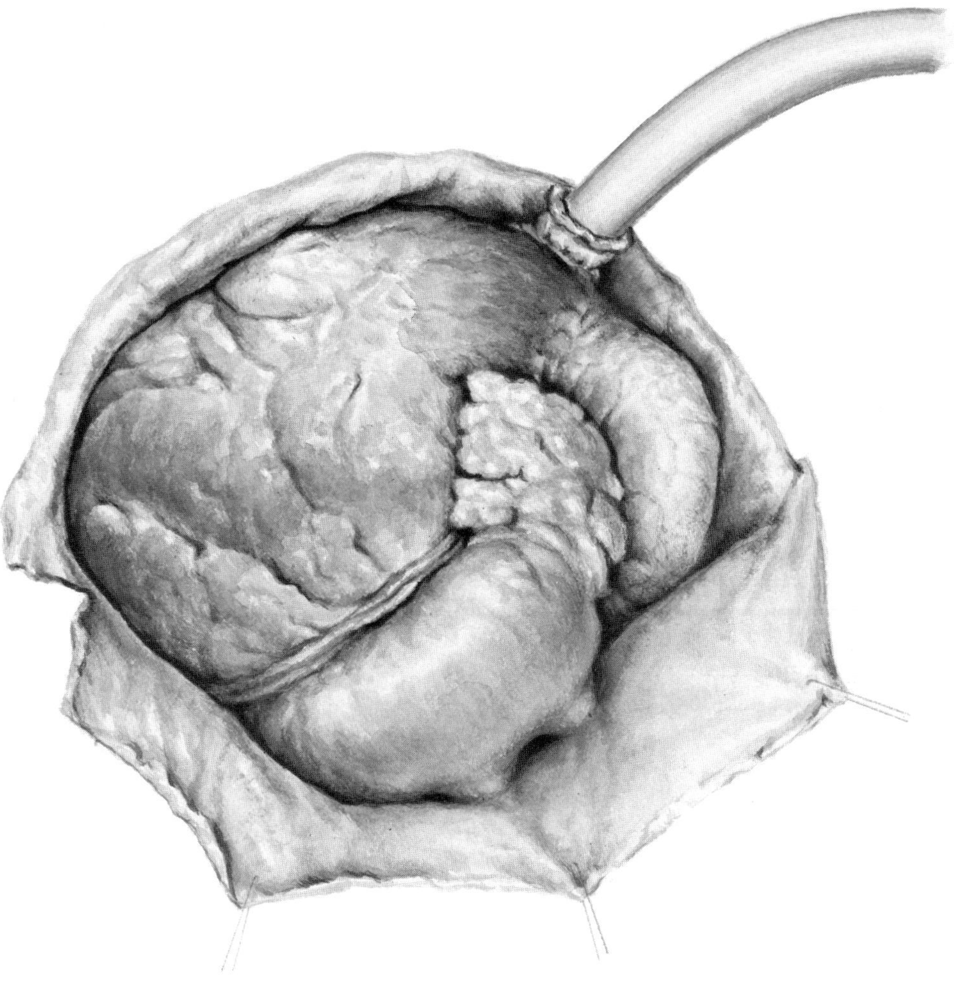

Fig. 409. Exposure of heart by left thoracotomy with connection of venous cannula device into right atrium.

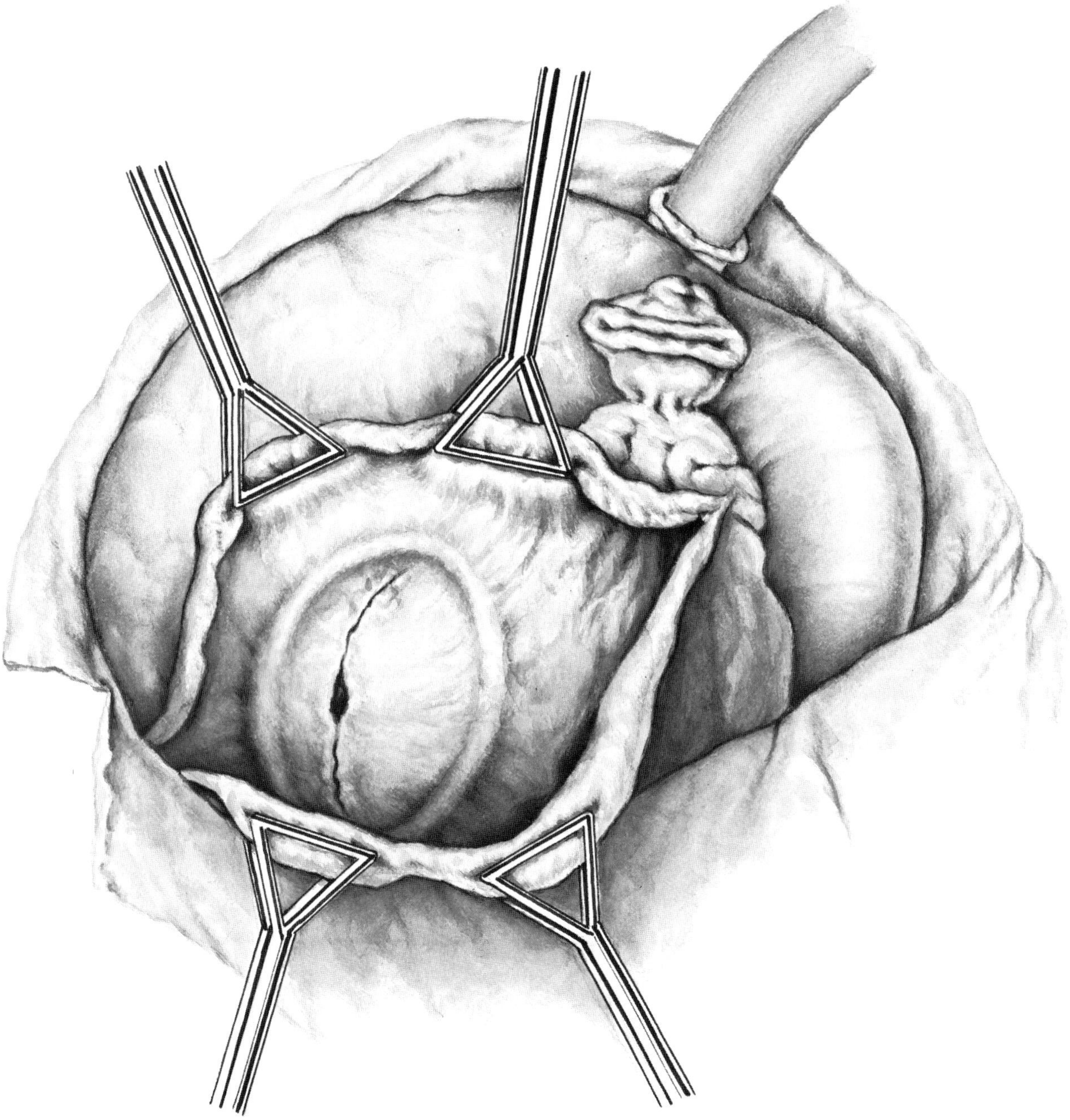

Fig. 410. Left atrium is opened along atrioventricular sulcus. Stenosed mitral valve viewed from left atrium.

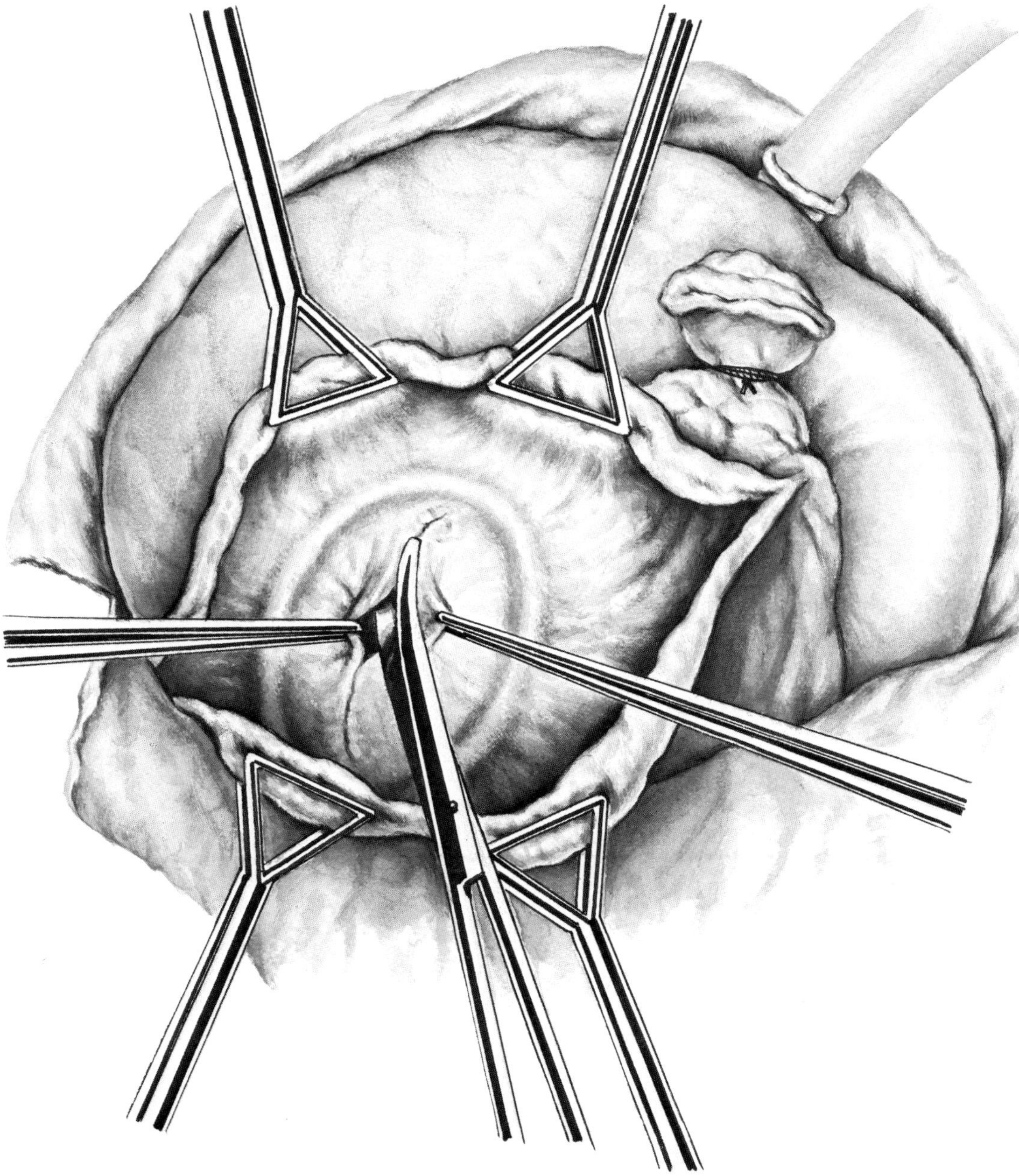

Fig. 411. Transection of anterior commissure.

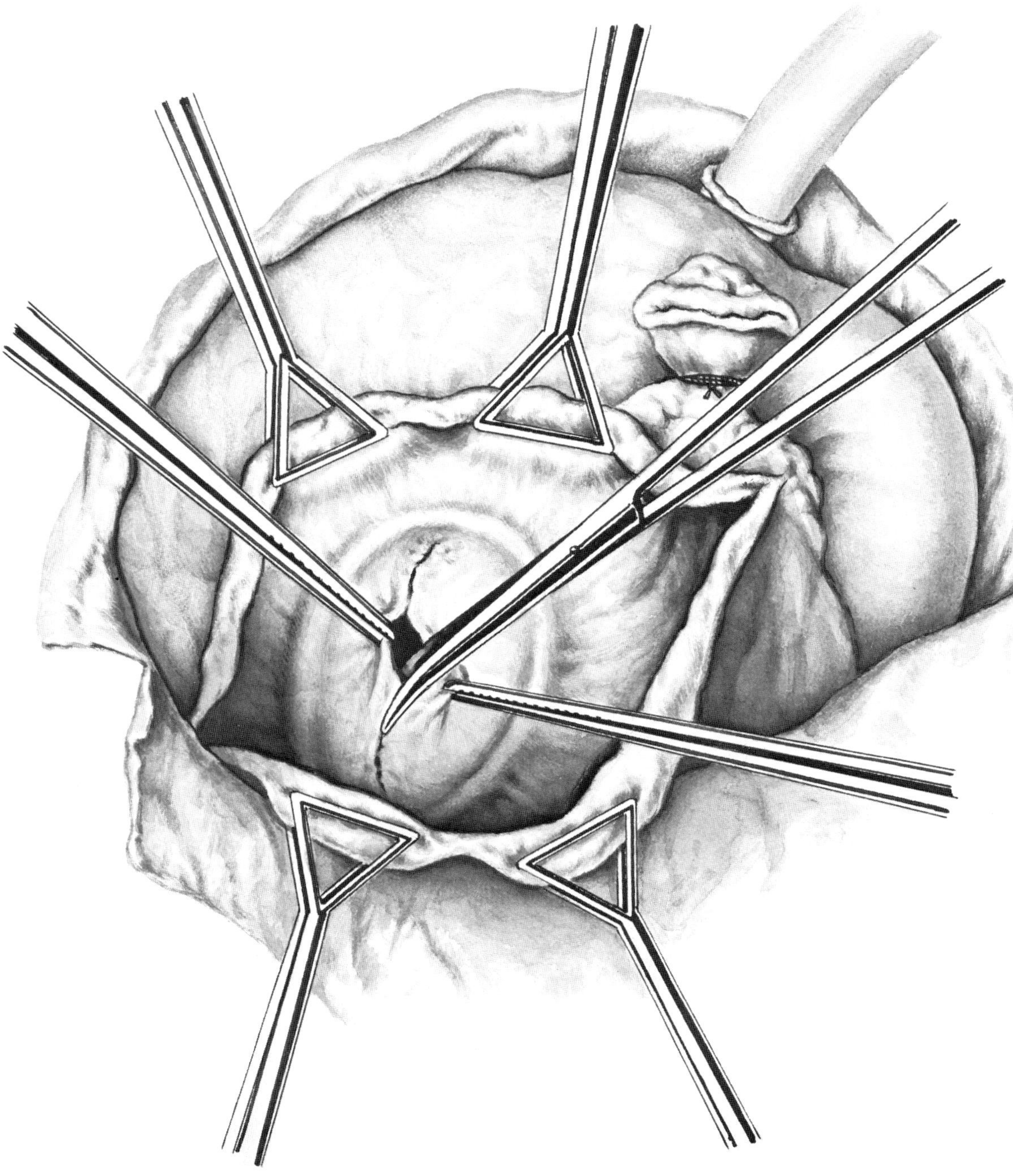

Fig. 412. Transection of posterior commissure.

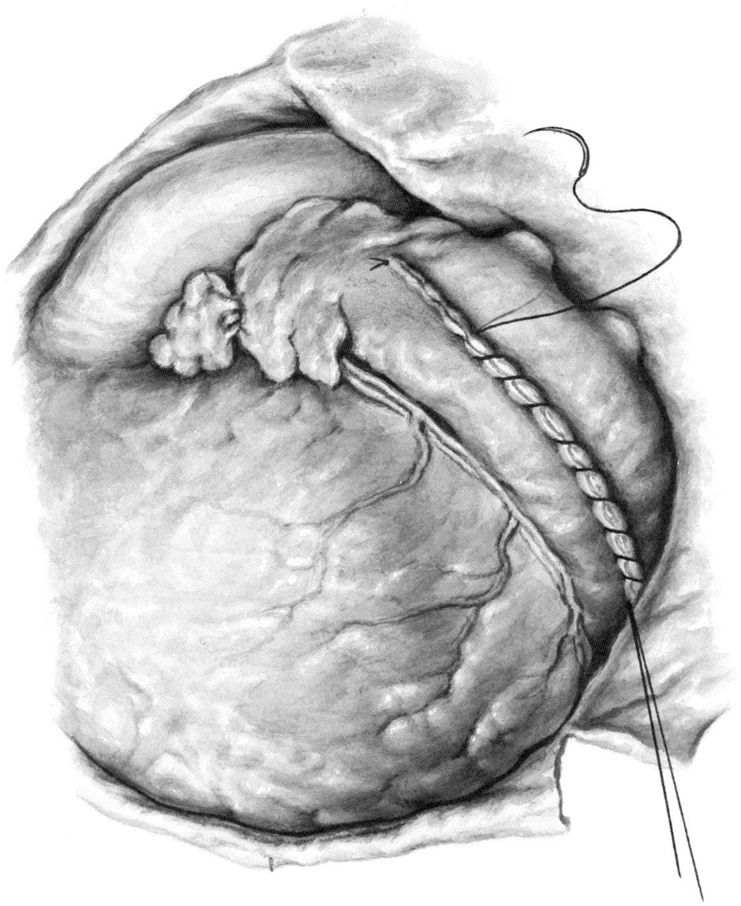

Fig. 413. Closure of wound in left atrium with Halsted and blanket sutures.

VALVE REPLACEMENT WITH BALL PROSTHESIS

The operation is carried out through longitudinal sternotomy or left or right thoracotomy. The heart-lung machine is connected, and the left atrium is opened wide (Fig. 414). The cusps of the mitral valve are held with clamps of the type of bullet forceps and pulled out into the cavity of the left atrium. About 3 or 4 mm from the fibrous ring the mitral valve is excised, beginning with a cut in the aortic cusp (Fig. 415). After circular incision of the cusps the valve is pulled into the left atrial cavity, and the apices of the papillary muscles are cut away with scissors (Figs. 416 and 417).

Halsted sutures are stitched through the fibrous ring of mitral valve with the ends of the threads brought out into the left ventricular cavity. To reduce pressure exerted on the tissue, it is expedient to space the Halsted sutures widely at an interval of 2 mm. Usually 10 to 12 sutures are enough for the whole circumference; their ends are successively passed through the base of the ball prosthesis held in place with a special retractor (Fig. 418). The ball prosthesis is lowered into the left atrioventricular orifice, and the sutures are tied one by one. The prosthesis is positioned so that its cage might not abut the interventricular septum (Fig. 419).

The wound in the left atrium is closed with a double-row suture. At the moment when the suture is being applied, the ball is drawn aside as far as possible by a thread brought around the struts of the prosthesis beforehand. In this manner distension of the left ventricle and the accumulation of air in it are avoided.

The ball prosthesis may be fastened in the fibrous ring

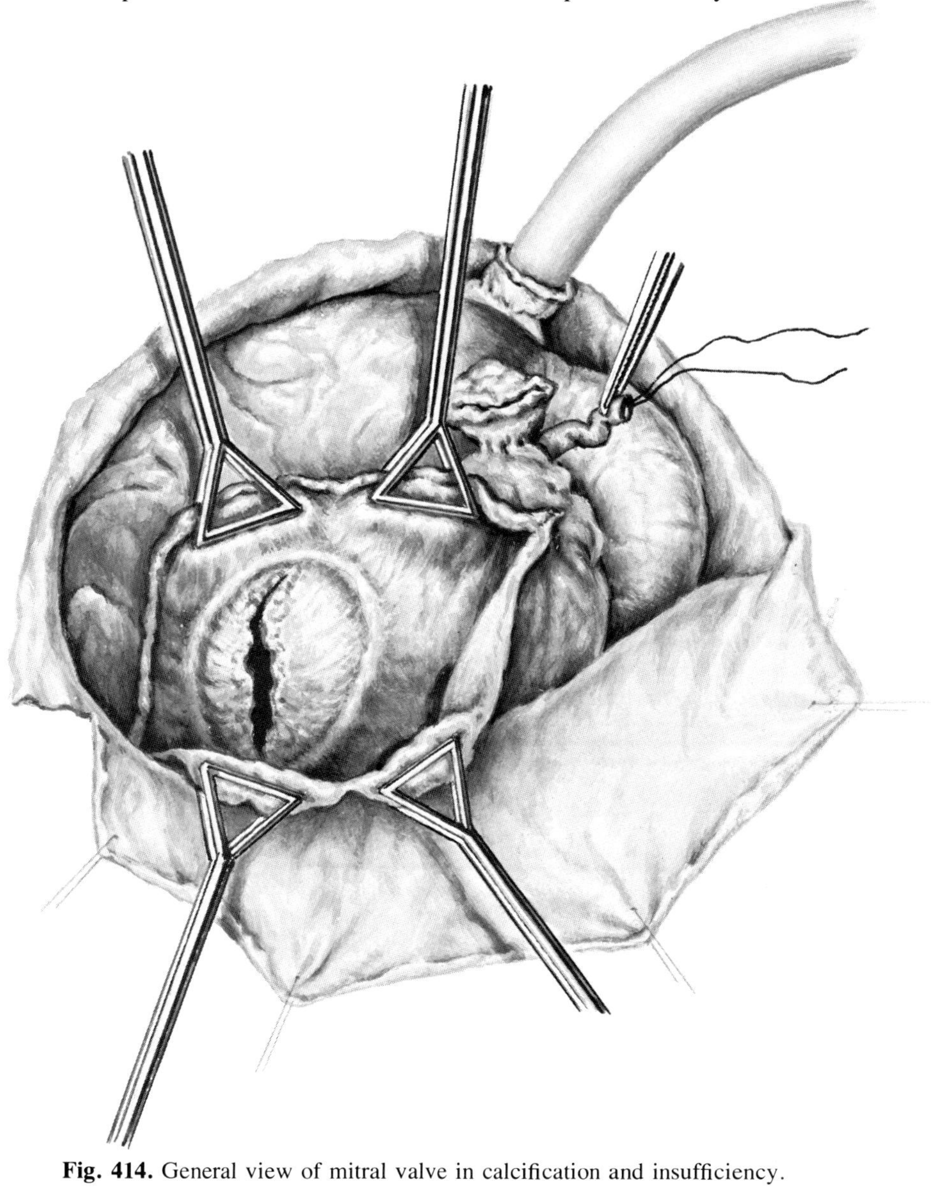

Fig. 414. General view of mitral valve in calcification and insufficiency.

by the nonsuture method. After the mitral valve has been excised, a purse-string suture is applied to the fibrous ring. The thread is not tightened in its middle part, but a loop is left free (Fig. 420). With the fibrous ring held back in a fixed position by this loop and the ends of the purse-string suture the diameter of the opening is measured with a gauge, and a corresponding prosthesis is chosen (Fig. 421). A mechanical mitral valve prosthesis secured on a handle is introduced into the orifice (Fig. 422). The purse-string suture is tied in the groove between the bushing of the prosthesis and the short needles of the duplex needle rim. When the handle of the holder is pressed, the needles pierce the rim of the tissue and fasten the prosthesis in the left atrioventricular orifice. The valve holder is removed, and the left atrium is closed by the method described above.

An operation by right thoracotomy is carried out through an incision made in the left atrium ventral to the entry of the right pulmonary veins (Fig. 423). With this approach the mitral valve is located deeper. To make manipulating easier, the edges of the valve cusps are held with tooth forceps and pulled out into the cavity of the left atrium (Figs. 424 and 425). With this operative method two venous cannulas are used, as a rule, for draining both venae cavae.

The operation may also be performed from the right atrial cavity with incision of the interatrial septum (Figs. 426 and 427). The mitral valve is excised, and a ball prosthesis stitched in by the method described above (Fig. 428). The interatrial septum is repaired with sutures (Fig. 429).

This method is applied in simultaneous replacement of the tricuspid and mitral valves with prostheses.

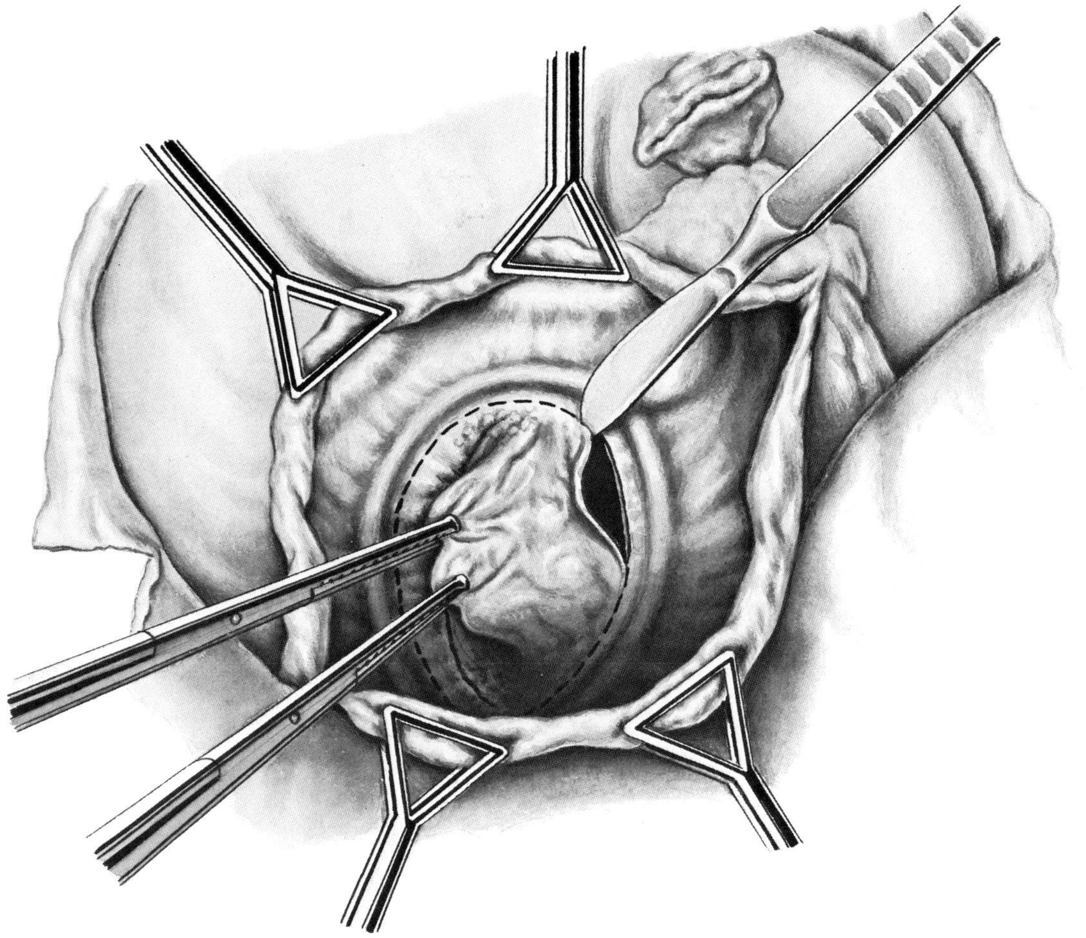

Fig. 415. Excision of mitral valve.

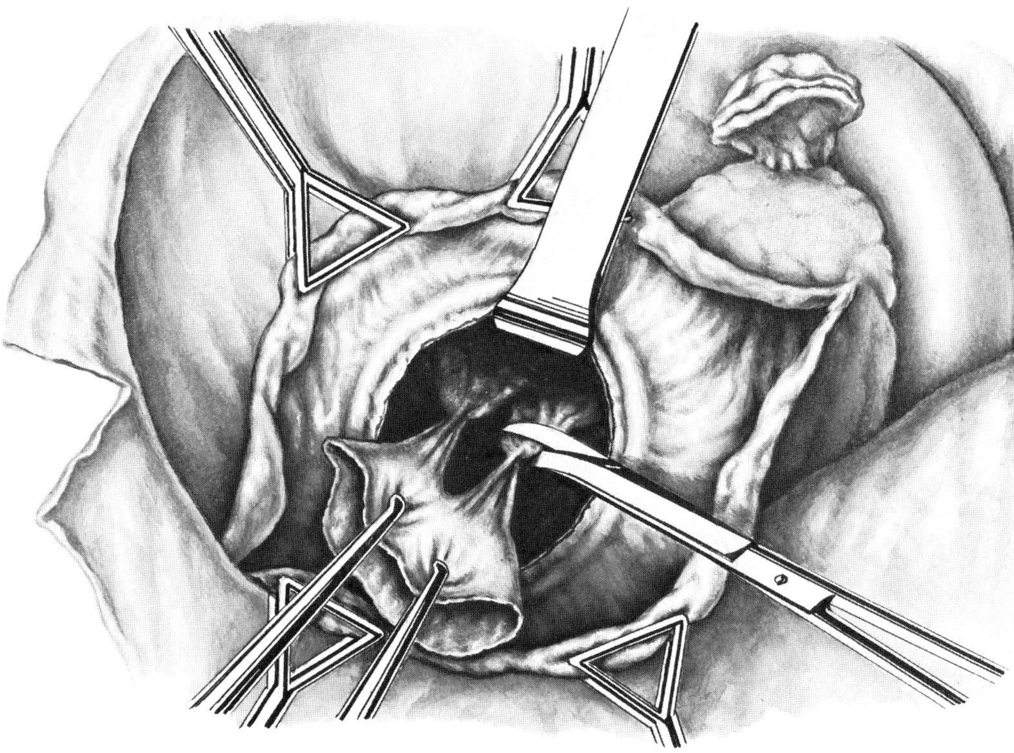

Fig. 416. Transection of apices of papillary muscles.

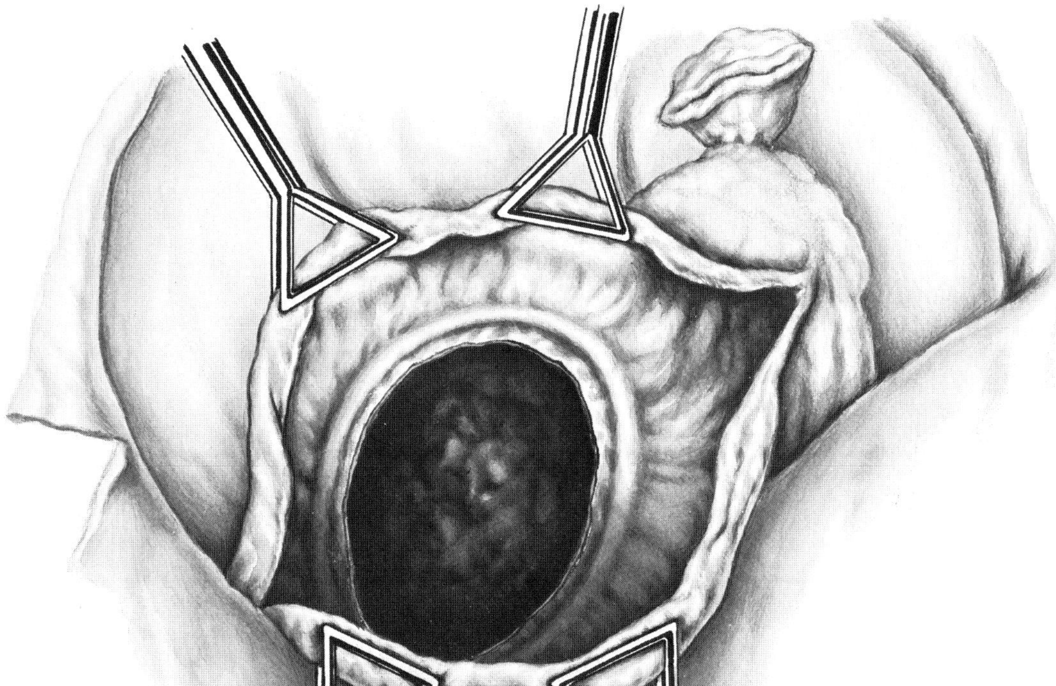

Fig. 417. View of fibrous ring after excision of valve.

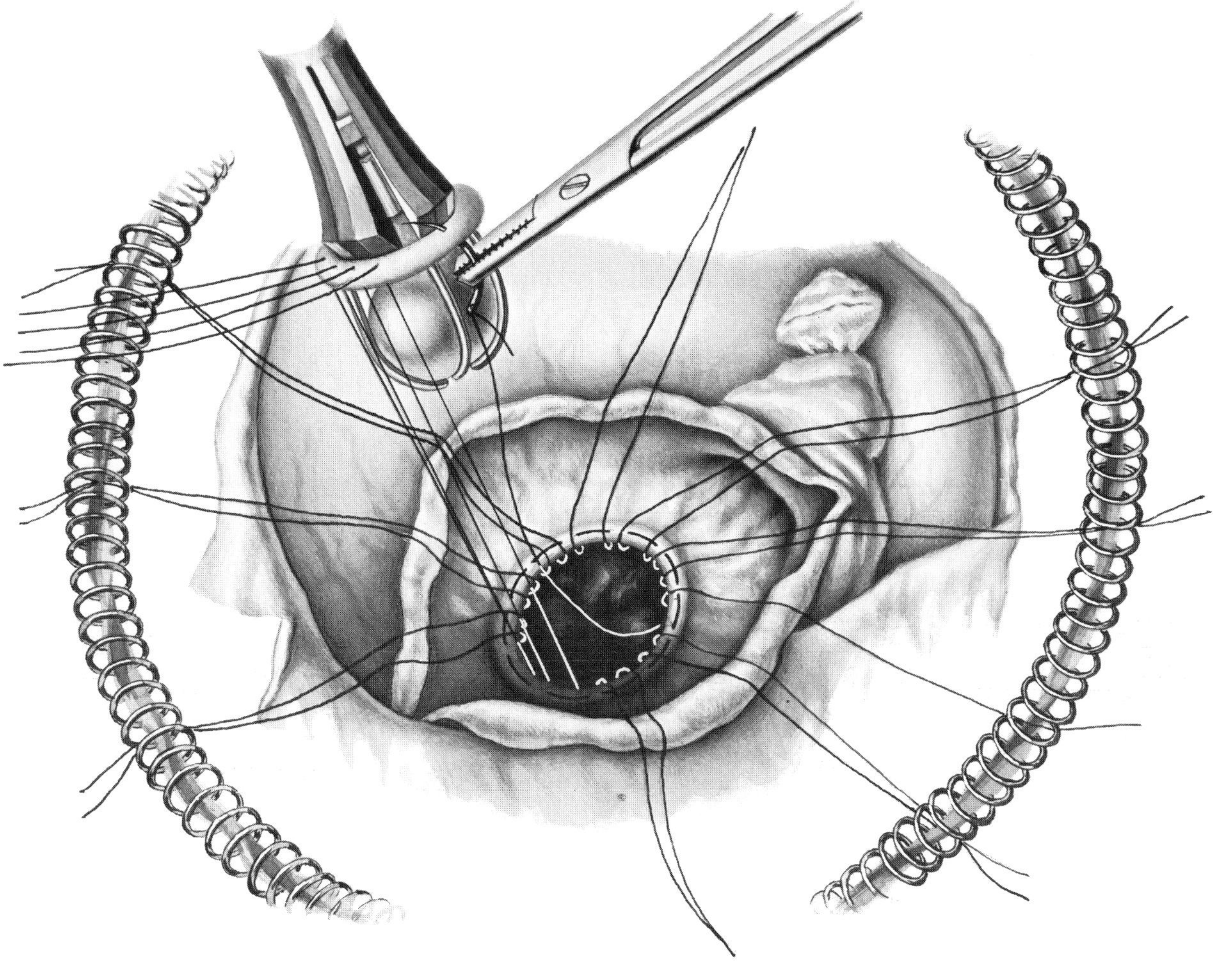

Fig. 418. Sutures are passed through ball prosthesis. Sutures are tied and prosthesis secured in left atrioventricular orifice.

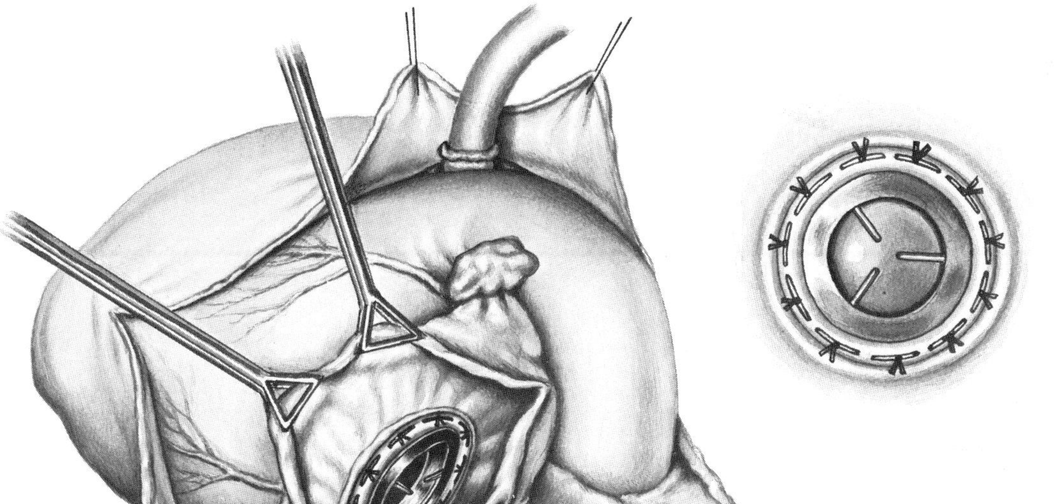

Fig. 419. View of prosthesis stitched into mitral position.

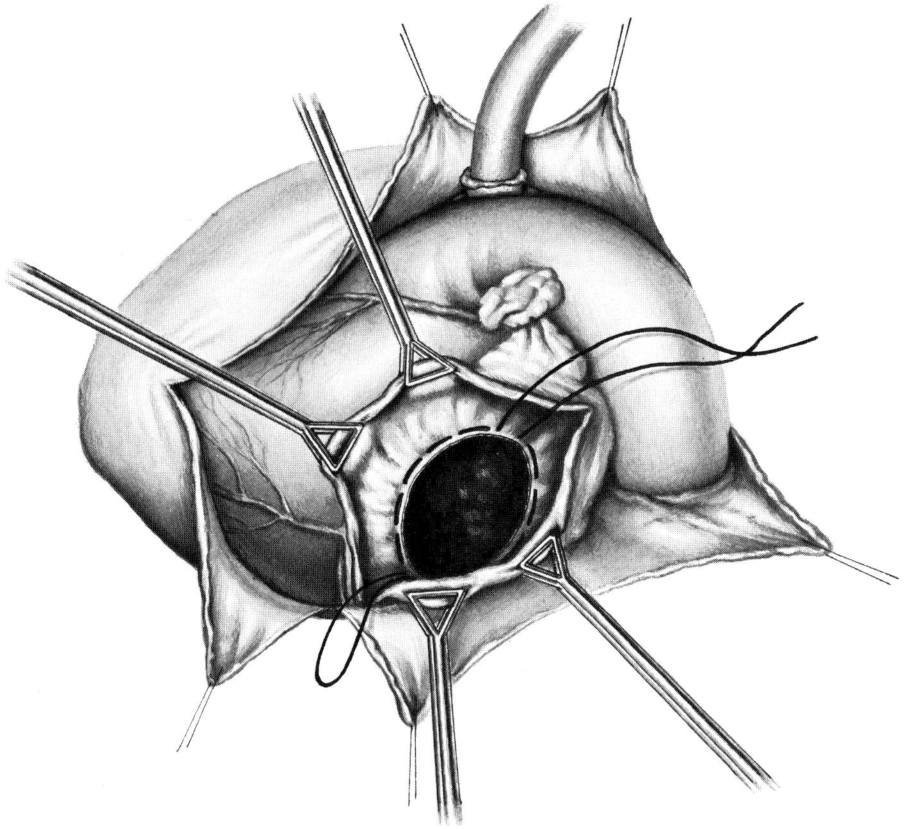

Fig. 420. Purse-string suture is applied to fibrous ring of mitral valve after resection of cusp and papillary muscles.

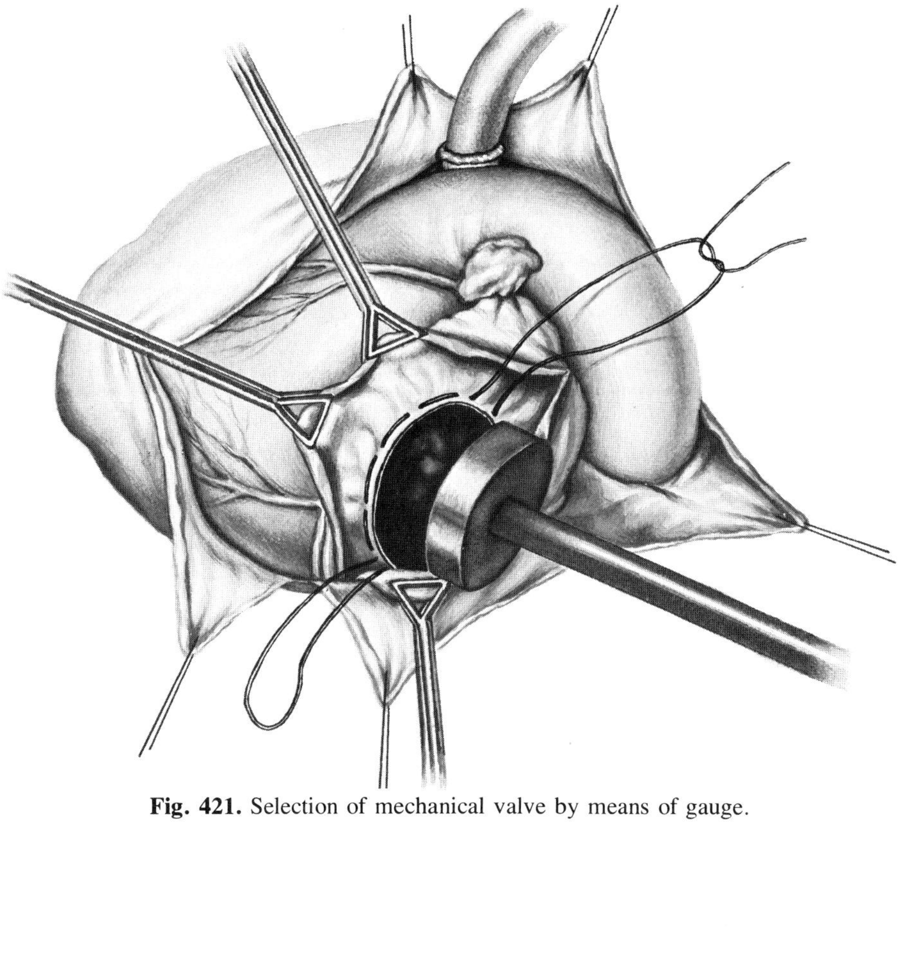

Fig. 421. Selection of mechanical valve by means of gauge.

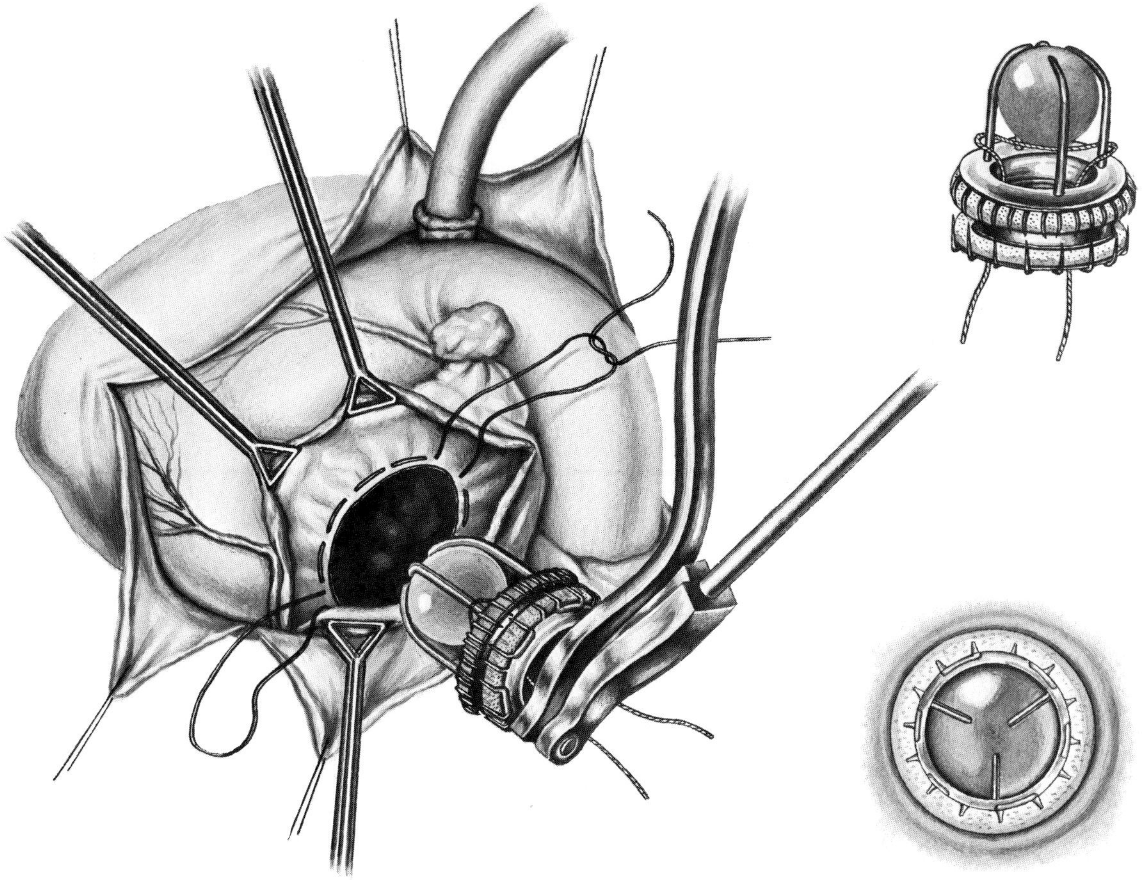

Fig. 422. Attachment of mechanical prosthesis. View of prosthesis after it has been stitched into left atrioventricular orifice.

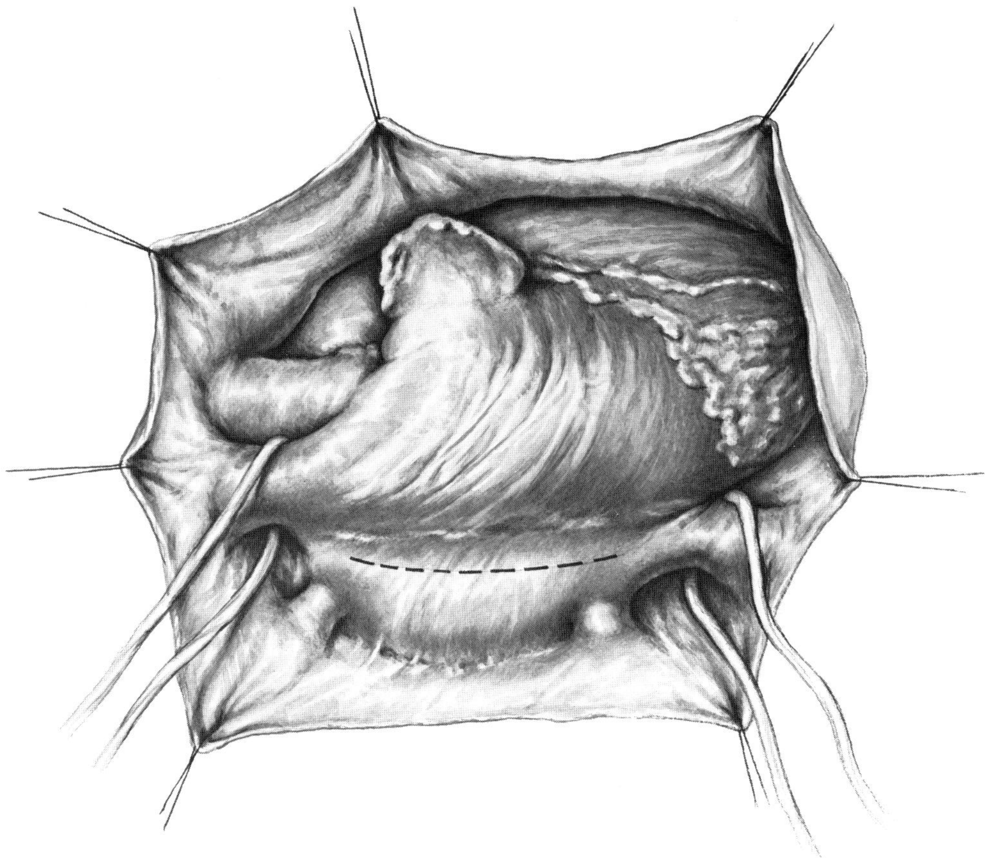

Fig. 423. Heart in mitral disease viewed on exposure through right thoracotomy in fifth intercostal space. Dashed line shows incision in left atrium.

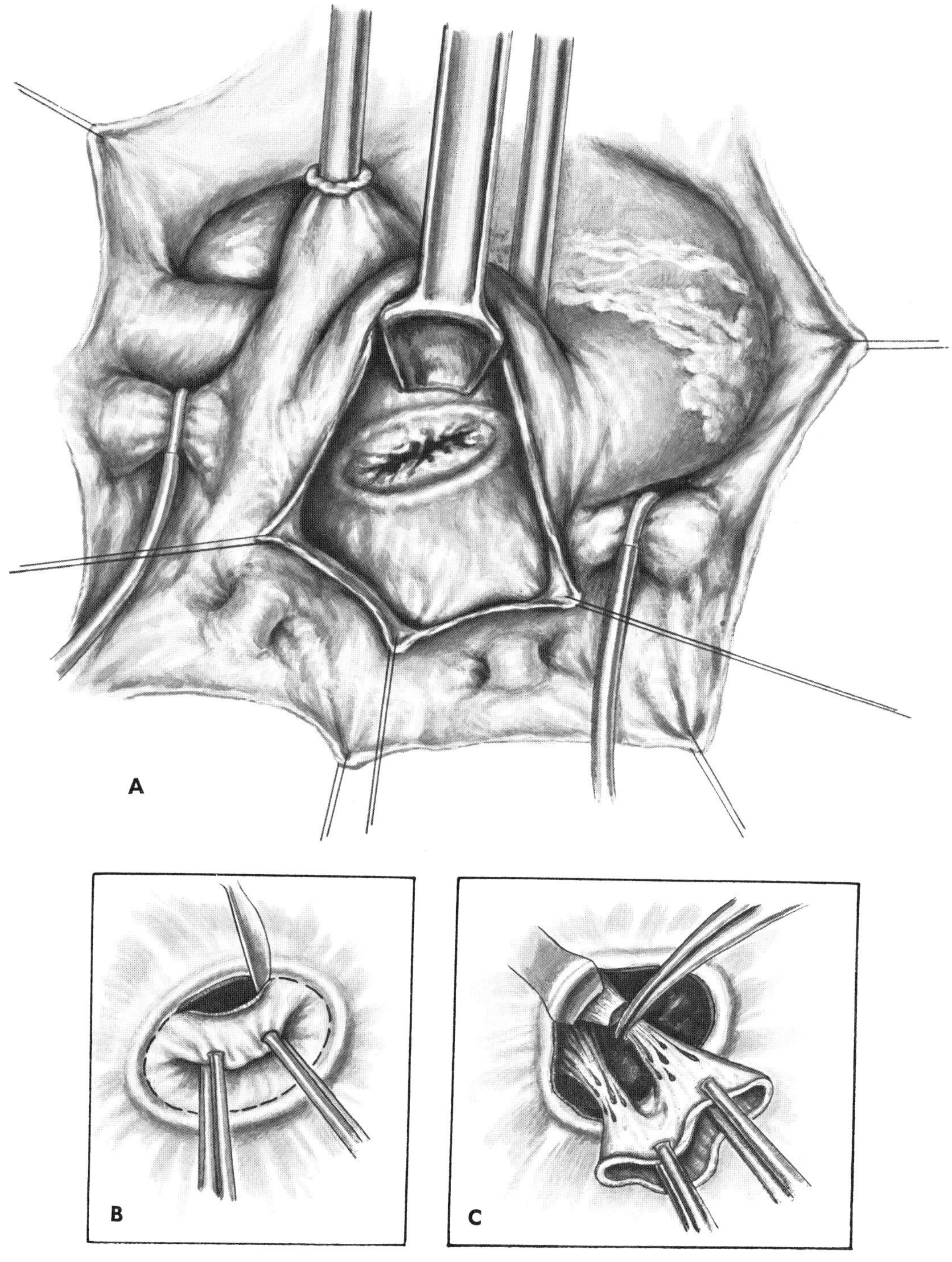

Fig. 424. A, Mitral valve in opened left atrial cavity viewed through right approach. **B,** Excision of valve. **C,**Transection of papillary muscles.

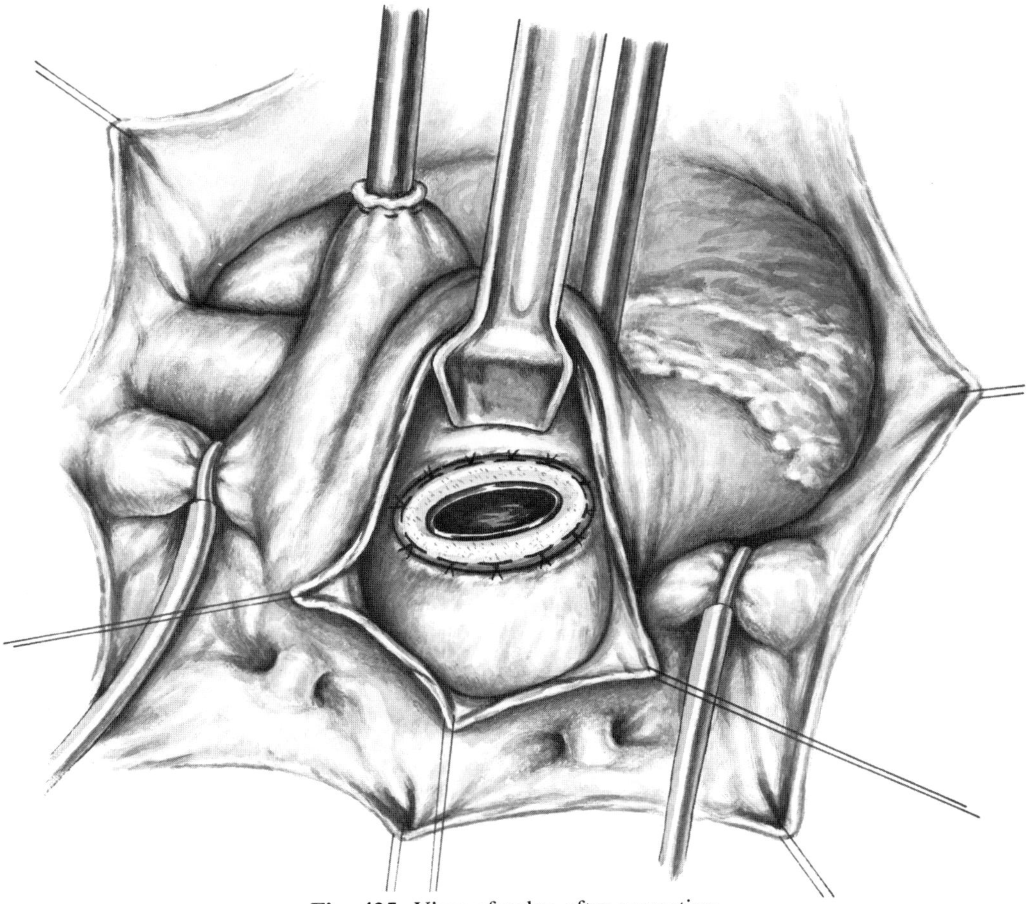

Fig. 425. View of valve after correction.

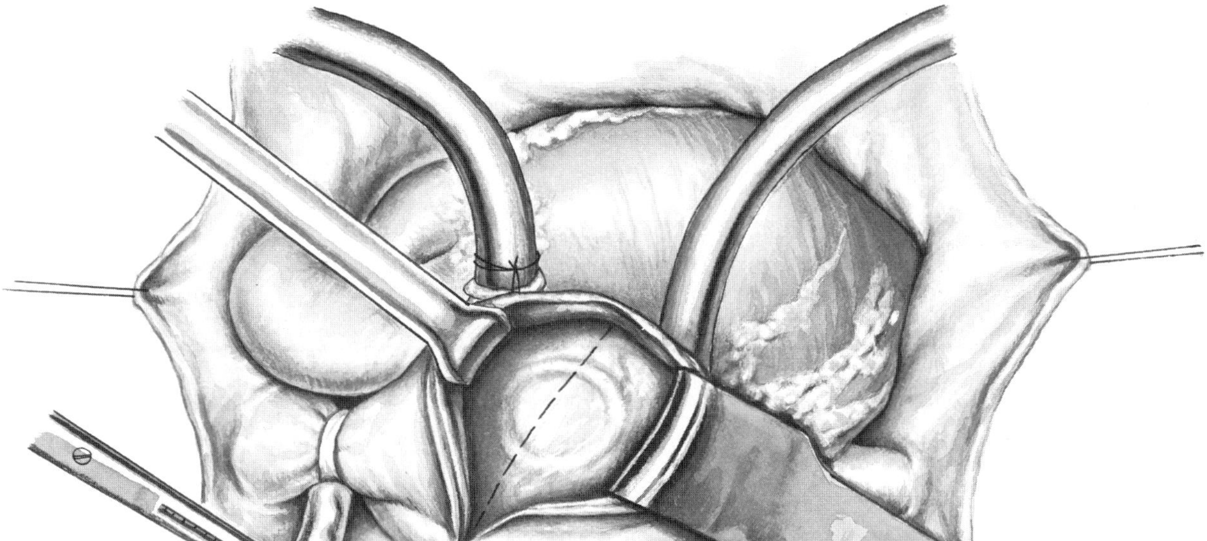

Fig. 426. Approach to left atrium by cutting interatrial septum from cavity of right atrium. Dashed line shows incision in interatrial septum.

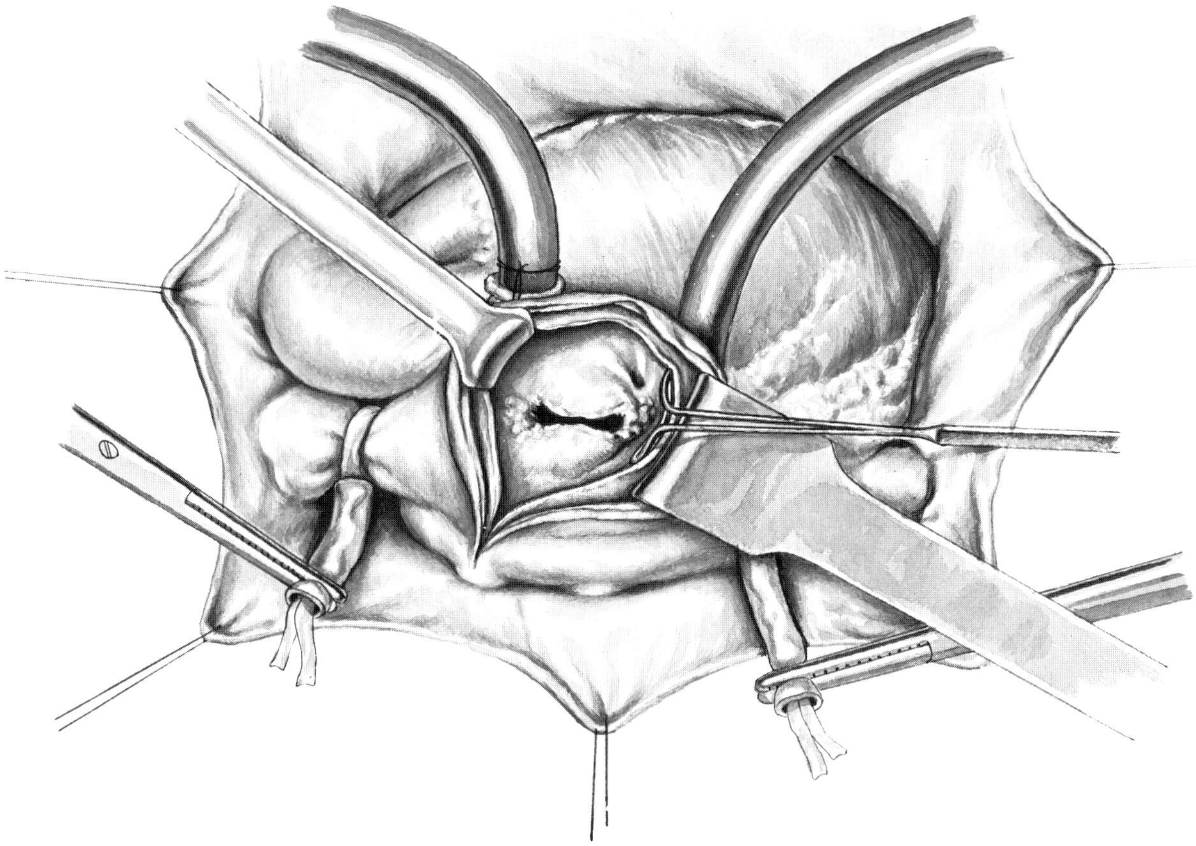

Fig. 427. Interatrial septum is cut. Mitral valve can be seen.

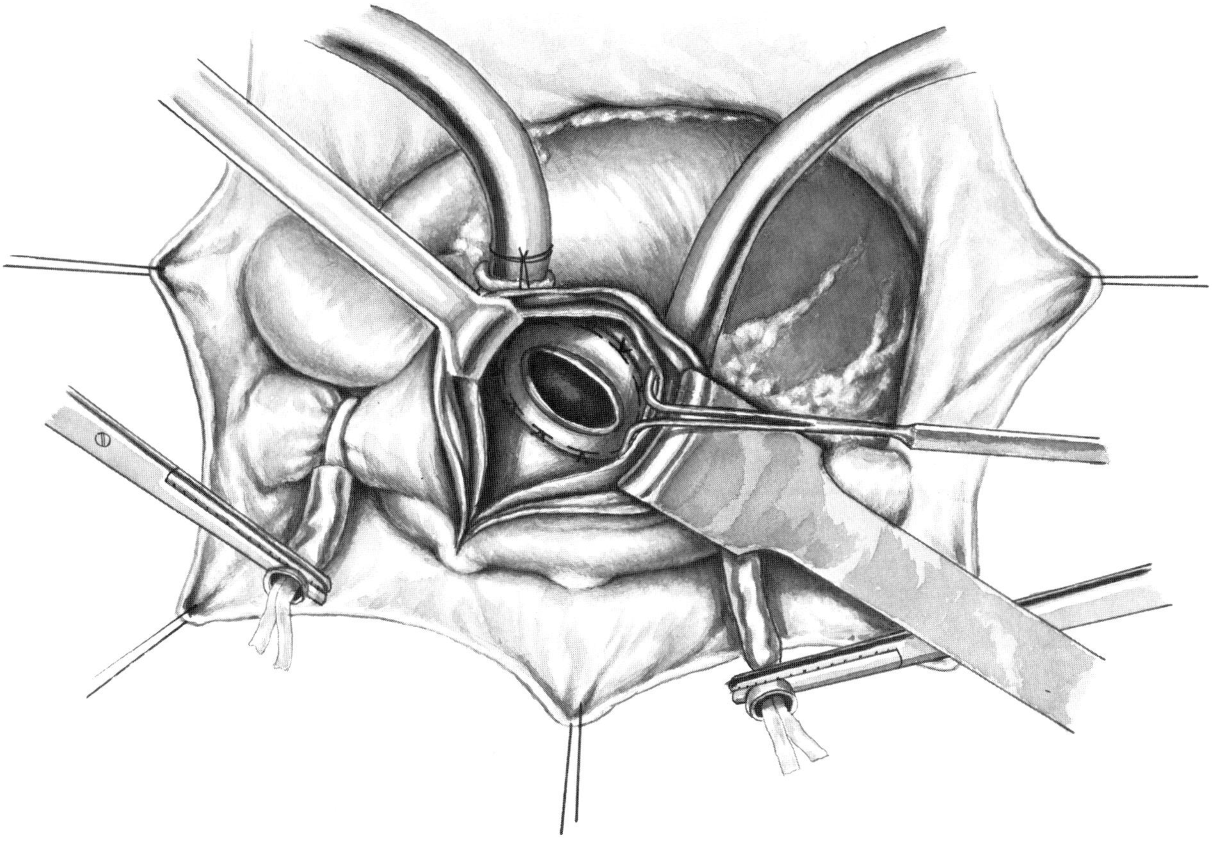

Fig. 428. Ball prosthesis is sutured in place.

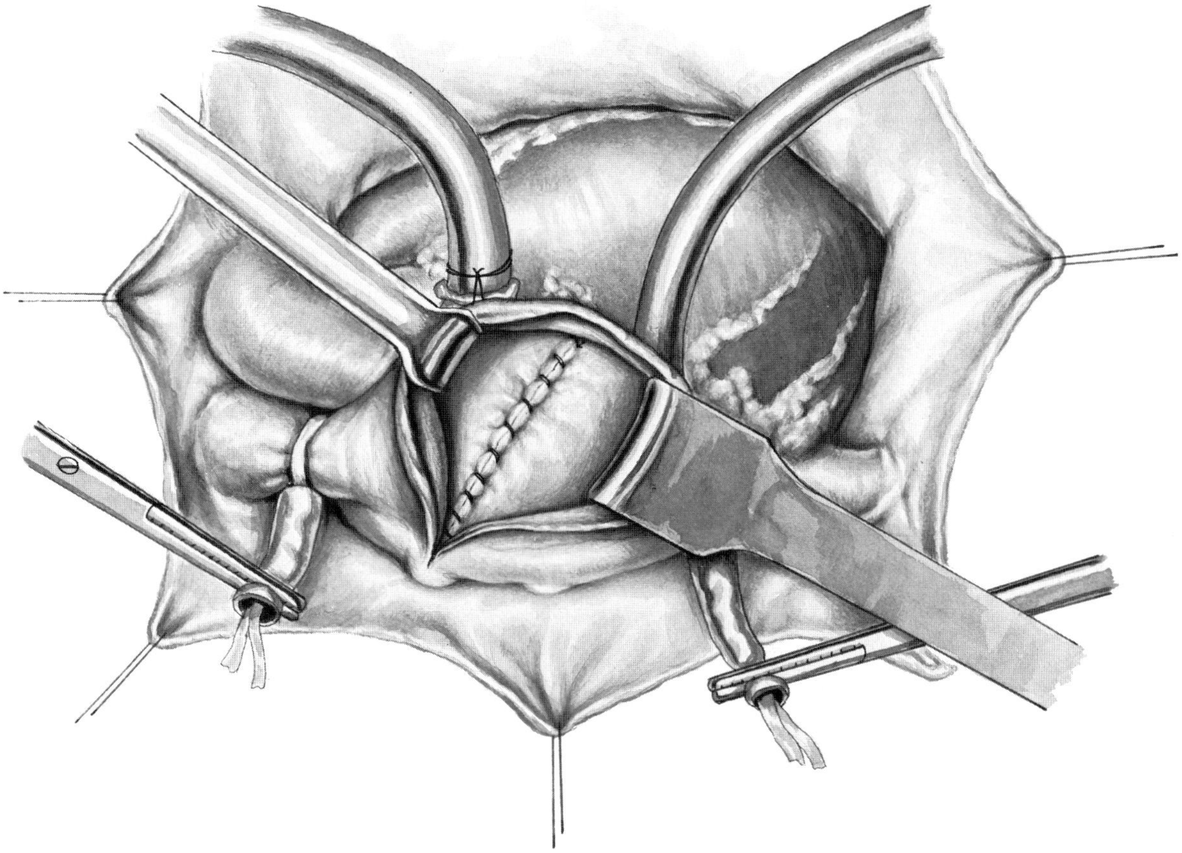

Fig. 429. Interatrial septum is sutured.

CORRECTION OF AORTIC VALVULAR DISEASE

The operation is conducted by longitudinal sternotomy. Intervention is also possible through right thoracotomy.

In some cases with stenosis of the aortic orifice, poststenotic dilatation of the aorta is encountered. In insufficiency of the aortic valve, intensified pulsation of the aorta is noted.

With the heart disconnected from circulation the ascending aorta, which had been mobilized previously, is clamped. It is opened transversely or with a hockey-stick incision extending into Valsalva's sinus of the noncoronary cusp of the aortic valve (Figs. 430 and 431). Both coronary arteries are cannulated for isolated coronary perfusion. To secure the cannulas, the aortic wall above the orifice of the coronary artery is stitched with an atraumatic thread, leaving its loop in the lumen of the aorta. The ends of the thread on the outer coat of the aorta are drawn through a fine plastic tourniquet.

The plastic coronary cannulas filled with blood are introduced into the orifice of the coronary artery through the fixation loop. The tourniquet is turned, fastening the coronary cannula to the aortic wall with the loop. Should

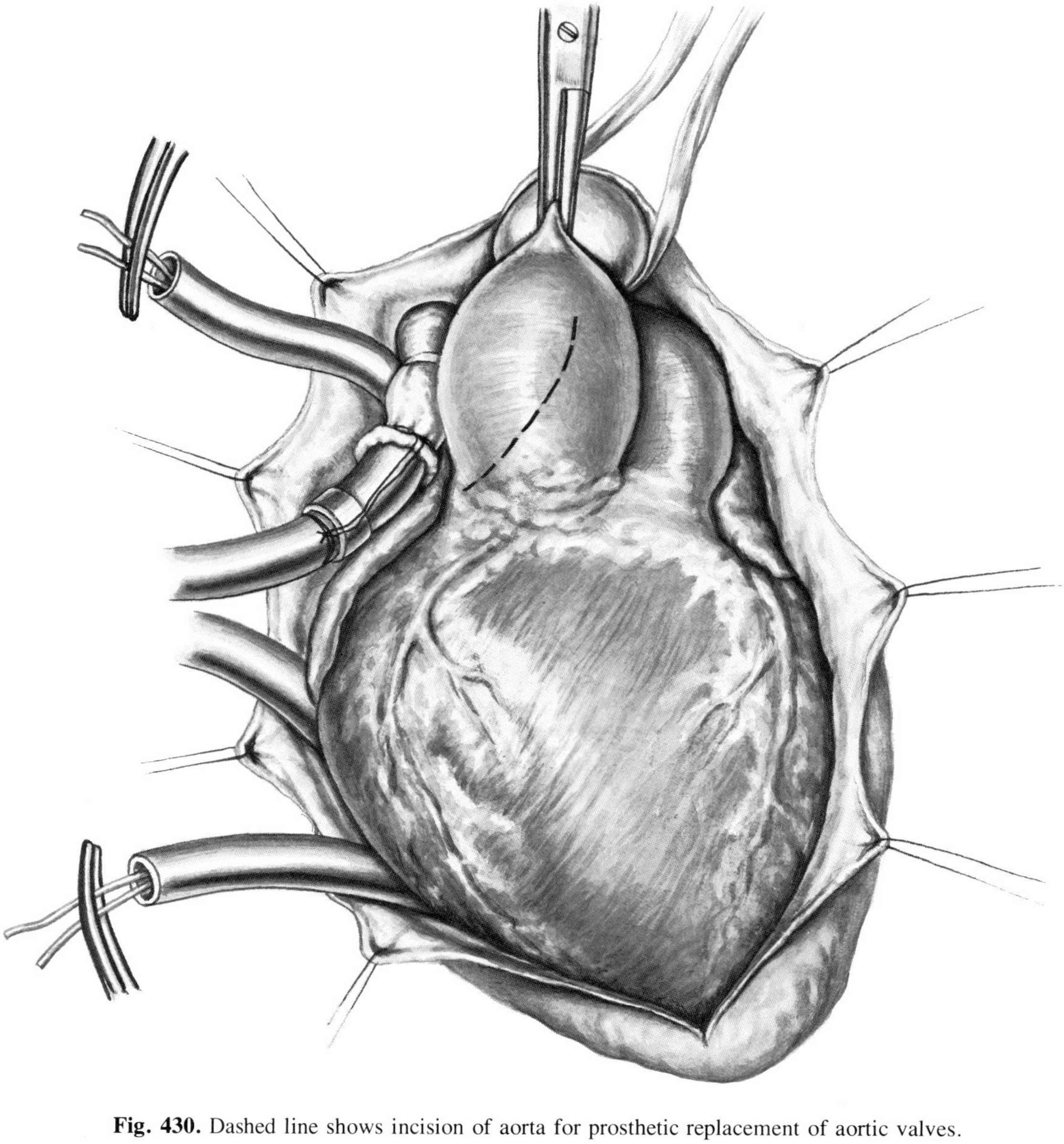

Fig. 430. Dashed line shows incision of aorta for prosthetic replacement of aortic valves.

any technical difficulties arise in cannulation of the right coronary artery, the manipulation may be limited to cannulating just the left coronary artery.

When coronary blood flow is arrested for no longer than 30 to 40 minutes and the implementation of coronary perfusion is technically difficult, it is permissible to operate without perfusion of the coronaries during anoxic arrest of the heart. In some cases cooling of the heart with ice placed around it is practiced. In this instance, however, the myocardium is cooled irregularly, which is fraught with the danger of small subepicardial necroses of the myocardium developing eventually.

Valvular stenosis of the aortic orifice is corrected by cutting along the commissures of the valve. To prevent the prolapse of the separated cusps the incision made with the scalpel in cutting their commissures does not reach the aortic wall, so that a mild degree of valvular

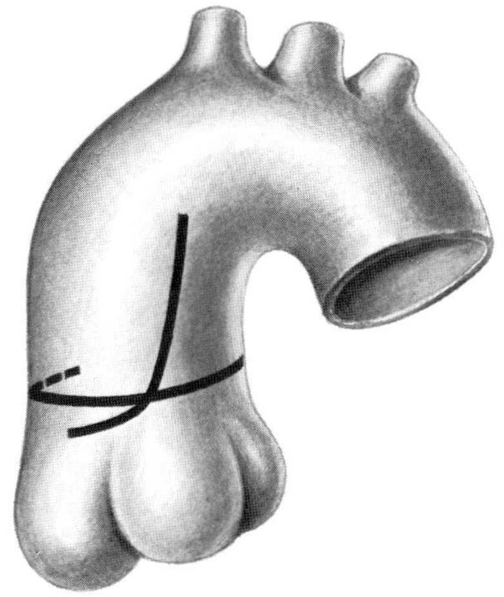

Fig. 431. Various incisions of aorta used in prosthetic replacement of aortic valves.

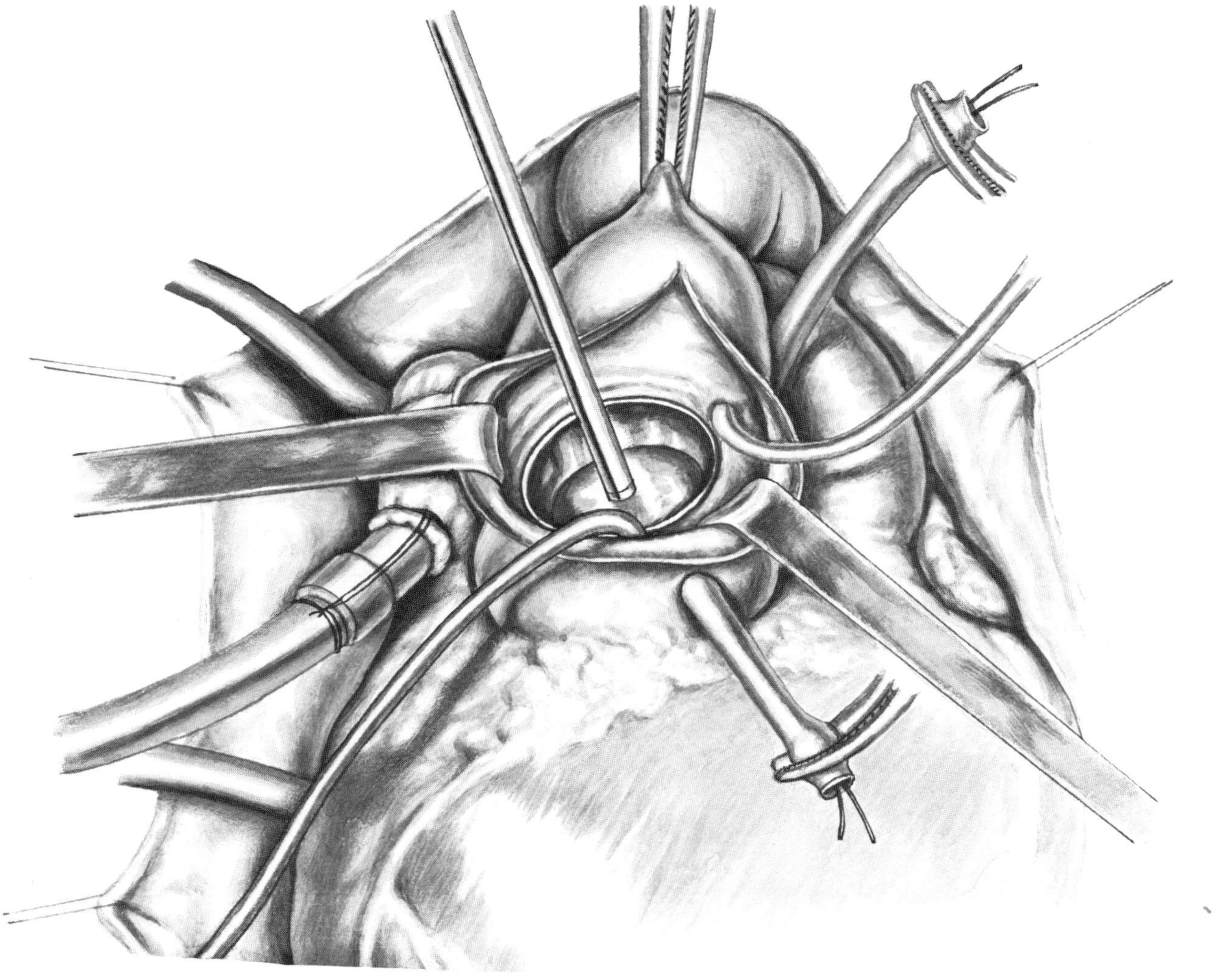

Fig. 432. Diameter of valvular ring is measured with gauge.

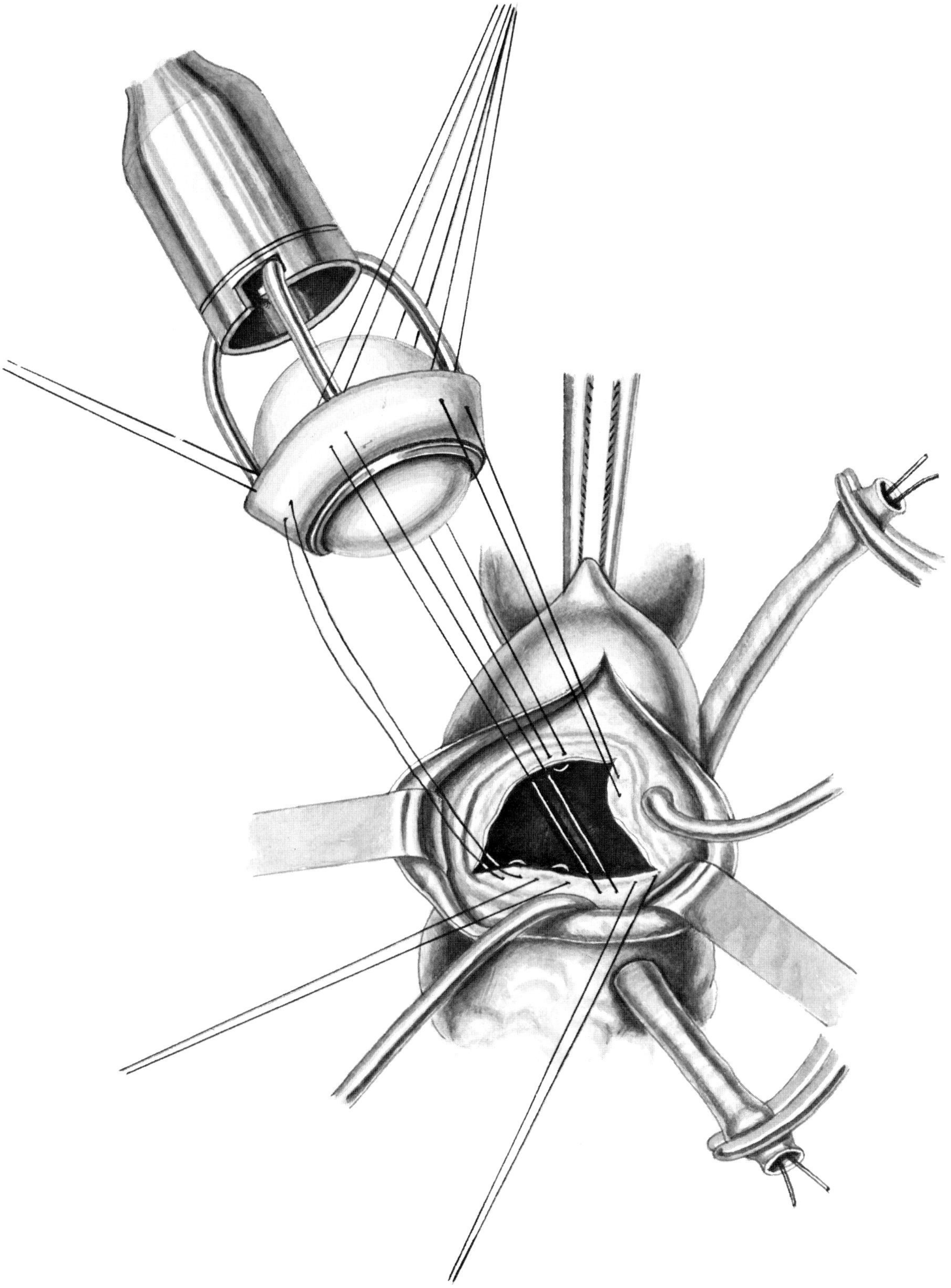

Fig. 433. Correction of aortic valvular defect with ball prosthesis. Sutures are applied to base of valvular cusps and base of prosthesis.

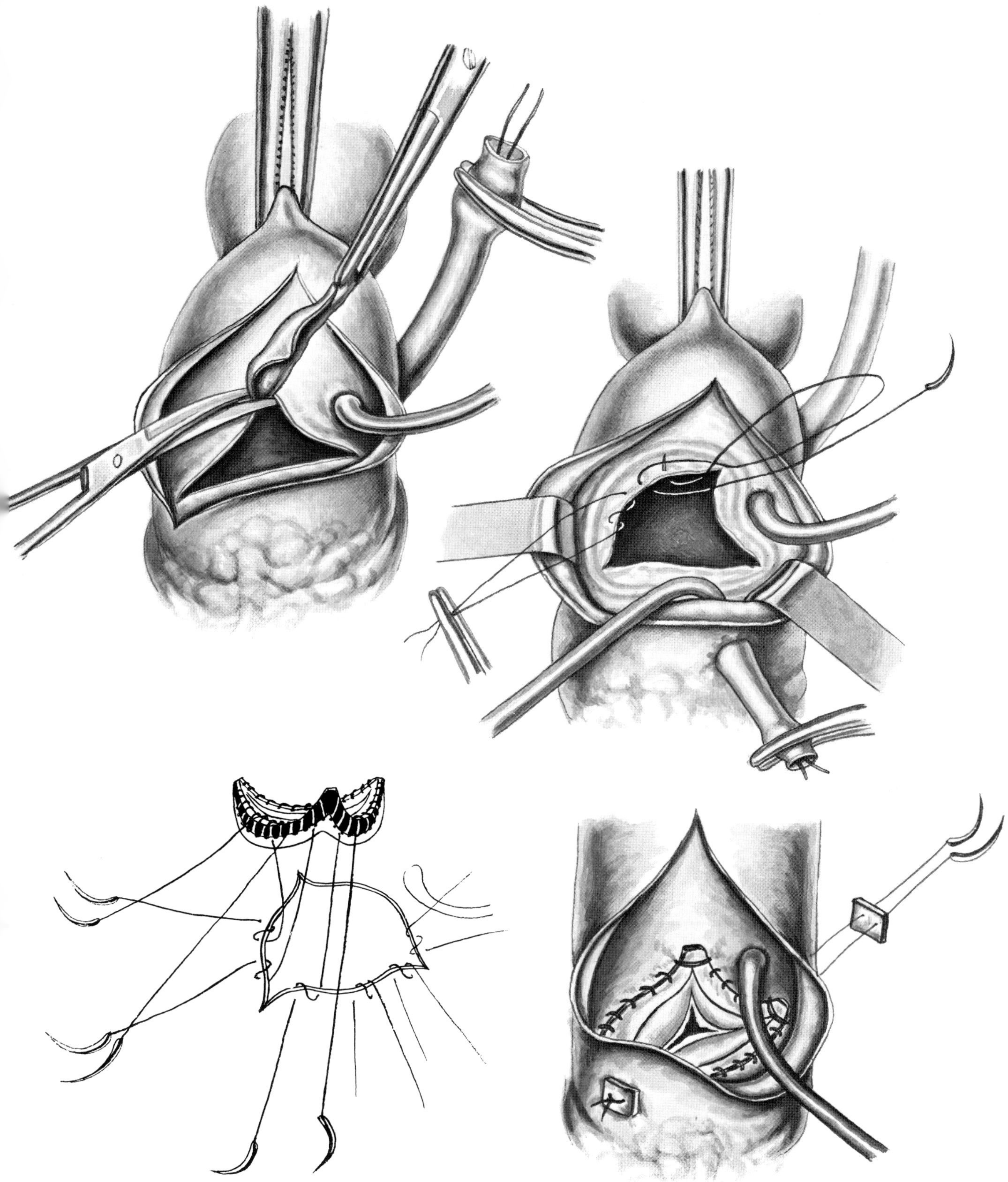

Fig. 434. Stage of plastic surgery of aortic valve by means of heterologous valves secured to rigid plastic frame.

stenosis remains. In calcified stenosis bits of calcium are cut away and cleaned to restore the mobility of the cusps.

In severe insufficiency of the semilunar aortic valves these are replaced with a ball prosthesis. The cups are excised with scissors, leaving a ridge of their tissue 1.5 to 2 mm high. The diameter of the aortic ring is measured with a gauge (Fig. 432). The ridge is stitched through with Halsted traction sutures in the region of the three commissures. With two neighboring commissures being pulled in succession into the aortic wound, Halsted or interrupted sutures are passed through the base of the cusp with inclusion of the aortic tissue. The same threads are stitched through the base of the ball prosthesis, which is then lowered on the base of the excised cusp, and the sutures are tied (Fig. 433).

If the aortic orifice is repaired with a homologous or heterologous valve armored on a plastic or metal frame, the sutures that had been applied beforehand on the ridge

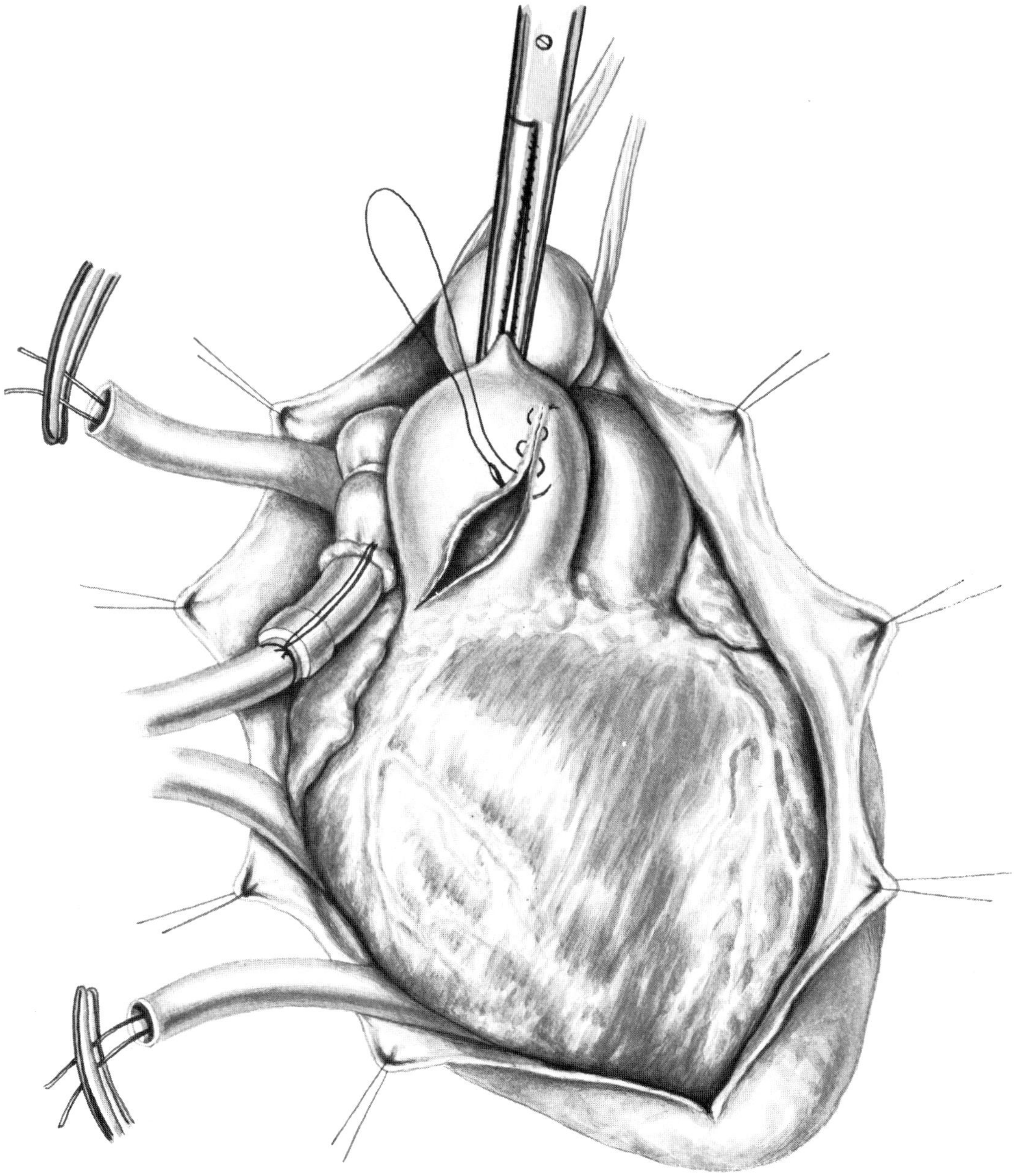

Fig. 435. After aortic valves have been replaced with prosthesis, incision in aorta is sutured.

or wall of the aorta are passed through the base of the cusps of the grafted valve (Fig. 434). The commissures of the valve are attached with additional Halsted sutures to the aortic wall. The ends of the sutures are brought outside and tied over plastic bolsters.

The aorta is closed with a double-row continuous Halsted and blanket sutures (Figs. 435 and 436). At the moment when the clamp is taken off the aorta, DuFeau's needle is inserted between the sutures for the removal of air and prevention of air embolism. The apex of the left ventricle is punctured in addition, with the heart dislocated from the pericardium (Fig. 437), or drained with a tube connected with a coronary aspirator.

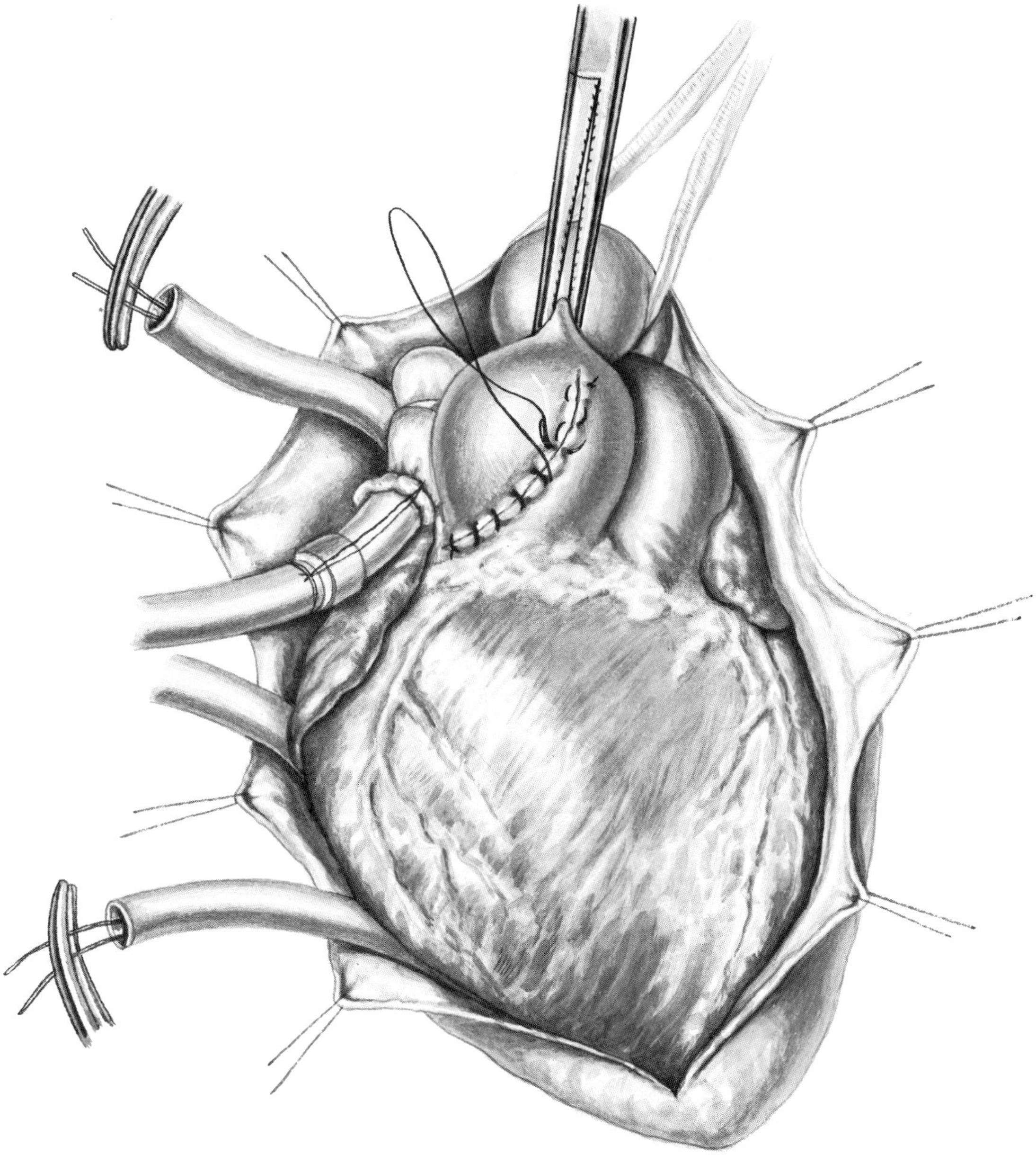

Fig. 436. Application of second row of sutures in closure of aortic wall.

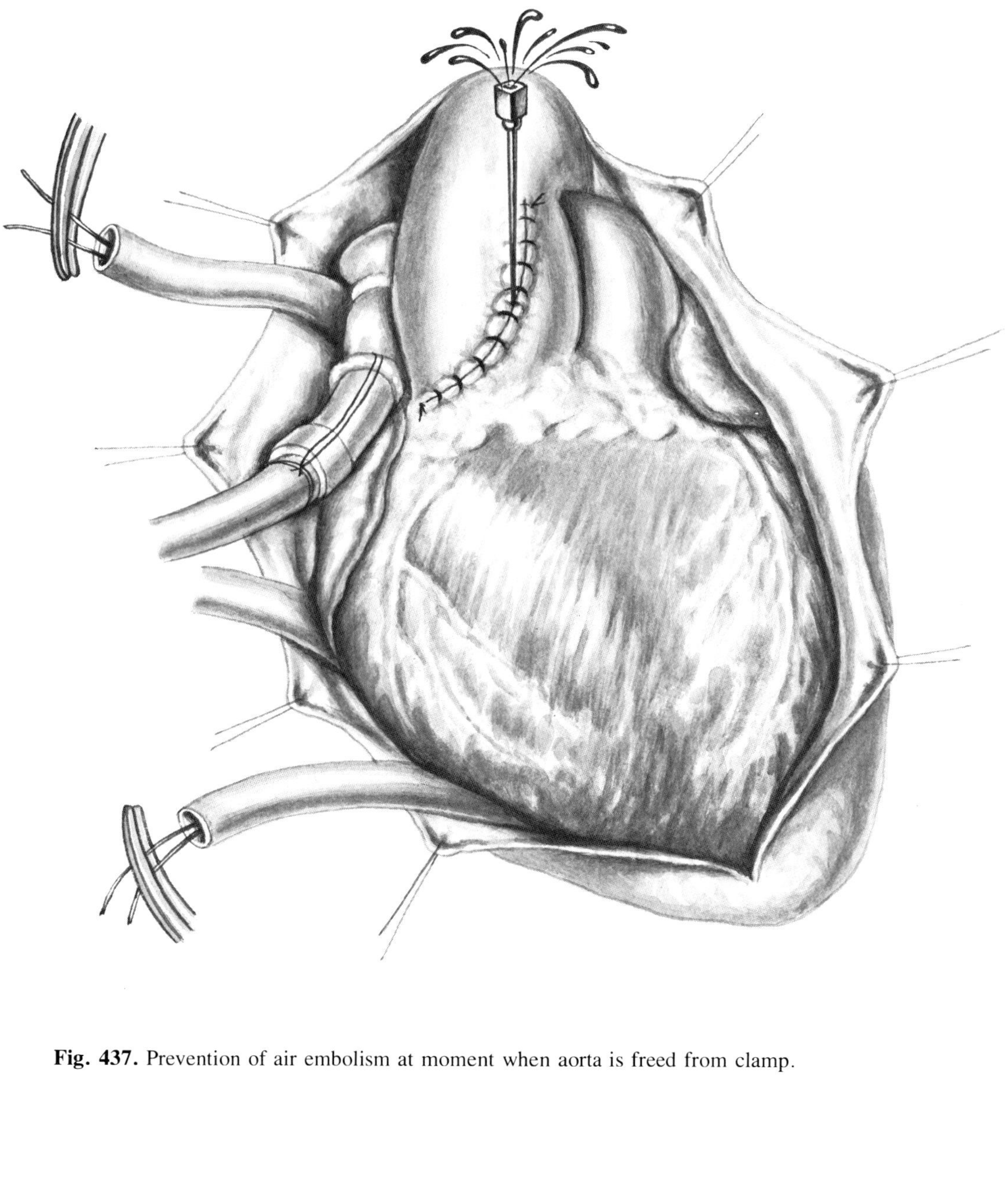

Fig. 437. Prevention of air embolism at moment when aorta is freed from clamp.

*RADICAL CORRECTION OF EBSTEIN'S ANOMALY

The operation is carried out by right thoracotomy or longitudinal sternotomy. In Ebstein's anomaly the right atrium and the right ventricle are drastically dilated. The wall of the right atrium is hypertrophied and cyanotic. The venae cavae are not dilated (Fig. 438).

In acute disorders of circulation after thoracotomy in this severe category of patients, an emergency need may arise for the connection to a heart-lung machine. This is accomplished by introducing a common venous cannula into the right atrium through its auricle (Fig. 439). Connection to the heart-lung machine leads to a reduction in the size of the right heart and makes it easier to mobilize the venae cavae and apply a purse-string suture to the right atrial wall for introducing a second venous cannula. The venous cannula inserted into the right atrium is advanced into one of the venae cavae, usually the inferior, and in favorable conditions the heart-lung machine is connected by the routine method.

With the heart disconnected from circulation the right atrium is opened wide with an incision made 2 to 3 cm above the atrioventricular sulcus and extended to the right auricle (Fig. 440).

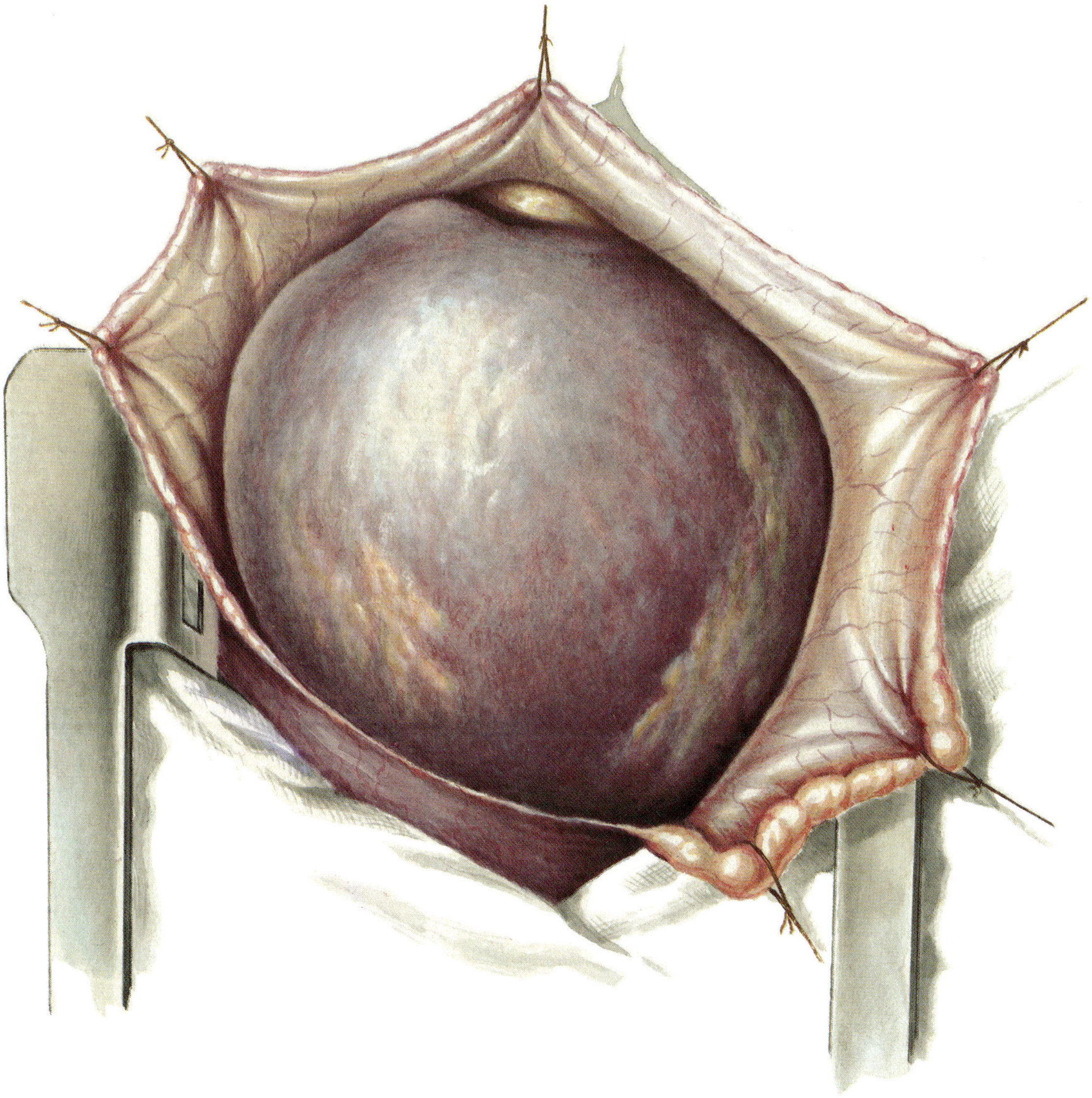

Fig. 438. General view of heart in Ebstein's anomaly exposed by longitudinal sternotomy.

The interatrial septal defect attendant to the anomaly is closed with a continuous suture (Fig. 441). The cavity of the right atrium is examined through the distended atrioventricular orifice to determine the condition of the cusps of the tricuspid valve and the right ventricular outflow tract. The latter may be constricted by a diaphragm located at the site of the subventricular crest, or by an abnormally located cusp of the tricuspid valve displaced into the depth of the ventricle. The diaphragm is usually excised. The cusps of the tricuspid valve are stretched along the walls of the right ventricle and therefore do not close. They do not hamper radical correction of Ebstein's anomaly and are not resected in most cases.

The distended right atrioventricular orifice is narrowed by means of a bolster semi-purse-string suture applied along the boundary between the right atrium and right ventricle (Fig. 442). The bolsters of the semi-purse-string suture remain on the outer wall of the right ventricle and between the aorta and the base of the right auricle. The threads in the atrial lumen are stitched from both sides to meet each other. By tying these threads the right atrioventricular orifice is narrowed on the gauge to the size of the largest ball prosthesis (Fig. 443).

Halsted sutures are applied along the projection of the fibrous ring and passed through the ball prosthesis. The prosthesis is lowered in place, and the sutures are tied. In

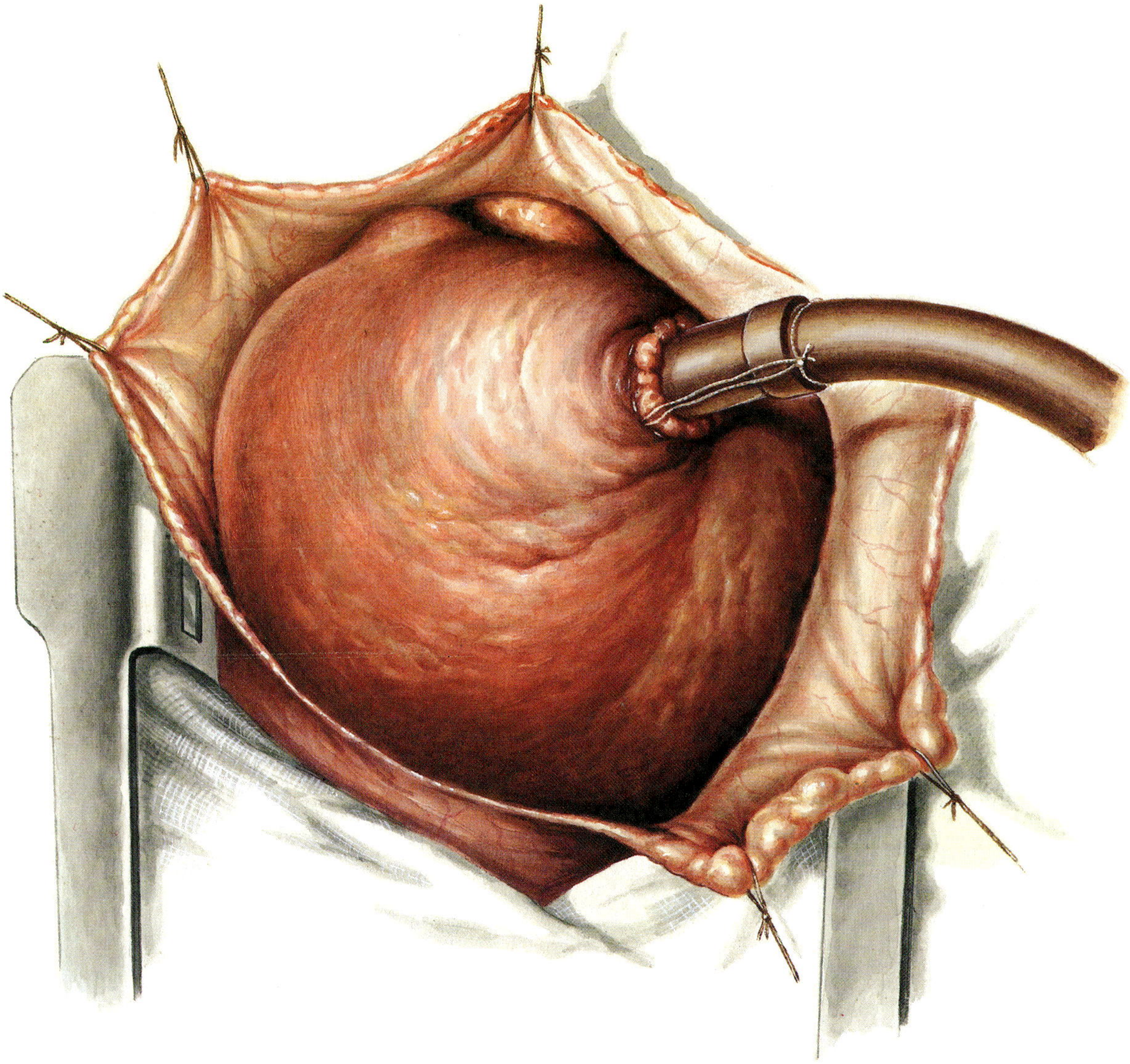

Fig. 439. Emergency connection of heart-lung machine with common venous cannula in right atrium.

most patients with the cyanotic form of Ebstein's anomaly, atrialization of the right ventricle is observed in the part between the base of the lateral cusp of the tricuspid valve and the projection of the fibrous ring, which is identified on the outside by the atrioventricular sulcus.

In marked atrialization, plication of the right ventricle with crimping Halsted sutures is performed. The sutures begin at the level of the fibrous ring and end at the base of the cusp of the tricuspid valve (Fig. 444). The ends of the sutures are passed through the base of the ball prosthesis. When these sutures are tied, plication of the atrialized part of the right ventricle occurs, and the ball prosthesis is secured (Fig. 445).

To prevent injury to the conducting pathways of the heart, the ball prosthesis is attached not along the projection of the fibrous ring, but directly to the interatrial septum above the orifice of the venous coronary sinus, which, after the prosthesis has been secured, is located in the cavity of the right ventricle (Fig. 446).

The wound in the right atrium is sutured by the routine techniques (Fig. 447). If persistent disorders of the cardiac rhythm develop after correction of the anomaly, an electrode of an electric stimulator is stitched to the right ventricle (Fig. 448).

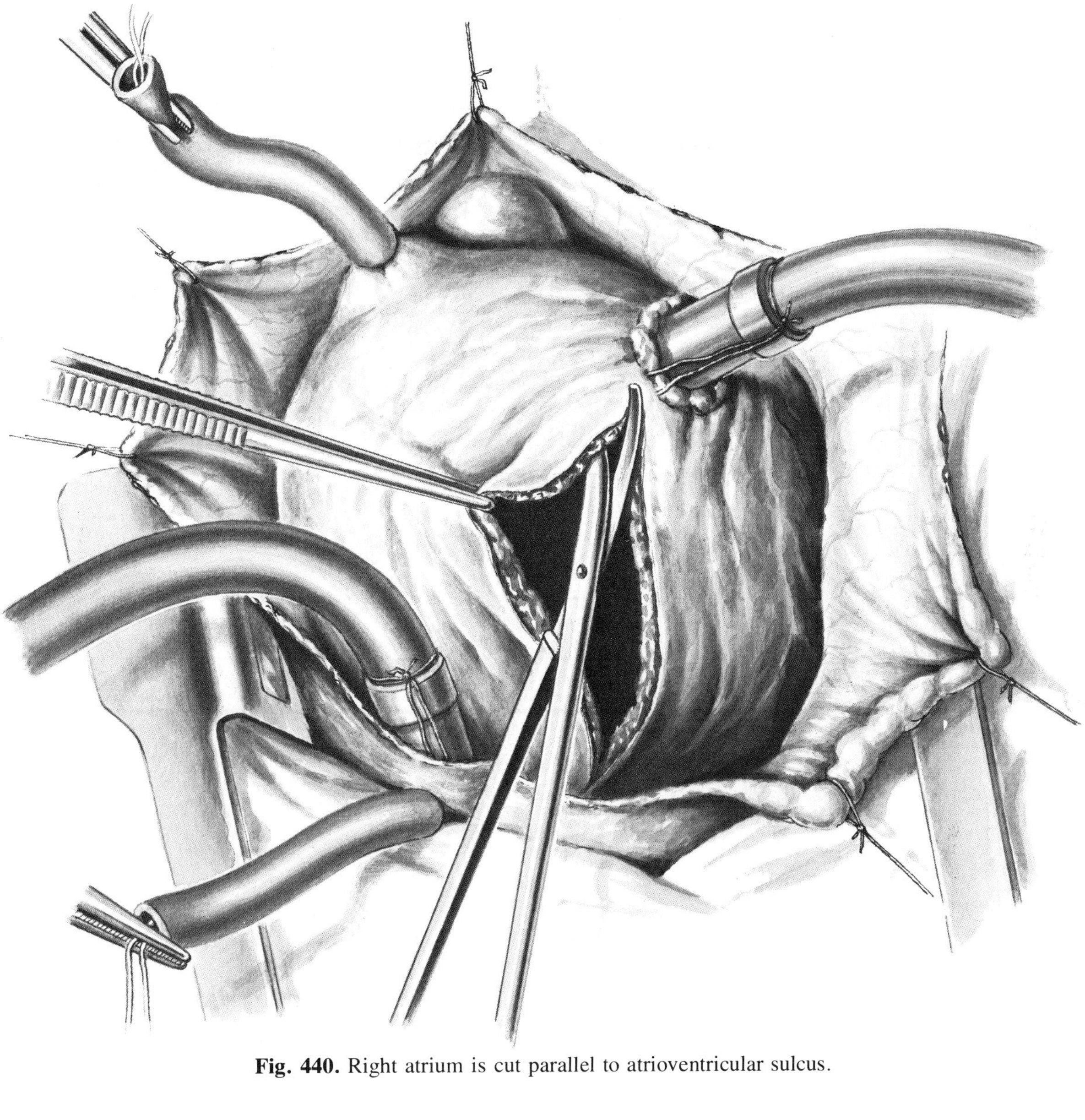

Fig. 440. Right atrium is cut parallel to atrioventricular sulcus.

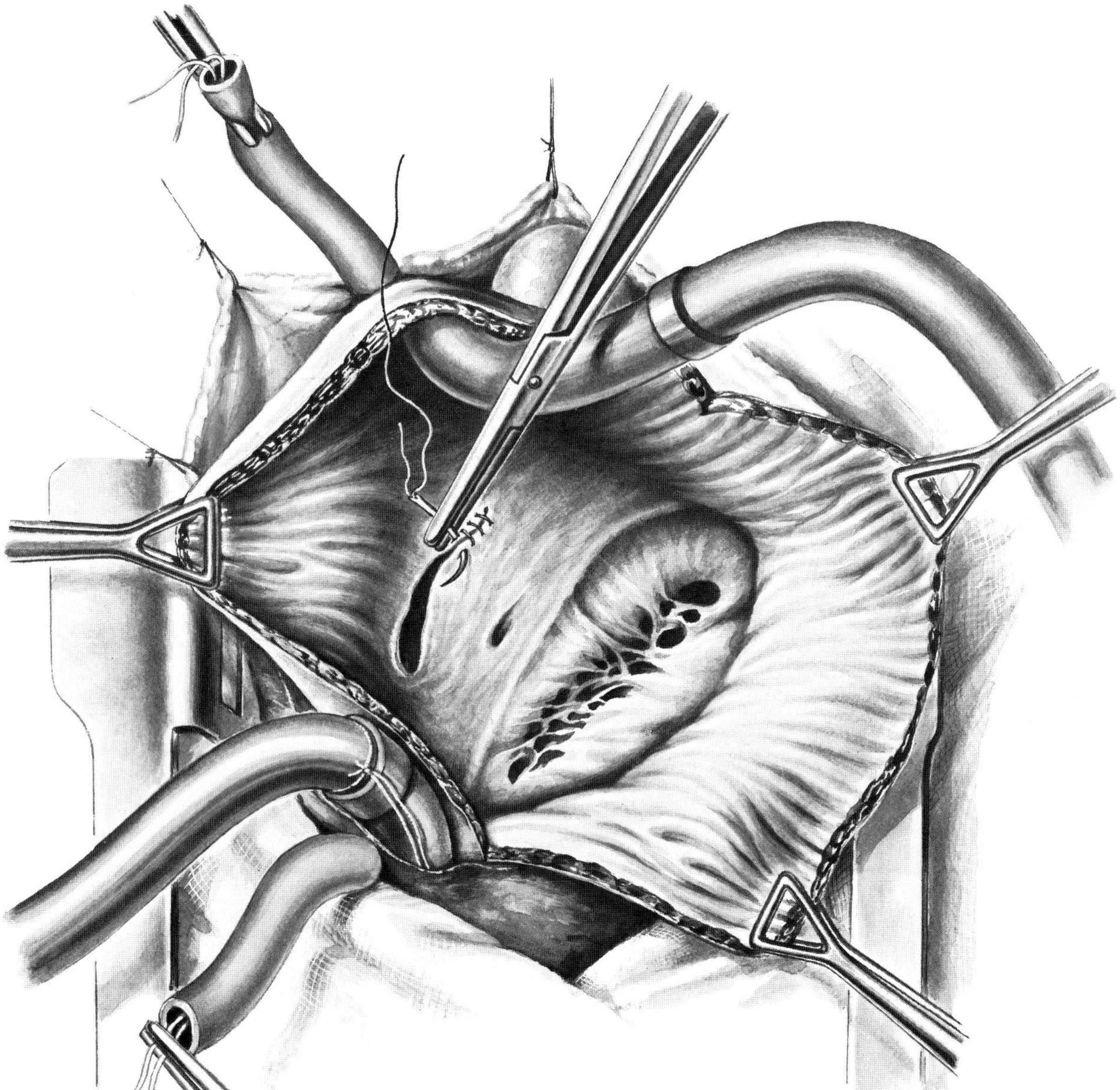

Fig. 441. Closure of interatrial septal defect with sutures.

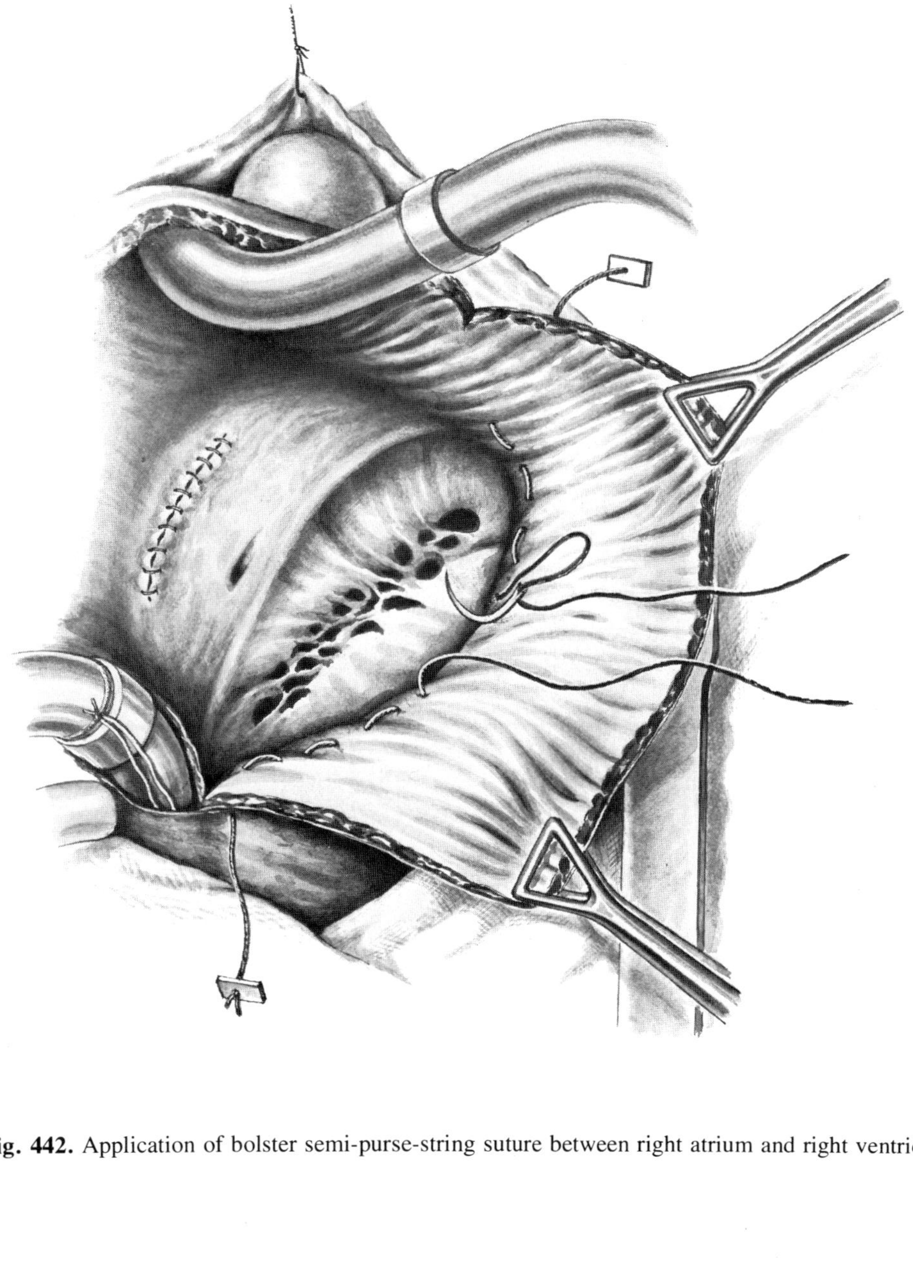

Fig. 442. Application of bolster semi-purse-string suture between right atrium and right ventricle.

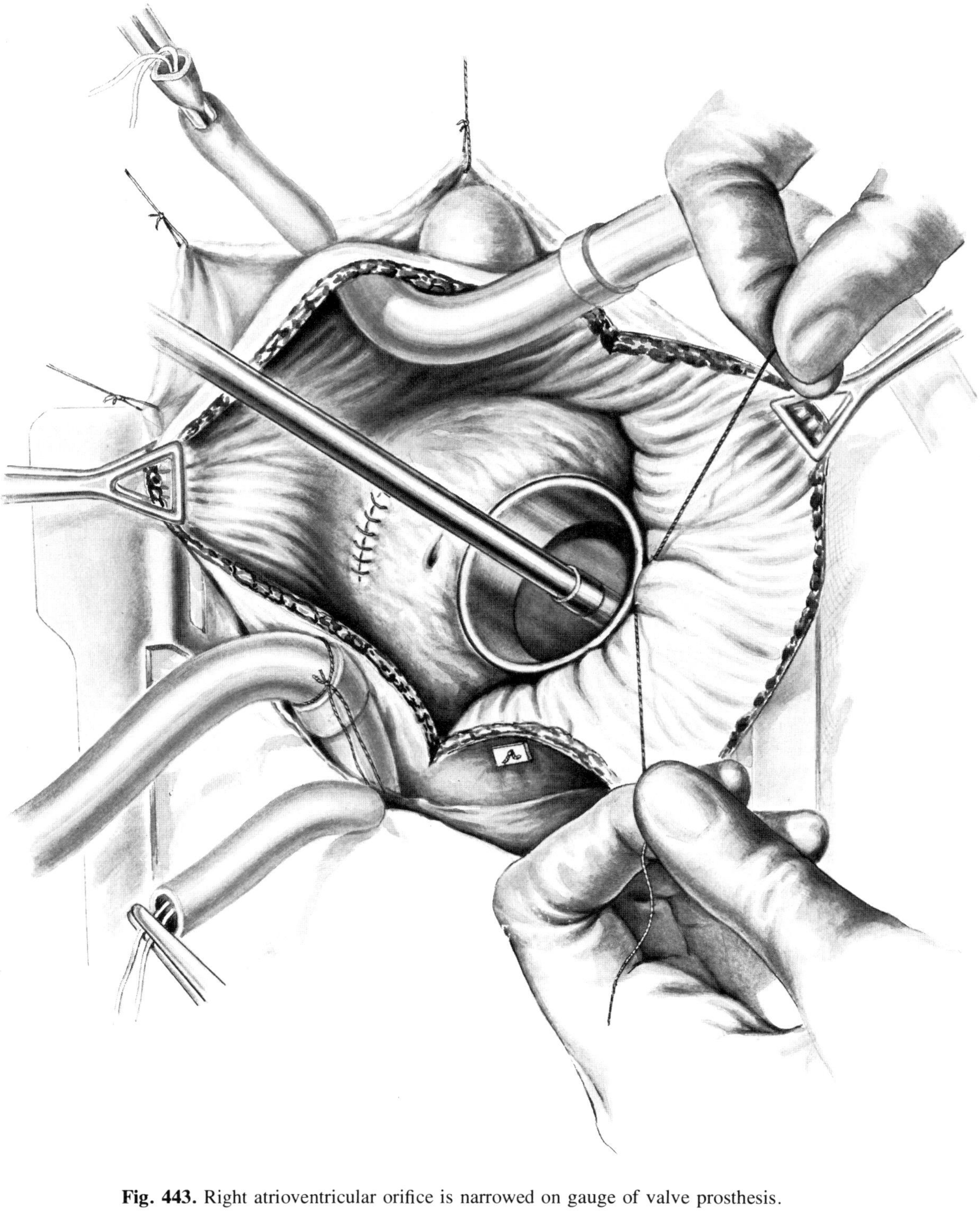

Fig. 443. Right atrioventricular orifice is narrowed on gauge of valve prosthesis.

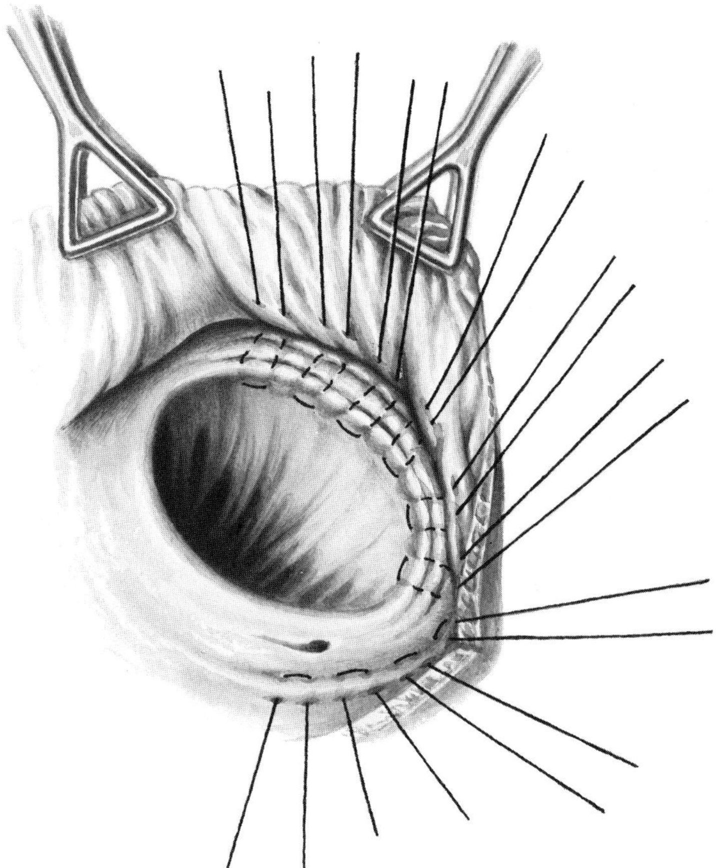

Fig. 444. Plication of atrialized part of right ventricular wall.

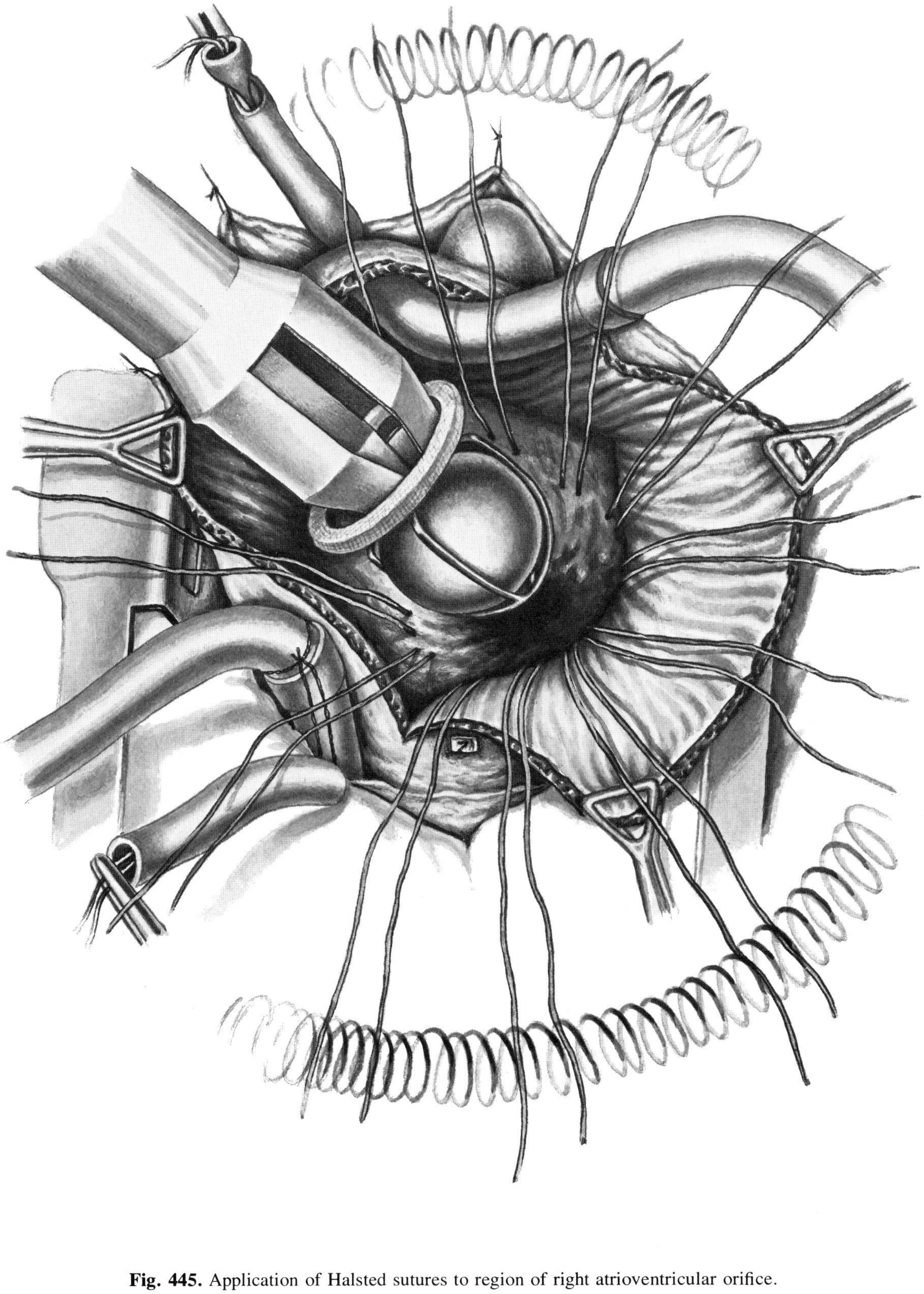

Fig. 445. Application of Halsted sutures to region of right atrioventricular orifice.

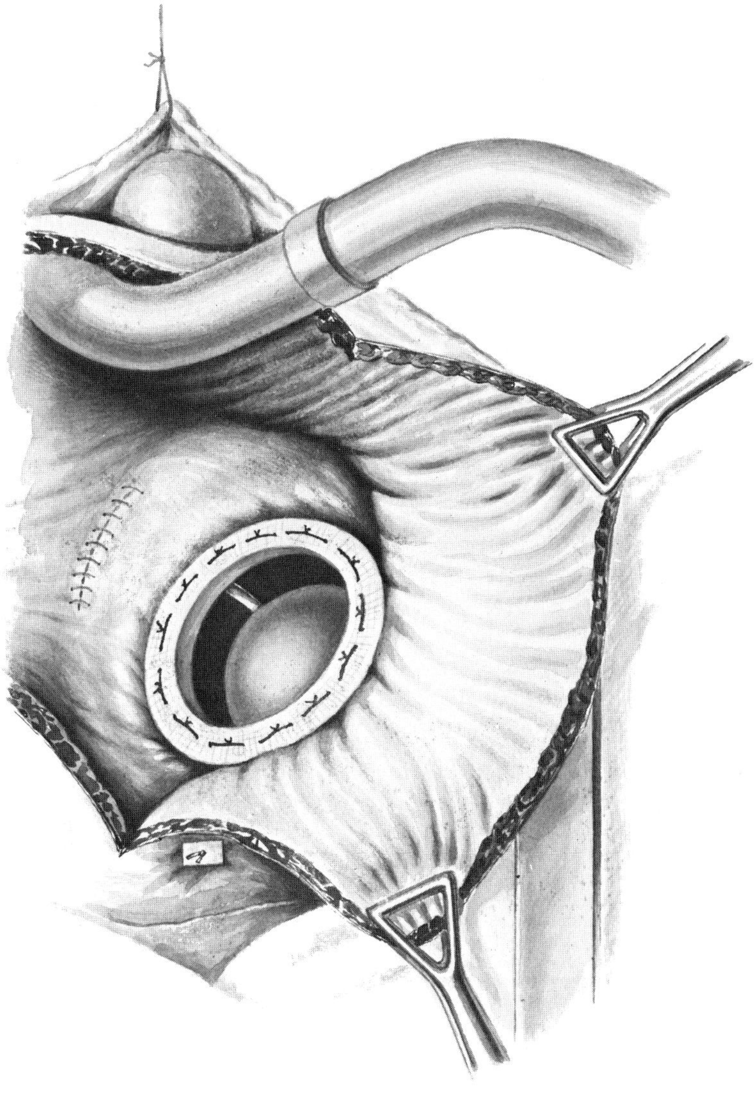

Fig. 446. View of ball prosthesis sutured into right atrioventricular orifice.

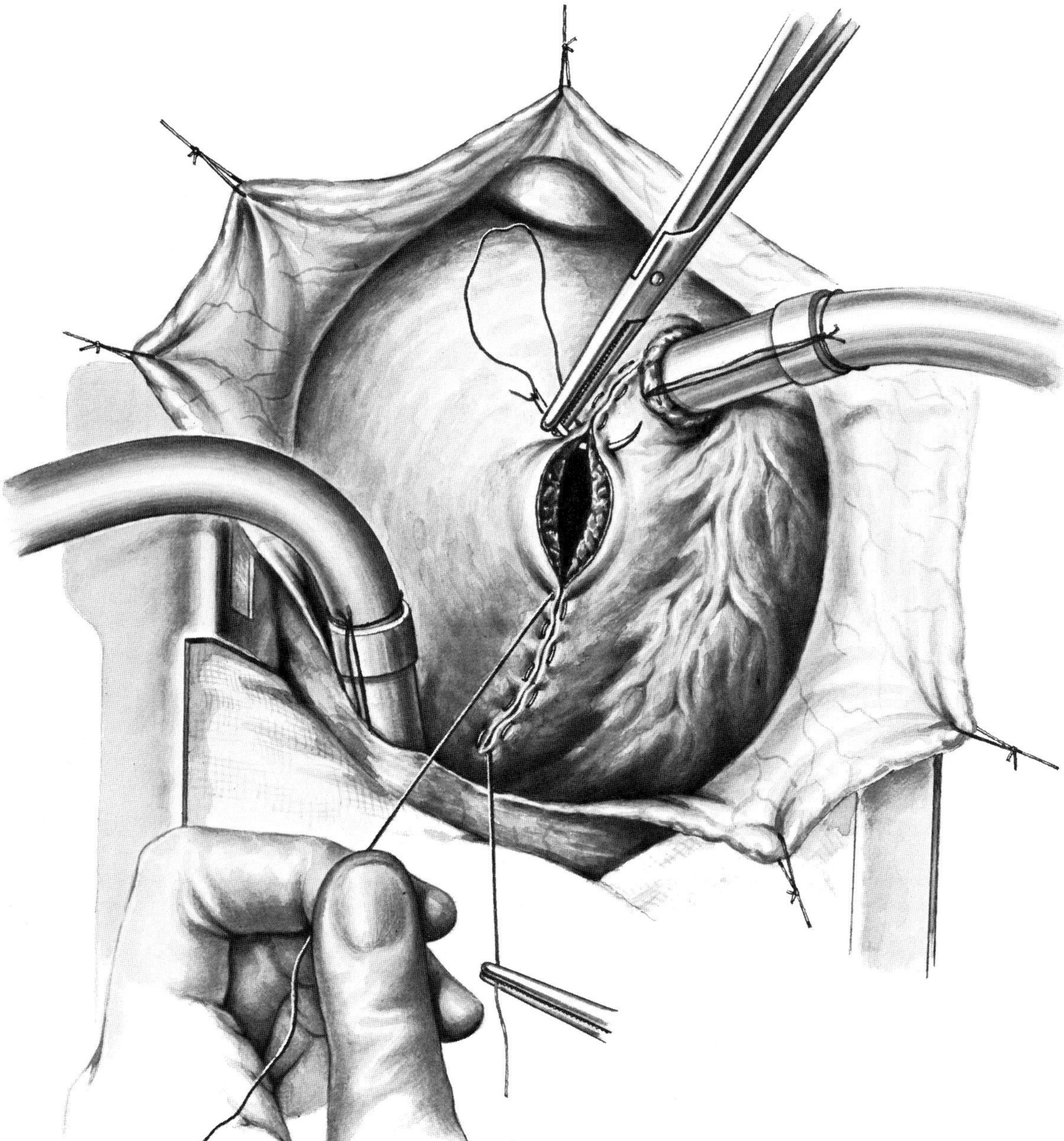

Fig. 447. Wound in right atrium is sutured.

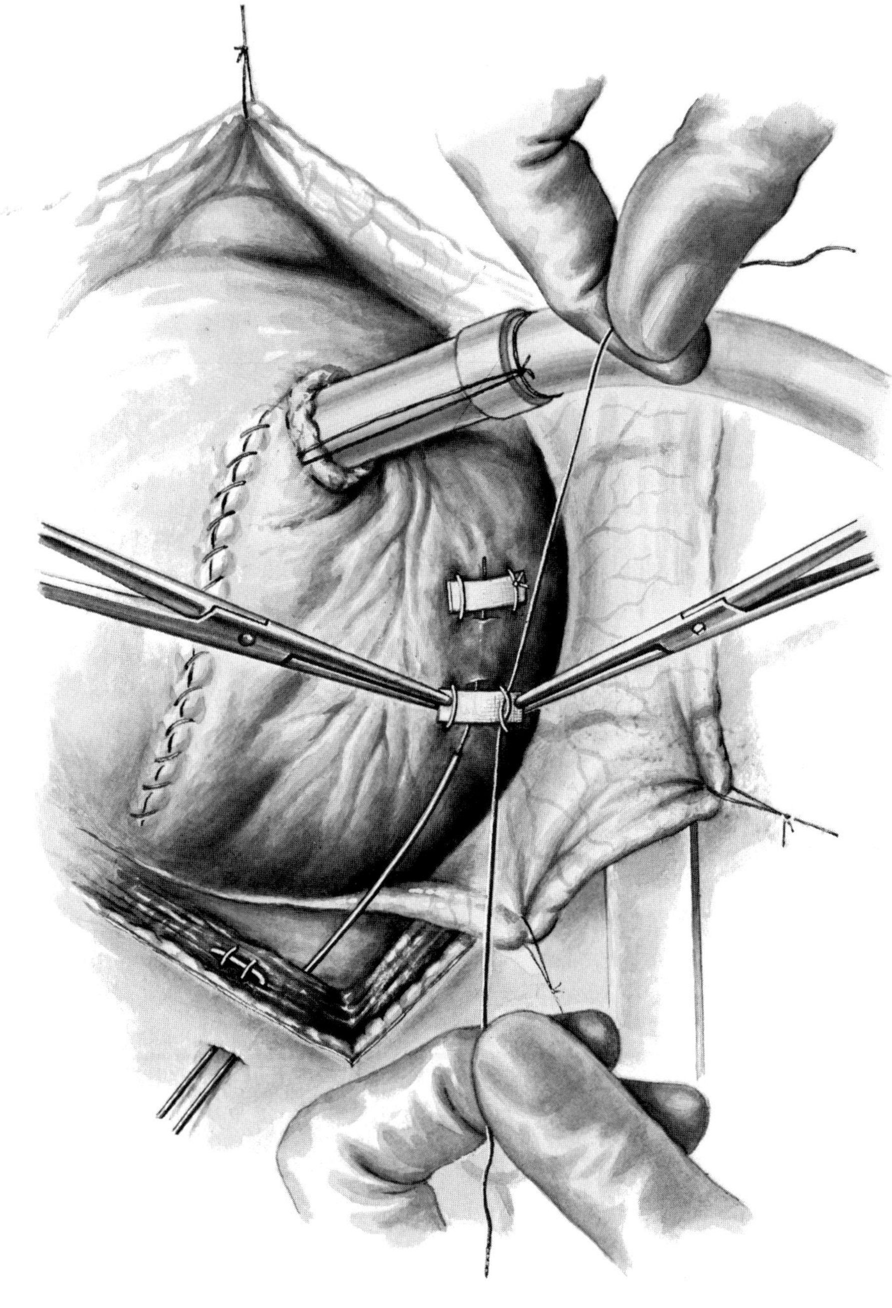

Fig. 448. Electrode of electrostimulator is stitched to right ventricle for stimulation of heart in event of block.

CORRECTION OF TOTAL TRANSPOSITION OF THE MAJOR VESSELS

The operative technique proposed by Mustard may be used in this anomaly.

The operation is performed by means of medial sternotomy (Fig. 449).

Radical correction consists in resecting the interatrial septum for the purpose of widening the existing defect and shaping a canal from a rectangular pericardial graft or a piece of plastic material to direct the orifice of the venae cavae and venous sinus toward the mitral valve.

The right atrium is opened by a vertical incision dorsal to the cannulas introduced into the venae cavae (Fig. 450). An area of the interatrial septum is resected, and a pericardial graft formed (Fig. 451). The widened entrance into the left atrium is separated with the pericardial graft in such a way as to channel blood from the pulmonary veins into the right atrium. The first suture applied attaches the middle of the graft to the fibrous ring of the mitral valve. Subsequent sutures secure the graft in such a manner that it divides the widened interatrial septal defect into two: a ventral part for the stream of venous blood to the mitral valve, and a dorsal part for the flow of arterial blood to the tricuspid valve. The orifice

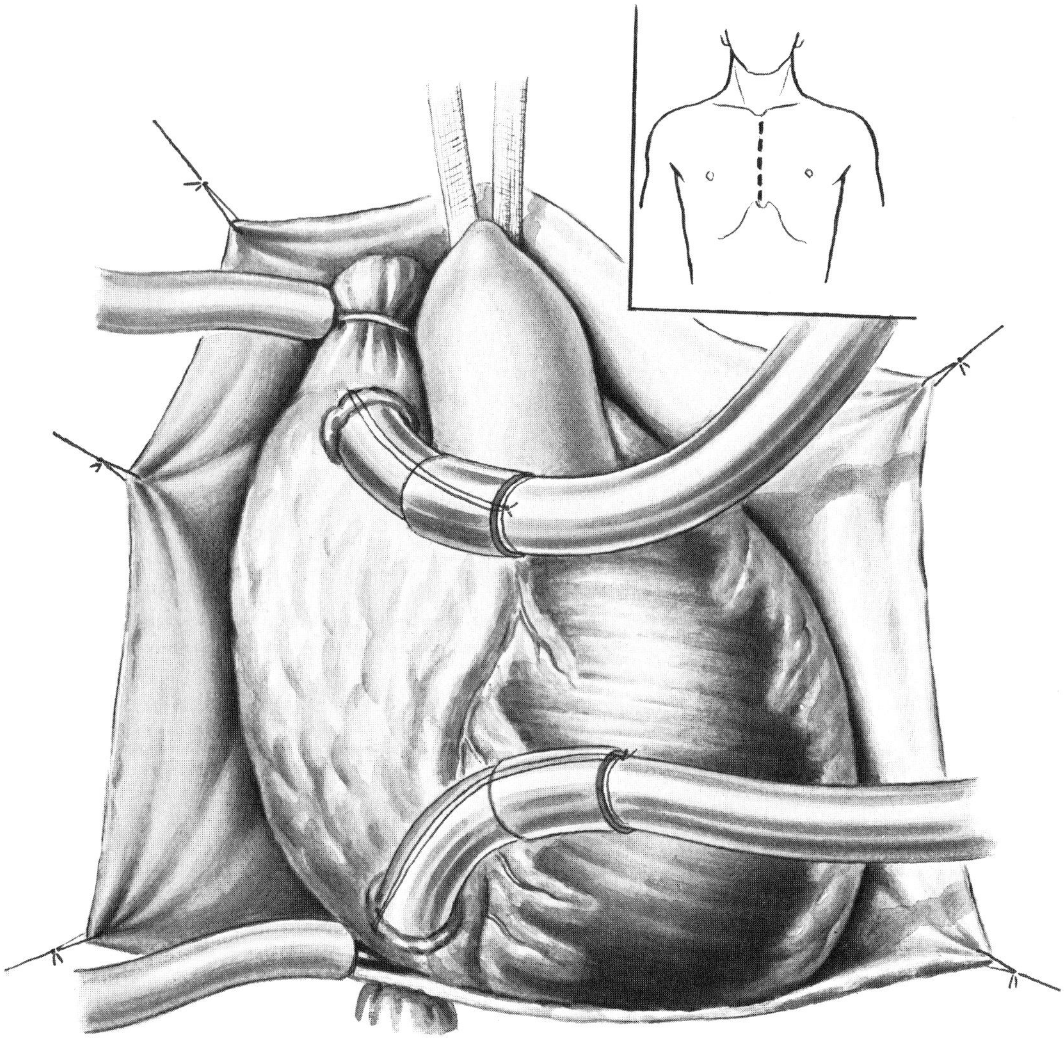

Fig. 449. Approach to and general view of heart in total transposition of major vessels.

of the venous coronary sinus is dilated by cutting the left atrial wall adjoining it.

The next step is to separate the orifice of the superior vena cava from the right atrium. For this purpose the septum and the left wall of the left atrium are sutured ventrally to the left pulmonary veins. The suture is continued on the wall of the right atrium, separating the orifices of the venae cavae (Fig. 452). The ventral edge of the graft is stitched to the wall of the right atrium (Fig. 453). In the long run, part of the right atrium with areas of the venae cavae and veins of the coronary sinus remains under the graft.

The cavity of the right atrium is closed, and air is carefully removed from it so as to avoid embolism of the vessels of the systemic circulation and the coronary vessels (Fig. 454).

It is expedient to conduct the operation on a fibrillating heart, clamp the aorta at the end of the operation, and check the presence of air in the aorta and in the right and left atria by puncture. The right atrium is sutured by the routine techniques.

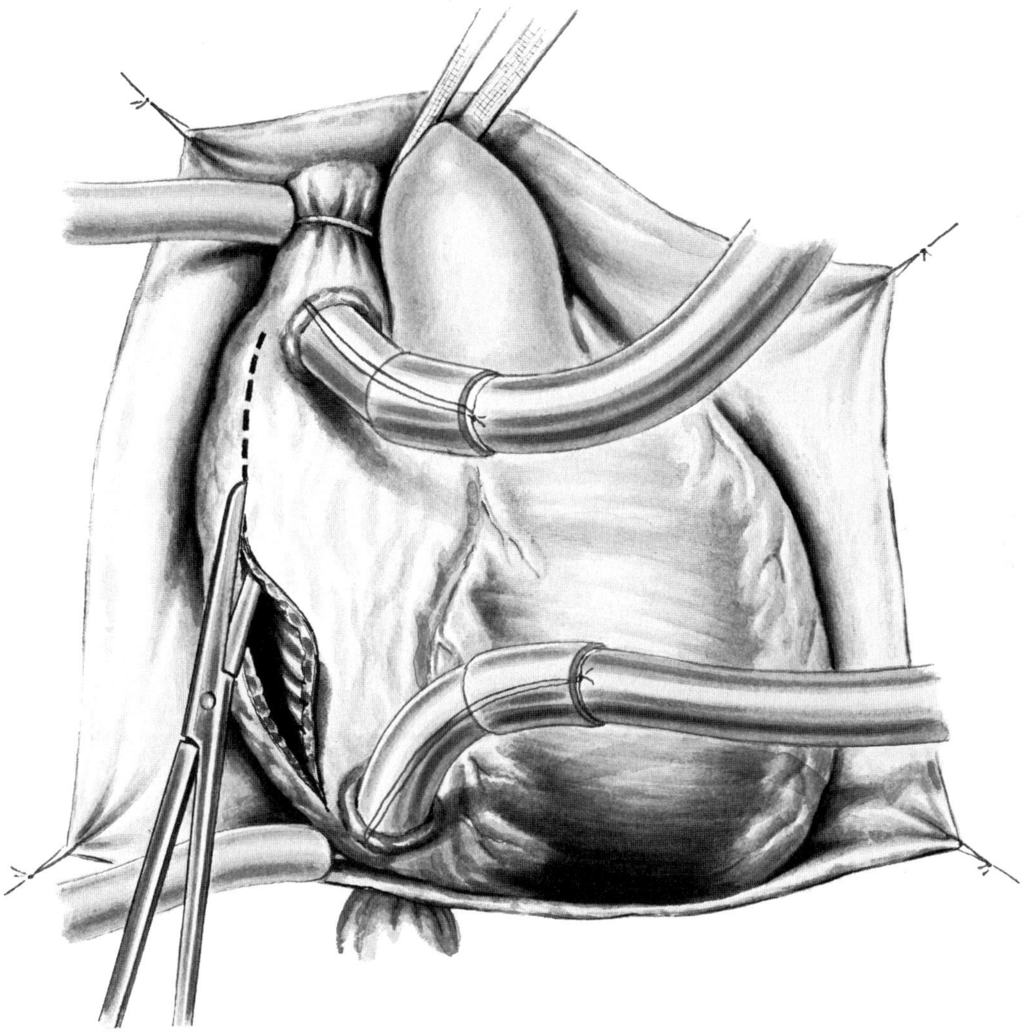

Fig. 450. Right atrium is cut.

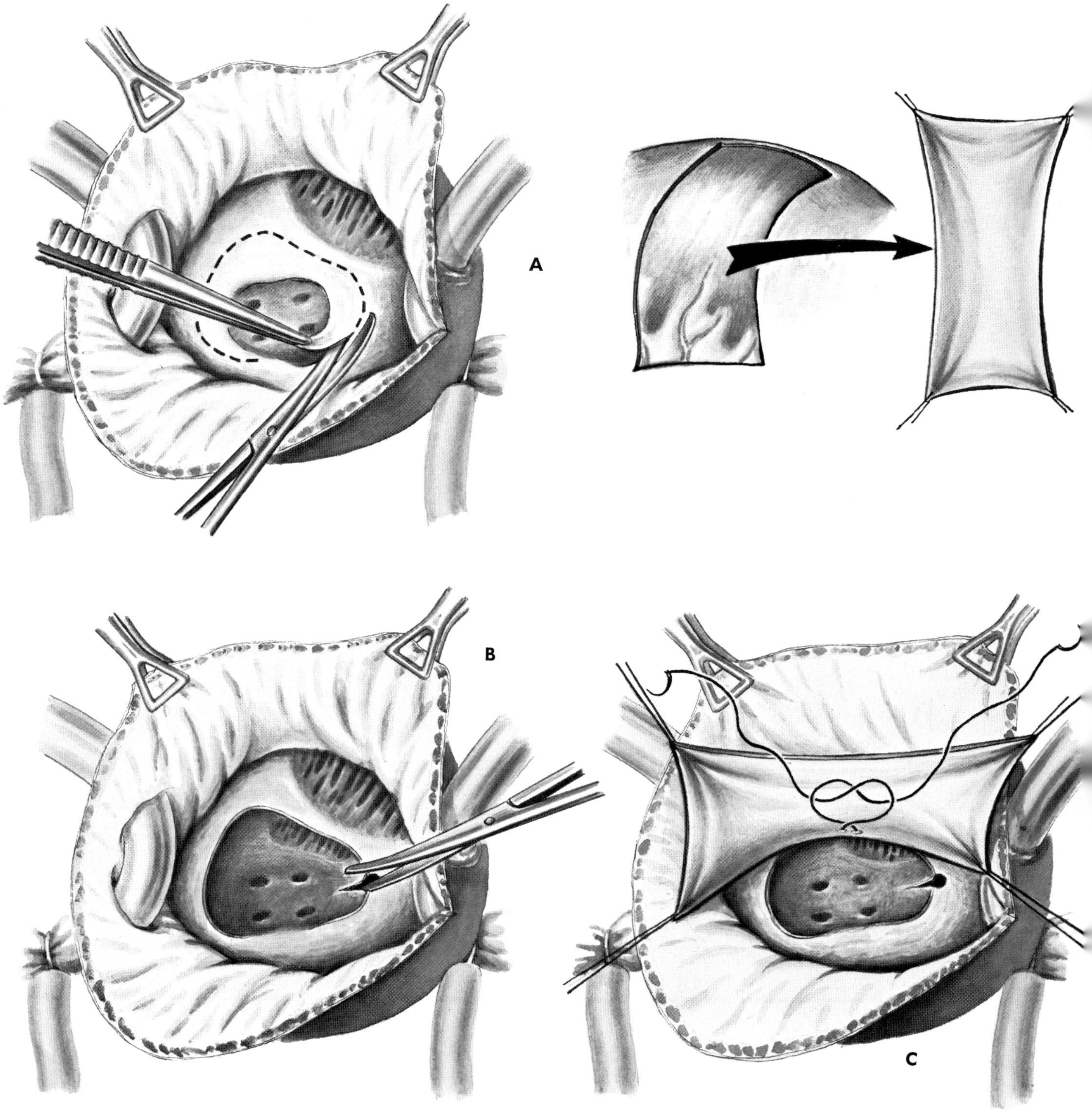

Fig. 451. Mustard's operation in total transposition of vessels. **A,** Area of interatrial septum is being resected and pericardial graft is formed. **B,** Interatrial septum has been resected; a cut is made in orifice of coronary sinus. **C,** Initial stage in attachment of periosteal graft.

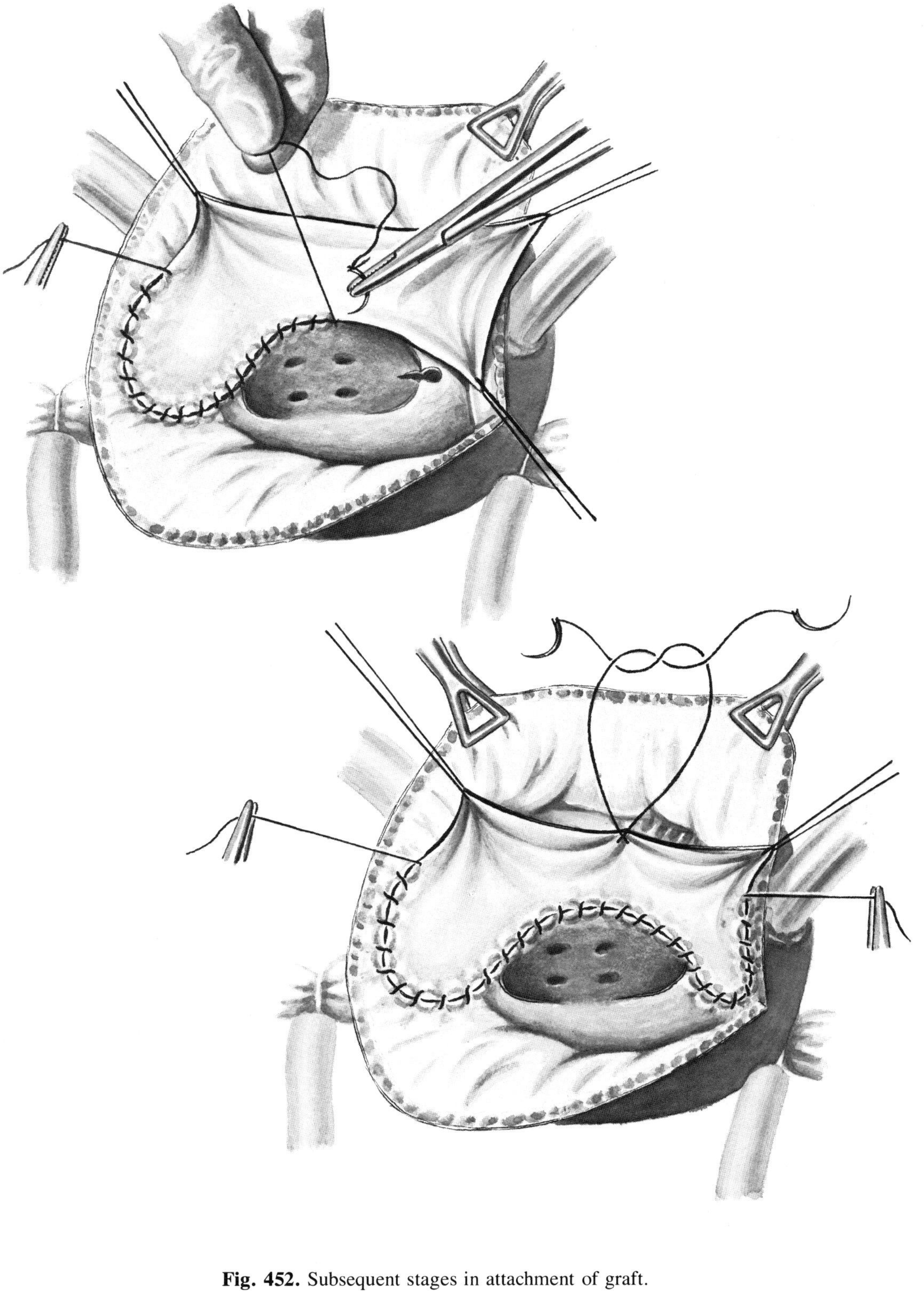

Fig. 452. Subsequent stages in attachment of graft.

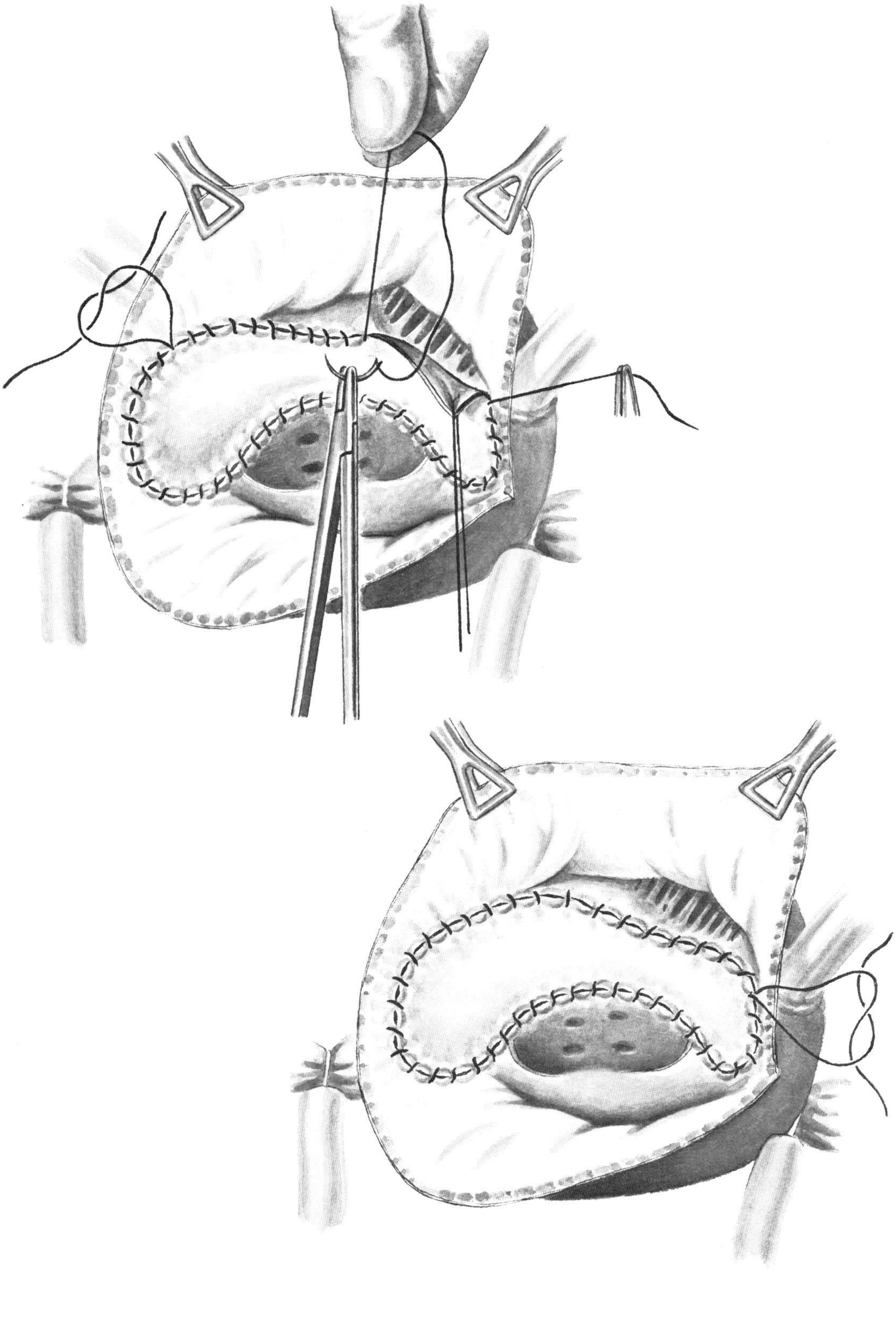

Fig. 453. Final stages in attachment of graft.

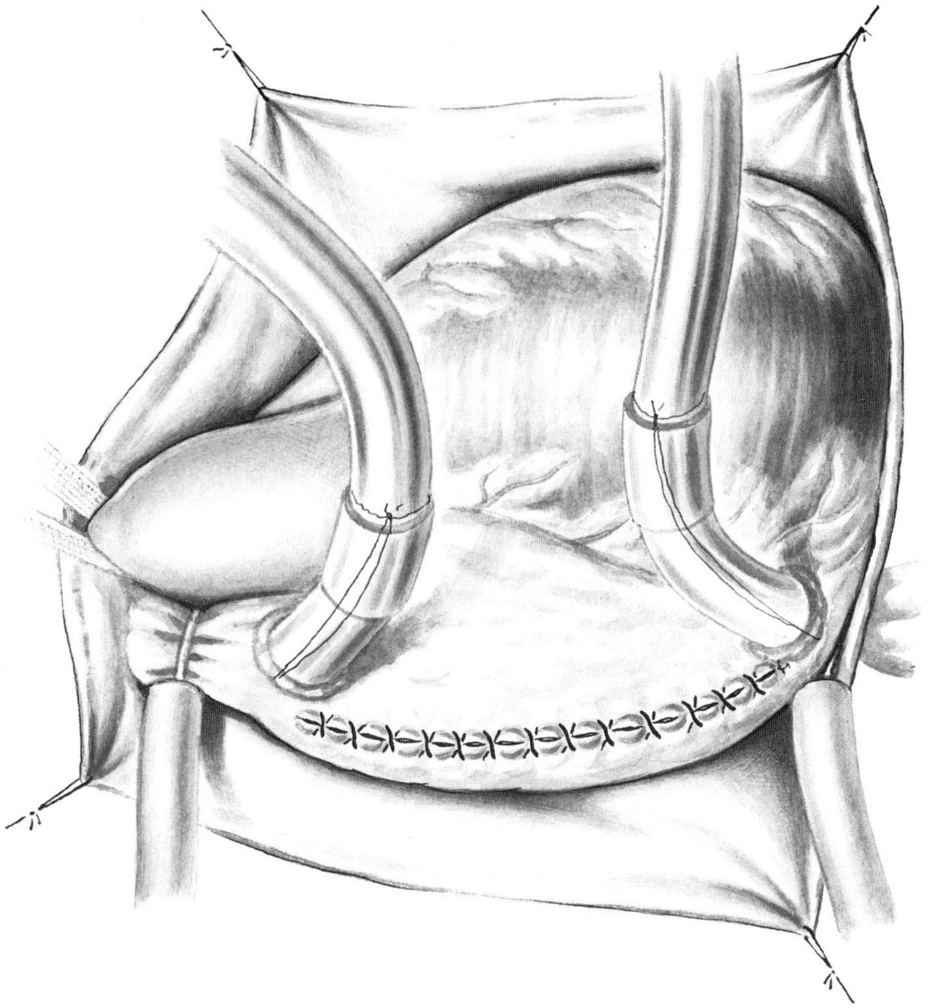

Fig. 454. Suture applied to right atrium.

*OPERATIONS IN ANEURYSM OF THE HEART

OPERATION BY THE CLOSED METHOD

Among postinfarction aneurysms of the heart there are diffuse, sacculated, and giant (aneurysm in an aneurysm) forms.

In diffuse aneurysm (Fig. 455) plastic surgery with a diaphragmatic pedicle graft is performed to reinforce its wall and revascularize the myocardium. A graft, 5 to 6 cm wide with the base at the apex of the heart, is formed from the diaphragm (Fig. 456). An aneurysm of the left

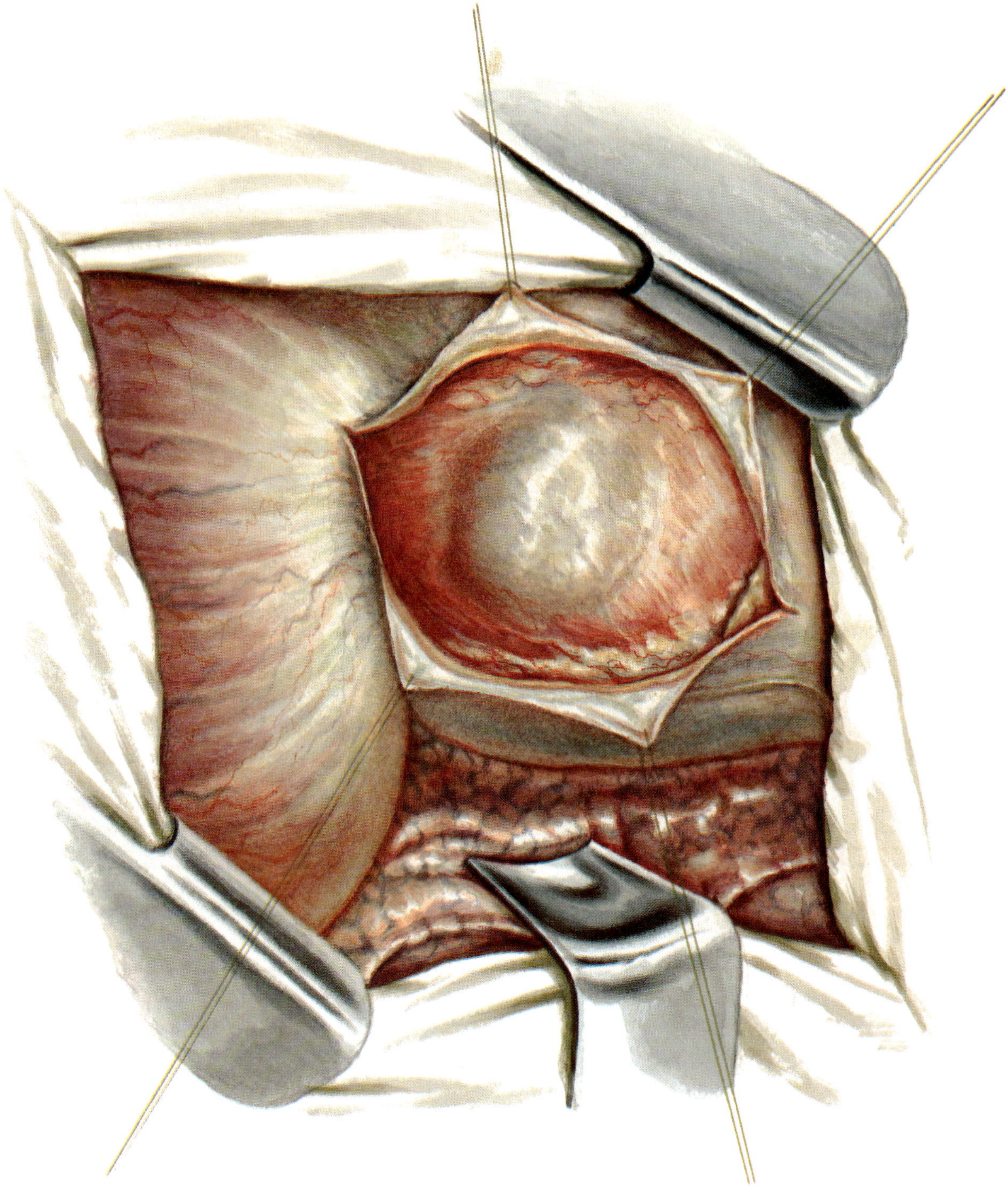

Fig. 455. View of diffuse aneurysm of heart exposed on opening pericardium.

ventricle is treated with a scarificator; the diaphragmatic graft is scarified in a similar manner (Fig. 457). The graft is slightly stretched and spread over the diffuse aneurysm and attached along its boundaries with interrupted sutures (Figs. 458 and 459).

The defect in the diaphragm is closed with thick silk sutures. Sometimes a triangular plastic graft is stitched into the defect in the diaphragm to prevent compression of the diaphragmatic graft. The edges of the divided pericardium are sutured over the diaphragmatic graft (Fig. 460).

In cases with large sacculated aneurysms the pericardium is usually fused with the epicardium in the region of the aneurysm and serves as its wall. In such instances

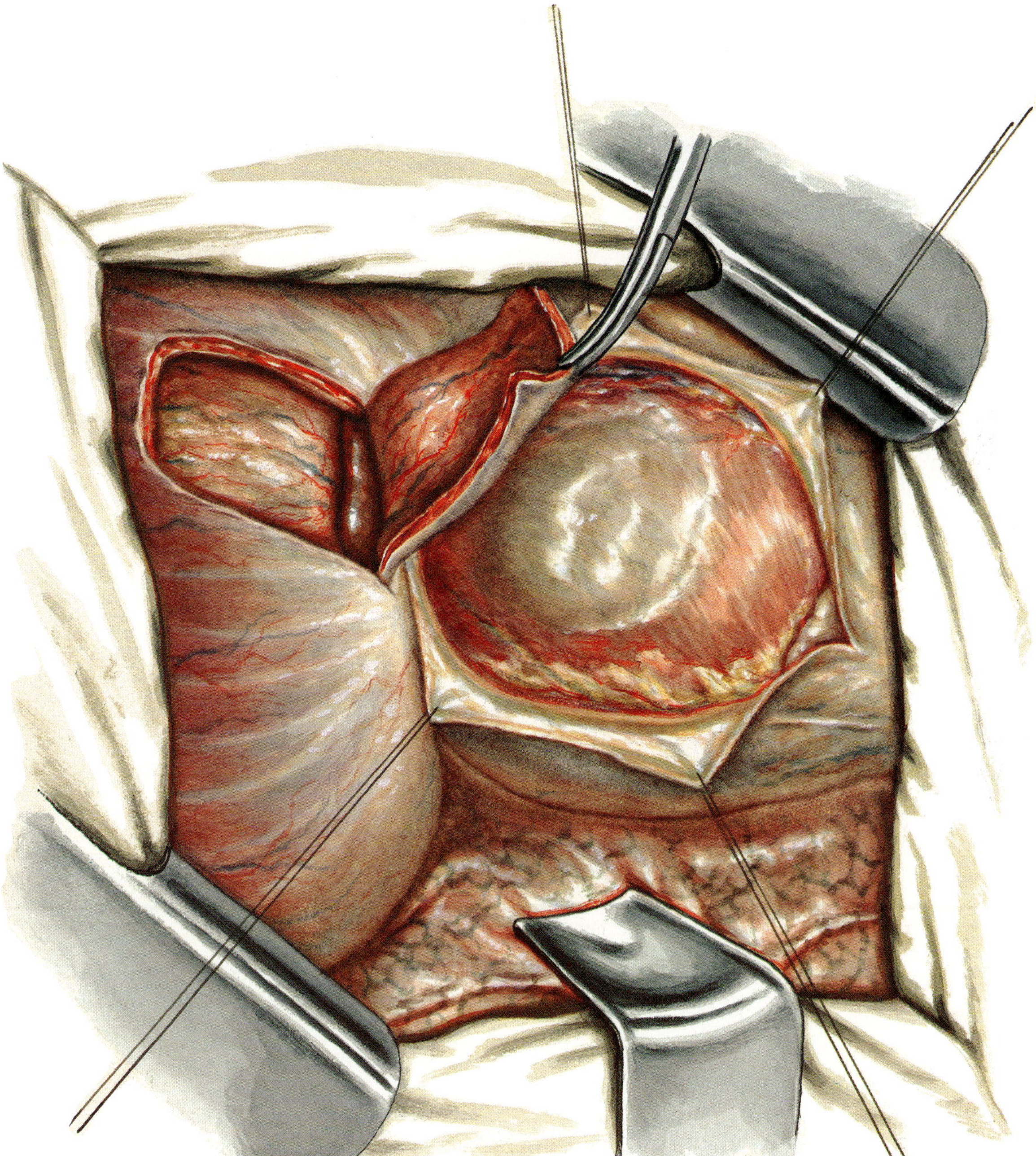

Fig. 456. Graft is formed from diaphragm.

circular resection of the pericardium in the region of the aneurysmal neck is performed (Fig. 461). Traction sutures are applied to the aneurysm along the circumference of the sac (Fig. 462). A needle-shaped clamp is applied to the neck of the sac by means of traction sutures so that the parts of the left ventricular wall involved in the aneurysm are clamped (Fig. 463). Several traction sutures are applied along the sides of the line of the intended incision between which the aneurysmal sac is opened. The mural thrombus is detached with a spade; the edges of the sac are held with two pairs of forceps (Figs. 464 and 465). The surgeon opens the needle-

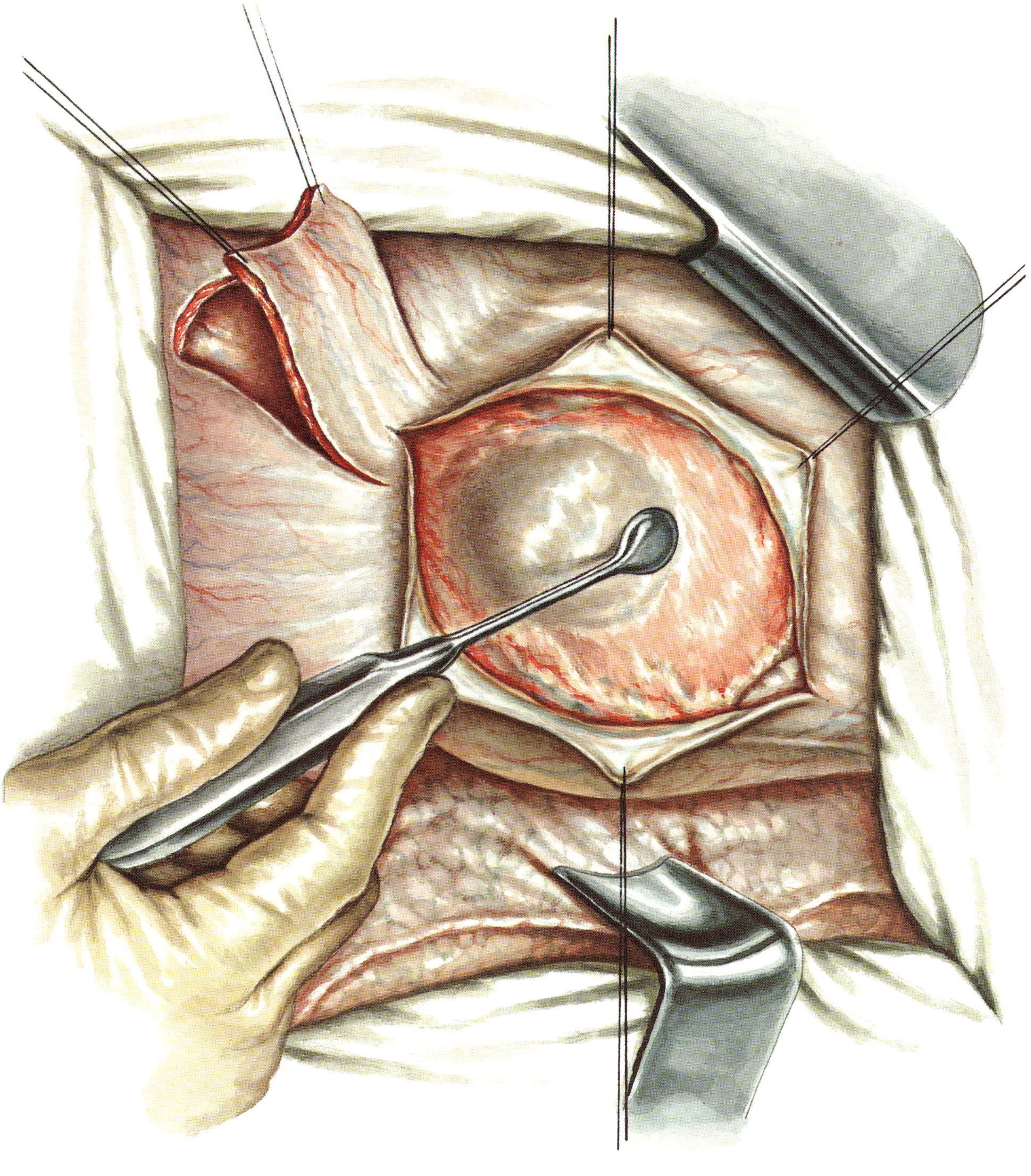

Fig. 457. Surface of aneurysm is treated with scarificator.

shaped clamp with the left hand and, while the assistant pulls the traction sutures on the edges of the incision apart, separates the thrombus from the left ventricle with the right index finger, which he then advances into the ventricular cavity (Fig. 466). The powerful jet of blood dislocates the thrombus from the left ventricle. Then the needle-shaped clamp is closed over the neck of the sac. The walls of the aneurysmal sac are excised with scissors. A continuous Halsted suture is stitched through the fibrous walls of the left ventricular sacculated aneurysm under the clamp (Fig. 467). With the continuous Halsted suture applied, the needle-shaped clamp is removed and the wound in the left ventricle is made airtight with a blanket suture (Fig. 468). A graft is formed out of the diaphragm, and the suture placed on the left ventricle after resection of the aneurysm is reinforced with it (Fig. 469).

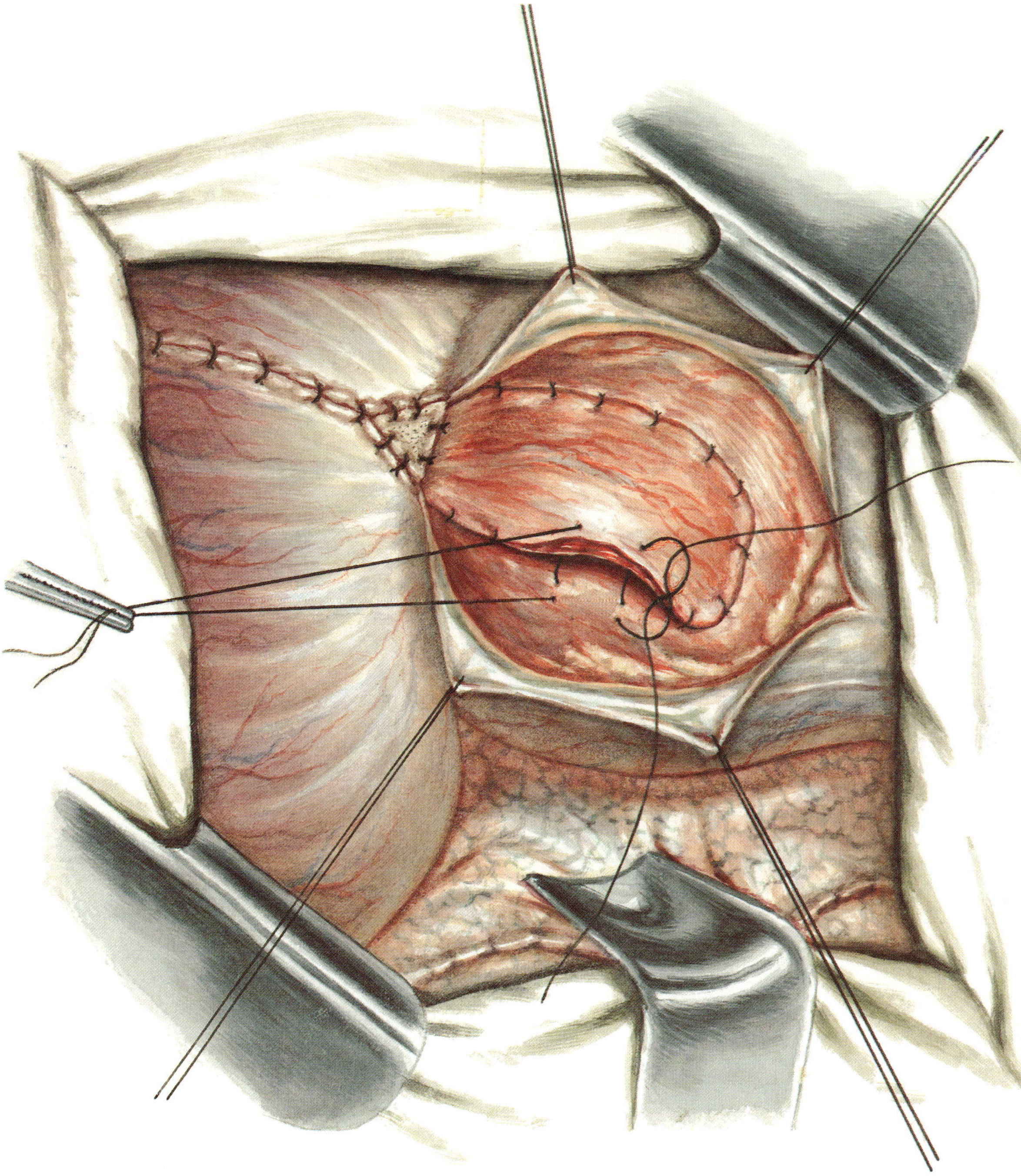

Fig. 458. Diaphragmatic graft is sutured in place.

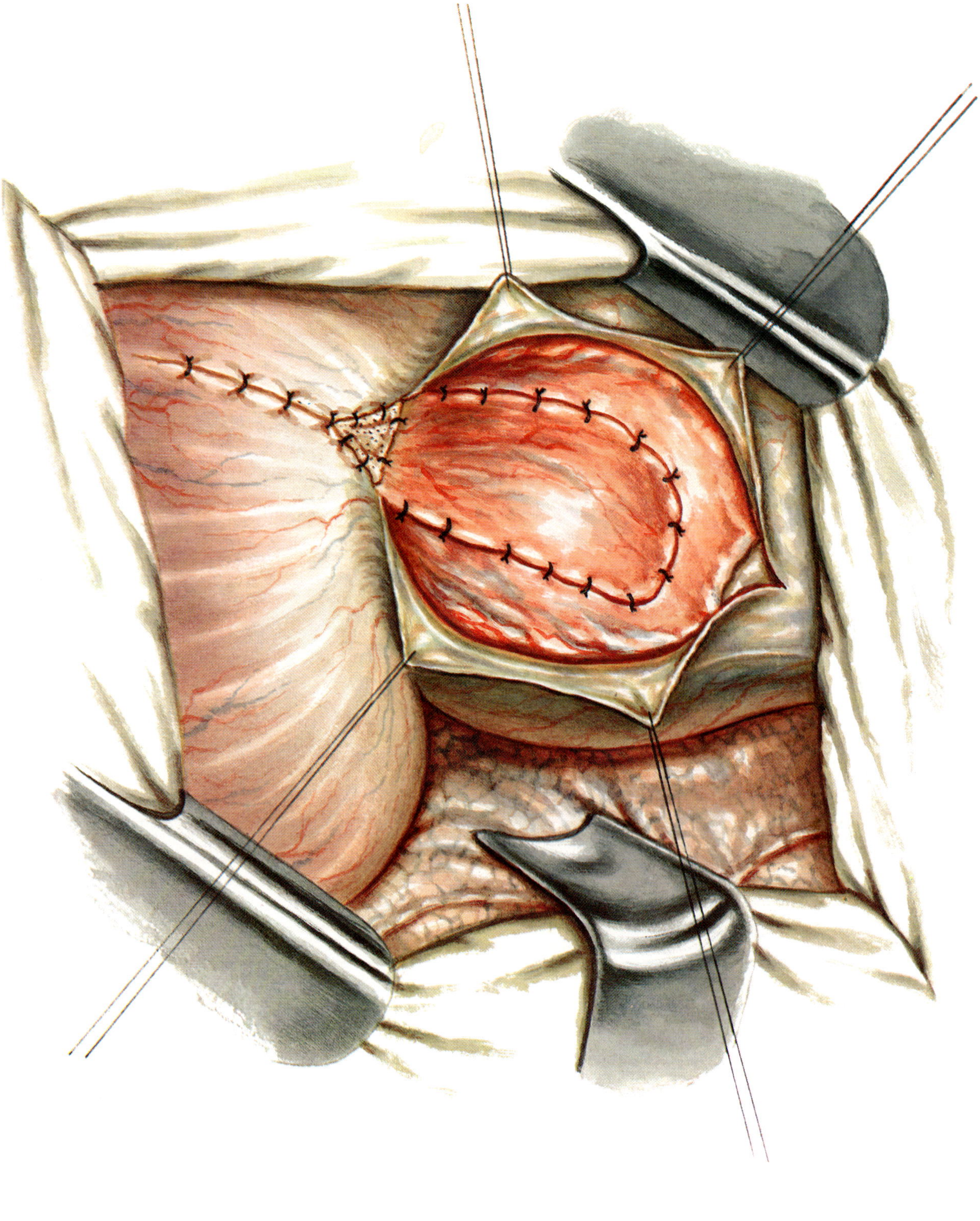

Fig. 459. Diaphragmatic graft has been sutured to myocardium.

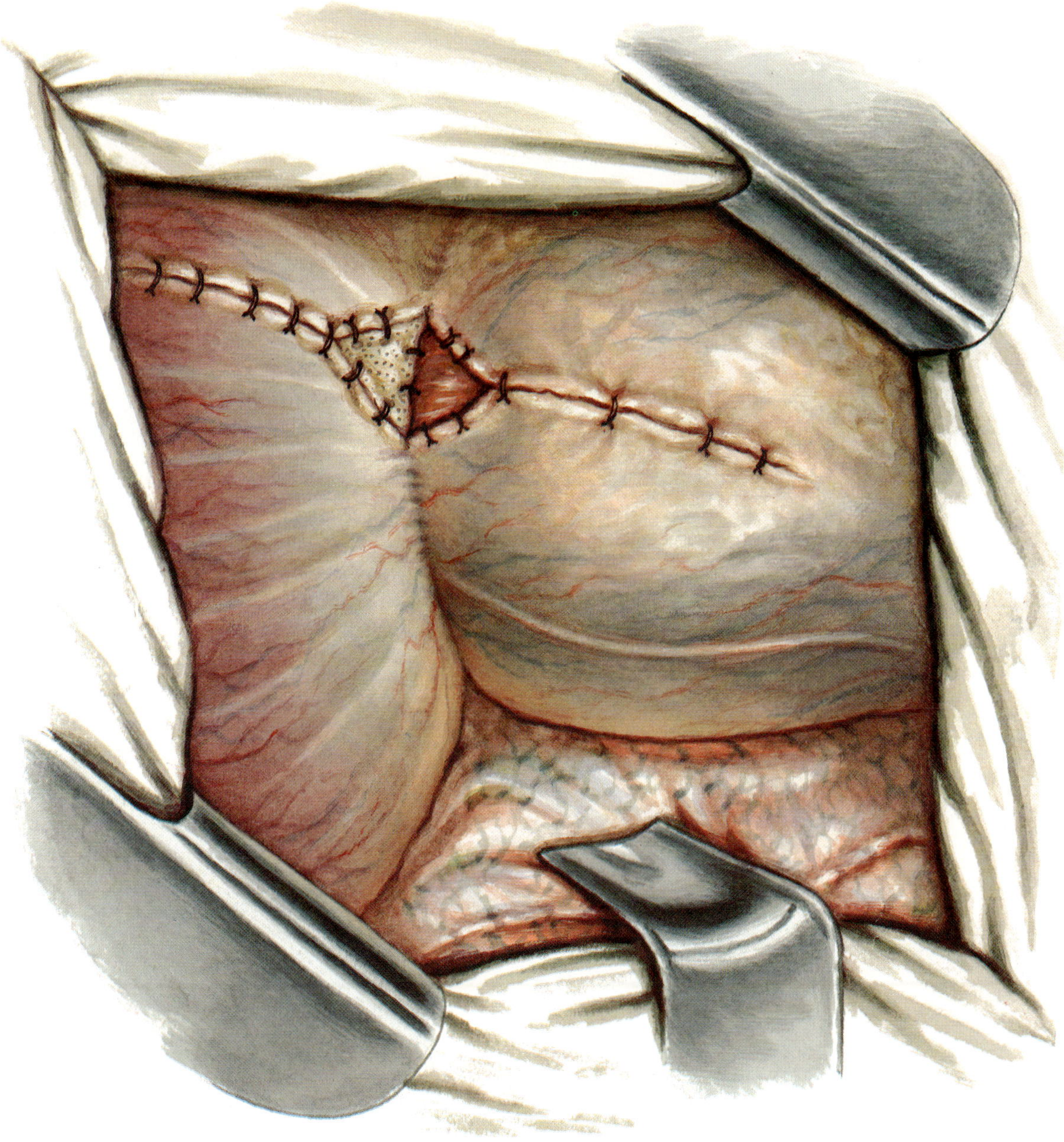

Fig. 460. Pericardium is sutured over diaphragmatic graft.

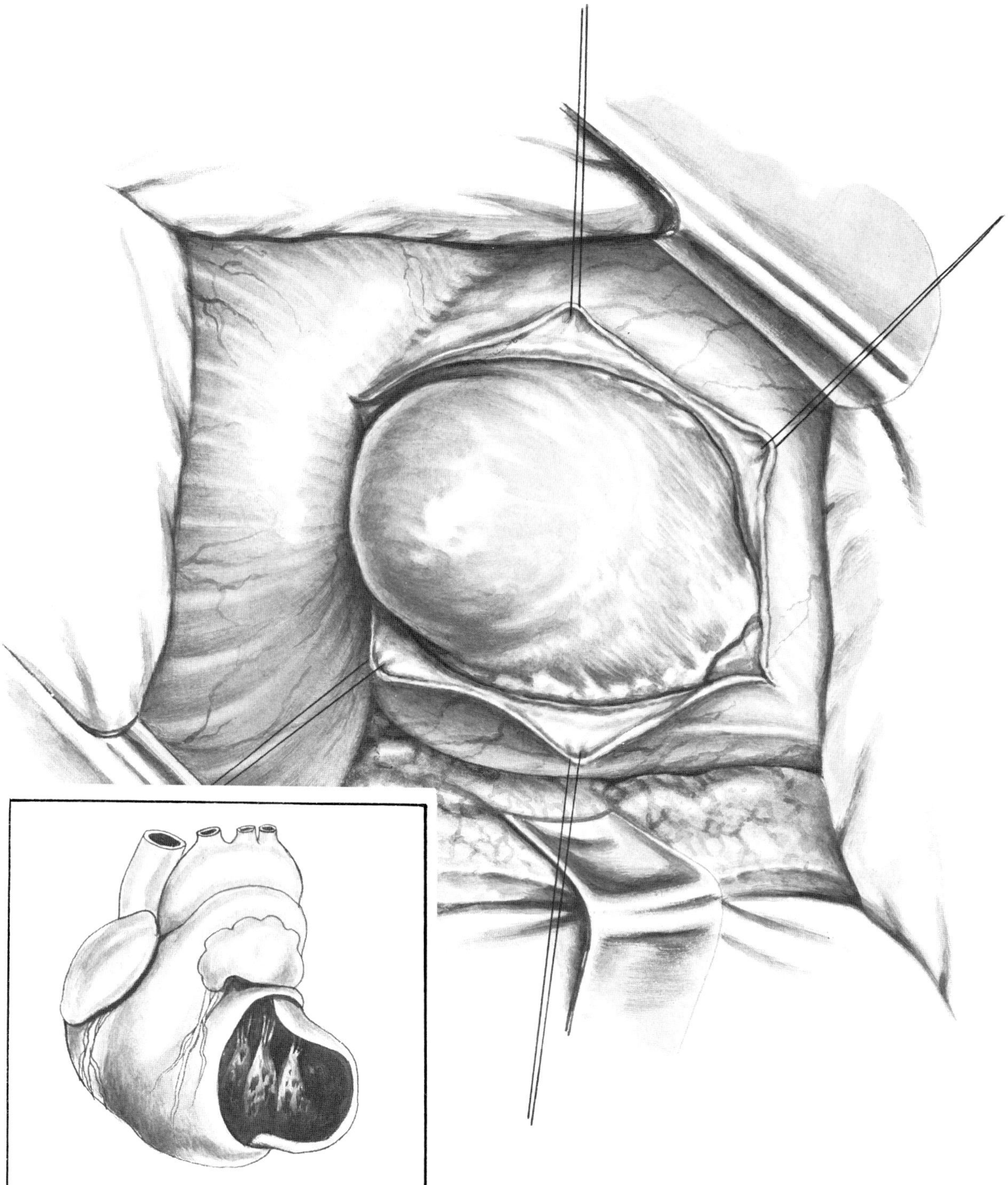

Fig. 461. View of sacculated aneurysm of left ventricle after separation of pericardium.

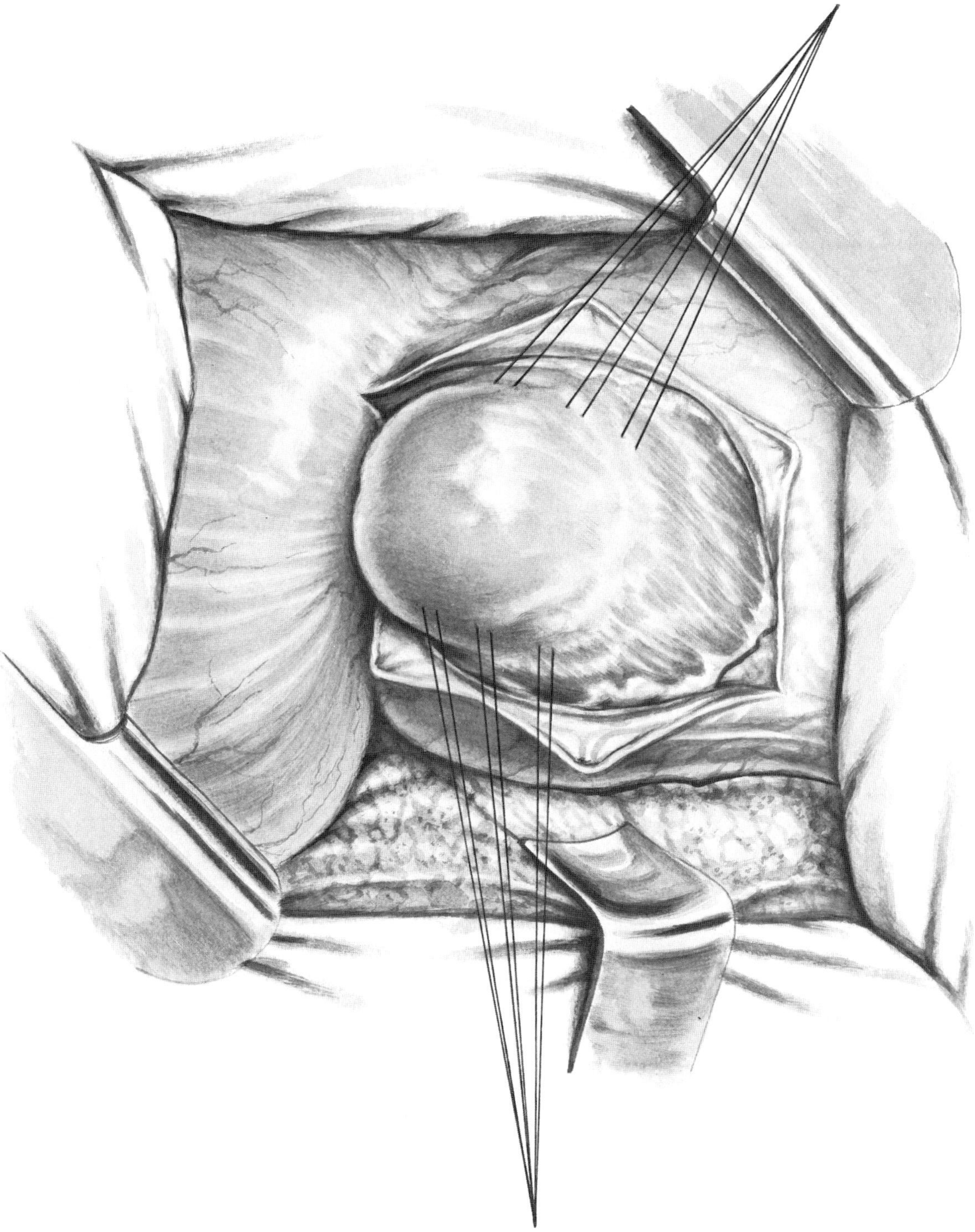

Fig. 462. Traction sutures are applied along circumference of aneurysmal sac.

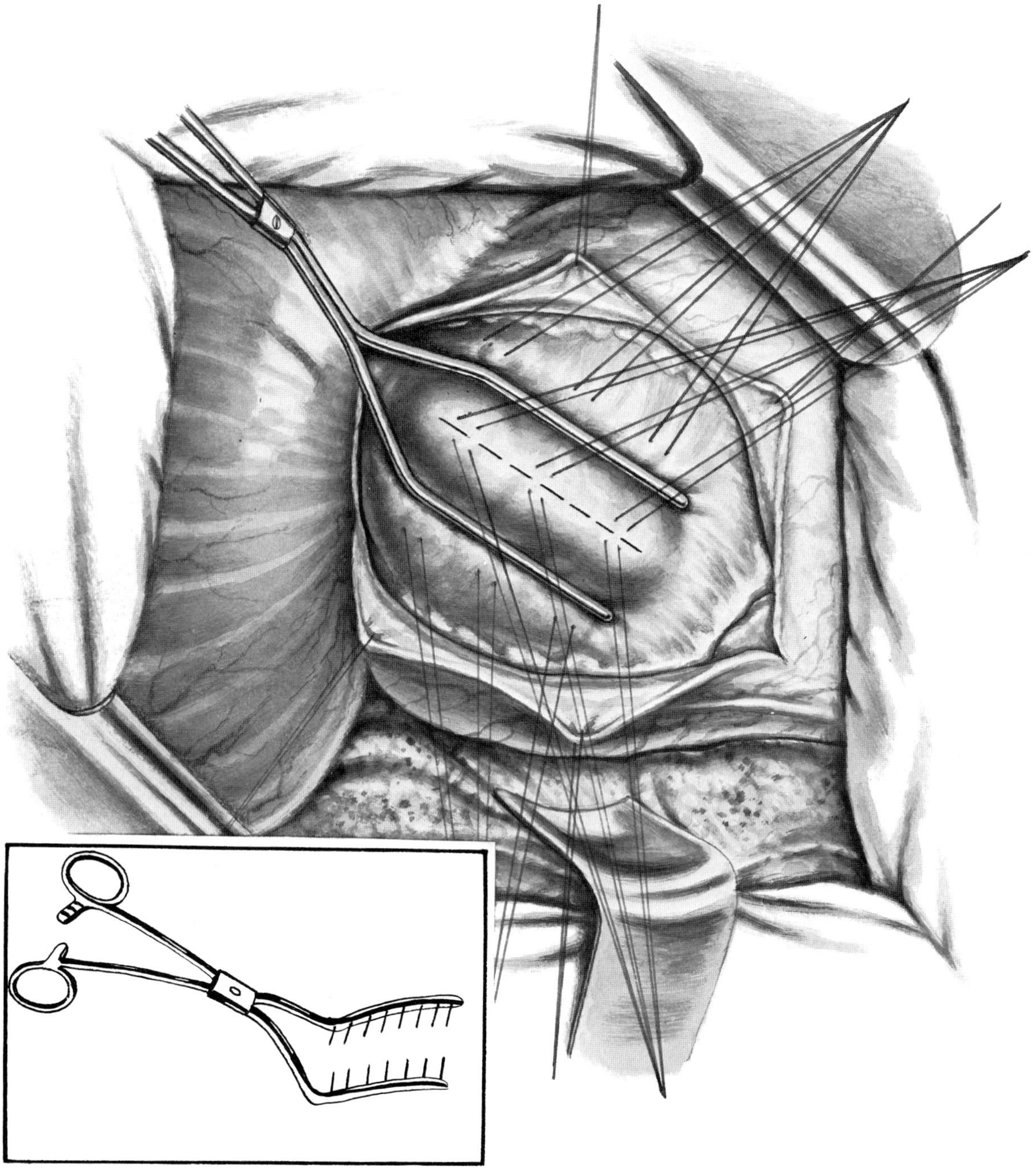

Fig. 463. Needle-shaped clamp is applied to neck of aneurysmal sac. Dashed line shows location of intended incision.

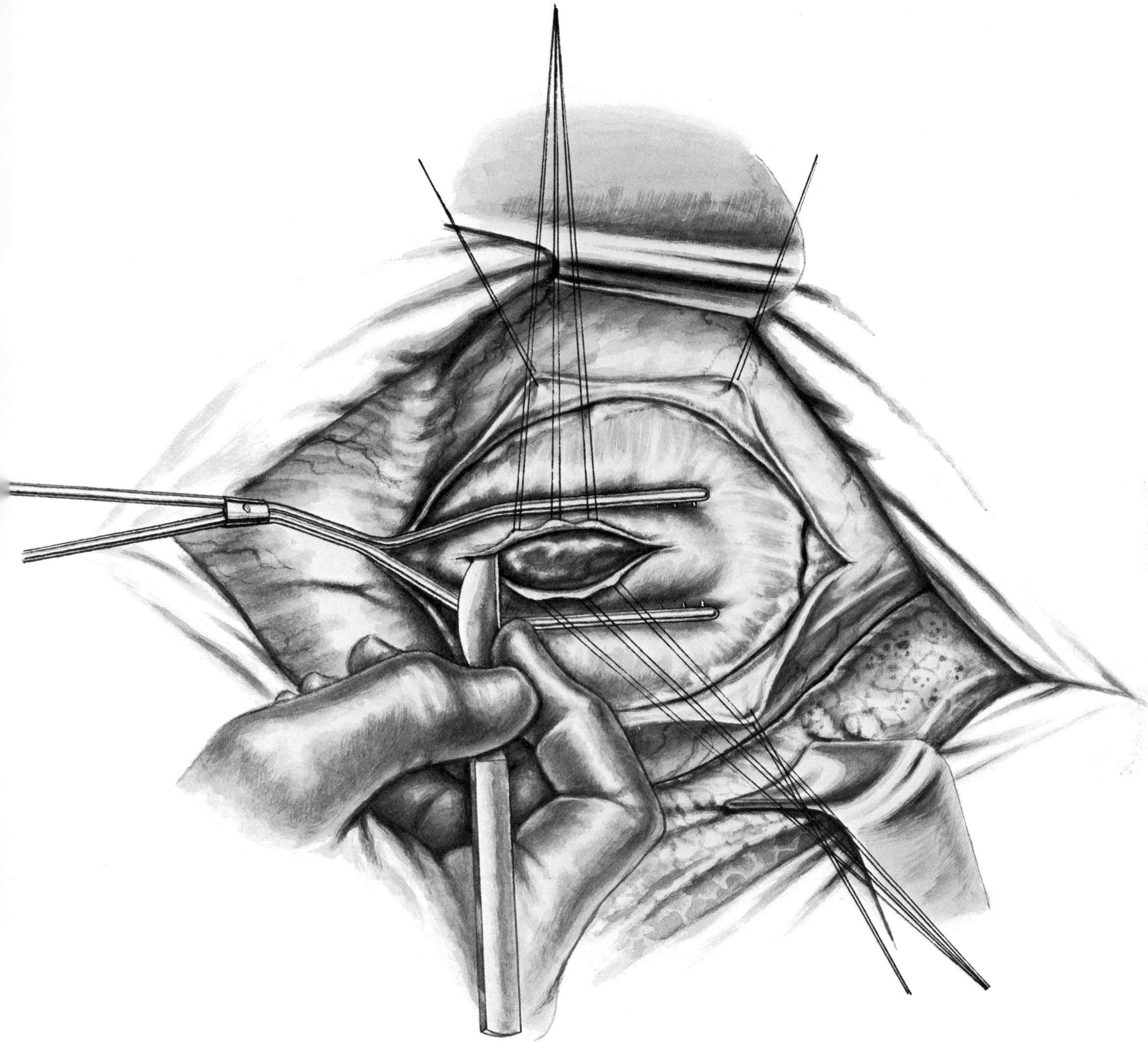

Fig. 464. Aneurysmal sac is opened.

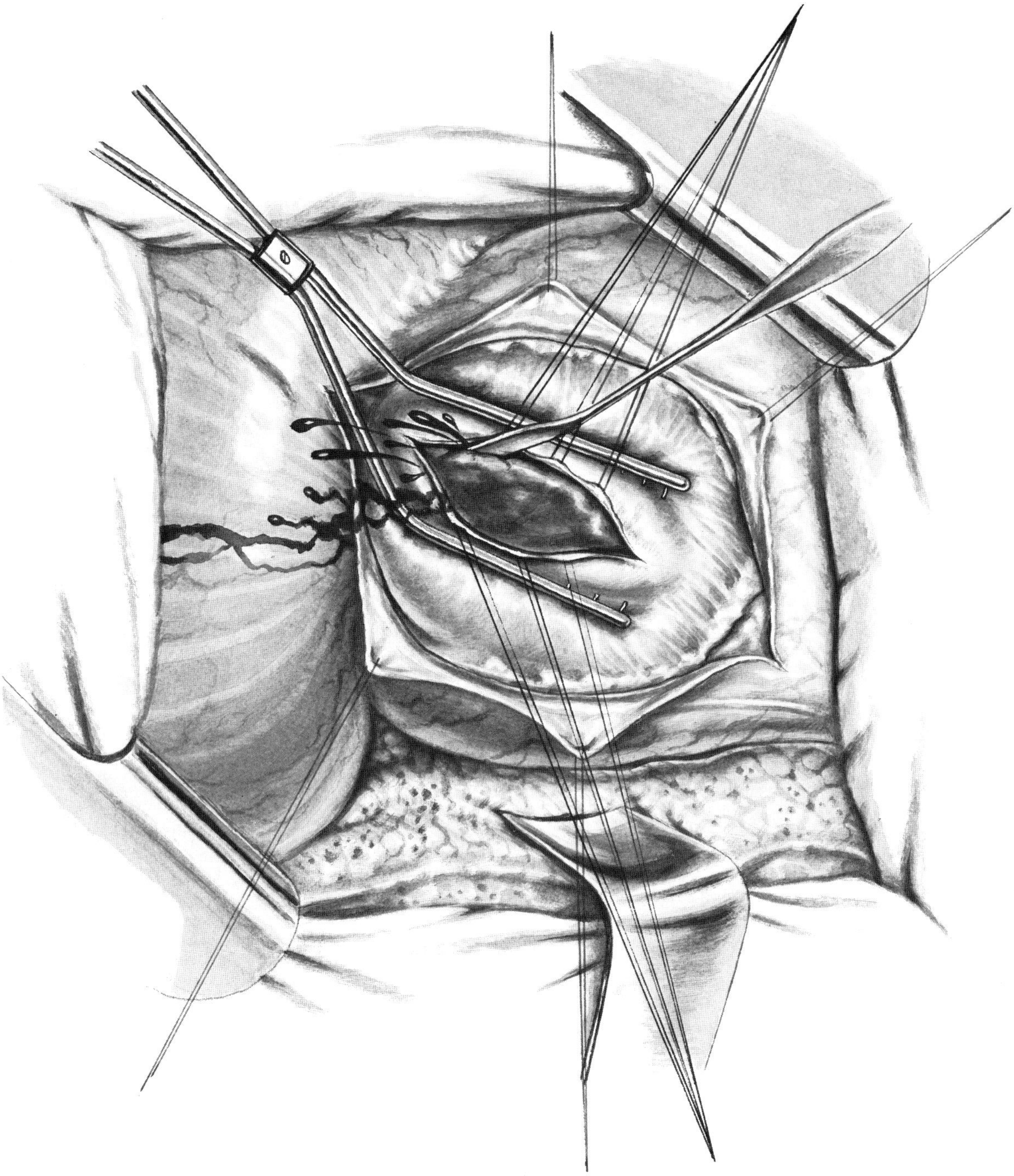

Fig. 465. Thrombotic masses (''cup'') are separated from aneurysmal sac.

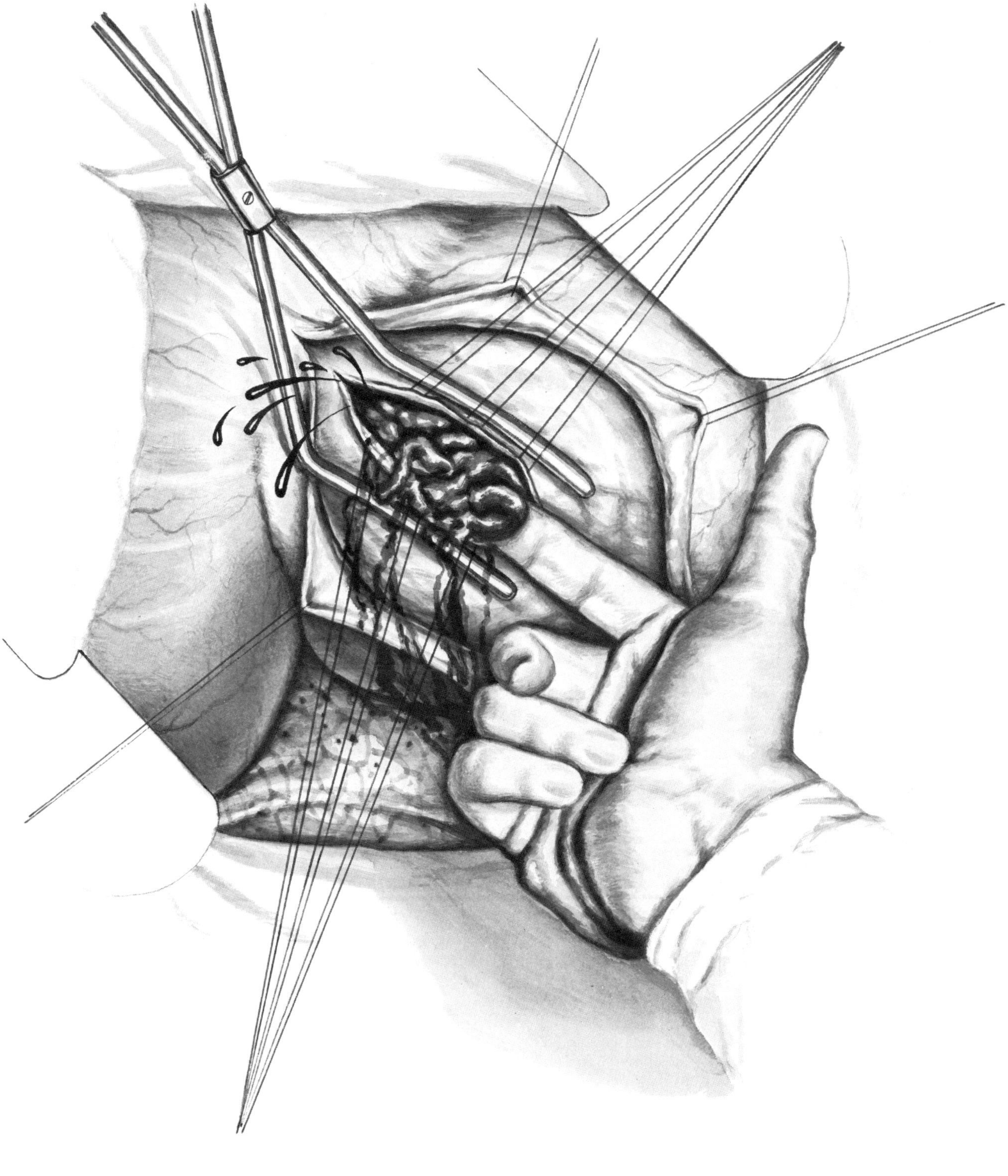

Fig. 466. Thrombotic masses are removed.

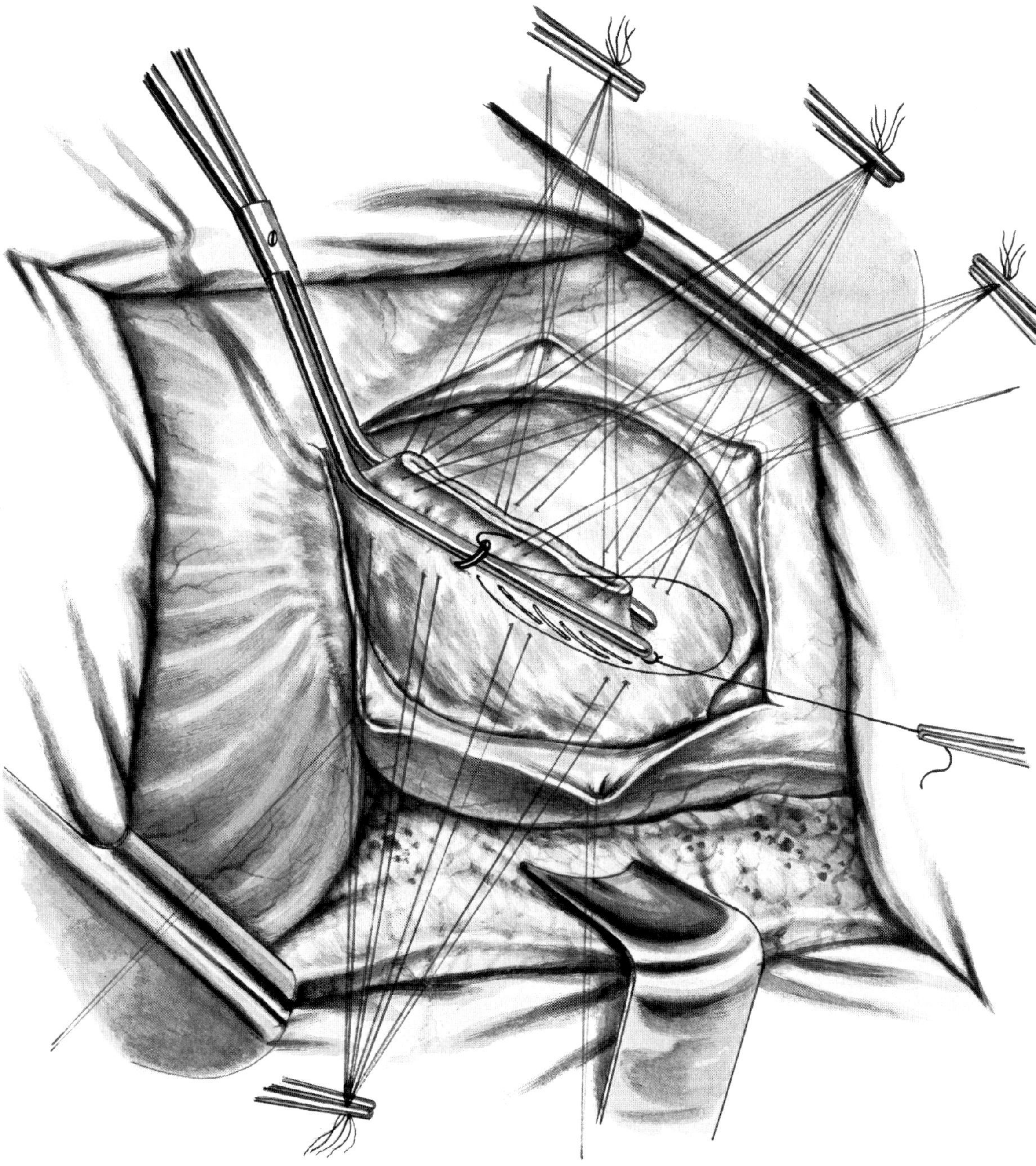

Fig. 467. Neck of sac is clamped with needle-shaped clamp, and continuous Halsted suture is applied to left ventricle below clamp.

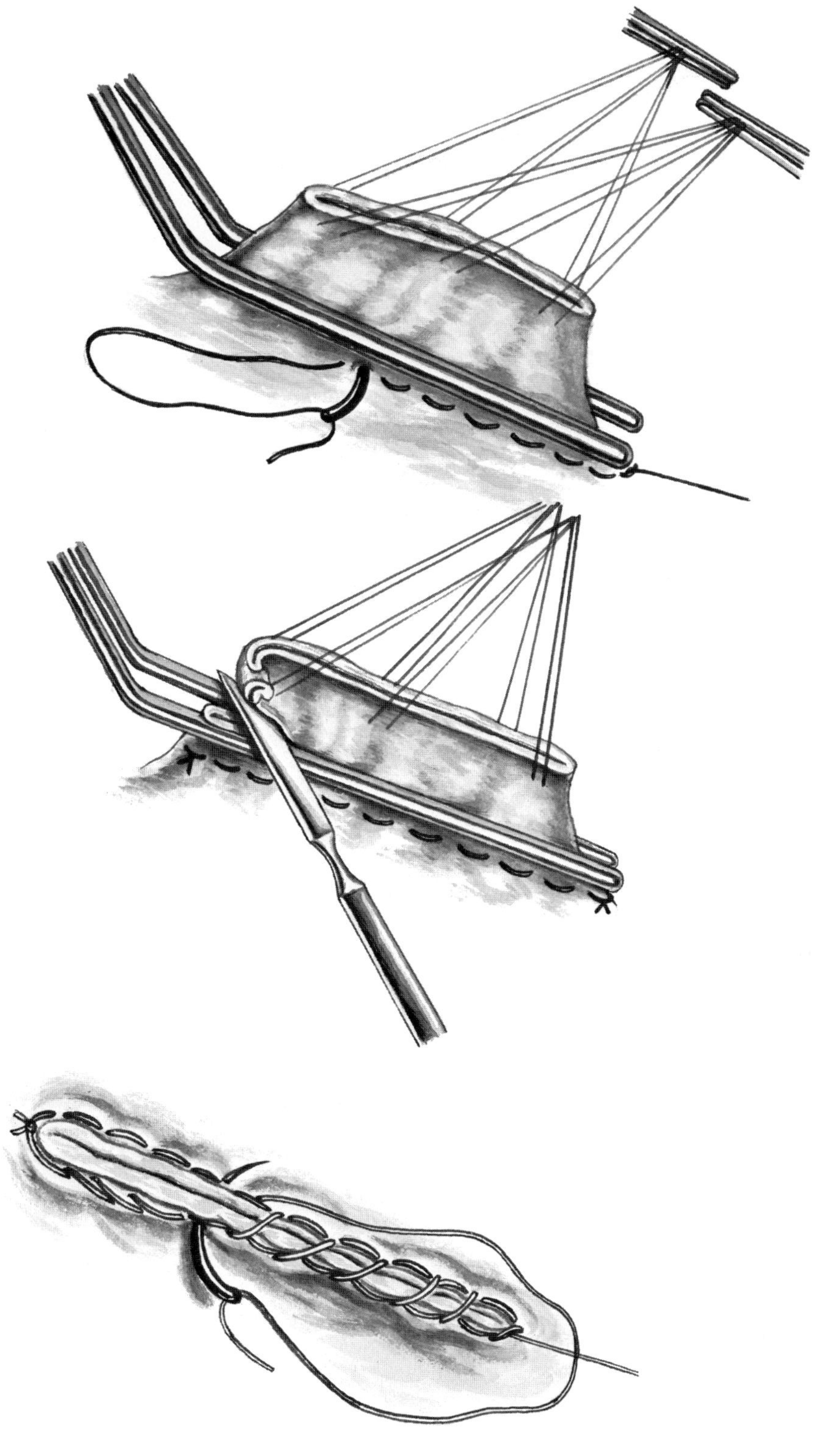

Fig. 468. Stages of resection of aneurysmal sac and closure of its base with sutures.

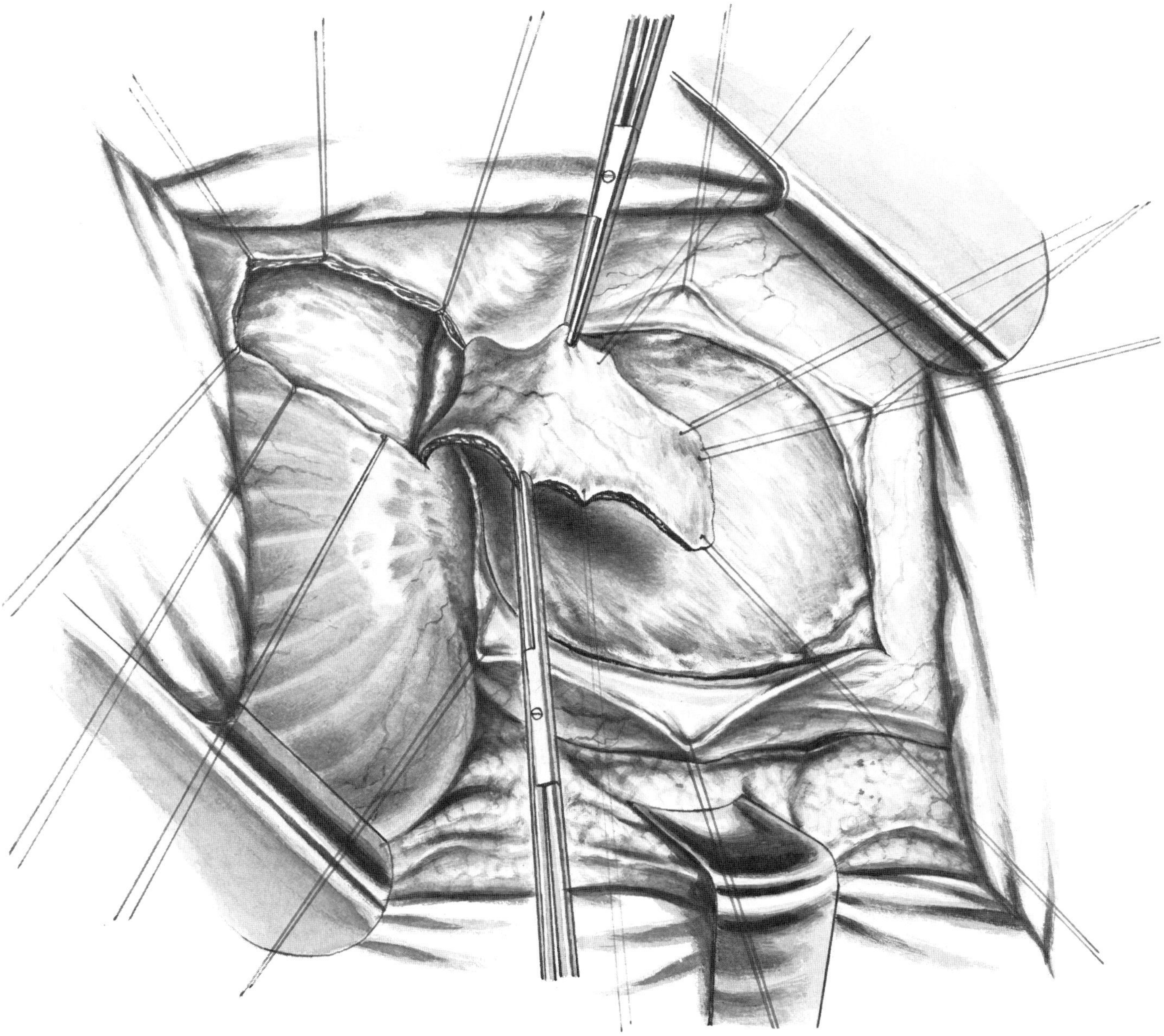

Fig. 469. Diaphragmatic graft used for repairing defect formed after resection of aneurysm of heart.

OPERATION BY THE OPEN METHOD

A large sacculated aneurysm of the left ventricle is resected by the open method under conditions of extracorporeal circulation.

The venous cannula of the heart-lung machine is introduced into the right cardiac auricle through a small right thoracotomy in the left intercostal space with tran-

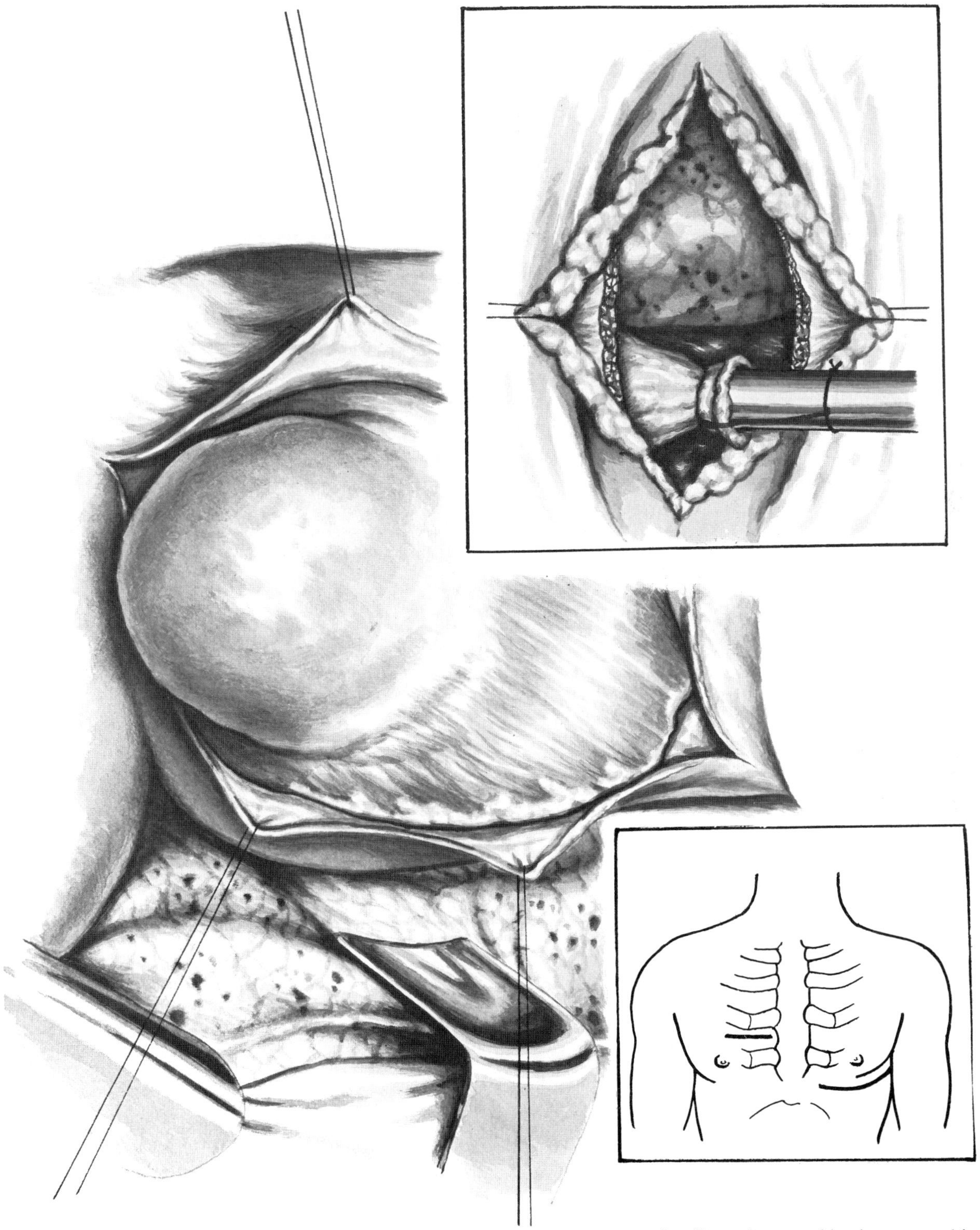

Fig. 470. View of sacculated aneurysm of heart. *Upper inset,* venous cannula of heart-lung machine is connected into right atrium through additional thoracotomy in third intercostal space. *Lower inset,* lines of incisions of thoracic cage.

section of one of the rib cartilages. The sacculated aneurysm of the left ventricle is exposed through left thoracotomy in the sixth intercostal space (Fig. 470). If necessary the cartilage of the next cranial rib is cut.

The pericardium is separated from the bottom of the aneurysm. The aneurysm is opened (Fig. 471). If its walls are thinned out, the incision is made through the pericardium without separating it from the aneurysm.

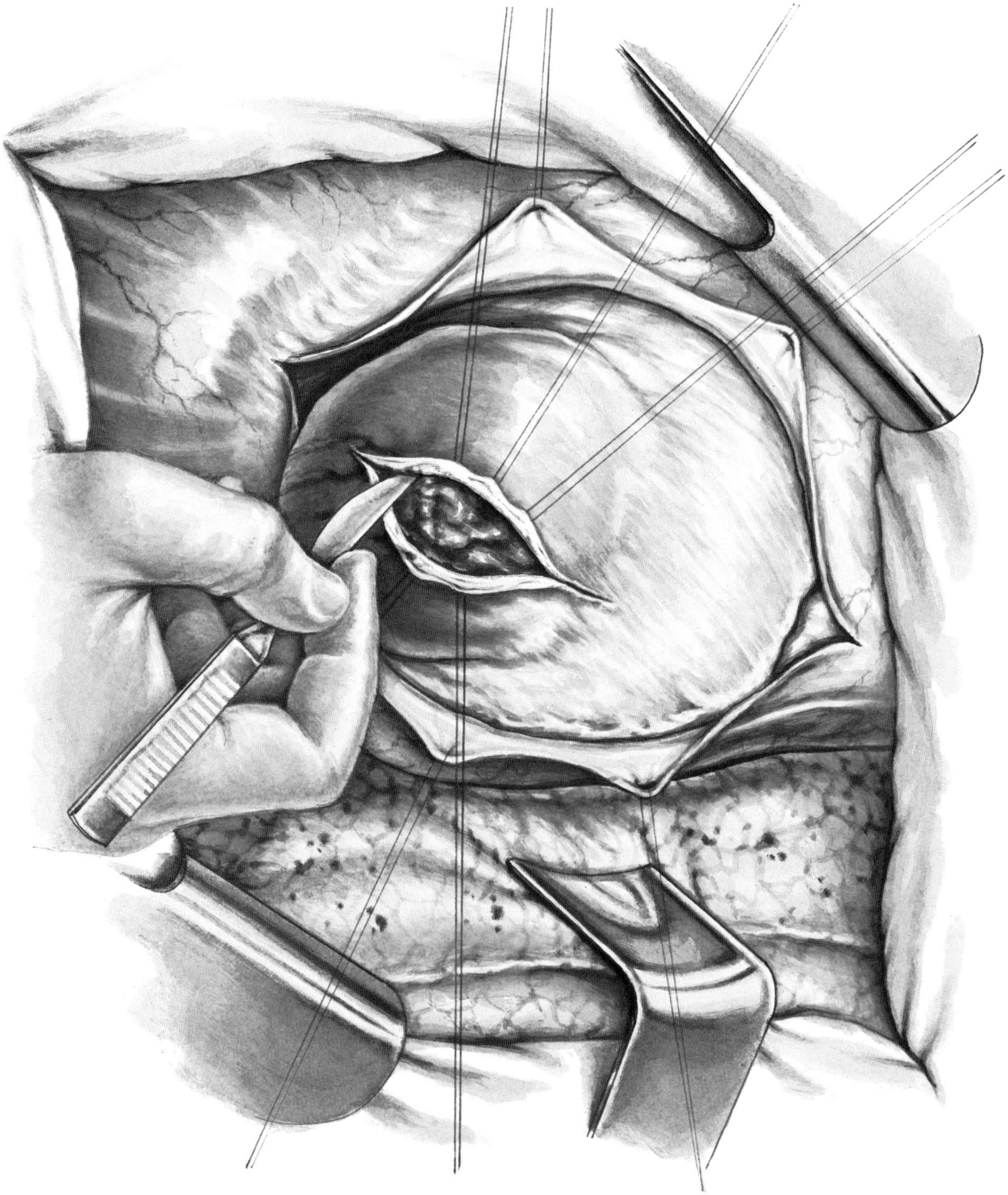

Fig. 471. Incision of aneurysm of heart under conditions of extracorporeal circulation.

Blood is aspirated from the cavity of the left ventricle; the thrombi are detached from the walls and removed. The aneurysmal cavity is examined and its boundaries from the side of the endocardium determined. The aneurysmal walls are excised, leaving a rim of fibrous tissue 1.5 cm high (Fig. 472).

The defect formed in the left ventricle is closed with a continuous mattress suture. To prevent the threads

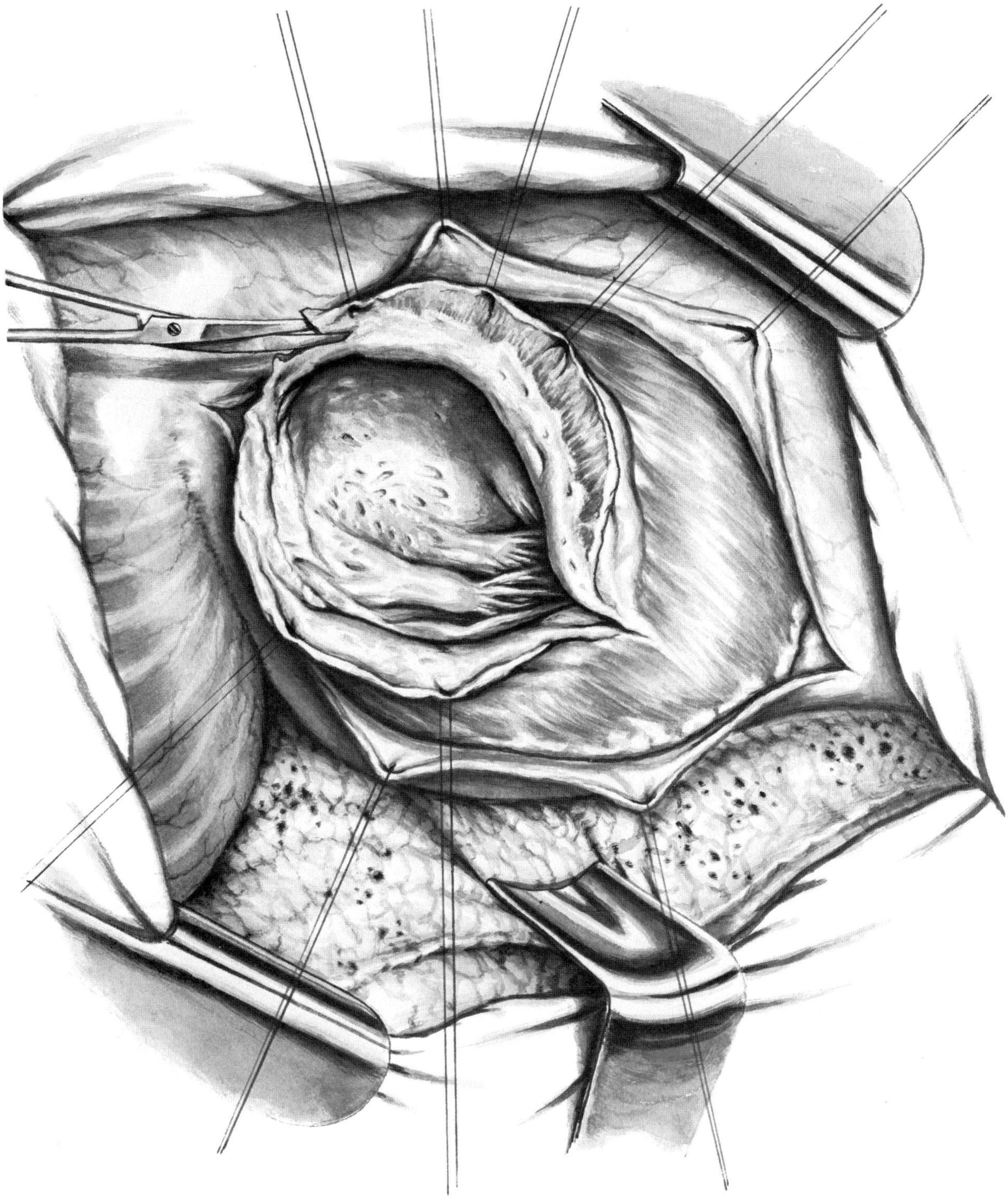

Fig. 472. Walls of aneurysm of heart are resected after thrombotic masses are removed.

from cutting through the tissues, plastic bolsters are applied on both sides of the suture line. The mattress suture is covered with a row of blanket sutures.

To remove air from the left ventricle, the suture in the region of the heart apex is tied "as the blood gushes out of the wound." This ends the operation performed under extracorporeal circulation. The machine is disconnected, the venous cannula removed, and the right auricle made airtight by tying the purse-string suture and applying a ligature to the base of the auricle. After heparin is neutralized with protamine sulfate in restoration of blood coagulation, a graft is formed from the diaphragm, and the suture of the left ventricle is covered with it (Fig. 473). The pericardium is sutured over the diaphragmatic graft.

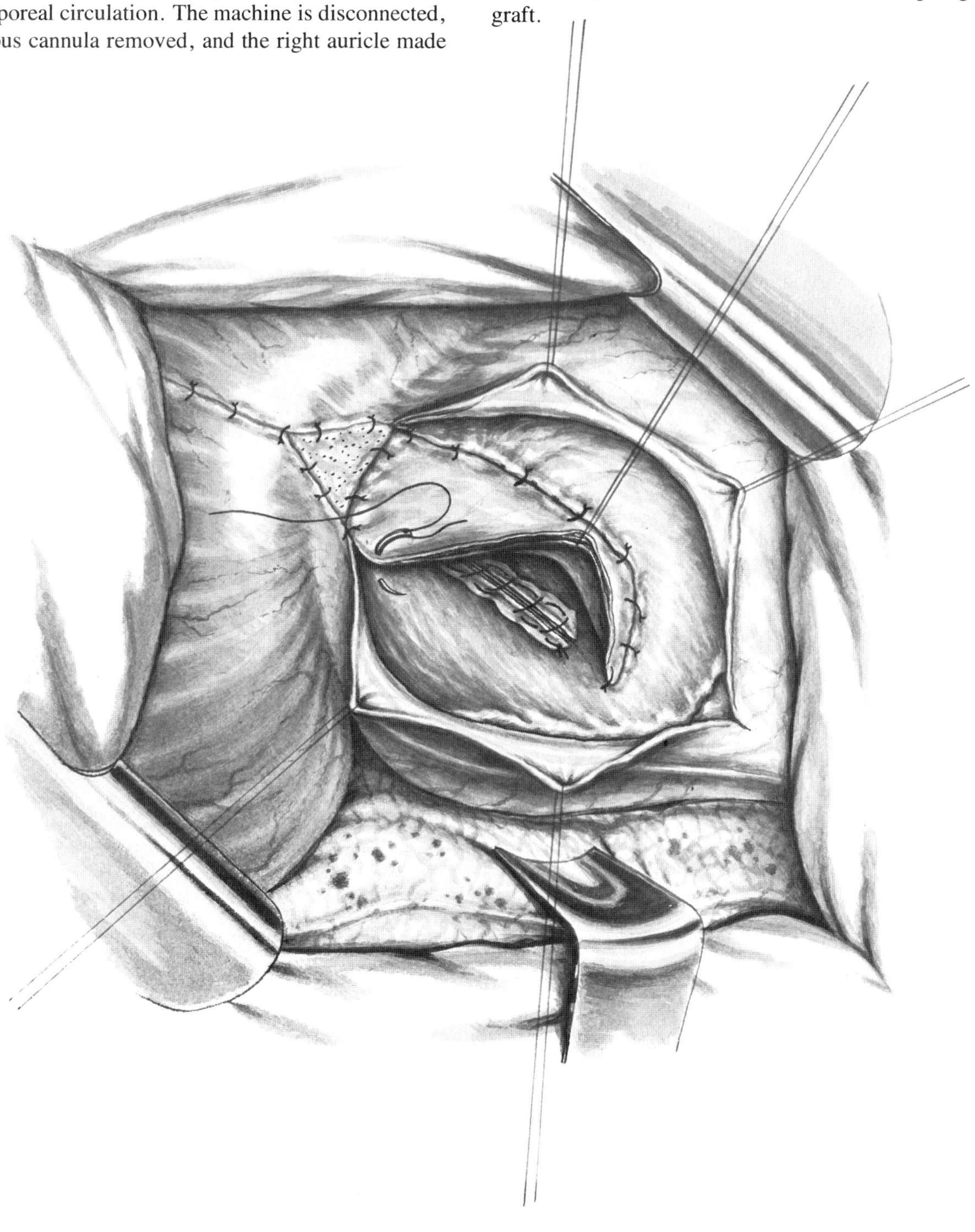

Fig. 473. Continuous Halsted suture with plastic bolsters is applied to left ventricle and then covered with diaphragmatic graft.